PRACTICAL

APPLICATION

of

COMPUTER-AIDED

DRUG DESIGN

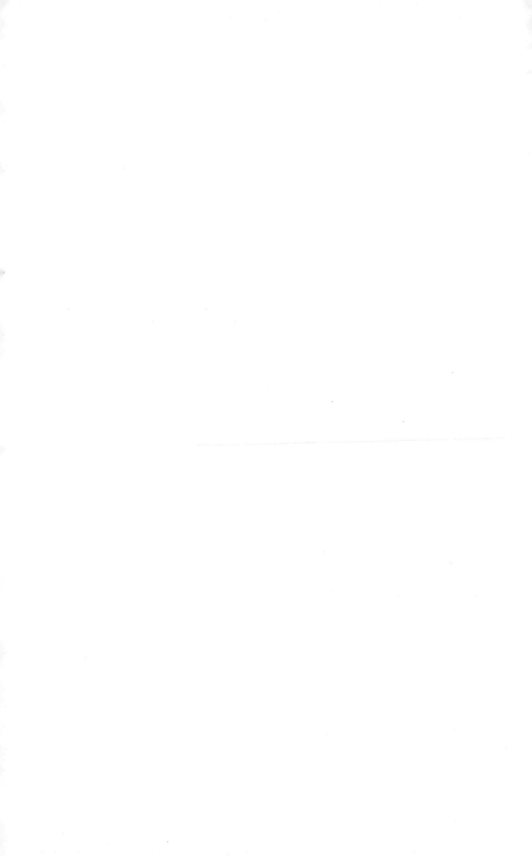

PRACTICAL

APPLICATION

of

COMPUTER-AIDED

DRUG DESIGN

edited by

Paul S. Charifson

Vertex Pharmaceuticals Incorporated
Cambridge, Massachusetts

MARCEL DEKKER, INC.   NEW YORK · BASEL · HONG KONG

Library of Congress Cataloging-in-Publication Data

Charifson, Paul S.
    Practical application of computer-aided drug design/Paul S. Charifson.
      p. cm.
    Includes index
    ISBN 0-8247-9885-6 (hc: alk. paper)
    1. Drugs—Design—Data processing. 2. Computer-aided design.
  I. Title.
  RS420.C47   1997
  615'.19'00285—dc21

                                              97-20897
                                              CIP

The publisher offers discounts on this book when ordered in bulk quantities. For more information, write to Special Sales/Professional Marketing at the address below.

This book is printed on acid-free paper.

MARCEL DEKKER, INC.
270 Madison Avenue, New York, New York 10016
http://www.dekker.com

Current printing (last digit):
10 9 8 7 6 5 4 3 2 1

PRINTED IN THE UNITED STATES OF AMERICA

To my wife, Nobuko and our daughters, Nikki and Mia

Preface

The usefulness of computational methods in the drug design process is no longer a point of debate. The contributions from this evolving field have become apparent to both pharmaceutical scientists and academic biomedical researchers. Because the nature of drug design is inherently multidisciplinary and involves the integration of vast amounts of complex information, it is clear that computational methods can aid in this process. From the statistical analysis of large data sets, to quantitative prediction, to simply sitting in front of a graphics terminal and using one's scientific intuition, success stories from these endeavors are appearing in the literature at an impressive rate.

With the exponential increase in structural information pertaining to biologically relevant targets, ligands, and their complexes, it is no coincidence that researchers from many previously distinct disciplines are crossing established barriers in an attempt to understand, develop, and utilize computational tools that will contribute regularly to the development of new medicinal agents. It is this convergence of scientific fields, ranging from molecular biology to physics, that necessitates the documentation of these methods and their practical application in a fashion that will minimize jargon and maximize comprehension.

It is the intent of this book to describe some of the recent advances in the computer-aided drug design field. Because the computational methods associated with the design of new pharmaceutical agents are constantly evolving, this book will provide essential information to active practitioners of computer-aided drug design. This book will also prove useful to graduate students aspiring to conduct rational drug design–related research. Each chapter covers a specific topic of current interest and presents a brief background, followed by an in-depth discussion of the most up-to-date techniques and applications.

The opening chapter sets the tone for the rest of the book by describing some of the successes and limitations of the technologies elaborated on in subsequent chapters. The remainder of the book is divided into three sections: methods that derive mainly from consideration of the ligand as the starting design point; those that emanate from consideration of the receptor as the starting design point; and those that consider essential improvements in the underlying molecular mechanics framework on which many of the ligand- and receptor-based methods depend.

Considerable progress has been made in the ability of macromolecular X-ray crystallography and nuclear magnetic resonance (NMR) spectroscopy to provide structural information for biological targets; however, there are still many more potential drug targets that have not been structurally characterized. Therefore, chapters on 3D-QSAR, pharmacophore mapping, and 3D-database searching are as critical as those focused on structure-based approaches. Additionally, application of the computational methods to chemical libraries is another natural development, the influence of which is starting to be felt. With our improved ability to parameterize and develop molecular mechanics forcefields, more effort can be applied to some of the less well characterized aspects of molecular simulation such as long-range electrostatic effects, solvation, and proper consideration of metal ions.

However, even with all of the progress that has been made, some still consider the "holy grail" of computer-aided drug design to be the ability to correctly fold proteins starting with only sequence information, to derive ligands de novo that bind to these proteins, and then to accurately predict the in vitro activity of those ligands. Although we have not yet been able to consistently accomplish any one of these goals, it is clear that we have made much progress in recent years.

Finally, I would like to thank all the contributors to this book and all the researchers in computational chemistry and related fields who have contributed to a better understanding of how and when to apply these methods.

Paul S. Charifson

Contents

Contributors

Ajay, Ph.D. Department of Computational Chemistry and Molecular Modeling, Vertex Pharmaceuticals Incorporated, Cambridge, Massachusetts

Libero J. Bartolotti, Ph.D. Research Institute, North Carolina Supercomputing Center, Research Triangle Park, North Carolina

Jeffrey M. Blaney, Ph.D. Structure, Design and Informatics, Chiron Technologies, Chiron Corporation, Emeryville, California

J. Phillip Bowen, Ph.D. Computational Center for Molecular Structure and Design, Department of Chemistry, University of Georgia, Athens, Georgia

Mark G. Bures, Ph.D. Department of Computer-Assisted Molecular Design and Diversity, Abbott Laboratories, Abbott Park, Illinois

Paul S. Charifson*, Ph.D Department of Structural Chemistry, Glaxo Wellcome Inc., Research Triangle Park, North Carolina

Thomas A. Darden, Ph.D. Laboratory of Computational Biology, National Institute of Environmental Health Sciences, Research Triangle Park, North Carolina

Renée L. DesJarlais, Ph.D. Department of Physical and Structural Chemistry, SmithKline Beecham Pharmaceuticals, King of Prussia, Pennsylvania

---

*Current affiliation: Department of Computational Chemistry and Molecular Modeling, Vertex Pharmaceuticals Incorporated, Cambridge, Massachusetts

Ulrich Essmann*, Ph.D. Department of Chemistry, University of North Carolina, Chapel Hill, North Carolina

A. J. Hopfinger, Ph.D. Department of Medicinal Chemistry, Chemistry, and Chemical Engineering, College of Pharmacy, The University of Illinois at Chicago, Chicago, Illinois

Irwin D. Kuntz, Ph.D. Department of Pharmaceutical Chemistry and Molecular Design Institute, University of California, San Francisco, San Francisco, California

Millard H. Lambert, Ph.D. Department of Structural Chemistry, Glaxo Wellcome Inc., Research Triangle Park, North Carolina

Guyan Liang, Ph.D. Computational Center for Molecular Structure and Design, Department of Chemistry, University of Georgia, Athens, Georgia

Eric Martin, Ph.D. Structure and Design Group, Chiron Technologies, Chiron Corporation, Emeryville, California

Mark A. Murcko, Ph.D. Department of Computational Chemistry and Molecular Modeling, Vertex Pharmaceuticals Incorporated, Cambridge, Massachusetts

Lee G. Pedersen, Ph.D. National Institute of Environmental Health Sciences, Research Triangle Park, North Carolina and Department of Chemistry, University of North Carolina, Chapel Hill, North Carolina

Manuel C. Peitsch, Ph.D. Geneva Biomedical Research Institute, Glaxo Wellcome Research and Development S.A., Geneva, Switzerland

Brian K. Shoichet, Ph.D. Department of Molecular Pharmacology and Biological Chemistry, Northwestern University Medical School, Chicago, Illinois

David C. Spellmeyer, Ph.D. Structure and Design, Chiron Technologies, Chiron Corporation, Emeryville, California

Pieter F. W. Stouten, Ph.D. Computer-Aided Drug Design Group, The DuPont Merck Pharmaceutical Company, Wilmington, Delaware

John S. Tokarski, Ph.D. Laboratory of Molecular Modeling and Design, College of Pharmacy, The University of Chicago, Chicago, Illinois, and The Chem21 Group, Lake Forest, Illinois

---

*Current affiliation: German National Research Center for Information Technology, Schloss Birlinghoven, Sankt Augustin, Germany

1

Recent Successes and Continuing Limitations in Computer-Aided Drug Design

*Paul S. Charifson
Glaxo Wellcome Inc., Research Triangle Park, North Carolina

Irwin D. Kuntz
University of California, San Francisco, San Francisco, California

I. INTRODUCTION

This volume focuses on computational methods used in the design of biologically active molecules. Our aim in this chapter is to evaluate the usefullness of computational chemistry in drug design. We specifically want to discuss the successes and failures of this technology. While this discussion cannot be comprehensive, we will draw on the recent literature, other chapters in this volume, and unpublished material to provide a current assessment.

We begin with the assumption that computational methods have the potential to speed the discovery of novel compounds and to guide optimization of the properties of these compounds [1]. We ask the following questions: How much of this potential has been realized to date; What are

---

*Current affiliation: Vertex Pharmaceuticals Incorporated, Cambridge, Massachusetts.

the current limitations? In the pharmaceutical arena, the primary role for computational efforts has been in the discovery phase of drug development [2], usually focused on in vitro testing. Reduction of screening costs or of the time required to identify a candidate are important goals of computer-aided molecular design [1].

Lead discovery is basically a search process. With the advent of a thorough understanding of cellular biochemistry, it has been possible to target specific enzymes through modification of their substrates or cofactors. There are currently many ways to make use of this information. For example, conventional screening of corporate databases, the National Cancer Institute database, or of novel natural products is a route to more than half the best-selling drugs on the market. Alternatively, the search can proceed through a variety of computational methods both in the presence and absence of structural information of the target. Finally, the great advances in both chemistry and molecular biology have made it possible to create libraries of organic compounds, peptides, oligonucleotides, and even whole proteins for screening [3–7].

However, discovery is only the beginning stage of a long process. We will also consider what computation might be able to do in evaluating the pharmacological and biopharmaceutical properties of molecules that are critical to testing in vivo and, looking even farther ahead, to speculate briefly on the computational issues involved in evaluation of the metabolism and toxicology of drug candidates that often determine their clinical success. We will also report on the status of specific compounds through the developmental pipeline.

Computer-assisted molecular design has contributed to both the design and development of potent in vitro lead molecules and clinically useful agents (i.e., drugs) [8–17]. Identification of such "success stories" is not always straightforward because it is difficult to distill the "true story" from a few sentences in a scientific publication, abstracted news release, Food and Drug Administration (FDA) database, or scientific meeting. Additionally, by nature, much of the research done in industry is proprietary. Although we have attempted a candid assessment, we apologize in advance for any omissions or misinterpretations.

To frame our discussion of the current status of computer-assisted molecular design, we reiterate the procedures in common use [for more details see Chaps. 2–13]. There are several basic types of searching and discovery methods. Database-searching methods, such as the DOCK program developed at the University of California, San Francisco (UCSF), identify molecules that are complementary in shape and chemical interactions to a user-supplied receptor structure [18,19]. Three-dimensional substructure searches (pharmacophore searches) find molecules that include selected functional groups or types of groups in specified geometric relations [20; see Chaps. 2 and 3]. Similarity searches rank database molecules by the number of features they have in common with a query [21]. In addition to these searching procedures, interaction site-based modeling [22,23] and de novo compound design are becoming increasingly popular [24; see also Chap. 9]. Aligned with these searching and discovery methods are the more statistically derived methods, such as two-dimensional (2D) and three-dimensional quantitative structure–activity relationships (3D-QSAR), which attempt to correlate observed biological responses with some calculable molecular properties.

II. DEFINITION OF SUCCESS

The process from identification of target to entry of a drug into the marketplace has the following steps: (a) identification of a lead compound, (b) optimization of the lead compound, (c) evaluation of delivery and metabolic issues, (d) optimization of synthesis, and (e) animal and clinical testing.

In the present work, we will concentrate our attention on how present computational methods directly impinge on the first three steps. We are especially interested when, as a result of these methods, a molecule has progressed through discovery to an in vitro lead and thence, into clinical trials or the marketplace. We will not examine computer-assisted organic synthesis [25–27] nor the statistical issues in evaluation of clinical trials.

To further focus this discussion, we find it useful to classify the various computational methods into several categories: quantitative structure–activity relationship studies, conformational analysis, pharmacophore studies, database-searching studies, and structure-based design studies. From the discussions of these methods in some of the later chapters in this book, it is clear that more often than not, any success actually derives from a combination of these techniques, rather than from any technique, in isolation. For example, conformational analysis is often involved as the first step in any or all of the other techniques listed, and pharmacophore studies often precede 3D-QSAR studies and database searches.

We will proceed by describing successes according to computational methods employed, but we want to emphasize the multifaceted nature of these approaches. The insights gained during the past 20 years from applying computational methods to the problems of drug design has led to a more mature understanding of the appropriate uses and limitations of these tools. Improved algorithms and computing environments, combined with such a multifaceted and multidisciplinary approach, are largely responsible for the recent successes described.

III. QUANTITATIVE STRUCTURE–ACTIVITY RELATIONSHIP SUCCESSES

Quantitative structure–activity relationship (QSAR) studies, based on 2D or 3D descriptors, have traditionally shown promise when the descriptors chosen were accurate and appropriate, the errors in the biological data were minimal, and the data were well-distributed. The problem is that, rarely, are all of these criteria met. Additionally, most molecular modelers are not necessarily well-versed in rigorous statistical analytical methods. Nonetheless, the traditional Hansch–Fujita QSAR approach has led to some successes in the realm of agrochemical and pharmaceutical agents [8]. An example begins with the 9-anilinoacridine antitumor agent, asulacrine [CI-921; (**1**)] which is an analogue of amsacrine [28]. This molecule resulted from a study of amsacrine analogues in which compounds with a defined set of physicochemical properties were chosen for synthesis in an attempt to optimize drug distribution. Specifically, in addition to desiring tight DNA-binding capabilities, Denny and co-workers wanted to improve aqueous solubility and lower the pKa. This study eventually resulted in asulacrine, which made it into phase II clinical trials [29] and showed activity against non–small-cell cancers and possibly breast cancers.

In the 3D-QSAR arena, there are many studies that attempt to rationalize a data set, but only a few of these studies are validated by predicting the in vitro activities of molecules outside the training set. Some recent examples of validated 3D-QSAR studies include some creative methods and study systems [30–35; see also Chap. 4].

Even for some of these validated 3D-QSAR studies, it is very difficult to find examples for which this information guided further synthetic efforts and led to a molecule that entered clinical trials. One example that does meet this criterion is the work done by Martin and co-workers at Abbott Laboratories in the development of D_1 dopamine agonists [36]. In work

{1}

{2}

spanning several years involving pharmacophore mapping, 3D database searching, and comparative molecular field analysis (CoMFA) studies, they developed a predictive CoMFA model that was able to distinguish active from inactive compounds among 170 molecules that were not used in the derivation of the CoMFA model. Later, this CoMFA model was extended to predict the D_1-binding affinities of 201 additional compounds. This study, which considered "all" conformers and stereoisomers, resulted in the synthesis of 19 compounds of which 10 had predicted pK_i values higher than 6.5. Five of the 10 compounds synthesized had pK_i values higher than 7.0, whereas another 4 had pK_i between 6.0 and 7.0. The prediction of the other 9 compounds with pK_i of less than 6.5 was also experimentally verified. This work ultimately guided the alkyl substitution pattern in the 2 position of the thiophene ring of A-86929 (**2**). One of the correctly predicted active molecules has been selected for clinical testing [Y. C. Martin, personal communication].

IV. PHARMACOPHORE–CONFORMATIONAL MODEL SUCCESSES

As with 3D-QSAR studies, most recent pharmacophore-mapping and conformational-modeling studies are rarely perfomed in isolation and are often a prelude to 3D-QSAR studies, 3D database searching, or de novo design studies. In Chapter 2, Bures emphasizes this point as well as the iterative incorporation of experimental data to refine an evolving pharmacophore model. Although there are many elegant examples in which pharmacophore generation has led to optimization of in vitro activities, there are fewer clear examples in which a pharmacophore or conformational model provided insight beyond this level. One recent example, however, did contribute to the discovery of a compound that is presently in clinical trials. This study involves a pharmacophore–conformational model derived from nuclear magnetic resonance (NMR) and crystallographic data of a cyclic peptide.

A. Fibrinogen Receptor Antagonists

Researchers at SmithKline Beecham were aware that peptides containing the sequence Arg–Gly–Asp (RGD) antagonized the binding of fibrinogen to its platelet GPIIb/IIIa receptor, thereby inhibiting platelet aggregation. These researchers had previously solved the NMR solution structures and X-ray crystal structures of various Arg–Gly–Asp-containing cyclic peptides [37,38]. These structures combined with other studies [39] indicated a C_7 turn at the aspartic acid residue of these cyclic peptides. The ^{1}H-NMR data for the cyclic RGD peptide, [Structure (**3**)] was used in the present study. The design process focused on identifying a nonpeptide scaffold that would maintain the critical positioning of the arginine and aspartic acid side chains, while additionally placing a lipophilic group next to the position occupied by aspartic acid [40]. These workers hypothesized that these requirements might be met by a 1,4-benzodiazepine nucleus and began a detailed "atom by atom, torsion by torsion" comparison of the 1,4-benzodiazepine nucleus with the NMR-derived structural information. Modeling suggested that the 2-position of the 1,4-benzodiazepine was equivalent to the aspartic acid C-α position and that substitution at this position with a carboxymethyl should be in the equatorial orientation. This analysis further suggested that to maintain the appropriate Arg-to-Asp spatial relation observed in the cyclic peptide, an amide group at position 8 of the 1,4-benzodiazepine might suffice. The carbonyl of this amide group could also potentially mimic the corresponding arginine backbone carbonyl. To complete the design, the amidinophenethyl group was chosen to

{3}

{4}

mimic the arginine side chain and the lipophilic phenethyl group was suggested at N-4. The resultant 1,4-benzodiazepine (4), displayed a K_i of 1–2 nM in competition radioligand-binding assays and represents a low molecular weight antagonist that employs the key three-dimensional features of a high-affinity peptide ligand. A close structural analogue of (4) has been chosen as a candidate for development and is currently undergoing clinical trials [C. E. Peishoff, personal communication].

Researchers at Genentech independently arrived at a benzodiazepine-type scaffold in the form of a benzodiazepinedione [41,42]. These workers also started with a structural model derived from NMR studies of potent cyclic peptides. They then employed ensemble molecular dynamics on related active analogues to produce a consistent model of the essential binding determinants. These pharmacophoric elements were then successfully reproduced in the context of the benzodiazepinedione scaffold. Molecules from this series are presently being optimized for consideration as preclinical candidates.

Additionally, Merck scientists were able to design low molecular weight nonpeptide fibrinogen antagonists different from the benzodiazepine or benzodiazepinedione scaffolds by exploitation of NMR-derived structures of cyclic RGD peptides [43]. These workers were also successful in developing clinical candidates for development as antithrombotic agents by this approach.

V. PHARMACOPHORE AND DATABASE SEARCHING WITH STRUCTURE-BASED APPROACHES

Recent examples of using the combination of developing a pharmacophore hypothesis and then searching 2D or 3D databases have led to potent compounds. In the first example, the pharmacophore was derived from crystallographic information of the binding site, whereas in the second example, the pharmacophore hypothesis came from superimposition of a lead molecule on the NMR structures of peptides in solution.

A. HIV-Protease Inhibition

An elegant example of combining aspects of protein crystallography, molecular docking, pharmacophore generation, and database searching is that of the study of Lam and co-workers [44] at Dupont Merck, which is briefly described in Chapter 3 of this book. These researchers were trying to design nonpeptide human immunodeficiency virus (HIV) protease inhibitors using information from known crystallographic complexes of various inhibitors bound to HIV protease. A feature common to all of these crystal structures was a conserved structural water linking the bound inhibitors to the "flaps" of the C_2-symmetric HIV protease dimer. They hypothesized that displacing this water with some appropriate functionality would contribute favorably to the overall binding free-energy profile. They were also interested in the use of a C_2-symmetric diol that could also bind to the catalytic aspartates, Asp-25 and Asp-25'. Because no crystallographic structures of a bound C_2-symmetric diol existed at that time, they generated computer models by docking representatives of this class of compound into the crystal structure of a different bound inhibitor complex with the inhibitor removed. From this model, they defined a pharmacophore consisting of two hydrophobic groups at P1 and P1', a hydrogen bond donor, and a hydrogen bond acceptor to interact with the catalytic aspartates. The resultant pharmacophore was defined by the intramolecular distances between these groups in the docked complex of their model C_2-symmetric inhibitor. They then performed a 3D search on the Cambridge Crystallographic Database using this pharmacophore as a query. One "hit" contained not only the features of the query, but also possessed an oxygen in a position that might be able to displace the conserved water molecule. Superimposition of this compound into their original docking model led them to the idea of using cyclohexanone and cycloheptanone scaffolds. However, the cycloheptanone provided a better realization of a diol functionality and was further modified to the seven-member cyclic urea based on synthetic accessibility and the further possibility of strengthening hydrogen bonding to the flaps. Additional modeling studies were performed with other cyclic urea molecules to predict the optimal stereochemistry and conformation needed for complementarity. These predictions were borne out experimentally by synthesis, biological testing, and subsequent crystallographic studies of a cyclic urea bound to HIV protease. DMP323 (**5**) showed good initial oral bioavailability and entered phase I clinical trials.

{5}

Unfortunately, this compound was dropped from clinical trials because of variable blood levels caused by low aqueous solubility [P. Y. Lam, personal communication].

B. Endothelin Receptor Antagonists

The second example in this section involves work done in the design of potent and selective nonpeptide endothelin receptor antagonists. The endothelin receptors are members of the G protein-coupled receptor superfamily and are characterized by the presence of seven transmembrane-spanning helices. There is presently no direct structural information for any receptor of this class.

Researchers at SmithKline Beecham performed 2D searches of their corporate database for compounds that are similar to antagonists of other G protein-coupled receptors and that also contained features of the endogenous ligand, endothelin-1 (ET-1), which were known to be important for receptor binding [45]. From these efforts, an indene carboxylic acid with low micromolar affinity for the ET_A receptor was identified. This small-molecule antagonist was overlaid on NMR-derived structures of ET-1, leading to the suggestion that the 1- and 3-phenyl groups of this molecule might mimic certain aromatic side chains of ET-1, including a critical tyrosine. Thus, if one could incorporate electron-donating substituents onto either the 1- or 3-phenyls of the "lead" small molecule, this might better approximate the electron-rich tyrosine of the endogenous ligand. Because the indene nucleus exhibited some stability problems, an indane framework with comparable affinity was chosen and the substituted phenyl analogues were synthesized. Several of these compounds showed significantly improved affinity for the ET_A receptor and measurable affinity for the ET_B receptor, as well. Because the COOH-terminal section of ET-1 was not well-defined in the NMR-derived structures, a mimetic of this region of the peptide was not included in the initial peptidomimetic hypothesis. This

{6}

functionality of ET-1 was an important parameter in the database searches and additional efforts focused on refining the conformation in this region of the peptide. To accomplish this, these workers used the NMR-derived conformations of the more rigid cyclic pentapeptide antagonist BQ-123 (cyclo-D-Trp-D-Asp-Pro-D-Val-Leu), that is postulated to mimic the COOH-terminal residues of ET-1. They generated sets of superimposed conformers of ET-1, BQ-123, and an indane carboxylic acid, which were consistent with the NMR data and the peptidomimetic hypothesis of the indane carboxylic acid, by the ensemble-distance geometry technique. This extension to the pharmacophore model suggested that a carboxylic acid separated from the 3-phenyl ring by two or three atoms might mimic the COOH-terminus of ET-1. Synthetic considerations led to oxyacetic acid as the substituent at this position. Compound (**6**) was subsequently synthesized and possessed low nanomolar affinities for both the ET_A and ET_B receptors and also a potent inhibition of contractile response in isolated animal models. Compound (**6**) is presently in clinical trials as an agent to treat acute renal failure, and a close structural analogue is under development for the treatment of pulmonary hypertension [C. E. Peishoff, personal communication].

It should also be noted that Texas Biotechnology Corporation has recently moved a small molecule ET_A antagonist, TBC11251, which derived from structure-based modeling, into early clinical development [46].

VI. STRUCTURE-BASED APPROACHES

Judging from numerous personal communications probably no other technology contributing to the development of medicinal agents has undergone so much scrutiny and criticism as that of structure-based drug design. The promise of this approach was obvious early on, but the realization of reducing the lead time to clinical development has only recently become apparent. Furthermore, these methods are beginning to take into account bioavailability, pharmacokinetics, and metabolic issues by prospective inclusion of functionalities that possess desirable absorption, distribution, and metabolism profiles. The ability to predict aqueous solubilities [47] and pK_a' [48] has also improved substantially. The following examples illustrate specific aspects of employing structure-based approaches.

Because HIV protease inhibitors represent one of the better-studied systems, we have devoted a section specifically to this topic; we then provide a brief description of examples from other biological targets in Table 1. We also call to the readers attention several therapeutic areas or targets for which present efforts are likely to generate clinical candidates in the near future [46]. These areas include multidrug-resistant cancer, sickle cell anemia, selectin antagonists, interleukin-1β–converting enzyme inhibitors, glycinamide ribonucleotide formyl transferase inhibitors, matrix metalloprotease inhibitors, and inhibitors of viral uncoating.

A. HIV-Protease Inhibition

Although success is not always proportional to effort, in the use of structure-based approaches to design inhibitors of HIV protease, sheer determination has prevailed. This may be the most thoroughly studied crystallographic system [49] and the following four examples all use the information provided from the crystal structures in a very fundamental fashion.

The first example discussed involves the Abbott compound ritonavir [Norvir or ABT-538, Structure (7)] [50]. This compound was approved recently by the FDA for the treatment of acquired immunodeficiency syndrome (AIDS). Ritonavir resulted largely from work that attempted to understand the structural basis for antiviral activity, while at the same time maintaining oral bioavailability and reducing hepatic metabolism. Earlier studies of C_2 symmetry-based diol inhibitors led the Abbott workers to realize that some of these molecules that had reached clinical trials (e.g., A-77003) were not well understood relative to how the stereochemistry of the diol core influenced binding affinity and ultimately protease inhibition and antiviral activity. Crystallographic studies performed on a diastereomeric series of C_2-symmetric- and pseudosymmetric-based diols showed that diastereomers with similar binding affinities could bind in different, asymmetric and symmetric modes [51]. This information led to modeling studies on some smaller asymmetric candidates that might possess some of the same binding characteristics of A-77003. These researchers further

Table 1 Examples of the Successful Application of Computer-Aided Drug Design Approaches to Biological Targets

Drug design goal	Research group [ref.]	Methods employed	Outcome
Thrombin inhibition	Hoffmann-La Roche, Ltd. [123]	Iterative cycles of modeling, synthesis, and crystallography to optimize hydrophobic sites relative to catalytic center. Discovery of novel scaffold and substituents.	Ro 46-6240 (**12**) selected for clinical development as an antithrombotic agent
	Biogen, Inc. [124,125]	Based on a 3-dimensional model of thrombin, bifunctional peptide inhibitors (hirulogues) were designed to optimally span the enzyme active site and the anion binding exosite.	BG8967 (**13**) is in phase III clinical trials as a potential replacement of heparin during coronary angioplasty
Neuraminidase inhibition	Monash University/Glaxo Wellcome Inc. [126]	Use of primary amine probe from GRID [22] for the neuraminidase-binding site suggested replacement of 4-hydroxy group with amino substituent. Guanidino group led to even greater potency. Predictions of the bound conformations of analogues were validated crystallographically.	4-Guanidino Neu5Ac2en [GG167(**14**)] presently in phase II clinical trials as an agent to prevent influenza virus A infection
Purine nucleoside phosphorylase inhibition	Biocryst Pharmaceuticals, Inc. [127–131]	Iterative cycles of modeling, synthesis, and crystallography to screen synthetic candidates. Compounds docked to PNP-binding site via a	BCX-34 [130,131] (**15**) in multidisease clinical trials: T-cell cancers, RA, MS: phase I/II for oral administration; phase III for topical

		Monte Carlo–energy-minimization protocol [132,133]. Low-energy conformers wre evaluated by molecular graphics. Lowest-energy conformers compared quite well with the X-ray–derived structure. Docking with the native form of PNP was less successful because of conformational changes on inhibitor binding.	administration; Psoriasis: phase II, topical administration
Thymidylate synthase inhibition	Agouron Pharmaceuticals, Inc. [134–136]	Iterative cycles of modeling, synthesis, and crystallography combined with determination of energetically favorable positions of various probes in the TS binding site using GRID program [22].	Thymitaq (AG337) (16) in clinical trials as anticancer agent [137,138].
Carbonic anhydrase inhibition	Merck Research Laboratories [9,15,139]	Multiple crystal structure determinations combined with ab initio conformational analysis to explain stereochemical preference of the S-thienothiopyran-2-sulfonamides series guided choice of substitution pattern; allowed optimization of desired topical efficacy of the molecule without adversely affecting inhibition of CA II.	Trusopt [MK-507 (17)] marketed as an agent to reduce the elevated intraocular pressure associated with glaucoma.

Table 1 (*continued*)

Drug design goal	Research group [ref.]	Methods employed	Outcome
Human rhinoviris-14 inhibition	Sterling Winthrop	Multiple crystal structure determinations of disoxaril (**18**) analogues bound to HRV-14 led to a volume map analysis for active and inactive compounds [140,141]. Model helped explain inactive compounds as having excessive bulk around phenyl ring, whereas active compounds occupy space below the pore area of the compound-binding site. This model guided synthetic efforts away from phenyls.	Disoxaril made it into phase I clinical trials, but fell out owing to crystalurea. WIN 54954 (**19**) and compound (**20**) made it past phase I clinical trials as potential agents to treat the common cold [A. M. Treasurywala, personal communication].
Aldose reductase inhibition	Ayerst Laboratories Research, Inc. [142,143]	Several hundred analogues already synthesized; 100 centered around Alrestatin (**21**). Extended Huckel molecular orbital calculations used to determine electronic effects. Calculations agreed with the SAR that electron-donating groups were desirable at the 6-position and electron withdrawing groups were desirable at the 5-position. Two compounds synthesized based on this model, including tolrestat (**22**) [A. M. Treasurywala, personal communication].	Tolrestat is marketed as an agent to treat some of the opthalmalogical complications of diabetes.

{15}

{14}

{13} [D-Phe-Pro-Arg-Pro-(Gly)₄-Asn-Gly-Asp-Phe-Glu-Glu-Ile-Pro-Glu-Glu-Tyr-Leu]

{19}

{18}

{22}

{21}

{12}

{17}

{16}

{20}

15

{7}

speculated that the rate of metabolism could be diminished by reducing the oxidation potential of the electron-rich pyridinyl groups with thiazole. This resulted in ABT-538, which was modeled into the A-77003 crystallographic complex and suggested that additional hydrophobic interactions between the isopropyl substituent on the P3 thiazolyl group with the side chains of Pro-81 and Val-82 of HIV protease might be established. The contributions of these new interactions to the low K_i of 15 pM for this molecule was validated crystallographically [49].

A second example involves work done at Merck Research Laboratories [52,53] that ultimately lead to the compound, indinavir [Crixivan; MK-639, L-735,524; Structure (8)], which was also recently approved by the FDA. In this work, Holloway and co-workers used the crystallographic complexes of HIV protease bound to acetylpepstatin or L-689,502 as their starting structures. They manually docked inhibitors into the binding site where either acetylpepstatin or L-689,502 had been and minimized the inhibitors keeping the protein fixed. They were able to show a high correlation between calculated intermolecular interaction energies and observed in vitro enzyme inhibition data for an initial training set of 33 inhibitors. They then made a priori predictions on new potential candidates

{8}

{9}

to guide synthetic efforts based on one of these regression models. One of the compounds predicted in advance of synthesis was a key precursor (**9**) of indinavir. The authors point out that even though they neglected key factors for binding, such as enzyme flexibility, inhibitor conformational energy, and solvation–desolvation characteristics of the system, their methods were predictive; successful predictions were made even for molecules that were not close structural analogues of those in the training set. The prime restrictions on attaining a predictive model were that the molecules had to be roughly the same size, occupy similar positions of the enzyme active site (i.e., span the P2–P2′-binding pockets), and that they had to be "charged" in a similar fashion (i.e., all neutral or all protonated). This work emphasizes the need for close collaboration between crystallographers, molecular modelers, and medicinal chemists.

The approach incorporated by the Vertex group in the design of their protease inhibitor, VX-478 [Structure (**10**)], is also an example of straightforward and focused methodology. These researchers prospectively incorporated synthetic accessibility, desirability of low molecular weight, and aqueous solubility, without obligate charges from the outset of their design [54]. They further wanted to avoid unfavorable strain energy by favoring

{10}

compounds for which the conformation would require minimal reorganization on enzyme binding. Thus, their overall strategy was to perform structure-based design employing conformational analysis calculations on potential inhibitors as well as aqueous solubility predictions. They calculated ab initio rotational barriers for the variable benzenesulfonamide nitrogen substituent of these molecules (intended for the P1' pocket), assuring themselves that docked conformations of compounds containing these fragments were close to these ab initio minima. This analysis suggested that branched aliphatics (e.g., N-isobutyl) would incur less strain energy on binding, relative to the prototypical benzyl group at this position. One lesson learned from this exercise was that any gain in binding free energy obtained by the larger benzyl group making more contacts and burying more lipophilic surface area relative to the isobutyl group were offset by a larger conformational strain energy cost.

They also performed a series of aqueous solubility calculations on the partially solvent-exposed P2' sulfonamide portion of these molecules using a variety of techniques [55] to rank their relative solvation free energies. The protease structural information was used in this context to ensure that any substitution that might increase aqueous solubility would not adversely affect binding affinity. Their efforts culminated in VX-478 which possessed all of their design criteria: molecular mass 506 Da, K_i of 0.6 and 19 nM, respectively for HIV-1 and HIV-2 proteases, effective in viral assays, and orally bioavailable. This compound is presently in phase II clinical trials and is being codeveloped by Vertex and GlaxoWellcome.

As a final example in this section, the Agouron group has successfully used crystallographic analysis to help arrive at their protease inhibitor, nelfinavir [Viracept or AG-1343; Structure (11)], which is presently in phase II/III clinical trials [56]. These researchers used mainly molecular graphics to generate ideas from known crystal structures. Nelfinavir was, thus, arrived at by iterative cycles of molecular graphics analysis, chemical synthesis, and crystallographic evaluation of the original design ideas [57].

{11}

The structure-based design cycles were largely aimed at optimizing the left-hand side (2″-methyl-3″-hydroxyphenylamide moiety) of the molecule.

VII. CURRENT ISSUES

What are the critical issues that are currently under study? The dominant ones are the evaluation of the strength of ligand–receptor interactions; the choices of databases to be searched; and methods for searching the conformation space of the ligand and receptor.

Evaluation of ligand–receptor interactions (scoring) is clearly a crucial aspect of selecting compounds [for a complete discussion of scoring functions see Chap. 10]. The most fundamental approach, based on quantum mechanics, has rarely been used for routine studies because of the amount of computational resources required. As computer speed and memory availability continue to improve, ab initio calculations are becoming feasible for host–guest problems [58] and may one day extend to appropriately limited ligand–macromolecule interactions [59]. The standard method used today for calculating interaction energies uses molecular force fields. These equations describe both intra- and intermolecular forces including bonding, van der Waals interactions, and coulombic interactions [60,61]. Good correlations with experimental binding energies have been reported [52,53], but they are usually limited to families of related compounds in one physical setting. Although the usual formulations lead directly to the internal energy of the system, entropic and free-energy terms can be obtained, in principle, using molecular dynamics or Monte Carlo techniques [62]. The cost and precision vary widely with the level of detail in the calculation. It is not easy to guess the accuracy of these approximate force-field calculations for molecular interactions in which one component is a macromolecule. Estimates of ± 4 kcal have been made [19]. Free-energy perturbation methods have in the best cases led to much more accurate results of about ± 1 kcal [19].

A second approach to evaluating molecular interactions uses heuristic models, either independently or in concert with the force-field terms [63]. The goal is to represent aspects of the system that might not be well-captured by the force-field approximations. For example, hydrogen-bonding, strain energy, and the hydrophobic effect are often accounted for in an ad hoc manner. Heuristic methods are especially useful when a complex concept can be approximated by a simple function, as in the use of buried surface area as a measure of the configurational entropy of the solvent [63].

Finally, one can make use of statistical procedures, the terms of which often include those mentioned in the foregoing discussion, but in which the importance of each term is adjusted to give the best-fit to a "training" data set. Statistical methods have the advantage that precise knowledge of the interaction coefficients or even of the "correct" equations themselves is not needed. They are often excellent interpolative procedures. Recent results have standard deviations in the free energy of binding of $\pm 1–2$ kcal [64; G. Marshall, personal communiction] over limited data sets. However, they have little or no physical rigor and are difficult to extrapolate to new systems.

Scoring is especially important in database searching when large numbers of diverse compounds are compared with each other. In our work, we have used a truncated molecular mechanics force field, evaluated on a grid, to achieve some balance of accuracy and speed [65].

Good quality structures of small molecules are important both as the foundation from which pharmacophore models are created and as the raw material for the database searching. The best starting point is experimental data, when available [66]. The most popular computational approaches are rule-based [67–69], although distance geometry [70] and molecular mechanics optimization [71] are also used. An unresolved issue is how extensive a set of ligand conformations should be generated. For database searching, it is frequently assumed that a single low-energy conformation is sufficient (see following discussion).

The databases of most interest are the Cambridge Structural File [72]; the Available Chemical Directory distributed by MDL Information Systems, San Leandro CA; the National Institute of Cancer Database [73]; and sections of the Chemical Abstracts Registry.

In the last few years, three-dimensional search methods [74–76] have begun to explore the conformational flexibility of potential ligands. Although storing multiple conformations of a single molecule is conceptually simple, it is limited by the amount of storage space available and by the linear increase in search time with the number of molecules to be searched. It is also impossible to ensure that the conformation being sought will be among those stored, even with systematic search algorithms, because of the chance that the conformation of the bound ligand is not a minimum-energy structure in the absence of the receptor. Instead of storing multiple conformations, some approaches [76] encode the distances accessible to pairs of atom centers. These accessible distances are used during the search to select molecules that could match a particular query, and the matching conformations are generated for only those compounds. Other approaches [74,75] adjust torsional angles to match the query. Flexible searching can significantly increase the amount of computer time required for searching. Because more hits are produced in a given search, the amount of human time required for screening the results also increases.

In our own work, we have used fragment-joining algorithms [77,78], and a procedure in which the largest rigid fragment in a molecule is docked and the rest of the molecule is attached while exploring conformational choices [79]. More recently, we have used a genetic algorithm to optimize conformations of compounds during docking [80].

To this point, little attention has been paid to macromolecular flexibility in database searching, although there are some indications on how to begin such an effort [81–83]. However, a very recent paper includes full flexibility of ligands and limited flexibility of the protein target [84].

In searching for a pharmacophore, it is sufficient to determine whether a molecule contains a specified set of distances and angles. Docking methods must go further to explore the orientational and translational space established by the receptor geometry. Studies with single ligands, for which bound geometries are known, have demonstrated that DOCK is capable of locating the correct binding orientations [65]. In searching databases, care is required to balance the number of orientations sampled for each molecule against the computer time available to search all desired molecules. The time required for such searches to be successful has recently been studied by Gschwend and co-workers [64,85], who concluded that the use of a simplex minimizer to adjust orientations improved performance. We are continuing to experiment with minimization in database searching because it allows us to sample fewer orientations and to use the computer time saved to optimize the best ones.

De novo design methods present an alternative to database searching, and they allow template selection, lead optimization, and the design of totally novel molecules. De novo design is advancing rapidly [24,86,87; see also Chap. 9]. Even though these approaches require a commitment to synthetic chemistry, they can immediately generate novel compounds of a proprietary nature.

Finding new leads is a demonstrated strength of database-searching methods, but these leads must usually be optimized to improve their activity, increase bioavailability, or reduce toxicity. These needs offer an opportunity to develop computer methods that will guide medicinal chemists in choosing chemical modifications. Structure-based approaches are most likely to be useful when the ligand-binding mode is well understood [88]. Improved functions for evaluating molecular interactions, or sampling procedures such as GRID [22] or multicopy simultaneous search [23] can be used to locate sites for modification. Considerations of solvation, counterions, and specific hydrogen-bonding are often of crucial importance. Some successes in such optimization of lead compounds have been reported [52,53,89,90, and other chapters in this book].

VIII. CURRENT ASSESSMENT

How shall we judge the contributions of computer-aided molecular design to drug discovery? It is too early to make a direct statement about the number of compounds that have reached the marketplace. This may not even be the most productive way to consider complex undertakings in which many components contribute to a final result. Instead, computer-aided molecular design should be judged on the same basis as any discovery technique: correct identification of compounds that bind to the target; correlation of structure and activity; accuracy of geometric hypotheses associated with pharmacophore models; predictability of statistical models; and correct ligand placement, ligand conformation, and macromolecular conformation in docking calculations. Practical considerations, such as cost and speed, are also important.

Present programs are relatively successful at lead identification [52,53,89,90]. This is the easiest task, because false-positive hits are acceptable and false-negative ones are not recognized. Typical hit rates of 1–10% are competitive with high-throughput experimental screens, and computer screening is much less expensive. An important issue is to determine the false-negative rate in computer screening. An appropriate test would be to run a substantial, diverse database of compounds through both computer and experimental screenings. Searches for antagonists of molecular recognition or macromolecular conformation changes have been more difficult, but some successes have been reported [91]. Nucleic acid targets have also been studied [92–94].

Structure–activity predictions in which the binding free energy has been calculated for diverse ligands bound to a common receptor have been in line with the foregoing expectations. Average errors are typically a few kilocalories per mole when only force-field terms are used. A comparison of scores with K_i or IC_{50} data spanning many orders of magnitude for a set of diverse inhibitor–receptor complexes would provide a stringent test of current scoring functions. Use of the most computationally intensive techniques, limiting attention to a family of analogues can yield much better agreement [52,53]. The present computational methods are better-suited for extracting the more active compounds from a database than for guiding the fine details of analogue synthesis. Compounds retrieved using these techniques have shown selectivity for the target [95–97].

The hardest task to ask of a docking computation is to predict the binding geometry (or geometries) of a ligand, for this involves assessing the relative free energy of several alternative binding modes. In our work, the computer methods have been good at suggesting plausible binding geometries [98,99], but as expected, they do not always select the dominant-binding mode or forecast the conformational rearrangements that occur. The most difficult task is to propose accurate (± 1 Å rms) geometric models. With DOCK, the best cases have shown displacements of 1–2 Å from the predicted geometry. In the worst cases, the displacements are about 5 Å [98,99]. Complications include the conformational freedom of the ligand and the receptor, the possibility of alternative-binding modes (configurational freedom), and the inclusion of water molecules and ions as part of the binding complex [100]. We have had problems with all of these phenomena. The obvious design or test protocol is to combine structural experiments with computations to provide rapid assessment of the degrees of freedom of a particular system of interest [99]. Some successful efforts at structure-based design have used one X-ray structure for each one to two compounds synthesized [101].

An important issue that is curiously difficult to resolve is the appropriate control for database searching. Ideally, comparing comprehensive screening with a rank-ordering obtained computationally would provide the necessary information to evaluate the performance of the program. A complete effort is probably not feasible because it would involve determining the chemical and chiral purity of all the compounds used, establishing the equilibrium binding constant of each compound, and adjusting the computation to match the assay conditions. Aspects of this experiment in which activities are measured and a list of false-positive and false-negative hits is generated have probably been carried out in industrial laboratories, but we are unaware of published analyses. For directed combinatorial libraries, in which only a limited set of compounds are chosen for synthesis, the comparison is even more difficult.

Overall, the current state of computer-aided molecular design can be summarized by saying that the methods meet the same standard of performance as other discovery methods: they identify molecules that can move forward into the clinics. It has proved most effective, to this point, for enzyme inhibitors. From anecdotal experiences, it offers some speedup and cost reductions (once the capital costs of the structural determinations are allowed for) because fewer syntheses are required for each clinical candidate. It is an attractive scientific approach because it offers testable structural hypotheses to guide the project.

IX. FUTURE ISSUES

Clearly, over the next decade, we can expect technical improvements in database searching, especially in the exploration of conformations and in the calculation of $\Delta G_{binding}$. Historically, these improvements have come by two routes: better algorithms and improvements in computers. Both will remain important in the future. We can anticipate that incorporation of the Ewald sums technology, and improvements in Poisson–Boltzmann treatments will lead to a better understanding of electrostatics and solvation [102; see also Chap. 11]. Second- and third-generation force fields will have moved from the current development phase into general usage [60,103–107; see also Chap. 13]. Increased processor speeds will extend the scope of free-energy perturbation computations. Within a single target system, a reasonable goal is an accuracy of ± 1 kcal, which implies routine searches of both the ligand and the side-chain conformational space. Finally, the availability of increased amounts of physical memory will permit greatly improved database searches by reducing the necessary amount of time-consuming disk input and output.

The improved engineering of user interfaces to computer-aided discovery programs should allow better access to the results in the future. The molecules retrieved by the database searches are determined only by the searching method and by the contents of the database. Hits are returned without consideration of availability, cost, synthetic accessibility, solubility, toxicity profiles, known impurities, or other parameters. The efforts of the chemist to examine the output could be made much more efficient if the final list included only those compounds that met user-determined criteria. Removing compounds because they are in chemical classes deemed to be uninteresting or because they contain biologically undesirable groups should be a straightforward procedure. An expert system to evaluate synthetic prospects could be used in de novo design as well as database searching [108,109].

The recent introduction of solid-phase methods for the simultaneous synthesis of many compounds with a common skeleton [110], now called combinatorial chemistry, provides an exciting meeting ground for the melding of chemistry and computation. Advances have already been made in optimal design for diversity and for directed libraries [111]. Docking procedures can be used to assist in the selection of scaffolds and side chains. Large libraries of "virtual" compounds can be examined before synthesis.

A crucial biological challenge to structure-based design has emerged in virulent resistance to even subnanomolar inhibitors of retroviral enzymes [112]. The expectation that mutations will generally produce less efficient enzymes [113] holds for point mutations of the HIV protease [114]. However, the virus explores a wide range of multiple mutations located away from the active site that appear to restore wild-type activity while reducing sensitivity to any single protease inhibitor. Even inhibitors designed to interact primarily with backbone atoms [115] have generated significant resistance. This challenge goes to the heart of structure–based design: that drugs and the substrates are competing for the same enzyme pockets. No strategy has yet been developed that clearly enunciates the rules of this competition. We may have to extend the vision of design from increasing the affinity of inhibitors to exploring large-scale kinetic barriers for the entire enzyme.

Another important issue is the use of structure-based methods to design agonists. This is a much more difficult problem than the design of antagonists. Antagonists can block processes in many ways, whereas agonist design generally requires some knowledge of the underlying mechanism. One exciting set of targets is the family of pharmacological receptors that use dimerization to generate a signal. An example, human growth hormone receptor (hGHr), has been crystallized bound to its ligand, human growth hormone (hGH) [116]. An examination of the structure immediately suggests that small-molecule agonists might be designed that encourage association of the hGHr dimer in the absence of hGH.

X. CONCLUSIONS

A perusal of the computer-assisted drug design success stories presented in this chapter gives one the impression that most of the examples rely on fairly fundamental methods such as molecular graphics, interaction energies, and molecular-docking, coupled with medicinal chemistry intuition. The reason that these more "simplistic methods" have been the most successful is the promotion of multidisciplinary "buy-in" from the outset of any design cycle [9,13,15,52,53]. This often affords a rapid evaluation of ideas and allows the early incorporation of synthetic and bioavailability considerations. Although all of the methods discussed in this chapter have shown documented contributions toward potent "drug-like" molecules, it is clearly our bias that the structure-based approaches possess the greatest overall potential.

Certain aspects of the docking problem have been solved. Both known and novel binding sites can be identified through automatic procedures, such as the negative-imaging approach used with DOCK [1]. Many of the programs discussed can reassemble the components of a known complex within 1-Å rms of the experimental structure. That is, the problem of constructing a "three-dimensional jigsaw puzzle" from rigid pieces of proper conformation has been solved. However, multiple-binding geometries, plausible on steric and chemical grounds, are routinely seen in docking studies [117]. The number of alternatives increases when conformational freedom is introduced. To sort among these states requires quite accurate determinations of free energy (e.g., ± 1 kcal/mol). Nevertheless, as we have documented in this chapter, there are now many examples of "proof-of-concept" in which lead development and lead optimization have been based on macromolecular structures.

There should be little doubt, however, that methods steeped in a more rigorous theoretical framework will also have their day in the sun, given the caveats of ameliorating some of the limitations cited in the foregoing. There are already clear examples in which methods, such as free-energy perturbation, have allowed the prioritization of design ideas for synthesis [118]. Also, note that in many of the examples presented, the word *iterative* is used to describe the design process. This is quite important, in that it should remove any misconceptions that a single piece of structural information or that a single model of any type is a static entity. These models must evolve toward the direction set by high-quality experimental data as it becomes available.

Calculations serve many purposes in the drug design effort. Four goals of structure-driven design are screening for new leads, rank-ordering similar and diverse compounds, proposing preferred ligand–receptor geometries, and rapid, semiautomatic optimization of a lead compound. A refinement of this last goal is coupling calculations to combinatorial chemistry [110].

One issue that has been only briefly discussed in this chapter is successes of computational methods as applied to combinatorial chemistry. Chapter 5 discusses the various computational tools that have been developed to aid in the design of chemical libraries, monomer selection, and analyses, which have led to in vitro successes [119,120]. Others have also reported examples in which computational methods have aided in the optimization of chemical libraries [121,122]. It will likely be a relatively short time before clear clinical successes can be traced to computational–combinatorial roots.

In sum, this is an exciting time in pharmaceutical science. Basic research into molecular interactions is being rapidly converted into practical procedures for drug discovery and optimization. Although much remains to be done, an important beginning has been made.

ACKNOWLEDGMENTS

We thank our many colleagues whose work has been discussed in this review. We would particularly like to thank the following individuals for their frank discussions: M. Katharine Holloway, Steven R. Jordan, Patrick Y. Lam, Yvonne C. Martin, Catherine E. Peishoff, Kent D. Stewart, and Adi M. Treasurywala. IDK's software projects have been funded by the

National Institutes of Health, the Department of Energy, and gifts from SmithKline Beecham, Glaxo Wellcome, Parke-Davis, and Procept.

REFERENCES

1. I. D. Kuntz, Structure-based strategies for drug design and discovery, *Science* *257*:1078–1082 (1992).
2. J. A. DiMasi, N. R. Bryant, and L. Lasagna, New drug development in the United States from 1963 to 1990, *Clin. Pharmacol. Ther. 50*:471–486 (1991).
3. H. M. Geysen, R. H. Meloen, and S. J. Barteling, Use of peptide synthesis to probe viral antigens for epitopes to a resolution of a single amino acid, *Proc. Natl. Acad. Sci. USA 81*:3998–4002 (1984).
4. E. M. Gordon, R. W. Barrett, W. J. Dower, S. P. A. Fodor, and M. A. Gallop, Applications of combinatorial technologies to drug discovery. 2. Combinatorial organic synthesis, library screening strategies, and future directions, *J. Med. Chem. 37*:1385–1400 (1994).
5. P. G. Schultz and R. A. Lerner, From molecular diversity to catalysis: Lessons from the immune system, *Science 269*:1835–1842 (1995).
6. E. Perez-Paya, R. A. Houghten, and S. E. Blondelle, Functionalized protein-like structures from conformationally defined synthetic combinatorial libraries, *J. Biol. Chem. 271*:4120–4126 (1996).
7. L. A. Thompson and J. A. Ellman, Synthesis and applications of small molecule libraries, *Chem. Rev. 96*:555–600 (1996).
8. D. B. Boyd, Successes of computer-assisted molecular design, *Rev. Comput. Chem. 1*:355–371 (1990).
9. M. A. Navia and M. A. Murcko, Use of structural information in drug design, *Curr. Opin. Struct. Biol. 2*:202–210 (1992).
10. J. W. Erickson and S. W. Fesik, Macromolecular X-ray crystallography and NMR as tools for structure-based drug design, *Annu. Rep. Med. Chem. 27*: 271–289 (1992).
11. C. E. Bugg, W. M. Carson, and and J. A. Montgomery, Drugs by design, *Sci. Am.* 92–98, (Dec., 1993).
12. R. Peters and R. C. McKinstry, Three-dimensional modeling and drug development: Has rational drug design arrived? *Biotechnology 12*:147–150 (1994).
13. P. J. Whittle and T. L. Blundell, Protein structure-based drug design, *Annu. Rev. Biophys. Biomol. Struct. 23*:349–375 (1994).
14. W. G. J. Hol and C. L. M. J. Verlinde, Structure-based drug design: Progress, results, and challenges, *Structure 2*: 577–587 (1994).
15. J. Greer, J. W. Erickson, J. L. Baldwin, and M. D. Varney, Application of the three-dimensional structures of protein target molecules in structure-based drug design, *J. Med. Chem. 37*:1035–1054 (1994).
16. W. C. Guida, Software for structure-based drug design, *Curr. Opin. Struct. Biol. 4*:777–781 (1994).

17. R. C. Jackson, Update on computer-aided drug design, *Curr. Opin. Biotechnol. 6*:646–651 (1995).
18. R. DesJarlais, R. P. Sheridan, G. L. Seibel, J. S. Dixon, I. D. Kuntz, and R. Venkataraghavan, Using shape complementarity as an initial screen in designing ligands for a receptor binding site of known three-dimensional structure, *J. Med. Chem. 31*:722–729 (1988).
19. I. D. Kuntz, E. C. Meng, and B. K. Shoichet, Structure-based molecular design, *Acc. Chem. Res. 27*:117–123 (1994).
20. Y. C. Martin, 3D database searching in drug design, *J. Med. Chem. 35*: 2145–2154 (1992).
21. P. J. Artymiuk, P. A. Bath, H. M. Grindley, et al., Similarity searching in databases of 3-dimensional molecules and macromolecules, *J. Chem. Inf. Comput. Sci. 32*:617–630 (1992).
22. P. J. Goodford, A computational procedure for determining energetically favorable binding sites on biologically important macromolecules, *J. Med. Chem. 28*:849–857 (1985).
23. A. Miranker and M. Karplus, Functionality maps of binding sites—a multiple copy simultaneous search method, *Proteins Struct. Funct. Genet. 11*: 29–34 (1991).
24. R. S. Bohacek and C. McMartin, Multiple highly diverse structures complementary to enzyme binding sites—results of extensive application of de novo design method incorporating combinatorial growth, *J. Am. Chem. Soc. 116*: 5560–5571 (1994).
25. E. J. Corey and W. T. Wipke, Automated computer program for organic synthesis, *Science 166*:178 (1969).
26. A. P. Johnson, C. Marshall and P. N. Judson, Starting material oriented retrosynthetic analysis in the LHASA program. 1. General description, *J. Chem. Inf. Comput. Sci. 32*:411–417 (1992).
27. W. T. Wipke and T. M. Dyott, Simulation and evaluation of chemical synthesis. Computer representation and manipulation of stereochemistry, *J. Am. Chem. Soc. 96*:4825–4834 (1974).
28. W. A. Denny, Amsacrine, *Chronicles of Drug Discovery* Vol. 3 (D. Lednicer, ed.), American Chemical Society, Washington DC, 1993, pp. 381–404.
29. V. J. Harvey, J. R. Hardy, P. C. Evans, J. W. Paxton, W. Grove, A. Grillo-Lopez, and B. C. Baguley, *Proc. Am. Soc. Clin. Oncol. 5*:204 (1988).
30. H. Kubinyi, ed., *3D-QSAR in Drug Design: Theory, Methods and Applications*, ESCOM Science Publishers, Leiden, 1993.
31. A. K. Ghose and G. M. Crippen, Modeling the benzodiazepine receptor binding site by the general three-dimensional structure-directed quantitative structure-activity relationship method REMOTEDISC, *Mol. Pharmacol. 37*: 725–734 (1990).
32. A. N. Jain, K. Koile, and D. Chapman, Compass: Predicting biological activities from molecular surface properties. Performance comparisons on a steroid benchmark, *J. Med. Chem. 37*:2315–2327 (1994).

33. A. N. Jain, N. L. Harris, and J. Y. Park, Quantitative binding site model generation: Compass applied to multiple chemotypes targeting 5-HT$_{1a}$ receptor, *J. Med. Chem. 38*:1295–1308 (1995).

34. T. I. Oprea, C. L. Waller, and G. L. Marshall, 3-D QSAR of HIV-1 protease inhibitors. 2. Predictive power using limited exploration of alternate binding modes, *J. Med. Chem. 37*:2206–2215 (1994).

35. J. S. Tokarski and A. J. Hopfinger, 3-D molecular shape analysis—QSAR of a series of cholecystokinin-A receptor antagonists, *J. Med. Chem. 37*: 3639–3654 (1994).

36. Y. C. Martin, C. T. Lin, and J. Wu , Application of CoMFA to D$_1$ dopaminergic agonists: A case study, *3D-QSAR in Drug Design: Theory, Methods and Applications* (H. Kubinyi, ed.), ESCOM Science Publishers, Leiden, 1993, pp. 643–660.

37. C. E. Peishoff, F. E. Ali, J. W. Bean, R. Calvo, C. A. D'Ambrosio, D. S. Eggleston, S. M. Hwang, T. P. Kline, P. F. Koster, A. Nichols, D. Powers, T. Romoff, J. M. Samanen, J. Stadel, J. A. Vasko, and K. D. Kopple, Investigation of conformational specificity at GPIIb/IIIa: Evaluation of conformationally constrained RGD peptide, *J. Med. Chem. 35*:3962–3969 (1992).

38. K. D. Kopple, P. W. Baures, J. W. Bean, C. A. D'Ambrosio, J. L. Hughes, C. E. Peishoff, and D. S. Eggleston, *J. Am. Chem. Soc. 114*:9615–9623 (1992).

39. J. F. Callahan, J. W. Bean, J. L. Burgess, D. S. Eggleston, K. D. Kopple, A. Nichols, C. E. Peishoff, J. M. Samanen, A. Wong, and W. F. Huffman, Design and synthesis of a C$_7$ mimetic for the predicted γ-turn conformation found in several constrained RGD antagonists, *J. Med. Chem. 35*:3970–3972 (1992).

40. T. W. Ku, F. E. Ali, L. S. Barton, J. W. Bean, W. E. Bondinell, J. L. Burgess, J. F. Callahan, R. R. Calvo, L. Chen, D. S. Eggleston, J. G. Gleason, W. F. Huffman, S. M. Hwang, D. R. Jakas, C. B. Karash, R. M. Keenan, K. D. Kopple, W. H. Miller, K. A. Newlander, A. Nichols, M. F. Parker, C. E. Peishoff, J. M. Samanen, I. Uzinskas, and J. W. Venslavsky, Direct design of a potent non-peptide fibrinogen receptor antagonist based on the structure and conformation of a highly constrained cyclic RGD peptide, *J. Am. Chem. Soc. 115*:8861–8862 (1993).

41. R. S. McDowell, T. R. Gadek, P. L. Barker, et al., From peptide to nonpeptide. 1. The elucidation of a bioactive conformation of the arginineglycine-aspartic acid recognition sequence, *J. Am. Chem. Soc. 116*: 5069–5076 (1994).

42. R. S. McDowell, B. K. Blackburn, T. R. Gadek, et al., From peptide to nonpeptide. 2. The de novo design of potent, non-peptidal inhibitors of platelet aggregation based on a benzodiazepinedione scaffold, *J. Am. Chem. Soc. 116*:5077–5083 (1994).

43. M. E. Duggan, A. M. Naylor-Olsen, J. J. Perkins, P. S. Anderson, C. T.-C. Chang, J. L. Cook, R. J. Gould, N. C. Ihle, G. D. Hartman, J. L. Lynch, R. L. Lynch, P. D. Manno, L. W. Schaffer, and R. L. Smith, Non-peptide

fibrinogen receptor antagonists. 7. Design and synthesis of a potent, orally active fibrinogen receptor antagonist, *J. Med. Chem. 38*:3332–3341 (1995).

44. P. Y. S. Lam, P. K. Jadhav, C. J. Eyermann, C. N. Hodge, Y. Ru, L. T., Bacheler, J. L. Meek, M. L. Otto, M. M. Rayner, Y. N. Wong, C. -H. Chang, P. C. Weber, D. A. Jackson, T. R. Sharpe, and S. Erickson-Viitanen, Rational design of potent, bioavailable, nonpeptide cyclic ureas as HIV protease inhibitors, *Science 263*:380–384 (1994).

45. J. D. Elliott, M. A. Lago, R. D. Cousins, A. Gao, J. D. Leber, K. F. Erhard, P. Nambi, N. A. Elshourbagy, C. Kumar, J. A. Lee, J. W. Bean, C. W. BeBrosse, D. S. Eggleston, D. P. Brooks, G, Feuerstein, R. R. Ruffolo, Jr., J. Weinstock, J. G. Gleason, C. E. Peishoff, and E. H. Ohlstein, 1,3-Diarylindan-2-carboxylic acids, potent and selective non-peptide endothelin receptor antagonists, *J. Med. Chem. 37*:1553–1557 (1994).

46. V. Glaser, Structure-based drug design remains a key method for drug discovery and optimization, *Genet. Eng. News 16(12)*:1,20,33 (1996).

47. G. Klopman, S. Wang, and D. M. Balthasar, Estimation of aqueous solubility of organic molecules by the group contribution approach. Application to the study of biodegradation *J. Chem. Inf. Comput. Sci. 32*:474–82 (1992).

48. L. A. Carreira, S. H. Hilal, and S. W. Karickhoff, Calculation of ionization pK_a for complex molecules. Book of Abstracts, 210th ACS National Meeting, Chicago IL, August 20–24 (1995), Issue Pt. 1, ENVR-052, American Chemical Society, Washington DC.

49. A. Wlodawer and J. W. Erickson, Structure-based inhibitors of HIV-1 protease, *Annu. Rev. Biochem. 62*:543–585 (1993).

50. D. J. Kempf, K. C. Marsh, J. F. Denissen, E. McDonald, S. Vasavanonda, C. A. Flentge, B. E. Green, L. Fino, C. H. Park, X. -P. Kong, N. E. Wideburg, A. Saldivar, L. Ruiz, W. M. Kati, H. L. Sham, T. Robbins, K. D. Stewart, A. Hsu, J. J. Plattner, J. M. Leonard, and D. W. Norbeck, ABT-538 is a potent inhibitor of human immunodeficiency virus protease and has high oral bioavailability in humans, *Proc. Natl. Acad. Sci. USA 92*:2484–2488 (1995).

51. M. V. Hosur, T. N. Bhat, D. J. Kempf, E. T. Baldwin, B. Liu, S. Gulnik, N. E. Wideburg, D. W. Norbeck, K. Appelt, and J. W. Erickson, Influence of stereochemistry on activity and binding modes for C_2 symmetry-based diol inhibitors of HIV-1 protease, *J. Am. Chem. Soc. 116*:847–855 (1994).

52. M. K. Holloway, J. M. Wai, T. A. Halgren, P. M. D. Fitzgerald, J. P. Vacca, B. D. Dorsey, R. B. Levin, W. J. Thompson, L. J. Chen, S. J. DeSolms, N. Gaffin, A. K. Ghosh, E. A. Giuliani, S. L. Graham, J. P. Guare, R. W. Hungate, T. A. Lyle, W. M. Sanders, T. J. Tucker, M. Wiggins, C. M. Wiscount, O. W. Woltersdorf, S. D. Young, P. L. Darke, and J. A. Zugay, A priori prediction of activity for HIV-1 protease inhibitors employing energy minimization in the active site, *J. Med. Chem. 38*:305–317 (1995).

53. M. K. Holloway and J. M. Wai, Structure-based design of human immunodeficiency virus-1 protease inhibitors. Correlating calculated energy with activity. *ACS Symp. Ser. Comput. Aided Mol. Design 589*:36–50 (1995).

54. E. E., Kim, C. T. Baker, M. D. Dwyer, M. A. Murcko, B. G, Rao, R. D. Tung, and M. A. Navia, Crystal structure of HIV-1 protease in complex with VX-478, a potent and orally bioavailable inhibitor of the enzyme, *J. Am. Chem. Soc. 117*:1181–1182 (1995).

55. B. G. Rao, E. E. Kim, and M. A. Murcko, Calculation of solvation and binding free energy differences between VX-478 and its analogs by free energy perturbation and AMSOL methods, *J. Comput. Aided Mol. Desgn.10*: 23–30 (1996).

56. A. K. Patick, H. Mo, M. Markowitz, et al., Antiviral and resistance studies of AG1343, an orally bioavailable inhibitor of human immunodeficiency virus protease, *Antimicrob. Agents Chemother. 40*:292–297 (1996).

57. S. W. Kaldor, V. J. Kalish, J. F. Davies, II, B. V. Shetty, J. E. Fritz, B. A. Dressman, J. H. Tatlock, K. Appelt, K. S. Su, K. M. Campanale, J. A. Burgess, P. L. Lubbehusen, M. A. Muesing, S. D. Hatch, N. Y. Chirgadze, D. A. Clawson, A. K. Patick, M. B. Kosa, and D. A. Khalil, AG1343: A potent, orally bioavailable inhibitor of HIV-1 protease. (manuscript in preparation; 1996).

58. M. Badertscher, M. Welti, P. Portmann, and E. Pretsch, Calculation of interaction energies in host–guest systems, *Curr. Chem. (Biomimetic Bioorg. Chem. 3)136*:17–80 (1986).

59. R. V. Stanton, S. L. Dixon, K. M. Merz, Jr., Free energy perturbation calculations within quantum mechanical methodologies, *ACS Symp. Ser. (Chemical Applications of Density-Functional Theory) 629*:142–153 (1996).

60. W. D. Cornell, P. Cieplak, C. I. Bayly, and P. A. Kollman, Application of RESP charges to calculate conformational energies, hydrogen bond energies and free energies of solvation, *J. Am. Chem. Soc. 115*:9620–9631 (1993).

61. S. J. Weiner, P. A. Kollman, D. A. Case, U. C. Singh, C. Ghio, G. Alagona, S. Profeta, and P. A. Weiner, A new force field for molecular mechanical simulation of nucleic acids and proteins, *J. Am. Chem. Soc. 106*:765–784 (1984).

62. W. L. Jorgensen and T. B. Nguyen, Monte Carlo simulations of the hydration of substituted benzenes, *J. Comput. Chem. 14*:195–205 (1993).

63. D. Eisenberg and A. D. McLachlan, Solvation energy in protein folding and binding, *Nature 319*:199–203 (1986).

64. D. Gschwend, Molecular Docking, PhD. dissertation, University of California, San Francisco, 1995.

65. E. C. Meng, B. K. Shoichet, and I. D. Kuntz, Automated docking with grid-based energy evaluation. *J. Comput. Chem. 13*:505–524 (1992).

66. F. H. Allen and O. Kennard, 3D search and research using the Cambridge Structural Database, *Chem. Design Automat. News 8 (1)*:1,31–37 (1993).

67. D. P. Dolata, A. R. Leach, and K. Prout, WIZARD: AI in conformational analysis, *J. Comput-Aided Mol. Design 1*:73–85 (1987).

68. A. R. Leach and K. Prout, Automated conformational analysis—directed conformational search using the A* algorithm, *J. Comput. Chem. 11*: 1193–1205 (1990).

69. A. Rusinko, R. P. Sheridan, R. Nilakatan, K. S. Haraki, N. Bauman, and R. Venkataghavan, Using CONCORD to construct a large database of 3-dimensional coordinates from connection tables, *J. Chem. Inf. Comput. Sci.* 29:251–255 (1989).

70. Rubicon, Daylight Chemical Information Systems, Mission Viejo CA.

71. N. L. Allinger, Y. H. Yuh, and J. J. Lii, Molecular mechanics in the MM3 force field for hydrocarbons, *J. Am. Chem. Soc.* 111:8551–8566 (1989).

72. F. H. Allen, S. Bellard, M. D. Brice, B. A. Cartwright, A. Doubleday, H. Higgs, T. Hummelink, B. G. Hummelink-Peters, O. Kennard, W. D. S. Motherwell, J. R. Rodgers, and D. G. Watson, The Cambridge Crystallographic Data Centre: Computer-based search retrieval, analysis, and display of information, *Acta Crystallogr. Sect. B* 35:2331–2339 (1979).

73. G. W. A. Milne, M. C. Nicklaus, J. S. Driscoll, and S. Wang. National Cancer Institute Drug Information System 3D Database, *J. Chem. Inf. Comput. Sci.* 34:1219–1224 (1994).

74. T. J. Hurst, Flexible 3D searching—the directed tweak technique, *J. Chem. Inf. Comput. Sci.* 34:190–196 (1994).

75. T. E. Moock, D. R. Henry, A. G. Ozkabak, and M. Alamgir, Conformational searching in ISIS/3D databases, *J. Chem. Inf. Comput. Sci.* 34:184 (1994).

76. N. W. Murrall and E. K. Davies, Conformational freedom in 3D databases. 1. Techniques, *J. Chem. Inf. Comput. Sci.* 30:312–316 (1990).

77. R. L. DesJarlais, R. P. Sheridan, J. S. Dixon, I. D. Kuntz, and R. Venkataraghavan, Docking flexible ligands to macromolecular receptors by molecular shape, *J. Med. Chem.* 29:2149–2153 (1986).

78. R. A. Lewis, D. C. Roe, C. Huang, T. E. Ferrin, R. Langridge, and I. D. Kuntz, Automated site-directed drug design using molecular lattices, *J. Mol. Graph.* 10:66–78 (1992).

79. A. R. Leach and I. D. Kuntz, Conformational analysis of flexible ligands in macromolecular receptor sites, *J. Comput. Chem.* 13:730–748 (1992).

80. C. M. Oshiro, I. D. Kuntz, and J. S. Dixon, Flexible ligand docking using a genetic algorithm, *J. Comput.-Aided Mol. Design* 9:113–130 (1995).

81. J. W. Ponder and F. M. Richards, Tertiary templates for proteins: Use of packing criteria in the enumeration of allowed sequences for different structural classes, *J. Mol. Biol.* 193:775–791 (1987).

82. C. Wilson, L. M. Gregoret, and D. A. Agard, Modeling side-chain conformation for homologous proteins using an energy-based rotamer search, *J. Mol. Biol.* 229:996–1006 (1993).

83. A. R. Leach, Ligand docking to proteins with discrete side-chain flexibility, *J. Mol. Biol.* 235:345–356 (1994).

84. G. Jones, P. Willett, and R. C. Glen, Molecular recognition of receptor sites using a genetic algorithm with a description of desolvation, *J. Mol. Biol.* 245:43–53 (1995).

85. E. C. Meng, D. A. Gschwend, J. M. Blaney, and I. D. Kuntz, Orientational sampling and rigid-body minimization in molecular docking, *Proteins Struct. Funct. Genet.* 17:266–278 (1993).

86. H. -J. Bohm, The computer program LUDI: A new method for the de novo design of enzyme inhibitors, *J. Comput.-Aided Mol. Design 6*:61–78 (1992).
87. H. -J. Bohm, LUDI: A rule-based automatic design of new substituents for enzyme inhibitor leads, *J. Comput.-Aided Mol. Design 6*:593–606 (1992).
88. K. Appelt, R. J. Bacquet, C. A. Bartlett, C. L. J. Booth, S. T. Freer, M. A. M. Fuhry, M. R. Gehring, S. M. Herrmann, E. F. Howland, C. A. Janson, T. R. Jones, C. -C. Kan, V. Kathardekar, K. K. Lewis, G. P. Marzoni, D. A. Matthews, C. Mohr, E. W. Moomaw, C. A. Morse, S. J. Oatley, R. C. Ogden, M. R. Reddy, S. H. Reich, W. S. Schoettlin, W. W. Smith, M. D. Varney, J. E. Villafranca, R. W. Ward, S. Webber, S. E. Webber, K. M. Welsh, and J. White, Design of enzyme inhibitors using iterative protein crystallographic analysis, *J. Med. Chem. 34*:1925–1934 (1991).
89. S. S. Abdel Meguid, B. W. Metcalf, T. J. Carr, et al., An orally bioavailable HIV-1 protease inhibitor containing an imidazole-derived peptide bond replacement—crystallographic and pharmacokinetic analysis, *Biochemistry 33*:11671–11677 (1994).
90. B. D. Dorsey, R. B. Levin, J. P. Vacca, et al., L-735,524—the design of a potent and orally bioavailable HIV protease inhibitor, *J. Med. Chem. 37*: 3443–3451 (1994).
91. D. L. Bodian, R. B. Yamasaki, R. L. Buswell, J. F. Stearns, J. M. White, and I. D. Kuntz, Inhibition of the fusion-inducing conformational change of influenza hemagglutinin by 1,4-benzoquinones and hydroquinones, *Biochemistry 32*:2967–2978 (1993).
92. P. D. J. Grootenhuis, D. C. Roe, P. A. Kollman, and I. D. Kuntz, Finding potential DNA binding compounds by using molecular shape, *J. Comput. Aided Mol. Design 8*:731–750 (1994).
93. S. M. Kerwin, I. D. Kuntz, and G. L. Kenyon, The design of a DNA binding compound using an automated procedure for screening potential ligands, *Med. Chem. Res. 1*:361–368 (1991).
94. Qi Chen, I. D. Kuntz, and R. H. Shafer, Spectroscopic recognition of guanine dimeric hairpin quadruplexes by a carbocyanine dye, *Proc. Natl. Acad. Sci. USA 93*:2635–2639 (1996).
95. R. L. DesJarlais, G. L. Seibel, I. D. Kuntz, P. R. Ortiz de Montellano, P. S. Furth, J. C. Alvarez, D. L. DeCamp, L. M. Babé, and C. S. Craik, Structure-based design of nonpeptide inhibitors specific for the human immunodeficiency virus 1 protease, *Proc. Natl. Acad. Sci. USA 87*:6644–6648 (1990).
96. Z. Li, X. Chen, E. Davidson, O. Zwang, C. Mendis, C. S. Ring, W. R. Roush, G. Fegley, R. Li, P. J. Rosenthal, G. K. Lee, G. L. Kenyon, I. D. Kuntz, and F. E. Cohen, Anti-malarial drug development using models of enzyme structure, *Chem. Biol. 1* (in press; 1994).
97. C. S. Ring, E. Sun, J. H. McKerrow, G. K. Lee, P. J. Rosenthal, I. D. Kuntz, and F. E. Cohen, Structure-based inhibitor design using protein models for the development of antiparasitic agents, *Proc. Natl. Acad. Sci. USA 90*: 3583–3587 (1993).

98. E. Rutenber, E. B. Fauman, R. J. Keenan, S. Fong, P. S. Furth, P. R. Ortiz de Montellano, E. Meng, I. D. Kuntz, D. L. DeCamp, R. Salto, J. R. Rosé, C. Craik, and R. M. Stroud, Structure of a non-peptide inhibitor complexed with HIV-1 protease, *J. Biol. Chem.* *268*:15343–15346 (1993).

99. B. K. Shoichet, R. M. Stroud, D. V. Santi, I. D. Kuntz, and K. M. Perry, Structure-based discovery of inhibitors of thymidylate synthase, *Science 259*: 1445–1450 (1993).

100. P. A. Karplus and C. Faerman, Ordered water in macromolecular structure, *Curr. Opin. Struct. Biol.* *4*:770–776 (1994).

101. S. H. Reich M. A. M. Fuhry, D. Nguyen, M. J. Pino, K. M. Welsh, S. Webber, C. A. Janson, S. R. Jordan, D. A. Matthews, W. W. Smith, C. A. Bartlett, C. L. J. Booth, S. M. Herrmann, E. F. Howland, C. A. Morse, R. W. Ward, and J. White, Design and synthesis of novel 6,7-imidazotetra-hydroquinoline inhibitors of thymidylate synthase using iterative protein crystal structure analysis, *J. Med. Chem.* *35*:847–858 (1992).

102. D. J. Tannor, B. Marten, R. Murphy, et al., Accurate first principle calculation of molecular charge distributions and solvation energies from ab initio quantum mechanics and continuum dielectric theory, *J. Am. Chem. Soc.* *116*: 11875–11882 (1994).

103. T. A. Halgren, Merck molecular force field. I. Basis, form, scope, parameterization, and performance of MMFF94, *J. Comput. Chem.* *17*:490–519 (1996).

104. T. A. Halgren, Merck molecular force field. II. MMFF94 van der Waals and electrostatic parameters for intermolecular interactions, *J. Comput. Chem 17*: 520–552 (1996).

105. T. A. Halgren, Merck molecular force field. III. Molecular geometries and vibrational frequencies for MMFF94, *J. Comput. Chem.* *17*:553–86 (1996).

106. T. A. Halgren and R. B. Nachbar, Merck molecular force field. IV. Conformational energies and geometries for MMFF94, *J. Comput. Chem.* *17*: 587–615 (1996).

107. T. A. Halgren, Merck molecular force field. V. Extension of MMFF94 using experimental data, additional computational data, and empirical rules, *J. Comput. Chem.* *17*:616–41 (1996).

108. V. Gillet, A. P. Johnson, P. Mata, S. Sike, and P. Williams, SPROUT: A program for structure generation, *J. Comput. Aided Mol. Design.* *7*:127–153 (1993).

109. V. J. Gillet, W. Newell, P. Mata, G. Myatt, S. SIke, Z. Zsoldos, and A. P. Johnson, SPROUT—recent developments in the de novo design of molecules, *J. Chem. Inf. Comput. Sci.* *34*:207–217 (1994).

110. B. A. Bunin and J. A. Ellman, A general and expedient method for the solid-phase synthesis of 1,4-benzodiazopenes. *J. Am. Chem. Soc.* *114*: 10997–10998 (1993).

111. E. J. Martin, J. M. Blaney, M. A. Siani, D. C. Spellmeyer, A. K. Wong, and W. H. Moos, Measuring diversity: Experimental design of combinatorial libraries for drug discovery, *J. Med. Chem 38*:1431–1436 (1995).

112. T. Ridky and J. Leis, Development of drug resistance to HIV-1 protease inhibitors, *J. Biol. Chem. 270*:29621–29623 (1995).

113. J. D. Hermes, S. C. Blacklow, and J. R. Knowles, Searching sequence space by definably random mutagenesis: Improving the catalytic potential of an enzyme, *Proc. Natl. Acad. Sci. USA 87*:696–700 (1990).

114. M. J. Kuroda, M. A. el-Farrash, S. Choudhury, and S. Harada, Impaired infectivity of HIV-1 after a single point mutation in the *POL* gene to escape the effect of a protease inhibitor in vitro, *Virology 210*:212–216 (1995).

115. J. A. Partaledis, K. Yamaguchi, M. Tisdale, et al., In vitro selection and characterization of human immunodeficiency virus type 1 (HIV-1) isolates with reduced sensitivity to hydroxyethylamino sulfonamide inhibitors of HIV-1 aspartyl protease, *J. Virol. 69*:5228–5235 (1995).

116. A. M. DeVos, M. Ultsch, and A. A. Kossiakoff, Human growth hormone and extracellular domain of its receptor—crystal structure of the complex, *Science 255*:306–312 (1992).

117. B. K. Shoichet and I. D. Kuntz, Protein docking and complementarity, *J. Mol. Biol. 221*:327–346 (1991).

118. M. R. Reddy, M. D. Varney, V. Kalish, V. N. Viswanadhan, and K. Appelt, Calculation of relative differences in the binding free energies of HIV1 protease inhibitors: A thermodynamic cycle perturbation approach, *J. Med. Chem. 37*:1145–52 (1994).

119. R. N. Zuckermann, E. J. Martin, D. C. Spellmeyer, et al. Discovery of nanomolar ligands for 7-transmembrane G-protein-coupled receptors from a diverse *N*-(substituted)glycine peptoid library, *J. Med. Chem. 37*:2678–85 (1994).

120. R. P. Sheridan and S. K. Kearsley, Using a genetic algorithm to suggest combinatorial libraries, *J. Chem. Inf. Comput. Sci. 35*:310 (1995).

121. L. Weber, S. Wallbaum, C. Broger, and K. Gubernator, Optimization of the biological activity of combinatorial compound libraries by a genetic algorithm, *Angew. Chem., Int. Ed. Engl. 34*:2280–2282 (1995).

122. J. Singh, M. A. Ator, E. P. Jaeger, M. P. Allen, D. A. Whipple, J. E. Soloweij, S. Chowdhary, and A. M. Treasurywala, Application of genetic algorithms to combinatorial synthesis: A computational approach to lead identification and lead optimization, *J. Am. Chem. Soc. 118*:1669–1676 (1996).

123. K. Hilpert, J. Ackermann, D. W. Banner, A. Gast, K. Gubernator, P. Hadvary, L. Labler, K. Muller, G. Schmid, T. B. Tschopp, and H. van de Waterbeemd, Design and synthesis of potent and highly selective thrombin inhibitors, *J. Med. Chem. 37*:3889–3901 (1994).

124. J. M. Maraganore, P. Bourdon, J. Jablonski, K. L. Ramachandran, and J. W. Fenton II, Design and charaterization of hirulogs: A novel class of bivalent peptide inhibitors of thrombin, *Biochemistry 29*:7095–7101 (1990).

125. E. J. Topol, R, Bonan, D. Jewitt, U. Sigwart, V. V. Kakkar, M. Rothman, D. de Bono, J. Ferguson, J. T. Willerson, J. Strony, P. Ganz, M. D. Cohen, R. Raymond, I. Fox, J. Maraganore, and B. Adelman, Use of a direct anti-

thrombin, hirulog, in place of heparin during coronary angioplasty, *Circulation 87*:1622–1629 (1993).

126. M. von Itzstein, W. -Y. Wu, G. B. Kok, M. S. Pegg, J. C. Dyason, B. Jin, T. V. Phan, M. L. Smythe, H. F. White, S. W. Oliver, P. M. Colman, J. N. Varghese, D. M. Ryan, J. M. Woods, R. C. Bethell, V. J. Hotham, J. M. Cameron, and C. R. Penn, Rational design of potent sialidase-based inhibitors of influenza virus replication, *Nature 363*:418–423 (1993).

127. J. A. Montgomery, S. Niwas, J. D. Rose, J. A. Secrist, Y. S. Babu, C. E. Bugg, M. D. Erion, W. C. Guida, and S. E. Ealick, Structure-based design of inhibitors of purine nucleoside phosphorylase. 1. 9-(Aryl-methyl) derivatives of 9-deazaguanidine, *J. Med. Chem. 36*:55–69 (1993).

128. J. A. Secrist, S. Niwas, J. D. Rose, Y. S. Babu, C. E. Bugg, M. D. Erion, W. C. Guida, S. E. Ealick, and J. A. Montgomery, Structure-based design of inhibitors of purine nucleoside phosphorylase. 2. 9-Alicyclic and 9-heteroalicyclic derivatives of 9-deazaguanidine, *J. Med. Chem. 36*: 1847–1854 (1993).

129. M. D. Erion, S. Niwas, J. D. Rose, S. Ananthan, M. Allen, J. A. Secrist, Y. S. Babu, C. E. Bugg, W. C. Guida, S. E. Ealick, and J. A. Montgomery, Structure-based design of inhibitors of purine nucleoside phosphorylase. 2. 9-Arylmethyl derivatives of 9-deazaguanidine substituted on the methylene group, *J. Med. Chem. 36*:3771–3783 (1993).

130. J. A. Montgomery and J. A. Secrist III, PNP inhibitors, *Perspect. Drug Discov. Design 2*:205–220 (1994).

131. J. A. Montgomery, H. W. Snyder, Jr., D. A. Walsh, and G. M. Walsh, *Drugs Future 18*:887 (1993).

132. F. Mohamadi, N. G. J. Richards, W. C Guida, R. Liskamp, M. Lipton, C. Caufield, G. Chang, T. Hendrickson, and W. C. Still, Macromodel—an integrated software system for modeling organic and bioorganic molecules using molecular mechanics, *J. Comput. Chem. 11*:440–467 (1990).

133. G. Chang, W. C. Guida, and W. C. Still, An internal coordinate Monte Carlo method for searching conformational space, *J. Am. Chem. Soc. 111*: 4379–4386 (1989).

134. K. Appelt, R. J. Bacquet, C. A. Bartlett, C. L. J. Booth, S. T. Freer, M. A. M. Fuhry, M. R. Gehring, S. M. Herrmann, E. F. Howland, C. A. Janson, T. R. Jones, C. Kan, V. Kathardekar, K. K. Lewis, G. P. Marzoni, D. A. Matthews, C. Mohr, E. W. Moomwaw, C. A. Mores, S. J. Oatley, R. C. Ogden, M. R. Reddy, S. Reich, W. S. Schoettlin, W. W. Smith, M. D. Varney, J. E. Villafranca, R. W. Ward. S. Webber, S. E. Webber, K. M. Welsh, and J. White, Design of enzyme inhibitors using iterative protein crystallographic analysis, *J. Med. Chem. 34*:1925–1934 (1991).

135. M. D. Varney, G. P. Marzoni, C. L. Palmer, J. G. Deal, S. Webber, K. M. Welsh, R. J. Bacquet, C. A. Bartlett, C. A. Morse, C. L. J. Booth, S. M. Herrmann, E. F. Howland, R. W. Ward, and J. White, Crystal-structure-based design and synthesis of benz[cd]indole-containing inhibitors of thymidylate synthase, *J. Med. Chem. 35*:663–676 (1992).

136. S. E. Webber, T. M. Bleckman, J. Attard, J. G. Deal, V. Kathardekar, K. M. Welsh, S. Webber, C. A. Janson, D. A. Matthews, W. W. Smith, S. T. Freer, S. R. Jordan, R. J. Bacquet, E. Howland, C. L. J. Booth, R. W. Ward, S. M. Herrmann, J. White, C. A. Morse, J. A. Hilliard, and C. A. Bartlett, Design of thymidylate synthase inhibitors using protein crystal structures: The synthesis and biological evaluation of a novel class of 5-substituted quinazolinones, *J. Med. Chem. 36*:733–746 (1993).

137. I. Rafi, G. A. Taylor, J. A. Calvete, et al., Clinical pharmacokinetic and pharmacodynamic studies with the nonclassical antifolate thymidylate synthase inhibitor 3,4-dihydro-2-amino-6-methyl-4-oxo-5-(4-pyridylthio)-quinazolone dihydrochloride (AG337) given by 24-hour continuous intravenous infusion. *Clin. Cancer Res. 1*:1275–84 (1995).

138. N. Touroutoglou and R. Pazdur, Thymidylate synthase inhibitors, *Clin. Cancer Res. 2*: 227–43 (1996).

139. J. J. Baldwin, G. S. Ponticello, P. S. Anderson, M. E. Christy, M. A. Murcko, W. C. Randall, H. Schwam, M. F. Sugrue, J. P. Springer, P. Gautheron, J. Grove, P. Mallorga, M.-P. Viader, B. M. McKeever, and M. A. Navia, Thienothiopyran-2-sulfonamides: Novel topically active carbonic anhydrase inhibitors for the treatment of glaucoma, *J. Med. Chem. 32*: 2510–2513 (1989).

140. G. D. Diana, A. M. Treasurywala, T. R. Bailey, R. C. Oglesby, and D. C. Pevear, A model for compounds active against human rhinovirus-14 based on X-ray crystallography data, *J. Med. Chem. 33*:1306–1311 (1990).

141. G. D. Diana and A. M. Treasurywala, Design of compounds active against HRV-14, *Drug News Perspect. 4*:517–523 (1991).

142. K. Sestanj, F. Bellini, S. Fung, N. Abraham, A. Treasurywala, L. Humber, N. Simard-Dequesne, and D. Dvornik, *N*-[[5-(Trifluoromethyl)-6-methoxy-1-naphthalenyl] thioxomethyl]-*N*-methylglycine (Tolrestat), a potent, orally active aldose reductase inhibitor. *J. Med. Chem. 27*:255–256 (1984).

143. K. Sestanj, N. Abraham, F. Bellini, A. Treasurywala, and L. Humber, *N*-Naphthoylglycine derivatives. European Patent Application, 67 EP 59596 A1 820908; US patent 4439617.

2

Recent Techniques and Applications in Pharmacophore Mapping

Mark G. Bures
Abbott Laboratories, Abbott Park, Illinois

I. INTRODUCTION

For two decades, the concept of a pharmacophore has been one of the central tenets of rational drug design. The term *pharmacophore* has several related meanings, depending on the individual researcher. However, in a broad sense, a pharmacophore or pharmacophoric pattern is the set of "features" a compound must have to elicit a certain biological activity. These features are typically any combination of structural, chemical, and physical attributes of a molecular structure. For example, a description of a pharmacophore can be relatively simple and nonspecific such as "two lipophilic centers separated by 10–12 A." On the other side of the spectrum, a pharmacophoric description could comprise a three-dimensional (3D) array of specific functional groups and their geometric relation. Whatever the degree of complexity, a pharmacophore is used to help understand the range of biological activity observed in a series of compounds, as well as to help guide the design of new, potentially more potent, compounds. Several recent manuscripts that present an overview of concepts involved in pharmacophore mapping are available [1–6].

A wide range of experimental and theoretical data is routinely used to develop pharmacophoric patterns. This process is generally referred to as pharmacophore mapping and involves three main aspects: finding the features required for biological activity; determining the molecular conformation required (i.e., the "bioactive" conformation); and developing a superposition or alignment rule for the series of compounds. The primary information used in pharmacophore mapping is derived naturally from the compounds synthesized in a series and their measured biological acitvity. From this, structure–activity relations emerge and rudimentary pharmacophore hypotheses can begin to be formulated. If the structure of the macromolecular target or target–ligand complex is known, either as determined experimentally or as computationally modeled, this information is obviously very useful to the pharmacophore-mapping process. A variety of molecular-modeling and computational chemistry techniques can then be applied, in conjunction with the experimental data, to develop pharmacophore models. These techniques range from simple, qualitative molecular graphics comparisons of several members in a series to sophisticated, quantitative methodologies for generating pharmacophore maps and measuring their ability to reproduce experimental results.

The focus of this chapter is to highlight, in some detail, recent pharmacophore-mapping techniques and their application to a representative sampling of current medicinal chemistry problems. The first section discusses how experimental studies are used to help formulate putative pharmacophore maps. A representative sample of the wide variety of computational pharmacophore-mapping techinques that have been reported in the past 5 or so years will be presented next, followed by a discussion of selected pharmacophore-mapping studies. The chapter closes with a section on current directions in pharmacophore-mapping techniques and applications.

Allied with pharmacophore mapping is the field of three-dimensional *quantitative* structure–activity relations (3D-QSAR). This chapter deals with techniques for pharmacophore mapping and their application, largely a *qualitative* exercise. 3D-QSAR techniques attempt to derive and investigate quantitative models of biological activity; namely, models that fit the potency of the studied compounds and that can be used to predict the potency of compounds outside the study set. In fact, the application of many 3D-QSAR methods requires a proposed pharmacophore model. Thus, excellent companions to this chapter are a recent monograph on 3D-QSAR [7] and Chapter 4 in this book.

II. EXPERIMENTAL CHEMICAL ASPECTS OF PHARMACOPHORE MAPPING

Each year, numerous papers involving ligand design appear, and many of these have a component of at least the beginnings of pharmacophore de-

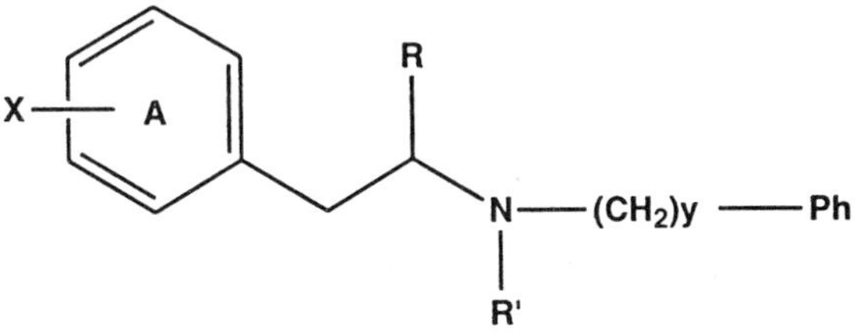

{1}

termination. Thus, pharmacophore mapping has its roots in traditional medicinal chemistry and the structure–activity relations derived from the synthesis and biological testing of series of compounds. From the relative measured potencies of individual members of a series, a picture of the types of functionality, and perhaps their spatial relations that are important for activity begins to emerge. More detailed molecular-modeling studies can then be used to formulate a more rigorous model (as discussed in the next section), but even in their absence proposed pharmacophore hypotheses can begin to take shape.

Several recent examples are illustrative of this process. Glennon and co-workers have been investigating structure–activity relations in several series of phenylalkylamine σ_1 receptor ligands [8]. One such series is represented by Structure (1). Synthesis and testing of various N-methylated and N,N-dimethylated derivatives of (1), showed that quaternary amines exhibited reduced affinity. Varying the y-chain length and substituent X, had a smaller effect, however. Replacing both phenyl rings with a 1-naphthyl or 2-naphthyl moiety showed that some bulk was tolerated in these two regions. In a related series, Structure (2), varying the y-chain length gave an affinity range of about two orders of magnitude. From these results and others [8], the authors were able to postulate a rudimentary model of features important for σ_1 binding. The model comprises a central nitrogen atom (functioning as a proton-acceptor) flanked by a hydrophobic

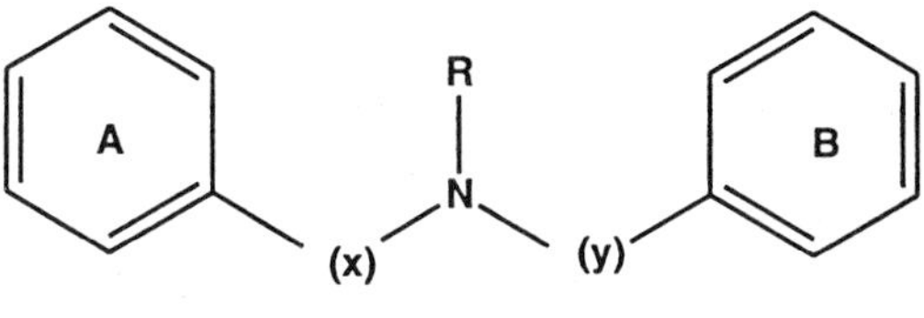

{2}

site [see ring B, structure (2)] and a secondary binding site [see ring A, structure (2)], and a set of distances between these sites [8]. This model is very typical of the types of pharmacophore maps that can be generated by systematic synthesis of analogues to probe structure–activity relations.

Additional representative examples of this are found throughout the medicinal chemistry literature. Structure–activity relations and pharmacophoric patterns in larger, more complicated structures, such as macrocyclic natural products, can be elucidated by investigating portions of the full structure [9]. A similar approach is often used when studying large peptides, whereby fragments of the full peptide are tested and selective residues are replaced with their D-isomer [10].

Many ligand-design studies employ molecular modeling as well as chemical synthesis to help elucidate pharmacophoric patterns. A representative example is the development of a pharmacophore model for the δ-opioid receptor, recently reported by Mosberg and colleagues [11]. The tactic used here is to prepare conformationally restrained analogues to help propose a bioactive conformation. A reference molecule in this study is the δ-opioid–selective, cyclic peptide, Tyr-c[D-Cys-Phe-D-Pen]OH (JOM-13; Pen; penicillamine, is β,β-dimethylcysteine). In JOM-13, the tyrosine residue was replaced by several conformationally restricted analogues, and their measured affinities and conformational analysis was used to help propose a bioactive conformation and superposition rule for this series.

For example, replacement of tyrosine by 6-hydroxy-2-aminotetralin-2-carboxylic acid (Hat) [11] or 6-hydroxy-2-aminoindan-2 carboxylic acid (Hai) [11] results in a 15- to 30-fold reduction in affinity relative to JOM-13. However, replacement of tyrosine by a more conformationally restricted analogue, such as 1,2,3,4-tetrahydro-7-hydroxyisoquinoline-3-carboxylic acid (OH-Tic) [11], results in an inactive compound (i.e., a 3200-fold loss in affinity). In contrast, replacement of tyrosine by *trans*-3-(4'-hydroxyphenyl)proline (*t*-Hpp) [11] gives a compound equipotent with JOM-13. To better understand these results, the authors used molecular mechanics calculations [11] to show that low-energy conformations available for the first residue are more limited in the Hat, Hai, and especially, the OH-Tic analogues, relative to the parent, JOM-13 and its *t*-Hpp analogue. The authors then used structure–activity data and the conformational analysis results to propose a bioactive conformation and superposition rule for the series. This was done by using molecular graphics to help find the best set of low-energy conformations that allowed good overlap of the functionality important for binding in the high- to moderate-affinity ligands. In addition, the model accounts for the inactivity of conformationally restricted compounds, such as the OH-Tic analogue, because the bioactive conformation is not energetically accessible. A report on refining the pharmacophore model for this series, focusing on a different residue, is also available [12].

Another common approach in pharmacophore mapping is the use of structurally rigid molecules to probe requirements for receptor binding. One of the advantages of using less conformationally flexible molecules is that they can more exactly define the bioactive conformation, provided that the rigid molecules selected show good affinity. Cook and colleagues recently reported on such a study involving six benzo-fused benzodiazepines (Fig. 1), which were used to further develop an agonist pharmacophore model for benzodiazepine receptors [13]. The compounds were selected to potentially occupy three different regions of a particular lipophilic pocket that is present in several proposed benzodiazepine receptor pharmacophore models [13]. Specifically, the authors hypothesized that the 7,8-benzo–fused ligand would fit well into a lipophilic pocket and function as an agonist, whereas the 6,7- and 8,9-benzo–fused analogues would protrude into regions occupied by the receptor; therefore, they would show little or no agonist activity. However, as is often true, the observed structure–activity profile was not this straightforward. All three nonfluorobenzene analogues exhibited in vitro potencies higher than 1000 nM. However, the 7,8-fluorobenzene analogue had an 50% inhibitory concentration (IC_{50}) of 55 nM, whereas the 8,9- and 6,7-fluorobenzene analogues gave IC_{50}s of 260 nM and more than 1000 nM, respectively. Thus, a 7,8-benzo–fused analogue was the most potent in the series, as expected from

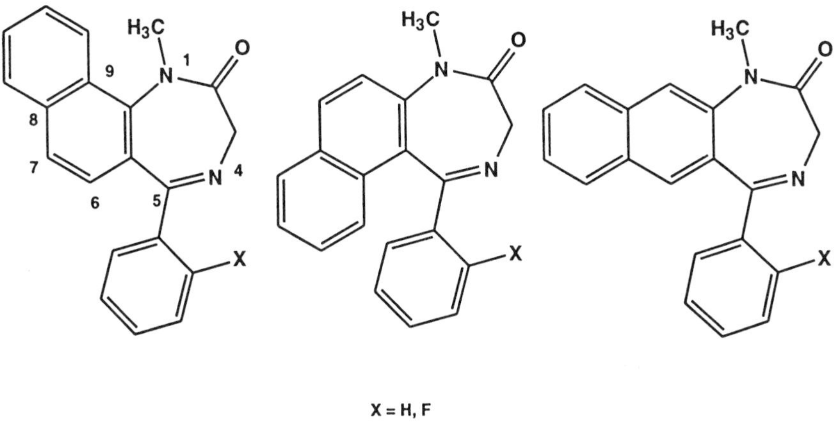

X = H, F

Figure 1 Six benzo-fused benzodiazepines studied by Cook and colleagues. (From Ref. 13.)

the model, but the fluorine substituent is also clearly playing an important role.

Use of rigidification to better define pharmacophore space has been used successfully in generating active nonpeptidic compounds from peptide leads. Ku and co-workers' recent work with nonpeptidic compounds [e.g., Structure (3)] based on cyclic RGD peptide analogues [e.g., Structure (4)] is a good example of this [14].

As is evident from the studies described in the foregoing, one of the major aspects of pharmacophore mapping is to develop a detailed picture of the three-dimensional requirements for activity. A recent investigation of piracetam-type nootropics, using X-ray diffraction, nuclear magnetic resonance (NMR) spectroscopy, and molecular dynamics, illustrates this point [15]. Two compounds studied were the bicyclic lactams, Structures (5) and (6). X-ray diffraction results showed that the six-membered ring of (5) adopts a boat conformation, whereas the six-membered ring of (6) is in a half-chair conformation. The five-membered ring of (6) is seen to be more puckered than that of (5). In addition, the N–C bond length in the piperidone ring of (6) is shorter than that observed in (5), whereas the C–O bond length in the piperidone ring of (6) is longer than that of (5).

{3}

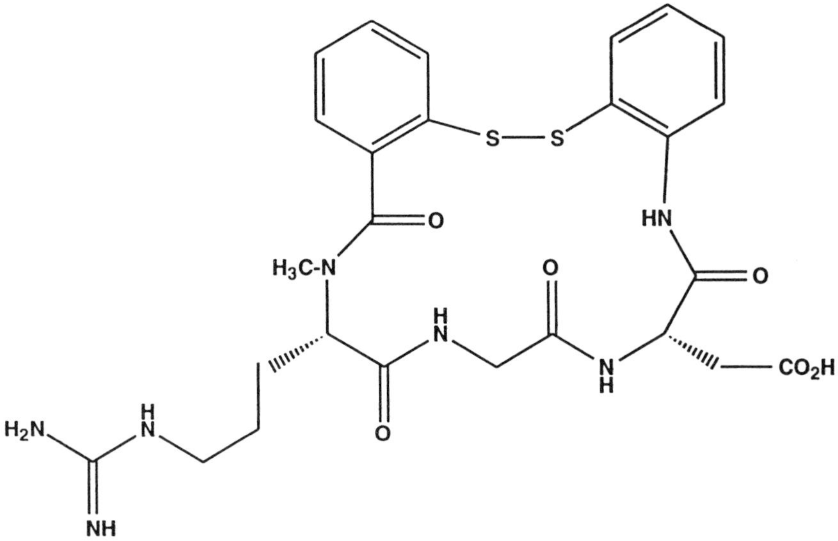

{4}

This difference in geometries of the two amide groups was evaluated using ab initio calculations to determine the amide's relative degrees of polarization, which may influence their biological activity. However, the results of these computations led the researchers to conclude that the different bond lengths were mainly due to differences in crystal packing [15]. Molecular dynamics was used to measure the conformational flexibility of Structures (5), (6), and two more flexible related compounds, (7) and (8).

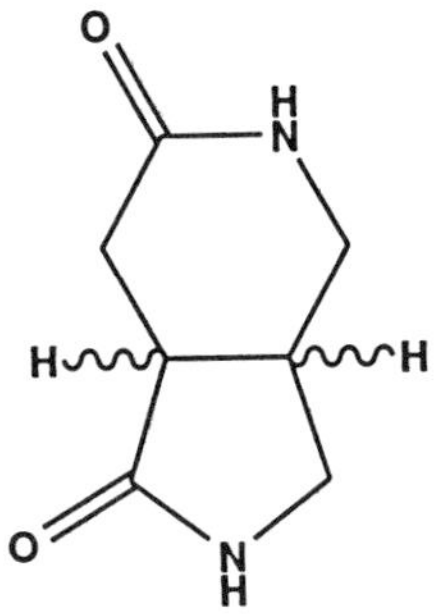

{5}

{6}

As expected, only a few conformers resulted for (**5**) and (**6**), whereas nearly 60 conformers were generated for (**7**) and (**8**). Representative low-energy conformations for the four compounds were compared with solution conformations obtained from NMR and with the X-ray defraction structures. The NMR results for (**6**), (**7**), and (**8**) were consistent with the X-ray defraction and molecular dynamic results. The solution conformation of the hydrogens attached to the ring junction in (**5**), however, was significantly different from the observed solid-state conformation.

The results discussed in the foregoing and previously proposed pharmacophore models for this class of compounds were used to further define important pharmacophoric features. For example, an inverse relation was observed between the distance separating the carbonyl oxygens in (**5–8**) and antiamnesic potency, in which optimal potency is achieved when this distance is less than 4 Å [15].

Small-molecule X-ray crystallography has also been used to help determine important pharmacophoric points in a series of compounds. For example, iron-chelating centers in (*S*)-deferrithiocin were determined using X-ray studies (Fig. 2), and this information was used to help explore the

{7} and {8}

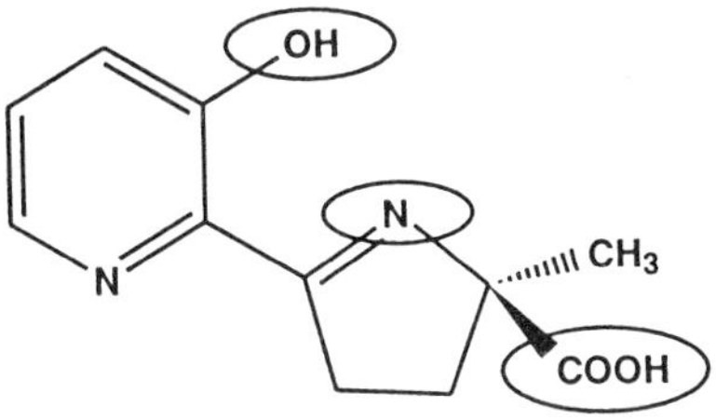

Figure 2 Iron-chelating centers in (*S*)-deferrithiocin. (From Ref. 16.)

pharmacophoric elements important for chelation in related compounds [16].

Another major aspect of pharmacophore mapping is developing superposition or alignment rules for the compounds of interest. Results from X-ray crystallography have also been used for this. A recent example involves the use of crystal structures for five different inhibitors complexed with human immunodeficiency virus type 1 (HIV-1) protease [17]. Crystal structures of seven complexes were superimposed by root mean-square fit of the backbone atoms of the enzyme. The coordinates of each inhibitor were then obtained from this overlay. This process generated both a bioactive conformation and a superposition rule for this set of compounds. An additional example of this type of work has also been reported [18]. These are specific examples of one approach to determining superposition rules; many other techniques are also used, as discussed in the following.

Several additional interesting examples of using structure–activity data to help elucidate pharmacophores have been reported, including allosteric modulators of muscarinic receptors [19] and a study of ligands for the histamine H_2-receptor [20].

III. COMPUTATIONAL METHODS FOR PHARMACOPHORE MAPPING

The work described in the previous section shows how experimental medicinal chemistry lays the foundation for pharmacophore-mapping exercises. Over the past 15 years several more formal, computational approaches to pharmacophore mapping have enjoyed continued development, as detailed in this section. Some of the methods focus on developing alignment rules (usually for pairs of molecules), whereas others treat the generation of bioactive conformations more heavily. Some of the more sophisticated approaches simultaneously consider both of these aspects. The methods rely on well-known molecular-modeling techniques, as well as more recently exploited tools, such as genetic algorithms and clique detection. One useful way to discuss the various approaches to pharmacophore mapping is to present them grouped by their primary focus. Hence, techniques concerned mainly with developing alignment or superposition rules [21–23] will be discussed first, followed by those that present a more complete treatment of the problem. Lastly, methods using less conventional techniques will be described.

A. Alignment or Bioactive Conformation Methods

One such alignment procedure, termed *steric and electrostatic alignment* (SEAL), uses steric and electrostatic features along with exhaustive searching to compare all possible orientations [24]. The method considers how these features affect ligand binding, without knowing the structure of the protein. Three assumptions (which are common to nearly all reported pharmacophore-mapping techniques) are made: all compounds in the set studied bind to the same site and groups within the site in the protein; the three-dimensional structure of the protein-binding site is similar for each ligand; therefore, the site can be held fixed; and several representative, low-energy conformations of each ligand can be used. Electrostatic features are represented by partial atomic charges, as calculated by several different methods [24]. The molecular volume, at the van der Waals radii, represents the steric or shape features. The heart of the method is the authors' scoring function, which measures the degree of similarity between two superimposed molecules. The function is a double sum over all atom pairs between two molecules, and contains terms for partial atomic charges and atomic radii, as well as several adjustable parameters [24]. Alignments are generated by random rotations and translations of one structure relative to the other, followed by minimization of the alignment function for each overlay. Multiple conformations for each structure are handled by comparing all pairs of low-energy, representative conformers for each molecule.

The SEAL method was used to generate alignments for two compounds that bind to dihydrofolate reductase (DHFR): the natural substrate dihydrofolic acid (DHF) and an inhibitor methotrexate (MTX). The best scoring alignment proposed by SEAL was in good agreement with that suggested by X-ray crystal structures for each compound complexed with DHFR [24]. The authors also presented SEAL results for two more flexible compounds, saxitoxin and tetrodotoxin, using several conformations for each. The examples required only 1–2 min of central processing unit (CPU) time on a modest computer. This work illustrates an important point for pharmacophore mapping: Even the superposition of two structures, although conceptually simple, is not a straightforward problem, owing to flexibility and the many possible ways to overlay molecules.

Recently, the SEAL work has been extended by a different group of researchers [25]. The SEAL approach was modified by the inclusion of terms in the alignment function [24] for atomic hydrophobicities and refractivities, which treat lipophilicity and polarizability. In addition, the authors performed a quite extensive calibration of several adjustable parameters found in the alignment function. The large test data set consisted of pairs of structurally diverse ligands for a variety of proteins, such as thrombin, trypsin, carbopeptidase, and HIV protease. As in the previous work [24], SEAL alignments were in general agreement with those observed from protein crystallography. However, both studies showed that the results were very sensitive to the value of the adjustable parameters, indicating that this approach would be more problematic when applied to situations for which experimental data are not available [25]. The authors also described extending the approach to align more than two molecules at a time. This method—and pharmacophore mapping, in general—is facilitated by having one or more rigid structures to help limit the number of possible conformations and potential alignments. For example, a rigid sterol structure, representing the putative transition state in ergosterol biosynthesis, was used in the simultaneous alignment of several flexible ergosterol biosynthesis inhibitors [25].

A significantly different technique for aligning sets of flexible molecules has been reported by Perkins and Dean [26]. An important feature of this strategy is the use of simulated annealing and cluster analysis to find a small set of very different conformers to represent the conformational space of each molecule in the set. All pairs of conformers are aligned by matching randomly selected sets of atoms and minimizing a difference distance metric (simulated-annealing techniques are also used here) [26]. Matches are then analyzed in three ways: clustering of all matched pairs to find representative conformers; matching of each representative conformation with each molecule as a reference; and determination of the best set of conformations independent of any reference molecule. A set of six representative angiotensin II antagonists was used as a test case. Representative conformers for each compound were obtained from a cluster analysis of thousands of conformers generated by simulated annealing (this step took about 10 min of CPU time). Match analysis was performed, as described earlier, and the best overall alignment, root mean square values of 1.5–2.9 A, for the six compounds was generated (required CPU time was several hours). Again, this work illustrates the challenge of developing unbiased (i.e., those not using predetermined feature correspondences) alignment rules for flexible molecules.

Another factor complicating pharmacophore mapping is the common observation that structurally similar molecules adopt very different receptor-binding modes. A good example of this is a set of antirhinovirus compounds bound to human rhinovirus 14 (HRV-14) [27]. The simulated annealing overlap approach described in the foregoing [26] was used to investigate potential alignments for this set of structures. First the researchers used only the conformation found in the crystal structure for 13 different analogues when bound to HRV-14. The crystal structures showed that these analogues had two modes of binding, differing by a 180° rotation of the long axis of the molecule. Alignments for all pairwise combinations of the 13 compounds were generated. Usually, at least one (and often most) of the top 10 alignments corresponded to the relative orientation found in the crystal structures. However, when the procedure was repeated using a generated low-energy conformation for each compound (instead of the crystal structure), all were predicted to have only one mode of binding; namely, the alignment is dependent on the starting conformation. Therefore, use of this method to help elucidate alternative-binding modes is somewhat problematic.

Pharmacophore mapping attempts to find features important for receptor binding. Therefore, researchers are developing alignment techniques that focus on deriving and comparing potential receptor-binding sites from ligands, rather than just using the atoms of the ligand (this is treated more fully in the next section). A good example of this is the AUTOFIT program developed by Itai and colleagues [28,29]. For each structure to be superimposed, hydrogen bond-accepting and bond-donating groups are assigned, and points representing interaction sites with heteroatoms in a receptor are generated. For example, a carbonyl oxygen in the ligand is perceived as a hydrogen bond-accepting atom, and two points at the locations of the lone pairs are generated; these points represent the position of a heteroatom in a hydrogen bond-donating group of a receptor (such as the oxygen atom of a hydroxy group in threonine). The program evaluates pairs of molecules, each having multiple representative conformers, by comparing all combinations of interaction site correspondences (for which donor must match donor and acceptor must match acceptor). A least-squares fit method is used to find the optimal superposition for each acceptable combination. A score, based on the root mean square value of the superimposed points and on the number of points in the superposition is also computed. AUTOFIT was able to reproduce the crystal structure-binding orientations of DHF and MTX, although a run that included conformational flexibility required about 6 h of CPU time on a workstation.

In contrast with considering specific sites within ligands as points of alignment, methods that use properties of the entire molecule have also been developed. One example is an alignment strategy based on the comparison of molecular shapes [30]. The shape of a molecule is represented by its van der Waals volume. The program evaluates pairs of superimposed molecules and measures their overlapping molecular volume. Rotation and translation of one molecule relative to the other is performed to maximize the overlap. In addition, the user may assign chemical types, such as hydrophobic or hydrogen bond donor, to selected atoms or groups in each molecule and require that the types match in the generated alignments. The algorithm also handles multiple low-energy conformations for each of the two molecules being compared. Thus, this method can be used to propose bioactive conformations for pairs of active compounds. The authors detail an example of the alignment of two angiotensin II receptor antagonists [Structures (**9**) and (**10**)]. The procedure involves evaluating all pairwise alignments of each low-energy conformation of the two compounds. In this example there were 192 pairs to evaluate, and each pair was allowed a maximum of 30 min of CPU time. With matching based only on shape

{**9**}

{10}

(no atom or group typing), the alignments with the best overlap (largest intersecting volume) had the biphenyl tetrazole moieties nearly perfectly superimposed. The quinoline and imidazole rings also exhibited a large amount of overlap, although their respective nitrogen atoms were not well aligned. A separate run, using shape and atom typing, in which these nitrogen atoms were assigned to the same class, provided overlays with good alignment of the nitrogen atoms, the quinoline and imidazole rings, and the biphenyl tetrazole groups.

A very recently reported (mid-1995) alignment method is embodied in a computer program called HipHop [31]. A wide range of structural features can be aligned, including hydrogen bond donors and acceptors, several classes of hydrophobic regions, and user-defined regions. The method is applicable to very flexible molecules and does not require the designation of a reference compound. In addition, HipHop can identify subsets of matching pharmacophoric points, rather than requiring that all regions match. Further details of the algorithms used in this approach were not available at the time of writing this chapter. The interested reader is encouraged to consult current literature for more information on this alignment method.

B. Pharmacophore Map Generation and Validation Methods

One of the first reported methods for pharmacophore or receptor mapping, which used structurally diverse active and inactive compounds, is known as the active analogue approach [32,33]. This approach begins by using observed structure–activity relations to propose functional groups important for bioactivity. For example, in a series of 28 potent angiotensin-converting enzyme (ACE) inhibitors, three requirements for binding were a terminal carboxyl group, a carbonyl oxygen (preferably in an amide group), and a good zinc-binding group (such as a carboxylic or hydroxamic acid) [32]. An initial pharmacophore map was constructed by evaluating the geometric relation of these proposed pharmacophoric points in several potent rigid analogues. A conformational search for each of the 28 compounds, using the systematic search facility in the molecular-modeling program SYBYL [34], was carried out to find the conformer that best matched the map. This is accomplished by defining a set of distances (with tolerances) between the potential pharmacophoric points, which are used as a guide when searching for low-energy conformations that fit the map. The proposed pharmacophore map was validated in two ways: by showing that there was a low-energy conformation of each of the 28 compounds that fit the map, and by showing that there are no low-energy compounds that fit the map for several inactive compounds that possess the necessary pharmacophoric groups. For an additional, more recent, application of the active analogue approach the interested reader should consult a study [35] involving a series of inhibitors of prolyl endopeptidase.

A related approach, used in identifying a pharmacophore for a series of cholesterol biosynthesis inhibitors, has been reported [36]. This is another example for which little is known structurally about the macromolecular target; thus, the pharmacophore must be deduced from the structural and physiochemical information contained within active and inactive ligands. As such, one of the preliminary tasks is a conformational analysis of the data set. In this work, a series of 11 3-hydroxy-3-methylglutaryl coenzyme A (HMG-CoA) reductase inhibitors were studied. The potencies of these compounds range from an IC_{50} of 5 nM (active) to an IC_{50} higher than 1000 nM (inactive). For each compound, a systematic conformational analysis was performed by varying key torsion angles and retaining all conformations within 6 kcal mol^{-1} of the global minimum. Previous structure–activity work on HMG-CoA reductase inhibitors provided several key features associated with activity [36]. This led to the selection of the following types of proposed pharmacophoric points: a point for the lactonic moiety, two lipophilic, one bulky, and one polar. The authors then defined ten distances between atoms corresponding to these points in each inhibitor and used these distances as conformational descriptors in the next step of the process. A principal components analysis identified that three distances were sufficient to describe the conformational flexibility of the 11 compounds. Low-energy conformations for each compound, derived from the three distances, were then subjected to a cluster analysis to determine if active compounds fall within the same group (cluster). The best clustering results had multiple conformations of four out of the five most active compounds grouped in the same cluster. However, conformations of two poorly active compounds were also present in this cluster, indicating that distance between important atoms alone is not enough to explain potency. As a means of further characterizing this data set, a molecular electrostatic potential (MEP) was calculated for the low-energy conformation of each compound contained in the cluster of active compounds and for several other representative compounds not in this cluster. Some trends in certain regions of the MEPs were observed. For example, one particular region of the MEP for most active compounds showed positive MEP values, whereas most weakly active and inactive compounds had negative values. This work shows that both geometric and electrostatic factors must often be taken into account in pharmacophore mapping.

    With the active analogue approach, it is also possible to investigate the molecular volume occupied by active compounds, regions of space occupied only by inactive compounds, and to draw inferences about the size and shape of the macromolecular-binding site. An example of this involving a series of active and inactive cannabinoids was recently reported [37]. The approach here is to attempt to determine the receptor essential volume (REV) (i.e., "that region of space occupied by the atoms of inactive analogs that is *not occupied* by atoms of active analogs" [37]). The REV was built by combining several computed molecular volumes of the low-energy conformers of the active and inactive analogues (using the Chem-X molecular-modeling program [38]). First, the union volume of active conformers is calculated. Next the unique volume, when compared with the union volume of active conformers, of each inactive compound is determined. Finally, these unique volumes are intersected to give the REV, which represents regions occupied by protein in the binding site. Before constructing the REV, the cannabinoids were aligned using pharmacophoric points proposed from previous structure–activity work and by application of the active analogue method. As a means of validation, the REV map was used to help rationalize the activity of several cannabinoids not used to make the map. For example, an active benzofuran cannabinoid, which is somewhat structurally different from the compounds used to make the map, fit well in the binding site and did not overlap the REV.

Several newer approaches to pharmacophore mapping incorporate the notion of calculating and treating potential receptor interaction sites as one of the features central to their technique. One such example is a program named DISCO (*dis*tance *co*mparisons) developed by Martin and co-workers [39]. DISCO simultaneously determines bioactive conformations and superposition rules (i.e., proposed pharmacophore maps). The first step of the process is to select a set of diverse, representative compounds that show good affinity (i.e., active ligands) for the biological target of interest. A conformational analysis, using any method desired, is then performed to give a set of low-energy, representative conformers for each compound. Next, all potential pharmacophoric elements are calculated for each compound. These elements are perceived using a substructure-searching language that can be controlled by the user [39]. Typically, one uses hydrogen bond-accepting and bond-donating sites, hydrophobic sites, and other key atoms of each compound as potential pharmacophoric points. An important feature of DISCO is the calculation of hydrogen bond-accepting and bond-donating sites. These points are automatically computed from atoms of interest in the compound and they represent putative sites of interaction with the biological target. For example, a carbonyl group would have two hydrogen bond-donating sites, at a distance of 2.9 A from the oxygen atom. These represent possible hydrogen–bond-interaction sites with a hydrogen bond-donating group in a protein. Finally, a reference compound (usually the one with the fewest conformations) is selected by the user.

Each conformation of all compounds (excluding the reference) is compared with the reference compound to find sets of pharmacophoric points that are common to at least one conformation of each compound. This is done by comparing corresponding interpoint distances of the reference with those in every other conformation. From this, a clique detection algorithm [39,40] finds the largest set (cliques) of common distances. Compared distances are considered to be within the same range if they differ by no more than a user-specified tolerance value. Finally, the cliques that meet any user-defined criteria, such as required number and type of pharmacophoric points, are output as proposed pharmacophore maps. Two examples are presented by the authors: a set of dopaminergic agonists [for readers interested in mapping investigations of dopaminergic antagonists, see Ref. 41] and a diverse collection of benzodiazepine agonists [for additional studies see Ref. 42]. The benzodiazepine study comprised seven structurally distinct agonists, with diazepam as the reference. Several pharmacophore maps were proposed, including two five-point models, each consisting of two ligand hydrogen bond acceptors, two site hydrogen bond donors, and a lipophilic region. Inclusion of the site points (protein interaction sites) provided better overall superpostitions than those models consisting of only ligand points. The CPU times for typical DISCO runs are approximately 1–5 min. Additional examples of DISCO applications, including two extensions to the algorithm, have recently been reported [43]. DISCO has been integrated into the SYBYL [34] molecular-modeling program.

As is evident, pharmacophore mapping typically involves searching several conformations of each compound for common sets of structural features. Because of the combinatorial nature of the problem, the algorithms used in the searching process (e.g., clique detection in DISCO [39]) are critical to the overall efficiency of the pharmacophore-mapping strategy. Clique detection is also used in another reported pharmacophore-mapping module, incorporated into the de novo molecular design program PRO_LIGAND [40]. The overall approach to pharmacophore mapping in PRO_LIGAND is essentially the same as that used in the DISCO strategy described earlier. In PRO_LIGAND, the proposed pharmacophore maps are used as starting points for the automated design of new ligands for the target of interest [40]. One pharmacophore-mapping test set for PRO_LIGAND was a series of seven dipeptide and tripeptide ACE inhibitors. Molecular dynamics, followed by energy minimization, were used to generate 50 conformations for each peptide. The most potent peptide in the set was used as a reference compound, and a proposed pharmacophore model with a tolerance of 1.5 A was generated. This four-point model, consisting of two lipophilic regions, an acceptor group, and a negatively charged group, concurred with other reported models [40].

An additional pharmacophore-mapping strategy that has been integrated in a commercially available molecular-modeling program is available in the Chem-X program [38]. The approach follows a familiar theme [44]. First, a conformational analysis is performed to identify low-energy conformers for the data set. The next step is automatic assignment of potential pharmacophore points, which are hydrogen bond acceptors, hydrogen bond donors, positively charged atoms, and aromatic ring centroids. During this process, distances between pairs of these points ("distance keys") and data on the number, types, and interpoint connectivity are stored ("formula keys"). Proposed pharmacophores are identified by searching the distance and formula keys for all possible three- or four-point pharmacophores. These pharmacophores must then be validated by checking that at least one conformation of each compound matches the pharmacophore. The pharmacophore-mapping function of Chem-X was recently used to generate a pharmacophore map for a set of eight serotonin (5-hydroxy-tryptamine; 5-HT_3) receptor antagonists [44].

Another example of a pharmacophore generation program incorporated into commercial molecular-modeling software is the program APEX-

3D [45,46]. Similar to other approaches to pharmacophore mapping, APEX-3D attempts to find sets of features common to low-energy conformations of each compound. These features (pharmacophoric points) can be ring centers, hydrophobic regions, and hydrogen-bonding sites. The program can evaluate two-dimensional (2D; topological) or three-dimensional (3D; topographical) relations between these points in generating proposed pharmacophore maps. Actually, the authors of APEX-3D have adopted the term *biophore* for pharmacophore, to denote pharmacological and toxicological activity [45]. Generation of biophores involves determining low-energy, representative conformers for each compound; calculation of descriptors for potential biophoric atoms; and searching (using a clique-detection algorithm) for maximal common 2D or 3D arrangements of biophoric centers. These arrangements or patterns are potential biophores, which are then evaluated for their statistical, quantitative correlation with biological activity [further discussion of this is beyond the scope of pharmacophore mapping; see Ref. 46 for more information]. A pharmacophore-mapping approach similar in concept to APEX-3D is a program called Catalyst [47]. The method uses potential pharmacophoric sites, such as hydrogen bond donors and acceptors, hydrophobic, positive and negative groups, along with a conformational model [48] and biological activity for each compound, to develop a quantitative pharmacophoric map or "hypothesis" [49].

Another pharmacophore-mapping strategy using entities related to protein interaction sites is the *h*ypothetical *a*ctive *s*ite *l*attice (HASL) methodology [50,51]. In this approach, a molecule is represented by a series of three-dimensional points in a lattice. The lattice is a three-dimensional grid of regularly spaced (typical spacing is 3.0 or 2.0 A) points, into which each molecule is placed. Grid points that lie within the van der Waals radius of the molecule are used to characterize the molecule. Each of these grid points has two values: an atom type of electron-rich, electron-poor, or electron-neutral; and partial-binding value. The remainder of the HASL process is best described by way of an example, such as a large series of HIV-1 protease inhibitors [50].

Crystal structures of two inhibitors bound to the protease were used as a template to build and overlay the remaining compounds in the set. Grid points for each compound are assigned as just described, and from this, a composite set of grid points for the entire set is determined. This process involves developing a highly self-consistent correlation between grid points and binding constants [50]. This resulted in a 899-point HASL describing the 84-compound set. Iterative removal of points from the HASL is then performed to obtain a model with as few points as possible, while retaining a good correlation ($r^2 > 0.8$). In this example, a so-called trimmed HASL contained 11 points, with an r^2 fo 0.83. The predictive ability of a HASL model was measured by creating a model with half of the compound set (784 points; self-consistency $r^2 = 1.00$) and predicting the binding constant of the remaining half (predictivity $r^2 = 0.73$). The 11-point HASL model represents a proposed pharmacophore map for this set of inhibitors. The five strongest and five weakest inhibitors were superimposed on the 11-point pharmacophore and there was good correspondence between inhibitor potency and grid-point partial-binding value, further indicating the relevance of this pharmacophore map. In addition, the map was used to corroborate the importance of several key hydrogen-bonding groups.

C. Less Conventional Methods

Recently, several groups of researchers have employed methods not commonly used in pharmacophore mapping. One such strategy uses a Monte Carlo search procedure, followed by energy minimization to generate proposed pharmacophore maps [52,53]. The procedure involves generating potential pharmacophoric sites for each compound and then using a Monte Carlo technique to simultaneously search conformational space and orientation space (how the molecules are superimposed). In the search, pharmacophoric sites of the same type are given "strong restraining potentials" which ensures that only equivalent pharmacophoric sites will be superimposed in the generated pharmacophore maps. In the Monte Carlo approach used, conformations and orientations are generated at random from a previous structure in an iterative process. If a conformation is lower in energy than its precursor, the conformation is used as a starting structure for the next generation. If the new conformation is higher in energy than its precursor, the conformation is selected with a probability that is inversely proportional to its change in energy relative to its precursor. In short, this technique helps ensure a good search of the entire conformational space by helping prevent the search from becoming trapped in a local energy minima [52]. Finally, pharmacophores generated by Monte Carlo are refined by energy minimization of all compounds in the map simultaneously, using the Multifit program [for recent application, see Ref. 54] in SYBYL [34]. Related work, using a novel conformational analysis method, has been reported [55].

Researchers applied the Monte Carlo approach to five compounds that bind to the platelet-activating factor (PAF) receptor [52]. Several atoms, thought to be important for binding and receptor interaction, sites derived from those atoms, were selected as potential pharmacophoric points and used in matching (as described earlier). Therefore, because the phar-

macophoric points were preselected, this example is an exercise in proposing bioactive conformations for a set of compounds. The Monte Carlo
approach plus refinement was applied for four separate runs, resulting in
40 pharmacophore maps. Two criteria were used to measure the quality of
the maps: the sum of the conformation energies (difference between the
energy of the conformation in the map and the global minima) of the five
compounds, and the highest conformation energy (HCE) of the five compounds. The seven maps with the smallest HCE (in the range of 5–8 kcal
mol^{-1}) were selected for further analysis. A view of the seven maps
showed that they were highly similar; that is, these solutions represented
the same pharmacophore map. In addition, four reference PAF antagonists,
structurally different from the five compounds studied, fit this pharmacophore map.

Genetic algorithms (GA) [56,57], an optimization technique that
mimics natural evolution, have recently been applied to several problems
in chemistry including 3D-QSAR and pharmacophore mapping [58–60].
Briefly, genetic algorithms work by generating random populations of solution to a problem, scoring the relative quality of the solutions, and carrying forward the most-fit solutions or analogues (generated through mutation and crossover) of other solutions to iteratively generate (and finally
converge on) new, more-fit solutions. One example of their use in pharmacophore mapping is the generation of proposed pharmacophores for a
series of three N-methyl-D-aspartate antagonists (NMDA) [59]. Sets of
equivalent pharmacophoric points were identified for the three compounds.
Distances between pairs of these equivalent points were used as constraints
in the optimization procedure. A GA approach was used to simultaneously
vary conformations and orientations, for many generations, until the resulting pharmacophore maps were of the desired fitness. The fitness of
generated maps was gauged by a combination of several measures: amount
of deviation in corresponding pharmacophore point–pharmacophore point
distances in different compounds; degree of shape similarity; overlap volume; similarity of charge distribution; and steric accessibility of the conformations of each compound. The GA was allowed to run for 1299 generations, with a population size (number of potential solutions or pharmacophore maps) of 8000. This required 10 days of CPU time on a
moderate workstation. The run converged to one particular pharmacophore
map which showed a good overall superimposition of each compound. In
a subsequent run, generation of random orientations was replaced by superimposing the compounds using the pharmacophoric points after each
new population was created. This greatly reduced the number of degrees
of freedom in the system and resulted in a run time of minutes (compared
with days for the previous run). Removing orientational freedom had pro-

duced a pharmacophore map with excellent overlap of the pharmacophore points, whereas the remaining portions of the molecules were less overlapped. Finally, increasing the weight of the volume overlap term in the scoring function, gave a pharmacophore map with a good overall superimposition and required about 4 h of CPU time.

As noted throughout this chapter, many pharmacophore-mapping approaches require the user to define the corresponding pharmacophoric points, groups, or sites for each compound in the set. Thus, the alignment rule is established before mapping takes place. This reduces the pharmacophore-mapping exercise to one of finding bioactive conformations or to one of pharmacophore validation. Several methods, as noted in this chapter, attempt to find pharmacophoric points (from a set of potential points), their alignment or superposition rule, and bioactive conformations simultaneously. The GA approach [59] has been extended to treat the entire pharmacophore-mapping problem [60].

The more recent GA strategy searches both conformational space and mappings between pharmacophoric sites. The types of pharmacophoric sites or features considered are points extending from hydrogen bond-donor protons, lone pairs (representing hydrogen bond-acceptors), and ring centers. In the GA procedure, each molecule is overlaid onto a base molecule, which typically is the molecule with the fewest features. During the search, all freely rotatable bonds were randomly varied and each structure was randomly translated before superimposition. Before calculating the fitness, each ensemble of conformations was superimposed onto the base molecule, using a one-to-one correspondence of similar pharmacophoric points. Terms in the fitness function were as follows: internal steric energy of each compound; overlap volume between each compound and the base molecule; and a similarity score measuring the number of features in common to all compounds in the overlay. The similarity score also included a calculation of the relative strength of similar hydrogen bond-acceptors and bond-donors. The fitness score was a weighted average of the sum of these terms.

The authors present a large number of examples using this GA strategy, including proposed pharmacophore maps for angiotensin II receptor antagonists, 5-HT_{1D} agonists, benzodiazepine ligands, and dopamine agonists. The reported example with the largest number of compounds is a study of seven dopamine-reuptake inhibitors. The GA method was run ten times and the average CPU time per run was about 6 min on a moderate workstation. All of these runs generated a two-point pharmacophore map that comprised points derived from an aromatic ring and a protonated nitrogen. A higher-scoring three-point model, containing the two previous points and an additional aromatic ring, was also generated. The highest-scoring map showed very good superimposition of the pharmacophoric points and a overall volume overlay that was much better than any of the other generated maps. The three-point model was also in good agreement with a literature pharmacophore map developed for five of the seven compounds [60].

The foregoing work shows that GA approaches to pharmacophore mapping show promise for becoming more useful with further development. There are several recent reports on the use of genetic algorithms in problems related to pharmacophore mapping. Walters and Hinds have published their work [58] on using structure–activity relations and genetic algorithms to build models of receptor sites, embodied in an approach called *genetically evolved receptor models* (GERM) [58].

A quite different approach to pharmacophore investigation involving the concept of a "hypermolecule," has been reported [61]. This method hypothesizes that the binding potency of a series of related active site inhibitors can be explained using specific regions of each compound and that these regions can be determined by combining the common portion and structural variations present in each compound into one structure, known as a *hypermolecule*. In the present work, one data set was a well-studied collection of 127 *ortho*-, *meta*-, and *para*-substituted phenyl-*N*-methylcarbamate inhibitors of acetylcholinesterase (AChE). The atom positions in the hypermolecule were characterized using several classes of descriptors to evaluate lipophilic interactions, polarizability, electronegativity, sterics, and hydrogen-bonding. A two-dimensional hypermolecule was constructed from the largest substructure common to the set of analogues plus an enumeration of each substituent [61]. Regression analysis of the measured biological activity against the hypermolecule provided insight about specific atoms and substructures of the substituents that are correlated with binding potency. For example, several regions favored lipophilic substituent atoms, whereas other regions showed strong steric interference. This method can give detailed information about the binding of active ligands which, in turn, can provide insight into the pharmacophore.

IV. SELECTED PHARMACOPHORE-MAPPING STUDIES

Highlights of recent pharmacophore-mapping investigations of special interest or usefulness are presented in this section. This discussion is intended to give the interested reader additional examples (over those presented in the foregoing) of how computer-aided pharmacophore-mapping strategies can be an integral part of current molecular design efforts.

Kovar and co-workers [62] recently reported on their efforts to develop and explain a pharmacophore map for 5-HT-reuptake inhibitors, using the active analogue approach, electrostatic potential, and molecular volume. This report is especially useful because the authors present, in simple terms, the background behind the methodology used and why the techniques were selected. The study involves the investigation of 25 active and 7 inactive structurally diverse 5-HT-reuptake inhibitors. The active analogue approach (as described earlier) was used to generate a pharmacophore map for the active compounds. A low-energy conformation of one of the most potent and somewhat rigid compounds of this set was used as the reference compound; that, is the compound used to define the distance constraints. The proposed pharmacophoric points used to define the distance constraints were a nitrogen atom and the endpoints of a normal through the center of an aromatic ring. Representative low-energy conformations (using the X-ray crystallographic structure when available as the starting conformation) of the active compounds were searched to find those that met the distance constraints of the reference. A map including the foregoing points and at least one conformation of each active compound was generated. From the overlay of all the active compounds onto the map, two additional pharmacophoric regions were proposed, an electronegative group and a second aromatic ring. With each active compound superimposed on the map, further analyses, such as volume and molecular electrostatic potential comparisons, can be performed. For example, the authors used differences in volumes of certain active compounds to rationalize differences in selectivity observed for these compounds. Differences in charge distribution, as seen when viewing the molecular electrostatic potential of some of the compounds in the map, were used to help explain 5-HT–reuptake receptor versus norepinepherin (noradrenaline; NA)–reuptake receptor affinity. Superimposition of inactive compounds onto the pharmacophore map can also provide useful information. For example, inactive compounds often occupy regions of the map that are outside the union volume of all active compounds. Furthermore, when the structure of the macromolecular target is known, the regions occupied by inactive compounds (and not active compounds) correspond to regions of the target involved in binding [62]. Alternatively, inactive compounds can be sterically forbidden from achieving the bioactive conformation described by the pharmacophore map. In this study, the authors described examples of inactive compounds that illustrate these points. Finally, one method to help validate a pharmacophore model is an attempt to fit potent compounds not used to build the model. In this study, the bioactive conformation of the potent 5-HT–reuptake inhibitor citalopram was generated by finding a low-energy conformation that matched the pharmacophore map. In addition, the bioactive conformation was in good agreement with a conformation determined using ^{1}H-NMR and infrared (IR) spectroscopy.

A recent report on the conformational analysis and pharmacophore investigation of three sodium channel modulators [63] highlights some of the challenges of studying large, complicated, highly flexible molecules [64]. The compounds studied each contain several flexible rings, as depicted in Figure 3. The researchers decided to focus on conformational analysis of the medium-sized rings present in these structures, also noted in Figure 3. A Monte Carlo search method was used to investigate the conformational space by systematically varying dihedral angles of these

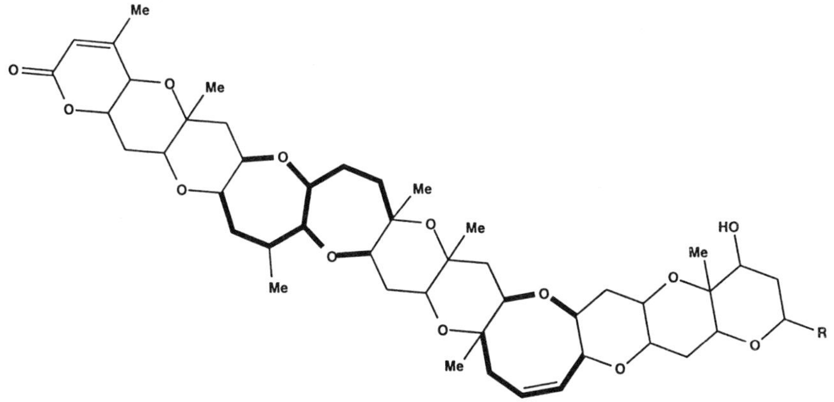

Brevetoxin B backbone

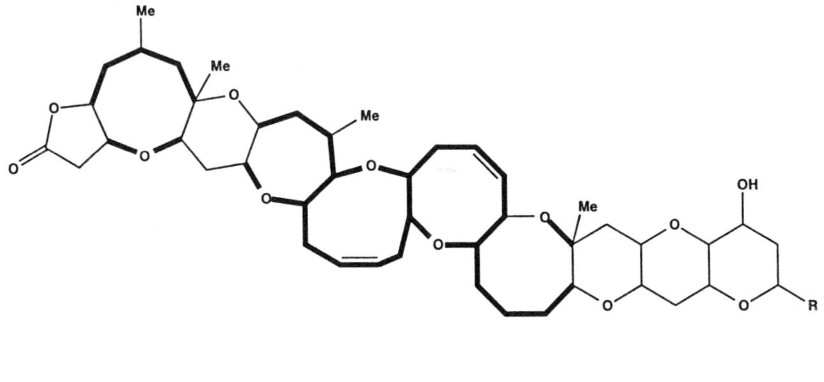

Brevetoxin A backbone

Figure 3 Backbones of brevetoxin A and B with rotatable bonds in boldface type. (From Ref. 64.)

rings. Several low-energy conformations were found for each of the rings; overall brevetoxin A was represented by 24 low-energy conformers and brevetoxin B by 7. Superimposition of these 31 conformers revealed similarities in the overall shape of the two compounds. The tail regions of both compounds are very tightly superimposed, whereas the head regions are more diffuse. Only four conformers of brevetoxin A and three conformers of brevetoxin B showed good overlap in the head region. In addition, the carbonyl oxygens of the lactone rings in the head region were also well superimposed, suggesting that this functionality is important for binding. These conformers represent a proposed model for the bioactive conformation of these two compounds. Additional pharmacophore investigations of highly flexible molecules include Hopfinger and Jin's recent work on thromboxane A_2 antagonists [65] and a report on protein phosphatase inhibitors [66].

Development of pharmacophore models, followed by experimental verification, is a powerful combination to aid in design of biologically active compounds. This point is illustrated by a recent report on pharmacophore mapping of a set of cytochrome P-450 inhibitors [67]. Six strong inhibitors of cytochrome P-450 2D6 were studied. A conformational analysis and search procedure was performed to identify low-energy conformers that were common to the set. Low-energy conformers were superimposed using a proposed four-point model: two points on the ends of a normal to an aromatic ring present in each inhibitor, and a protonated nitrogen atom and its proton. One of the most rigid compounds studied, raubasine (ajmalicine), was chosen as the reference compound, that is the compound on which the others were superimposed. Molecular dynamics showed that raubasine had two different low-energy conformations, and each was used as the reference structure. Only one of the conformers of the reference matched at least one low-energy conformer of the other inhibitors. Thus, a pharmacophore model that comprised a tertiary nitrogen atom and a flat hydrophobic region, such as an aromatic ring, was generated. In this model there is also a region that, when occupied with atoms containing lone pairs, leads to increased potency. Raubasine has two groups containing oxygen atoms in this region. The validity of the model was investigated by measuring the inhibition of a variety of structurally related compounds, and superimposing these compounds on the model. For example, compounds containing only part of the ring systems of raubasine and no tertiary basic nitrogen exhibit greatly diminished inhibitory potency. In another validation exercise, compounds that differ from raubasine in the orientation of the lone pairs just noted, were one to three orders of magnitude less potent than raubasine.

{11}

A topic of much interest over the past few years is computer-assisted modeling of solvation effects. Solvation is an important, although often untreated, issue in pharmacophore mapping, as evidenced by recent work of Testa and colleagues [68]. They studied a set of nine congeners of raclopride [Structure (11)], which block dopamine D_2 receptors. Specifically, the researchers were investigating the ionization state and intermolecular hydrogen-bonding ability of the hydroxy and amino groups in different solvents and in the gas phase and how this affected conformational preferences. At physiological pH (7.4) raclopride is predominantly in the zwitterionic form. However, two of the compounds studied are only 5% zwitterionic at pH 7.4. A molecular dynamics technique was used to sample the conformational space of the different ionic forms of the set of compounds. Two types of calculations were performed: one simulating gas-phase (in vacuo) conditions and the other in aqueous phase. The in vacuo and aqueous results show that the neutral form of raclopride has a planar, aromatic system, with two intermolecular hydrogen bonds. The zwitterionic form has a different behavior in the two phases studied. In vacuo, zwitterionic raclopride exhibited "internal salt" conformations (i.e., conformers where the phenolate and protonated amine groups are in close proximity). However, the low-energy conformations of zwitterionic raclopride in aqueous phase were similar to those of the neutral form (i.e., having intermolecular hydrogen bonds). The conformational analysis results were then used to help propose a conformation for this class of compounds when receptor-bound. Previous work has shown that the receptor-binding site for these compounds is a low-polarity environment [68]. Therefore, this implies that raclopride and its congeners would bind in the neutral form, suggesting a bioactive conformation, with a planar aromatic system and two intermolecular hydrogen bonds.

V. CURRENT DIRECTIONS

Most of the recent work in the area of pharmacophore mapping involves the use (rather than the generation) of pharmacophore maps in related molecular-modeling applications, such as database searching, 3D-QSAR, and de novo compound design. Because these areas are outside the scope of this chapter (indeed some are covered in other chapters in this monograph), only a brief mention of leading works will be presented here.

Pharmacophoric patterns can often be translated into queries for 3D database searching, as illustrated by the work of Sheridan and co-workers [69]. Evaluation and development of methods for pharmacophore pattern searching, including techniques for treating conformational flexibility, have recently been reported [70–72]. Two specific examples of using pharmacophoric pattern searching can be found in reports involving endothelin antagonists [73] and nootropic agents [74]. Finally, an entire issue of the electronic journal *Network Science* was devoted to 3D database searching and several of the articles discussed pharmacophore searching [75–79].

As mentioned in the introduction to this chapter, pharmacophore maps are often used to help develop 3D-QSAR in series of biologically active compounds. In fact, 3D-QSAR generation methods have been partly used to help validate pharmacophoric hypotheses [80]. Additional recent examples of 3D-QSAR studies include an evaluation of three superpositions of endothelin inhibitors [81]; investigation of several data-handling methods [82]; a comparison fo traditional QSAR and 3D-QSAR [83]; and work using DISCO [39] and 3D-QSAR to develop and evaluate pharmacophore models for σ_3 receptor ligands [84].

An important area in computer-aided molecular modeling is the development of methods for de novo compound design [85]. Several approaches in this field can use pharmacophore models as starting points for structure design. For example, in the program NEWLEAD, key fragments from bioactive conformations are joined with spacers to generate new structures to fit the model [86]. In the program SPROUT, templates, such as five- and six-membered rings and acyclic fragments are joined such that atoms in the resulting structure correspond to atoms in a pharmacophore model [87]. Finally, a program called ChemNovel has been used to generate a structurally diverse set of compounds to fit a pharmacophore model for 5-HT_3 receptor antagonists [88].

REFERENCES

1. V. E. Golender and E. R. Vorpagel, Computer-assisted pharmacophore identification, *3D QSAR in Drug Design* (H. Kubinyi, ed.), ESCOM, Leiden, 1993, pp. 137–149.

2. G. R. Marshall, C. D. Barry, H. E. Bosshard, R. A. Dammkoehler, and D. A. Dunn, The conformational parameter in drug design: the active analog approach, *Computer-Assisted Drug Design* (E. C. Olson and R. E. Christoffersen, eds.), *ACS Symp. Ser. 112*:205–226.

3. P. J. Goodford, A computational procedure for determining energetically favourable binding sites on biologically important macromolecules, *J. Med. Chem. 28*:849–857 (1985).

4. Y. C. Martin, Computer-assisted rational drug design, *Methods Enzymol. 203*: 587–613 (1991).

5. C.-G. Wermuth and T. Langer, Pharmacophore identification, *3D QSAR in Drug Design* (H. Kubinyi, ed.) ESCOM, Leiden, 1993, pp. 117–136.

6. L. M. Balbes, S. W. Mascarella, and D. B. Boyd, A perspective of modern methods in computer-aided drug design, *Rev. Comput. Chem. 5*:337–378 (1994).

7. H. Kubinyi, ed., *3D QSAR in Drug Design*, ESCOM, Leiden, 1993.

8. R. A. Glennon, S. Y. Ablordeppey, A. M. Ismaiel, M. B. El-Ashmawy, J. B. Fischer, and K. B. Howie, Structural features important for σ_1 receptor binding, *J. Med. Chem. 37*:1214–1219 (1994).

9. D. L. Boger and D. Yohannes, K-13 and OF4949: evaluation of key partial structures and pharmacophore delineation, *Bioorg. Med. Chem. Lett. 3*: 245–250 (1993).

10. T. L. Peeters, M. J. Macielag, I. Depoortere, Z. D. Konteatis, J. R. Florance, R. A. Lessor, and A. Galdes, D-Amino acid and alanine scans of the bioactive portion of porcine motilin, *Peptides 13*:1103–1107 (1992).

11. H. I. Mosberg, A. L. Lomize, C. Wang, K. Kroona, D. L. Heyl, K. Sobczyk-Kojiro, W. Ma, C. Mousigian, and F. Porreca, Development of a model for the δ opiod receptor pharmacophore. 1. Conformationally restricted Tyr1 replacements in the cyclic δ receptor selective tetrapeptide Tyr-c[D-Cys-Phe-D-Pen]OH (JOM-13), *J. Med. Chem. 37*:4371–4383 (1994).

12. H. I. Mosberg, J. R. Omnaas, A. Lomize, D. L. Heyl, I. Nordan, C. Mousigian, P. Davis, and F. Porreca, Development of a model for the δ opioid receptor pharmacophore. 2. Conformationally restricted Phe3 replacements in the cyclic δ receptor selective tetrapeptide Tyr-c[D-Cys-Phe-D-Pen]OH (JOM-13), *J. Med. Chem. 37*:4384–4391 (1994).

13. W. Zhang, K. F. Koehler, B. Harris, P. Skolnick, and J. M. Cook, Synthesis of benzo-fused benzodiazepines employed as probes of the agonist pharmacophore of benzodiazepine receptors, *J. Med. Chem. 37*:745–757 (1994).

14. T. W. Ku, W. H. Miller, W. E. Bondinell, K. F. Erhard, R. M. Keenan, A. J. Nicols, C. E. Peishoff, J. M. Samanen, A. S. Wong, and W. F. Huffman, Potent non-peptide fibrinogen receptor antagonists which present an alternative pharmacophore, *J. Med. Chem. 38*:9–12 (1995).

15. C. Altomare, A. C. Cellamare, G. Casini, and M. Ferappi, X-ray crystal structure, partitioning behavior, and molecular modeling study of piracetam-type nootropics: insights into the pharmacophore, *J. Med. Chem. 38*:170–179 (1995).

16. R. J. Bergeron, C. Z. Liu, J. S. McManis, M. X. B. Xia, S. E. Algee, and J. Wiegand, The desferrithiocin pharmacophore, *J. Med. Chem. 37*:1411–1417 (1994).

17. C. L. Waller, T. I. Oprea, A. Giolitti, and G. R. Marshall, Three-dimensional QSAR of human immunodeficiency virus (I) protease inhibitors. 1. A CoMFA study employing experimentally determined alignment rules, *J. Med. Chem. 36*:4152–4160 (1993).

18. S. A. De Priest, D. Mayer, C. B. Naylor, and G. R. Marshall, 3D-QSAR of angiotensin-converting enzyme an thermolysin inhibitors: a comparison of CoMFA models based on deduced and experimentally determined active-site geometries, *J. Am. Chem. Soc. 115*:5372–5384 (1993).

19. M. H. Botero Cid, U. Holzgrabe, E. Kostenis, K. Mohr, and C. Trankle, Search for the pharmacophore of bispyridinium-type allosteric modulators of muscarinic receptors, *J. Med. Chem. 37*:1439–1445 (1994).

20. E. E. J. Haaksma, H. P. Voss, G. M. Donne-Op den Kelder, and H. Timmerman, An interaction model for tiotidine and analogs with the histamine H_2-receptor, *Quant. Struct. Act. Relat. 11*:142–150 (1992).

21. G. Klebe, Structural alignment of molecules [review], *3D QSAR in Drug Design: Theory, Methods and Applications* (H. Kubinyi, ed.), ESCOM, Leiden, 1993, pp. 173–199.

22. A. Lagersted, E. Falch, B. Ebert, and P. Krogsgaard-Larsen, Conformational aspects of the muscarinic receptor interactions of bicyclic isoxazole ester bioisosteres of arecoline, *Drug Design Discov. 9*:237–250 (1993).

23. P. R. Kym, G. M. Anstead, K. G. Pinney, S. R. Wilson, and J. A. Katzenellenbogen, Molecular structures, conformational analysis, and preferred modes of binding of 3-aroyl-2-arylbenzo[*b*]thiophene estrogen receptor ligands: LY117018 and aryl azide photoaffinity labelling analogs, *J. Med. Chem. 36*: 3910–3922 (1993).

24. S. K. Kearsley and G. M. Smith, An alternative method for the alignment of molecular structures: maximizing electrostatic and steric overlap, *Tetrahedron Comput. Methodol. 3*:615–633 (1990).

25. G. Klebe, T. Mietzner, and F. Weber, Different approaches toward an automatic structural alignment of drug molecules: applications to sterol mimics, thrombin and thermolysin inhibitors, *J. Comput. Aided Mol. Design 8*: 751–778 (1994).

26. T. D. J. Perkins and P. M. Dean, An exploration of a novel strategy for superimposing several flexible molecules, *J. Comput. Aided Mol. Design 7*: 155–172 (1993).

27. G. Diana, E. P. Jaeger, M. L. Peterson, and A. M. Treasurywala, The use of an algorithmic method for small molecule superimpositions in the design of antiviral agents, *J. Comput. Aided Mol. Design 7*:325–335 (1993).

28. Y. Kato, A. Inoue, M. Yamada, N. Tomioka, and A. Itai, Automatic superposition of drug molecules based on their common receptor site, *J. Comput. Aided Mol. Design 6*:475–486 (1992).

29. A. Itai, N. Tomioka, M. Yamada, A. Inoue, and Y. Kato, Molecular super-position for rational drug design, *3D QSAR in Drug Design* (H. Kubinyi, ed.), ESCOM, Leiden, 1993, pp. 200–225.

30. B. B. Masek, A. Merchant, and J. B. Matthew, Molecular shape comparison of angiotensin II receptor antagonists, *J. Med. Chem. 36*:1230–1238 (1993).

31. HipHop is developed and distributed by Biosym-MSI, San Diego CA.

32. D. Mayer, C. B. Naylor, I. Motoc, and G. R. Marshall, A unique geometry of the active site of angiotensin-converting enzyme consistent with structure-activity studies, *J. Comput. Aided Mol. Design 1*:3–16 (1987).

33. J. R. Sufrin, D. A. Dunn, and G. R. Marshall, Steric mapping of the L-methionine binding site of ATP:L-methionine *S*-adenosyltransferase, *Mol. Pharmacol. 19*:307–313 (1981).

34. SYBYL is developed and distributed by Tripos Associates, St. Louis MI.

35. T. Langer and C. A. Wermuth, Inhibitors of prolyl endopeptidase; character-ization of the pharmacophric pattern using conformational analysis and 3D-QSAR, *J. Comput. Aided Mol. Design 7*:253–262 (1993).

36. U. Cosentino, G. Moro, D. Pitea, S. Scolastico, R. Todeschini, and C. Sco-lastico, Pharmacophore identification by molecular modeling and chemo-metrics: the case of HMG-CoA reductase inhibitors, *J. Comput. Aided Mol. Design 6*:47–60 (1992).

37. P. H. Reggio, A. M. Panu, and S. Miles, Characterization of a region of steric interference at the cannabinoid receptor using the active analog approach, *J. Med. Chem. 36*:1761–1771 (1993).

38. Chem-X is developed and distributed by Chemical Design Ltd, Oxon, UK and Mahwah NJ.

39. Y. C. Martin, M. G. Bures, E. A. Danaher, J. DeLazzer, I. Lico, and P. A. Pavlik, A fast new approach to pharmacophore mapping and its application of dopaminergic and benzodiazepine agonists, *J. Comput. Aided Mol. Design 7*:83–102 (1993).

40. B. Waszkowycz, D. E. Clark, D. Frenkel, J. Li, C. W. Murray, B. Robson, and D. R. Westhead, PRO_LIGAND: an approach to de novo molecular de-sign. 2. Design of novel molecules from molecular field analysis (MFA) mod-els and pharmacophores, *J. Med. Chem. 37*:3994–4002 (1994).

41. M. Froimowitz and V. Cody, Biologically active conformers of phenothiazines and thioxanthenes. Further evidence for a ligand model of dopamine D_2 re-ceptor antagonists, *J. Med. Chem. 36*:2219–2227 (1993).

42. G. Wong, K. F. Koehler, P. Skolnick, Z-Q. Gu, S. Ananthan, P. Schonholzer, W. Hunkeler, W. Zhang, and J. M. Cook, Synthetic and computer-assisted analysis of the structural requirements for selective, high-affinity ligand bind-ing to diazepam-insensitive benzodiazepine receptors, *J. Med. Chem 36*: 1820–1830 (1993).

43. M. G. Bures, E. Danaher, J. DeLazzer, and Y. C. Martin, New molecular modeling tools using three-dimensional chemical substructures, *J. Chem. Inf. Comput. Sci. 34*:218–223 (1994).

44. Applications in Chem-X. Lead Generation I: automatic pharmacophore identification for a set of compounds, Chemical Design, Ltd., Oxon, UK, 1995.
45. APEX-3D is integrated in the InsightII molecular-modeling program, developed and distributed by Biosym-MSI, San Diego CA.
46. APEX-3D User Guide, Version 1.3, DCL Systems International, Biosym-MSI, San Diego CA, 1993.
47. Hypotheses in Catalyst, Biosym-MSI, San Diego, CA, 1992.
48. A. Smellie, S. L. Teig, and Pl Towbin, Poling: promoting conformational variation, *J. Comp. Chem.* *16*:171–187 (1995).
49. A. Smellie, S. D. Kahn, and S. L. Teig, Analysis of conformational coverage. 2. Applications of conformational models, *J. Chem. Inf. Comput. Sci.* 35: 295–304 (1995).
50. A. Doweyko, Three-dimensional pharmacophores from binding data, *J. Med. Chem.* *37*:1769–1778 (1994).
51. A. K. Saxena, M. Saxena, H. Chi, and M. Wiese, Indentification of a pharmacophore by application of hypothetical active site lattice (HASL) approach, *Med. Chem. Res.* *3*:201–208 (1993).
52. E. E. Hodgkin, A. Miller, and M. Whittaker, A Monte Carlo pharmacophore generation procedure: application to the human PAF receptor, *J. Comput. Aided Mol. Design* *7*:515–534 (1993).
53. E. E. Hodgkin, A. Miller, and M. Whittaker, A partial pharmacophore for the platelet activating factor (PAF) receptor, *Bioorg. Med. Chem. Lett.* *2*:597–602 (1992).
54. J. P. Whitten, B. L. Harrison, J. R. Weintraub, and I. McDonald, Modeling of competitive phosphono amino acid NMDA receptor antagonists, *J. Med. Chem.* *35*:1509–1514 (1992).
55. A. K. Ghose, M. E. Logan, A. M. Treasurywala, H. Wang, R. C. Wahl, B. E. Tomczuk, M. R. Gowravaram, E. P. Jaeger, and J. J. Wendoloski, Determination of pharmacophoric geometry for collagenase inhibitors using a novel computational method and its verification using molecular dynamics, NMR, X-ray crystallography, *J. Am. Chem. Soc.* *117*:4671–4682 (1995).
56. J. H. Holland, Genetic algorithms, *Sci. Am.* *267*:66–72 (1992).
57. Z. Michalewicz, *Genetic Algorithms + Data Structures = Evolution Programs*, Springer-Verlag, Berlin, 1992.
58. D. E. Walters and R. M. Hinds, Genetically evolved receptor models: a computational approach to construction of receptor models, *J. Med. Chem.* *37*: 2527–2536 (1994).
59. A. W. R. Payne and R. C. Glen, Molecular recognition using a binary genetic search algorithm, *J. Mol. Graphics* *11*:74–91 (1993).
60. G. Jones, P. Willett, and R. C. Glen, A genetic algorithm for flexible molecular overlay and pharmacophore elucidation, *J. Comput. Aided Mol. Design* *9*: 532–549 (1995).
61. P. S. Magee, A new approach to active-site binding analysis. Inhibitors of acetylcholinesterase, *Quant. Struct. Act. Relat.* *9*:202–215 (1990).

62. A. Rupp, K.-A. Kovar, G. Beuerle, C. Rug, and G. Folkers, A new pharmacophoric model for 5-HT reuptake inhibitors: differentiation of amphetamine analogues, *Pharm. Acta Helv.* *68*:235–244 (1994).

63. H. Koga, M. Ohta, H. Sato, T. Ishizawa, and H. Nabata, Design of potent K^+ channel openers by pharmacophore model, *Bioorg. Med. Chem. Lett.* *3*: 625–631 (1993).

64. K. S. Rein, D. G. Baden, and R. E. Gawley, Conformational analysis of the sodium channel modulator, brevetoxin A, comparison with brevetoxin B conformations, and a hypothesis about the common pharmacophore of the "site 5" toxins, *J. Org. Chem.* *59*:2101–2106 (1994).

65. B. Jin and A. J. Hopfinger, A proposed common spatial pharmacophore and the corresponding active conformations of some TxA_2 receptor antagonists, *J. Chem. Inf. Comput. Sci.* *34*:1014–1021 (1994).

66. R. J. Quinn, C. Taylor, M. Suganuma, and H. Fujiki, The conserved acid binding domain model of inhibitors of protein phosphatases 1 and 2A: molecular modeling aspects, *Bioorg. Med. Chem. Lett.* *3*:1029–1034 (1993).

67. G. R. Strobl, S. von Kruedener, J. Stockigt, F. P. Guengerich, and T. Wolff, Development of a pharmacophore for inhibition of human liver cyctochrome P-450 2D6: molecular modeling and inhibition studies, *J. Med. Chem.* *36*: 1136–1145 (1993).

68. R.-S. Tsai, P.-A. Carrupt, B. Testa, P. Gaillard, N. El Tayar, and T. Hogberg, Effects of solvation on the ionization and conformation of raclopride and other antidopaminergic 6-methoxysalicylamides: insight into the pharmacophore, *J. Med. Chem.* *36*:196–204 (1993).

69. R. P. Sheridan, A. Rusinko III, R. Nilakantan, and R. Venkataraghavan, Searching for pharmacophores in large coordinate data bases and its use in drug design, *Proc. Natl. Acad. Sci. USA* *86*:8165–8169 (1989).

70. D. E. Clark, G. Jones, P. Willett, P. W. Kenny, and R. C. Glen, Pharmacophoric pattern matching in files of three-dimensional chemical structures: comparison of conformational searching algorithms for flexible searching, *J. Chem. Inf. Comput. Sci.* *34*:197–206 (1994).

71. D. E. Clark and P. Willett, Pharmacophoric pattern matching in files of three-dimensional chemical structures: implementation of flexible searching, *J. Mol. Graphics* *11*:146–156 (1993).

72. A. R. Poirrette, P. Willett, and F. H. Allen, Pharmacophoric pattern matching in files of three-dimensional chemical structures: characterization and use of generalized torsion angle screens, *J. Mol. Graphics* *11*:2–14 (1993).

73. M. F. Chan, I. Okun, F. L. Stavros, E. Hwang, M. E. Wolff, and V. N. Balaji, Identification of a new class of ET_A selective endothelin antagonists by pharmacophore directed screening, *Biochem. Biophys. Res. Commun.* *201*:228–234 (1994).

74. Y. Takahasi, T. Akagi, and S. Sasaki, Three-dimensional pharmacophoric pattern search using COMPASS: nootropic agents, *Tetrahedron Comput. Methodol.* *3*:27–35 (1990).

75. P. S. Charifson, A. R. Leach, and A. Rusinko III, The generation and use of large 3D databases in drug discovery, *Network Sci. 1*: http://edisto.awod.com/netsci/index.html (1995).

76. J. H. Van Drie, 3D database searching in drug discovery, *Network Sci. 1*: http://edisto.awod.com/netsci/index.html (1995).

77. D. Weininger, A note on the sense and nonsense of searching 3-D databases for pharmaceutical leads, *Network Sci. 1*: http://edisto.awod.com/netsci/index.html (1995).

78. D. R. Henry and O. F. Guner, Techniques for searching databases of three-dimensional (3D) sturctures with receptor-based queries, *Network Sci. 1*: http://edisto.awod.com/netsci/index.html (1995).

79. K. Davies and R. Upton, 3D pharmacophore searching, *Network Sci. 1*: http://edisto.awod.com/netsci/index.html (1995).

80. K. Prendergast, K. Adams, W. J. Greenlee, R. B. Nachbar, A. A. Patchett, and D. J. Underwood, Derivation of a 3D pharmacophore model for the angiotensin-II site one receptor, *J. Comput. Aided Mol. Design 8*:491–512 (1994).

81. S. R. Krystek, J. T. Hunt, P. D. Stein, and T. R. Stouch, Three-dimensional quantitative structure–activity relationships of sulfonamide endothelin inhibitors, *J. Med. Chem. 38*:659–668 (1995).

82. G. Cruciani and K. A. Watson, Comparative molecular field analysis using GRID force-field and GOLPE variable selection methods in a study of inhibitors of glycogen phosphorylase *b*, *J. Med. Chem. 37*:2589–2601 (1994).

83. A. Agarwal, P. P. Pearson, E. W. Taylor, H. B. Li, T. Dahlgren, M. Herslof, Y. Yang, G. Lambert, D. L. Nelson, J. W. Regan, and A. R. Martin, Three-dimensional quantitative structure–acitivity relationships of 5-HT receptor binding data for tetrahydropyridinylindole derivatives: a comparison of the Hansch and CoMFA methods, *J. Med. Chem. 36*:4006–4014 (1993).

84. A. M. Myers, P. S. Charifson, C. E. Owens, N. S. Kula, A. T. McPhail, R. J. Baldessarini, R. G. Booth, and S. D. Wyrick, Conformational analysis, pharmacophore identification, and comparative molecular field analysis of ligands for the neuromodulatory σ_3 receptor, *J. Med. Chem. 37*:4109–4117 (1994).

85. R. A. Lewis and A. R. Leach, Current methods for site-directed structure generation, *J. Comput. Aided Mol. Design 8*:467–475 (1994).

86. V. Tschinke and N. C. Cohen, The NEWLEAD program: a new mthod for the design of candidate structures from pharmacophoric hypotheses, *J. Med. Chem. 36*:3863–3870 (1993).

87. V. J. Gillet, W. Newell, P. Mata, G. Myatt, S. Sandor, Z. Zsoldos, and A. P. Johnson, SPROUT: recent developments in the de novo design of molecules, *J. Chem Inf. Comput. Sci 34*:207–217 (1994).

88. Applications in Chem-X. Lead generation II: novel structures from a pharmacophore, Chemical Design Ltd, Oxon, UK, 1995.

3

Generation and Use of Three-Dimensional Databases for Drug Discovery

Renée L. DesJarlais

SmithKline Beecham Pharmaceuticals,
King of Prussia, Pennsylvania

I. INTRODUCTION

In general, biologically active molecules exert their effect by binding to a receptor. The ability of a given molecule to bind to a receptor is determined by the presence of certain important functional groups and the three-dimensional (3D) presentation of these features by the molecule. A goal of molecular modeling in the context of designing bioactive molecules is to understand the determinants of receptor binding and to use this knowledge in the design or discovery of novel molecules with the desired activity. The availability of structure–activity data or the structure of a receptor enables the proposal of a pharmacophoric pattern which, in the best case, would include the functionality required for activity and the relative orientation of the functional groups [1]. In this chapter, such a proposal will be referred to as a 3D pharmacophore hypothesis, to emphasize the inclusion of spatial constraints. Recent advances in techniques for generating 3D molecular structures for typical drug-sized organic molecules and for searching databases of 3D structures combined with a 3D pharmacophore hypothesis give the medicinal chemist new tools that can assist in discovering novel active molecules. A 3D pharmacophore can be used as a query to search a database of molecules for those that are predicted to possess the desired activity if the pharmacophore hypothesis is correct. If a receptor structure or receptor site model is available, another type of 3D searching can be used. For this, molecules are selected based on their steric and chemical match to the receptor structure, without the need to propose which interactions might be most important. The methods are complementary and both have assisted in the discovery of active molecules. This work will review the generation of databases of 3D chemical structures, methods available for searching such databases, and examples of the successful use of these techniques in discovering active molecules.

II. SOURCES OF THREE-DIMENSIONAL STRUCTURES

A prerequisite for any 3D search is a chemical database that includes 3D structural information. The primary source of experimental structures for small organic molecules is X-ray crystallography, and these structures are collected in the Cambridge Structural Database (CSD) [2]. The CSD contains structures for about 140,000 molecules. There are much larger databases of molecules for which the 2D (connectivity) information is available, but experimental structures have not been determined for all molecules (e.g., the Available Chemicals Directory [3], Spresi [4], the Chemical Abstracts Database [5], the National Cancer Institute Database [6], and many corporate databases). For these databases, 3D structures can be generated with a variety of computational methods; for several others, either software vendors [7] or database vendors [8–10] have done the 2D to 3D conversion. Although this eliminates the need for the user to do this calculation, it is important to know the method used to generate the 3D structures to appropriately query a database and understand the results of a 3D search. A variety of methods for generating 3D structures from connectivity information are discussed in the following. Some of the important differences between methods include whether a single low-energy structure or many different conformations are generated, and whether the method is exclusively rule-based or incorporates an energy minimization step.

A. CONCORD™

The most commonly used method for converting a 2D database to a 3D database is the program CONCORD [11]. CONCORD is a fast (<1 s/structure), robust method for generating a single low-energy structure of a small molecule. CONCORD combines a rule-based algorithm with a pseudomolecular mechanics approach. An initial structure is generated based on rules derived from examination of experimental structures, and a univariate strain function is then optimized. Optionally, a torsion minimization can be carried out to improve structures with van der Waals overlap. Although CONCORD usually generates structures with good internal geometry and reasonable torsion angles, it does poorly on rings with more than ten members. For a series of molecules with a common core, CONCORD will generate the same conformation for this core.

B. CORINA

CORINA [12] is a 2D to 3D building program that first builds up a crude 3D structure from a standard set of bond lengths, angles, and torsion angles, and some special rules for dealing with cyclic systems. The molecule is then subjected to a pseudoforce-field calculation that includes only the bond-stretching, angle-bending, out-of-plane–bending, and torsion energies. This corrects any unfavorable bond lengths and angles and removes close van der Waals contacts. The method produces a single low-energy structure and requires several seconds per molecule on a SUN4 Space Station IPC.

C. Distance Geometry

There are several programs available that use the technique of distance geometry [13] to build 3D structures. Most of these programs use a starting 3D structure to determine bond length and bond angle constraints. The program RUBICON, from Daylight Chemical Information Systems [14], uses bond length and bond angle tables so that structures can be generated from connectivity information alone. In distance geometry, the bond length and bond angle information is used to build a matrix of upper- and lower-bounds on the distances between all atoms. A set of random distances from within these bounds is selected, ad the structure is embedded from this high-dimensional distance space into three dimensions. The resulting structure is then optimized versus the initial constraints. This procedure can be done for one set of random distances to obtain a single conformation, or many times with different sets of random distances to obtain a variety of conformations. Distance geometry is a relatively slow mechanism for generating structures and may be best suited for structure generation when a rule-based method has failed.

D. Artificial Intelligence Approaches

WIZARD [15] and COBRA [16] both use artificial intelligence techniques to generate a user-specified number of low-energy conformations for any given molecule. The general approach is similar for both programs. From the molecular connectivity, these programs analyze a molecule and divide it up into conformational units about which the program has some knowledge. Each conformational unit is assigned one or more "conformational templates," and heuristics are used to combine these templates. Each conformation is then criticized to discover inconsistencies and, if necessary, resolve any strain. The conformational templates are derived from a combination of the Cambridge Database and molecular mechanics-generated structures. COBRA incorporates the A* algorithm [16] to direct the conformation search to areas of low-energy structures without examining all template conformations, thereby decreasing the search times by a factor of 2–10 relative to the complete conformation search. COBRA requires on the order of 10s of seconds per molecule.

AIMB [17] and MIMUMBA [18] are two other knowledge-based approaches to generating multiple 3D conformations from 2D information. AIMB uses fragments derived from the Cambridge Crystallographic Database [2]. It attempts to use the largest appropriate fragments to assemble conformers. MIMUMBA uses torsion angle libraries, also derived from crystal structures.

E. MOLGEO

MOLGEO is a program for the rapid construction of a 3D model from the molecular connectivity and from bond length and bond angle tables [19]. Two different algorithms are implemented for building a 3D model: a distance geometry approach and a depth-first conformation search. The distance geometry method is based on the work of Crippen [20] and, in general, has the features described in Section II.C. The depth-first search method was implemented in an attempt to generate higher-quality structures more quickly than the distance geometry method. Conformations are built one torsion at a time, and the partial conformation is evaluated with a set of heuristics. Although these heuristics eliminate many branches of the search, this method was about 60-fold slower than CONCORD on a test set of 639 small molecules for which X-ray crystallographic structures were available [21].

F. Flexibases

Kearsley et al. have published a method [22] for generating databases that contain multiple conformations for each molecule, for which the conformations are chosen to be dissimilar. Initial 3D conformations are generated from minimization of the 2D structures. The minimization is carried out using IDEALIZE [22], a robust molecular mechanics program that does not require hydrogens and uses only the repulsive part of the nonbonded interactions.

Conformations are generated with distance geometry, using an empirically derived rule for the number of trials necessary to cover conformation space. The conformers are then reminimized with IDEALIZE and compared using a root mean square (RMS) deviation, calculated after least-squares fitting of nonhydrogen atoms. Structures that differ by more than a user-specified cutoff from any conformers already kept are added to the list. If this number is higher than the maximum number of conformers per structure, then the procedure is repeated using a larger RMS cutoff. This procedure takes 3–8 min of CPU on a Cray YMP for a typical drug-like molecule. An RMS cutoff of 1.2 A leads to an average of eight conformations selected from 40–80 energetically acceptable conformations.

G. Poling

Smellie et al. [23] have developed a method called poling that can assist in generating a diverse set of conformers. A random set of conformers is generated, and energy is minimized with a potential function that includes a term that derives the current conformation away from previously found conformations. This new term, the *poling energy*, uses the distances between features (e.g., heteroatoms) and the centroid of all features to define the conformation. The poling energy is defined in Eq. (1),

$$F_{\text{pole}} = W_{\text{pole}} \left(\sum_i \frac{1}{(D_i)^n} \right) \tag{1}$$

where D_i is the RMS deviation between the poling distances in the current conformation and previously encountered conformation i, n is a positive integer that controls the steepness of the function F, and W_{pole} is a scaling factor. When the poling function is properly scaled the conformers generated by using the poling function are energetically reasonable.

III. ASSESSING THE QUALITY OF A DATABASE OF CHEMICAL STRUCTURES

There are two distinct issues that are critical in assessing the quality of a database of three-dimensional structures: whether the structures stored are reasonable low-energy conformations, and the breadth of chemistry spanned by the collection. With the exception of databases of experimental structures, the energy and conformation will be determined by the structure-generation method used. In general, these methods can be expected to do well for bond lengths and angles, but the torsion angles chosen often result in structures with unreasonable van der Waals clashes. Such structures can be excluded from the database or handled with a different structure-generation algorithm. If such structures are excluded, this typically results in substantially fewer molecules in the final database. To some extent, CONCORD 3.0.1 addresses the issue of unreasonable van der Waals clashes by introducing a torsion optimization. The result has been a decrease in the number of structures with severe clashes. Minimizing the energetics for an entire database is conceivable, but the dilemma is whether the force field used in the evaluation will be better parameterized for the variety of chemistry in the database than the original structure-generation program. Most commercially available force fields are not general enough to deal with the wide variety of functionality in a large database of drug-like organic molecules.

Evaluating the chemistry present in a database is a topic that has received much attention recently [24,25]. Interest is particularly keen in the pharmaceutical companies, because corporate molecular databases are very much biased toward the chemistry of programs that have had long lifetimes. To assess the diversity of a chemical database, it is necessary to choose either a measure of diversity or similarity, and to define reasonable bounds for the space described by the measure. For instance, if part of the diversity measure is net charge, a database with polyanions and polycations would be quite diverse, but perhaps not so interesting in terms of molecules likely to be successful pharmaceuticals. To date, methods for assessing diversity have focused primarily on the similarity of molecular connection tables, without considering possible three-dimensional structures and conformations. The availability of databases containing three-dimensional structures is allowing the consideration of not only the presence or absence of a functional group, but also the disposition of different functional groups relative to each other [26]. As the research into measures of diversity continues, it is likely that several useful measures of diversity will emerge.

IV. SEARCH METHODS

A. Rigid Three-Dimensional Searching

The most straightforward 3D search is a rigid search for a 3D pharmacophore. A database of molecules that includes atom and connectivity information as well as 3D structures is required. The user specifies a 3D pharmacophore that comprises a set of functional groups and the geometric relations between them. The geometric relations might be based on single atoms from the functional groups, or centroids, lines, planes, or excluded volumes derived from the functional groups. The search, which typically includes a screening step and a matching step, is then carried out over the 3D structures stored in the database. The screening stage allows searches to be performed rapidly. Features, which might be functionality alone or distances between functional groups, are encoded as a bit string that can be quickly compared with the query to exclude molecules that lack the features of the query. This results in the exclusion of a large fraction of the database, leaving a much smaller number of molecules for the more time-consuming substructure matching step [27]. In a rigid 3D search, although there is no consideration of alternative conformations for any molecule, most search software allows many conformations of a given molecule to be stored.

3Dsearch

The program 3Dsearch [28] was developed by Sheridan and co-workers to allow quick searching of a database of 3D structures. For each nonhydrogen atom, five pieces of data are stored: element, the number of nonhydrogen neighbors, the number of π-electrons, the expected number of attached hydrogens, and the formal charge. In addition, four types of dummy atoms are also calculated and stored for each molecule. These are the centroid of planar five- and six-membered rings, positions 0.5 A above and below these rings along the normal to the ring, and the calculated positions of heteroatom-bound hydrogens and lone pairs. All queries are specified using these atom descriptions or as wild cards. The search is made rapid by the use of an inverted key scheme. For each entry in the database, keys are stored for all atom–atom pairs, and for each pair of atom types, the distances are divided into bins. The system allows for distance, three-point angle, four-point angle, and excluded volume constraints. In general, the use of atom descriptions may limit the users ability to specify the chemical substructure around any particular query element.

Aladdin

The program Aladdin [29] permits geometric, substructural, and steric queries of a database of 3D chemical structures. In the query, atoms or functional groups can be defined, and distances and angles can be specified between them. Features such as exclusion volumes can also be defined. A novel feature of Aladdin is the ability to specify the location of a hydrogen bond donor or acceptor with which an appropriate atom from each hit must interact. This permits one to find hits that will be able to make the desired hydrogen bond, but may do so by approaching the hydrogen bond site from different directions. Aladdin goes beyond simple database searching and can redesign molecules in the database to better or more simply fulfill the query. For example, Aladdin can strip off unnecessary substituents that might otherwise cause steric problems, or it can change atom types to provide the desired hydrogen-bonding characteristics. Such designed molecules will require a synthetic effort. The benefit of the design aspect will depend on the number and type of compounds available for direct screening and the abundance of synthetic resources that can be put toward a given project.

UNITY™

The UNITY package of programs is a database-searching package from Tripos, Inc. Query features are specified by element and connectivity and can include centroids, lines, planes, and normals. UNITY includes the capability for using Markush atoms, which could define generic hydrogen bond donors, for example. An advantage of this approach is that the user can define generic atom types that might be problem-specific and were not anticipated at the time the database was generated. A disadvantage is that the definition of Markush atoms is complicated enough that it is likely to be employed only by an experienced user. Three-dimensional features can include distance, angle, and either inclusion or exclusion volumes. The 3D search is divided into a 2D screen for the presence of the desired chemical functionality, and a 3D screen for distances between the functionality of interest, and finally a matching step to check that all constraints can be simultaneously met. Tools are supplied for viewing hit lists and performing Boolean operations on them. The database-searching programs are closely tied to the other Tripos products, making further modeling of a hit list convenient.

MACCS-3D™

MACCS-3D adds 3D search capability to the MACCS™ chemical database software. This program is similar in approach to UNITY, with key searches to eliminate molecules that do not contain the correct functionality within the specified distance ranges. MACCS does not store generic atom-type information. Atoms are specified by element and bonding patterns. The interface provides a convenient way to specify alternative elements that would be acceptable at a given position. The MACCS front-end is familiar to many medicinal chemists and many corporate databases are already stored in MACCS-2D form; thus, MACCS-3D may provide the quickest entrée into 3D pharmacophore searching.

Catalyst™

Catalyst is a database search system that allows rigid searching over a database of small molecules [30]. Catalyst queries are formulated based on the chemical function (e.g., hydrogen bond donation) desired. Hydrogen bond donors, hydrogen bond acceptors, charge centers, and hydrophobic regions are identified as part of the database-building procedure. The identification of these generic chemical functionalities includes checking that the group is sterically accessible in the stored conformation. Many queries are easily specified using these generic functionalities, but these definitions can be modified only by rebuilding the databases; hence, the definitions cannot be tailored to a specific problem, as is sometimes required. A unique feature of Catalyst is the use of target zones around the specified functions, as opposed to the distance between the specified functions. This can lead to more precise query specifications, with fewer parameters, and makes visual comparison of the query and the hits easier [30].

CAVEAT

CAVEAT [31,32] is a program that uses a database search to assist in the design of novel molecules. It is a special-purpose program that was written to aid in the design of small molecules that could mimic a protein loop important in a protein–protein interaction. The basic assumption of the program is that protein–protein recognition is based on specific positioning of amino acid side chains and that the backbone is not critical and could be replaced. The CAVEAT program attempts to find ring systems that can present the side chains in the desired orientation. A CAVEAT database consists of the distance and angle relations of vectors, defined by the exocyclic bonds of ring systems, and an index back to the 3D structure of the ring. A typical query might define the $C\alpha$–$C\beta$ vector relations that would be required to present the necessary side chain analogues. Such a vector search could be conducted by most generic database-searching programs discussed in this chapter; however, CAVEAT is optimized for this task. Although the initial CAVEAT applications were for protein mimicry, the program could be useful in any situation for which one needed a novel scaffold to present a set of functional groups in a defined orientation. The latest CAVEAT suite of programs includes the ability to cluster the hits, based on size or substructure similarity, and to rank hits by size, number of atoms at ring fusions, and whether the designed molecule would have eclipsing interactions. Two novel databases are available for use with CAVEAT: Triad, a computer-generated collection of all tricyclic hydrocarbons, and Iliad, a collection of acyclic molecules. Software is also available to create CAVEAT databases from the Cambridge Structural Database [2].

Cambridge Structural Database

The Cambridge Structural Database (CSD) has associated searching software that allows many types of 3D searching [33]. Although the CSD software can perform the same kinds of 3D searching as the aforedescribed programs, the database and software are probably most useful because they provide access to a large amount of experimental data. This data contains not only bond length, bond angle, and torsion information on a wide variety of molecules, but also information about intermolecular interaction that can be deduced from the interactions between molecules in the crystal. It should be remembered that the conformation and intermolecular interactions seen in the crystal may be influenced by the constraints of crystal packing and do not necessarily represent the minimum energy structure in solution. Nevertheless, this data has been, and continues to be, used in the development and validation of molecular mechanics methods and automated 3D structure-generation tools. It is the ability to search noncovalent crystal contact information that sets the CSD software apart from other software discussed here.

B. Flexible Three-Dimensional Searching

The consideration of a single, rigid conformation will certainly miss some molecules that could present the pharmacophore in a conformation other than the one stored in the database. There are two basic approaches for dealing with conformational flexibility: by storing information about multiple conformations at database generation time, or by evaluating conformations during the search. If conformations are to be generated at the start, then one must decide on the number of conformations to generate and which conformations to include. Methods for generating databases that include multiple conformations were discussed in Section II.

Several algorithms have been developed for examining conformations during a search. Typically, the molecules are first screened for those that contain the desired functionality, and then, the flexible search is performed. These methods have an advantage over searching pregenerated conformations, in that they are not restricted to minimum-energy conformations and will not miss conformations that might fit the query but, for various reasons, have not been stored in a multiconformer database. A corollary to this is that, typically, when conformations are explored during the search, they are not checked for energy; consequently, it is possible for the program to return structures with unreasonable geometries. Such structures would not be included in a database that stores pregenerated conformations. Depending on the number of hits retrieved and the tools available for postprocessing a hit list, the inclusion of high-energy structures could be considered a problem, or a feature.

Directed Tweak

Hurst has developed the "directed tweak" algorithm [34] that allows consideration of conformational flexibility at search time. The conformation search begins with the stored conformation, and its torsions are adjusted to minimize the sum of the squared deviations between the distances in the 3D query and the corresponding distances in the structure. This method is able to consider the flexibility of ring systems as well as acyclic systems. It is fast, taking hundredths of seconds per structure to seconds, depending on whether ring flexibility and bump checking were performed. The time per molecule increases rapidly with the size of the molecule. In tests of this method it produced more hits than searching a single conformation, or than searching a database containing 20 conformers for each molecule [34]. The directed tweak algorithm is implemented in UNITY from Tripos, Inc.

Torsion Optimization

Mook et al. [35] report a method for flexible searching that is available in MDL's MACCS and ISIS™ systems. They use either a simplex optimizer, in the general case, or derivative-based optimizer when only distances and angles are involved in the query. An optimization is carried out in torsion space to minimize the root mean square deviation between the constraints from the query and the values measured from the structure. Search times are 2–20 times longer than rigid 3D searches.

ChemDBS-3D

The ChemDBS-3D™ [36] module of CHEM-X™ provides the capability for searching a database of 3D structures. Although the search method is essentially a rigid search, it is specifically designed to work with a multi-conformer database. ChemDBS-3D uses generic atom types that are deduced at database-generation time from the molecular connectivity information. Typical generic atom types would be hydrogen bond-donors, hydrogen bond-acceptors, ring centroids, atoms with a formal charge of +1, atoms with a formal charge of −1, or others. These can be customized by the user at database-generation time. The initial search is a bit screen that involves a chemical formula screen to eliminate molecules that do not possess the correct atom types and a 3D screen to eliminate molecules that cannot place the desired pairs of centers at the appropriate distance. After the screening step, a conformational search must be performed to ensure

that a low-energy structure can simultaneously meet all the query constraints. This search is the same as that used to generate the database and
uses rules similar to those described by Dolata et al. for WIZARD [15].
The program can return all low-energy conformations that match the query,
or simply return a list of molecules with at least one low-energy conformation matching the query. The type of list requested will depend on
whether the user wishes to perform further modeling studies or simply to
supply a list of compounds for screening.

Distance Geometry

Willett and co-workers [37] describe a system that uses distance geometry
to generate a conformation of a candidate molecule that will fit the query.
Distance geometry calculations are relatively slow. Estimates of upper and
lower bounds of distances between query atoms are used to determine if
a particular structure should be subjected to the distance geometry calculation. Even with this screening procedure, the times for this type of search
would be 10–100 times longer than a rigid 3D search.

Other Flexible Search Methods

Various other methods have been applied to the flexible search problem.
A systematic search of conformation space in which rotatable bonds are
adjusted by a defined increment has been examined [38]. This method is
feasible only for molecules with a few rotatable bonds, otherwise the time
to explore conformations is prohibitive. Other optimization techniques that
have been tried include Monte Carlo and genetic algorithms [38].

Comparison of Flexible Search Methods

The most time-consuming part of a flexible 3D search is the conformation
search step. A comparison of distance geometry, systematic search, Monte
Carlo search, genetic algorithm, and the directed-tweak algorithm discussed earlier has been carried out [38]. Eight different pharmacophore
patterns, involving only distance constraints, were examined with the various search methods. Of the methods tested, the directed-tweak algorithm
performed best. The genetic algorithm found fewer hits and was somewhat slower. The other methods were all too slow to warrant serious
consideration.

C. Rigid Versus Flexible Pharmacophore Searching

The question of whether to conduct a flexible or a rigid 3D search is not
easily answered. The quick response is certainly to do the flexible search,

because otherwise potentially interesting molecules might be missed. In practice, flexible searches often require more resources and time than is feasible. Haraki et al. [39] have compared hit rates with flexible and rigid 3D searches and find that, as expected, the flexible search finds more active molecules. Usually, however, the percentage of active compounds is higher for the rigid search. Also, a rigid search is less likely to miss molecules with few degrees of freedom, and these may be more interesting in the end, because there will be lower entropic cost for binding such molecules to the receptor. For example, a long peptide that matches a query in a conformation that brings its end residues together is unlikely to prove an interesting lead. Both UNITY and MACCS-3D allow the user to specify a maximum number of rotatable bonds. This may provide a reasonable compromise.

Searches that generate structures as part of the search have the possibility for generating high-energy conformations. In general, the user must evaluate the energy, or must attempt to optimize the energy of the search hits in a separate calculation. An exception to this is the detection of close contacts. Both UNITY and MACCS can check conformations for close van der Waals contacts and attempt to relieve them with an energy-minimization process. This can be time-consuming, but it is a necessary step if energies are to be used in any prioritization or analysis of hits.

D. Rigid Searching Versus a Receptor Site

DOCK

When a structure or model of a receptor is available, it is possible to search a database for molecules that have shape or electrostatic complementarity to that receptor without developing a pharmacophore hypothesis. The most well-studied method for this type of searching is DOCK [40–43]. DOCK characterizes the receptor site using a set of spheres. A clique detection algorithm is then used to match sphere centers with atom centers from a small molecule. Each clique is used to define an orientation of the small molecule in the receptor site by least squares fitting the atom centers onto the matched sphere centers. Each orientation is then scored. Scoring schemes, including shape only [41], shape and electrostatics [43], and shape and hydrophobicity [44], have been used.

Several derivatives of DOCK have incorporated the ability to associated properties with spheres so that only atoms with complementary properties are allowed to match those spheres [45,46]. Such approaches can dramatically reduce search time and improve the chemical complementarity of the hits.

CLIX

CLIX is a program that combines elements of a 3D pharmacophore search and a DOCK search versus a receptor [47]. The user defines three positions in the receptor site of interest and the functionality that should occupy these sites. The program explores orientations of the small molecules from the database that fulfill the functionality requirements of these target sites. Hits are ranked by their energy of interaction with the receptor site.

Ellipsoid Searching

A different way in which to use receptor site information is to search for molecules that generally have the correct shape and size. Sudarasanam et al. [48] have developed a method in which small molecules are characterized as ellipsoids, and the shape of a binding site is characterized as an ellipsoid. The database can be rapidly screened for molecules that would be expected to fill the binding site, based on having similar ellipsoid dimensions. These molecules can then be examined by hand to determine whether the detailed shapes match as well. The database search part of such a procedure should be quick, but to the extent that hand examination is needed, this may be less desirable than an automatic procedure.

E. Flexible Searching Versus a Receptor Site

DOCK, CLIX, and the other methods discussed in the previous section are rigid searches in which both the small molecule and the protein site are held fixed. This limitation has been addressed in several ways by different groups. DesJarlais et al. added an element of flexibility by splitting small molecules up into fragments that could reasonably be considered rigid [49]. These were then examined for sets of fragments that could be joined to recreate the small molecule. Although this approach proved successful, it is not easily adapted to database searching because rules for fragmenting and rejoining would need to be defined for each molecule.

Leach and Kuntz [45] describe a method combining aspects of DOCK and aspects of COBRA to explore the orientational and conformational degrees of freedom of a single molecule in a binding site [45]. They expand the binding site characterization to include sites of potential hydrogen bonds. The method is fairly slow, requiring about 20 min of CPU to explore the binding of a single ligands. Although this would not be excessive for a molecule of particular interest, it is too long to be useful in searching large databases.

Oshiro et al. [50] describe the use of a genetic algorithm to fit conformationally flexible molecules into an active site. Their method uses ideas derived from DOCK to characterize the receptor site. The genetic algorithm optimizes both the orientation of the ligand and its conformation in the receptor site, using scores calculated by the force field scoring from DOCK [43]. The genetic algorithm is able to generate low-energy structures for the test systems, some of which are close to the crystallographically determined binding mode. Although many orientations or conformations can be examined per minute, the total time to generate a reasonable number of low-energy conformations (e.g., five structures within 20% of the energy of the crystal structure) requires 10 min or more per molecule on an R3000 SGI workstation. This makes it still too slow for examining a database of small molecules.

F. Three-Dimensional Similarity Searching

The similarity between two molecules has traditionally been compared by examination of their atom type and connectivity information. The 2D screens used in chemical database programs typically encode the presence of bonded fragments. Similarity can be calculated on the basis of screens in common between two molecules. Similarity in three dimensions can be approached in the same fashion, for which the focus is on specific atoms and distances between them, but it can also be thought of in a whole-molecule sense in which properties, such as shape, volume, electrostatics, and other molecular properties, are compared. Research is on-going using both approaches. To be useful, any similarity measure must be efficient to calculate and should classify molecules with similar biological activity as similar.

Several groups have used the size of the 3D maximum common substructure (MCS) of two compounds as a measure of their similarity [51–53]. The 3D-MCS is analogous to the 2D-MCS. The nodes of the graph are atom centers in both cases, and the edges of the graph are the interatomic distances for the 3D version, as opposed to the bonds in the 2D version. The calculation of the MCS for two molecules is quite time-consuming, but the use of an upperbound screen can speed things considerably [54]. To be useful in database searching, a 3D similarity measure needs to be effective at identifying molecules that possess similar properties and is efficient to calculate.

Molecules can also be compared based on properties of the molecule as a whole. Such a procedure requires a method for finding the optimal orientation of two molecules based on the property of interest. Van Geerestein et al. [55] have developed a program called SPERM. SPERM provides a means for mapping a molecular property (e.g., electrostatic potential) onto 32 points distributed on a sphere. The points are 12 vertices of an icosahedron and the 20 vertices of a dodecahedron, oriented such that the vertices of the dodecahedron are centered on the icosahedral faces. Once this is done, molecules can be compared by superimposing their centers of mass and testing the various orientations of their vertices for the best match of the properties. This corresponds to rotating one molecule relative to the other. Searches over 30,000 molecules were carried out in 24 h on a VAX 3100 model 76.

V. APPLICATIONS

A. Pharmacophore Searching

Human Immunodeficiency Virus Protease Inhibitors

The wealth of structural information about HIV-1 protease and its inhibitors has made this a fruitful area for the use of 3D database searching. Bures et al. [56] used a pharmacophore derived from examination of several HIV protease/inhibitor crystal structures as the basis of a 3D database search. Their pharmacophore included a hydroxyl to interact with the active site aspartates, a hydrogen bond acceptor to interact with the backbone NHs of I50 and I50′ from the flaps and center of a phenyl ring to occupy the S1 subsite (Fig. 1a). This pharmacophore was used in an Aladdin search over a database of compounds from the Abbott corporate database, the Fine Chemicals Directory (currently known as the Available Chemicals Database [3]) and the MedChem Database [57]. A total of 686 molecules met the pharmacophore criterion. These compounds were then evaluated by overlaying the pharmacophore elements with the HIV protease/A-74707 crystal structure [58]. Any molecules that collided with the S1 or S1′ subsites were removed from consideration. Thirty molecules were selected for evaluation as HIV protease inhibitors. Three compounds had IC_{50} between 10 and 100 μM. All three were related benzophenones and the most active ($IC_{50} = 11$ μM) is shown in Figure 1b.

Lam et al. [59] used MDL's MACCS-3D to search the Cambridge Crystallographic Database [2,33] for potential inhibitors of HIV protease. Their pharmacophore consisted of two hydrophobic groups to occupy the S1 and S1′ pockets of the enzyme and a hydrogen bond donor–acceptor to interact with the active site aspartates (Fig. 2a). One of their hits contained not only these features, but also an oxygen that could replace a conserved water molecule (see Fig. 2b). Modification of this interesting hit to better match the requirements of the binding site led to a series of cyclic seven-membered ureas (see Fig. 2c) that were synthesized and tested. These molecules are quite active in the low nanomolar range and are orally bioavailable. The identification of molecules with the expected activity proves the usefulness of database search methods, but, from a theoretical

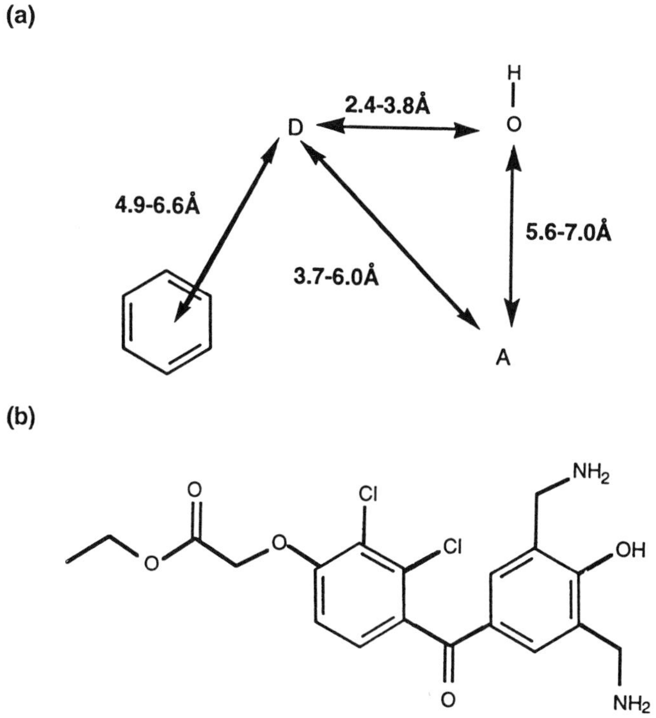

(a)

(b)

Figure 1 (a) The HIV-1 protease pharmacophore used by Bures et al. to search the Abbott corporate database; (b) the most active molecule found in the search (IC_{50} = 11 μM) [56].

point of view, one would like to know whether the molecules are active because of the features used in the search. In this example, the design implies a particular-binding mode in the HIV-1 protease active site. The crystal structure of the naphthyl derivative (see Fig. 2c) shows that the molecule does bind as expected, with the phenyl rings occupying the S1 and S1′ pockets, the naphthyl rings occupying the S2 and S2′ pockets, the OH groups interacting with the active site aspartates, and the urea carbonyl group interacting with the flaps [59].

Auxin Transport Inhibitors

Inhibitors for transport of the plant hormone auxin are potentially interesting as herbicides. These molecules bind to a site on the plant membrane that has an affinity for the herbicide N-1-naphthylphthalamic acid (NPA).

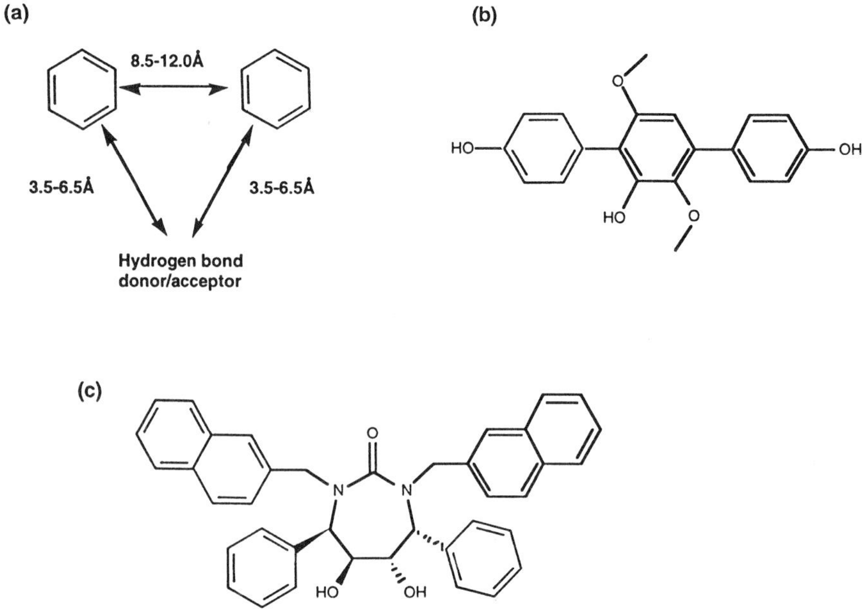

(a)

(b)

(c)

Figure 2 HIV-1 protease pharmacophore used by Lam et al. to search the CSD with MACCS-3D; (b) molecule retrieved by search of CSD; (c) most active derivative ($K_i = 2.14$ nM) achieved after several modifications based on modeling [59].

A pharmacophore was proposed after analysis of several known auxin transport inhibitors [60]. This three-point pharmacophore includes an acidic functionality, a sterically bulky group (which can be aromatic), connected to an aromatic system. Three different searches using slightly different representations of this pharmacophore were conducted using the Aladdin software. These searches retrieved 467 compounds from the Abbott corporate database, of which 77 were screened for inhibition of NPA binding. Of these, 19 had some inhibitory activity [60].

Protein Kinase C Inhibitors

Three-dimensional pharmacophore searching has been successfully applied to the discovery of molecules that bind to protein kinase C (PKC) [61]. The pharmacophore was derived from the structure of phorbol dibutyrate, a compound known to activate PKC. Features included in the search are illustrated in Figure 3a. Because of the relatively rigid ring structure, the distances were tightly constrained. ChemDBS-3D was used to search the NCI3D database [6,8]. Of the 206,876 compounds searched, 535 com-

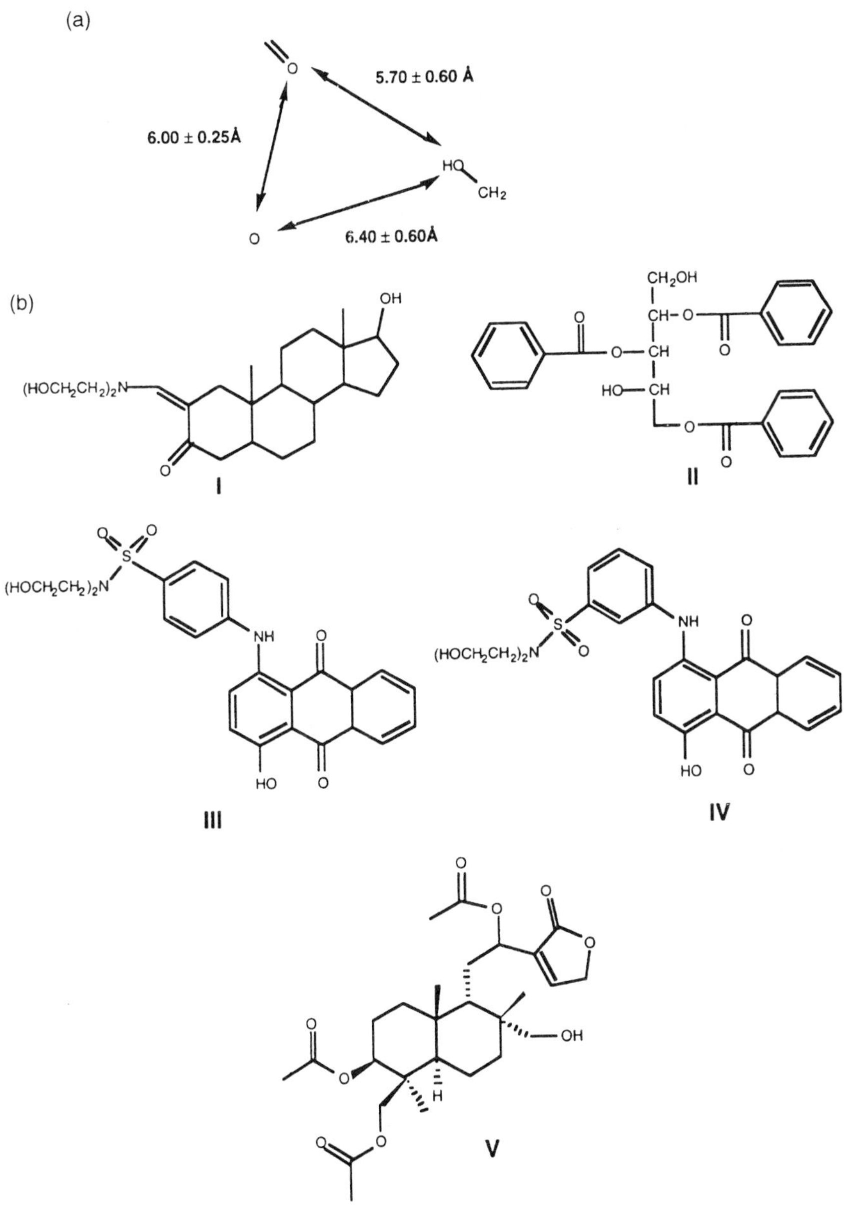

Figure 3 (a) Protein kinase C pharmacophore derived from phorbol dibutyrate and used by Wang, et al. to search the NCI-3D database with CHEM-X; (b) five active compounds from the NCI-3D search. All compounds have K_i of less than 40 μM, with the best compound (**III**) having a K_i of 7.8 μM [61].

pounds met the search criteria and, of these, 286 had samples. These compounds were further examined for the presence of the hydrophobic moiety considered necessary for PKC binding. A total of 125 compounds met this additional requirement and were tested for competitive PKC binding versus phorbol dibutyrate. Five compounds with K_i values less than 40 μM were found, with the best compound having a K_i of 7.8 μM (see Fig. 3b) [61]. The authors point out an important problem with the NCI3D database: many entries lack stereochemical data. When faced with no stereochemical information, the CHEM-X database-generation program arbitrarily chooses a configuration (as do most other 3D structure-generation programs). In this example, the NCI database includes some phorbol esters that do not have their stereochemistry specified and were missed in the search because the configuration chosen by CHEM-X happened to be incorrect.

B. CAVEAT

Cyclosporine Analogues

Because the conformation of cyclosporine (cyclosporin A) bound to cyclophilin differs significantly from the unbound conformation, it should be possible to design more potent cyclosporine analogues by introducing constraints that favor the bound conformation. Alberg and Schreiber [62] applied CAVEAT to this problem, and searched the Cambridge Structural Database for ring systems that could replace the dipeptide L-Ala^7-D-Ala^8 in the bound conformation. This particular region was chosen because these residues do not contact cyclophilin and can be mutated without significant loss of biological activity. The heterocycle shown in Figure 4 was identified as an appropriate replacement, and the corresponding cyclosporine ana-

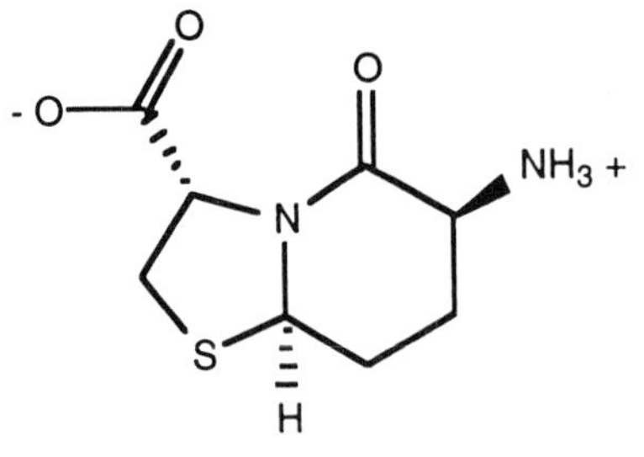

Figure 4   The heterocycle used to replace L-Ala^7-D-Ala^8 in cyclosporine (cyclosporin A) yielding an analogue with threefold greater ability to inhibit the rotamase activity of cyclophilin and two- to threefold greater activity in a number of cellular assays [62].

logue was synthesized. This analogue was threefold more potent than cyclosporine at inhibiting the rotamase activity of cyclophilin and was two-to threefold more potent in a number of cellular assays [62]. This data indicates some success in stabilizing the desired conformation.

Major Histocompatibility Complex Peptides

CAVEAT has been applied to the design of molecules to bind to major histocompatibility complex (MHC) class 1 proteins [63]. MHC proteins present peptides to the immune system. Different alleles of MHC class 1 molecules bind peptides with certain residues in common. These peptides are usually eight- to ten-residues long and the important amino acids for MHC binding occur at position 2 and the carboxy terminus. CAVEAT was used to find a cyclic system to replace the central residues, which are variable. The TRIAD database was searched using vectors derived from the $C\alpha$–N bond of the fourth residue and the $C\alpha$–carbonyl carbon bond of the seventh residue of the Flu-NP peptide bound to the MHC molecule HLA-Aw68. This search returned a number of 3,8-disubstituted tricyclic compounds. Although none of these systems were planar, molecular modeling indicated that a planar system could lead to a similar vector relation. This observation and synthetic considerations led to the choice of 3,8-diamino-6-phenylphenanthridine. When this linker is elaborated with the appropriate amino acids, the compounds bind to MHC molecules with the expected specificity, although somewhat lower affinity than the natural peptides.

C. Searches Targeting a Receptor Site

HIV-1 Protease

The first experimental test of DOCK was on the HIV-1 protease system [64]. DOCK was used to search a subset of the Cambridge Crystallographic Database [2] for molecules with a shape similar to HIV-1 protease. Molecules were examined graphically for those that had either an NH or an OH that could interact with the active site aspartates (a feature known to be important in peptide-based inhibitors of HIV-1 protease) and that could be easily obtained or synthesized. One such molecule retrieved by the search, bromperidol [molecule(**VI**), Fig. 5a], was recognized as a close analogue of haloperidol [molecule(**VII**), Fig. 5a], a compound that could be purchased. Haloperidol was tested and was a 100 μM inhibitor of HIV-1 protease. Subsequent synthesis of analogues yielded a compound with a K_i of 15 μM [see molecule(**VIII**), Fig. 5b) [65]. DOCK produces a particular binding mode for each molecule in the hit list. Crystallographic analysis was performed on a complex of HIV-1 protease and molecule(**VIII**)

(a)

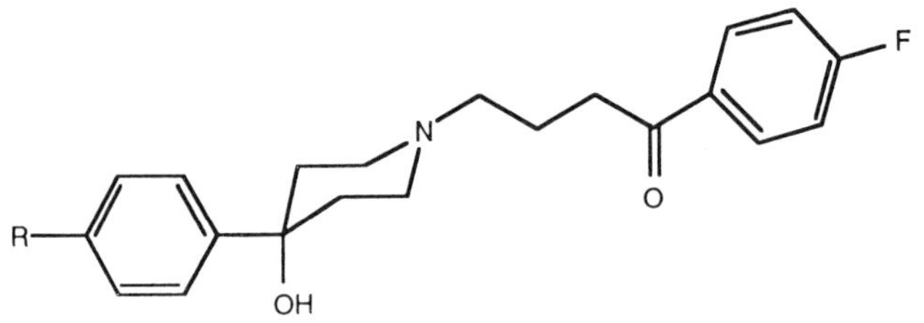

VI, R = Br
VII, R = Cl

(b)

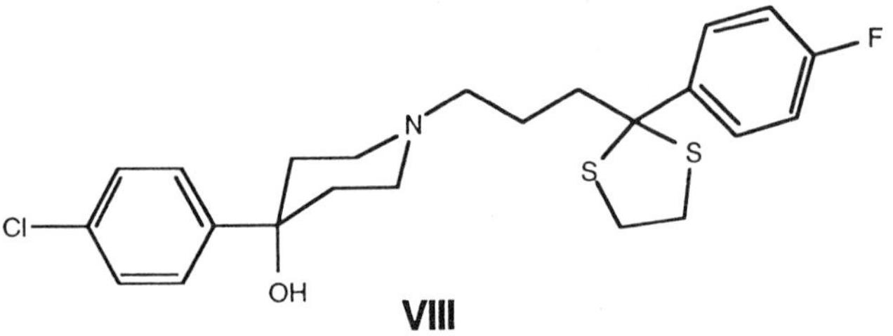

VIII

Figure 5 (a) The structure of bromperidol (**VI**, R = Br) identified in a DOCK search versus HIV-1 protease and an analogue, haloperidol (**VII**, R = Cl) [64]; (b) Thioketal derivative of haloperidol [65].

and the binding mode was quite distinct from the mode produced by DOCK and from the mode of known inhibitors [65]. The flap region of the protease was in a partially open form with molecule(**VIII**) binding under the flaps away from the active site aspartates (D25/D25'). A chloride ion binds between the inhibitor and the flaps. A second crystal structure with a mutant form of the enzyme (Q7K) complexed with molecule(**VIII**) produced a different crystal form, with the inhibitor bound in a mode very similar to that produced by DOCK, even though the site of mutation is not in contact with the inhibitor in either structure [65]. Given the crude shape-only score used in this study, it is perhaps not surprising that an inhibitor could bind in a manner different from that suggested by DOCK. The newer force-field DOCK-scoring method does improve the ability of DOCK to identify an experimental binding mode [65]. It should also be kept in mind that, with fairly weak inhibitors, there may be several binding modes that are similar in energy.

A modified version of DOCK, targeted-DOCK, was also used to discover inhibitors of HIV-1 protease [46,66]. In this example, all molecules

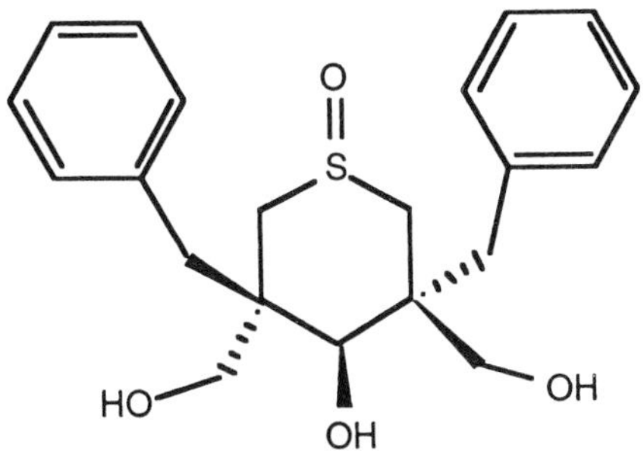

Figure 6 The structure of the cyclic sulfoxide inhibitor of HIV-1 protease (K_i = 7 μM) discovered with the aid of targeted-DOCK [46,66].

and orientations explored were forced to have oxygen or nitrogen atoms near the active site aspartates and in place of a tightly bound water molecule that bridges two inhibitor carbonyls and two backbone NHs from the flap region of the protease. This restriction severely limits the orientations explored. Targeted-DOCK was used to search the SmithKline Beecham corporate database for molecules that could place either a nitrogen or an oxygen near the aspartates and near the flaps (at the position of a conserved water molecule). This search demonstrated that a 1,4-dihydroxy six-membered ring could provide the required interaction. This was combined with hydrophobic substituents known to occupy the S1 and S1' subsites and hydrogen-bonding groups to mimic peptide amide bonds to give a series of HIV-1 protease inhibitors, with the most active having a K_i of 7 μM [66] (Fig. 6). Limited SAR supports the design hypothesis in which the phenyl rings occupy the S1 and S1' pockets, CH_2OH groups hydrogen-bond to G27/G27', the ring hydroxyl interacting with the active site aspartates (D25/D25'), and the sulfoxide oxygen interacting with the flaps [66]. Interestingly, these molecules are similar to the those designed by Lam et al. [59] from a pharmacophore search method.

Thymidylate Synthetase

The enzyme thymidylate synthetase is a target for antiproliferative and anticancer agents because of its crucial role in the synthesis of deoxythymidine monophosphate and thus the synthesis of DNA. The Fine Chemical Directory [3] was searched for molecules that would bind to the active site of thymidylate synthetase, using the program DOCK, with a score that included both sterics and electrostatics [67]. The top molecules were subsequently sorted by including a solvation correction. The DOCK search retrieved the substrate, some compounds related to known inhibitors, as

(a)   (b)

Figure 7   (a) The structure of sulisobenzone identified in a DOCK search against thymidylate synthetase; (b) the structure of phenolthymolphthalein identified in subsequent round of DOCK searching against thymidylate synthetase [67].

well as compounds not previously known to interact with the enzyme. Two crystal structures have been solved for the complex between thymidylate synthetase and sulisobenzone (Fig. 7a), one of the better novel compounds [67]. These structures both showed that, rather than being occupied by the sulfonate group, the enzyme's phosphate-binding site is occupied by an anion from the solvent. The two structures did provide insight into previously unexplored regions of the thymidylate active site, and DOCK searches of this region with compounds similar in structure to sulisobenzone retrieved molecules with higher activity; for example, phenolthymolphthalein (see Fig. 7b) with an IC_{50} of 7 μM.

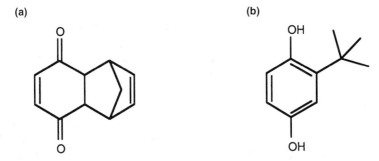

(a)   (b)

Figure 8   (a) The structure of the initial DOCK lead active in inhibition of the pH-induced conformational change of hemagglutinin; (b) the structure of an analogue of the initial lead versus hemagglutinin found by substructural searching which has antiviral activity in vitro [68].

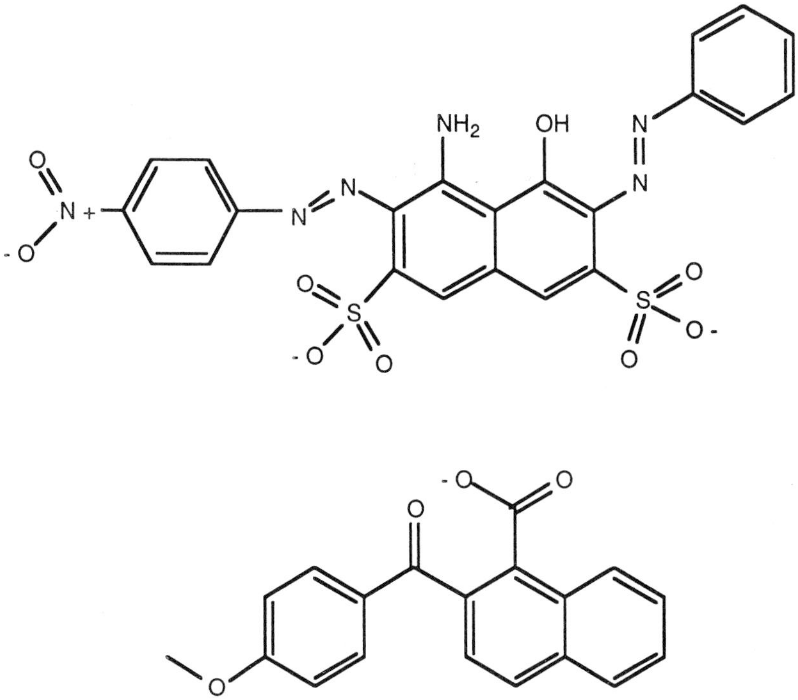

Figure 9 The structures of two molecules identified in a DOCK search against a homology model of a schistosomal protease, which is active at less than 10 μM [69].

Influenza Hemagglutinin

Entry of the influenza virus into a host cell is mediated by the viral glycoprotein hemagglutinin. Hemagglutinin undergoes a conformational change in the low-pH environment of the endosome, which results in fusion of the viral membrane with the endosomal membrane. It should be possible to prevent infection by the influenza virus with a compound that would block the hemagglutinin-mediated fusion. To identify such a compound, a DOCK search was carried out on the high-pH form of the hemagglutinin protein [68]. The site targeted by the search is not a classic binding site, but was chosen because of its proximity to the portion of the hemagglutinin protein known to be responsible for fusion. A shape-only score was used. An initial crude search was run to select the top 5000 of the approximately

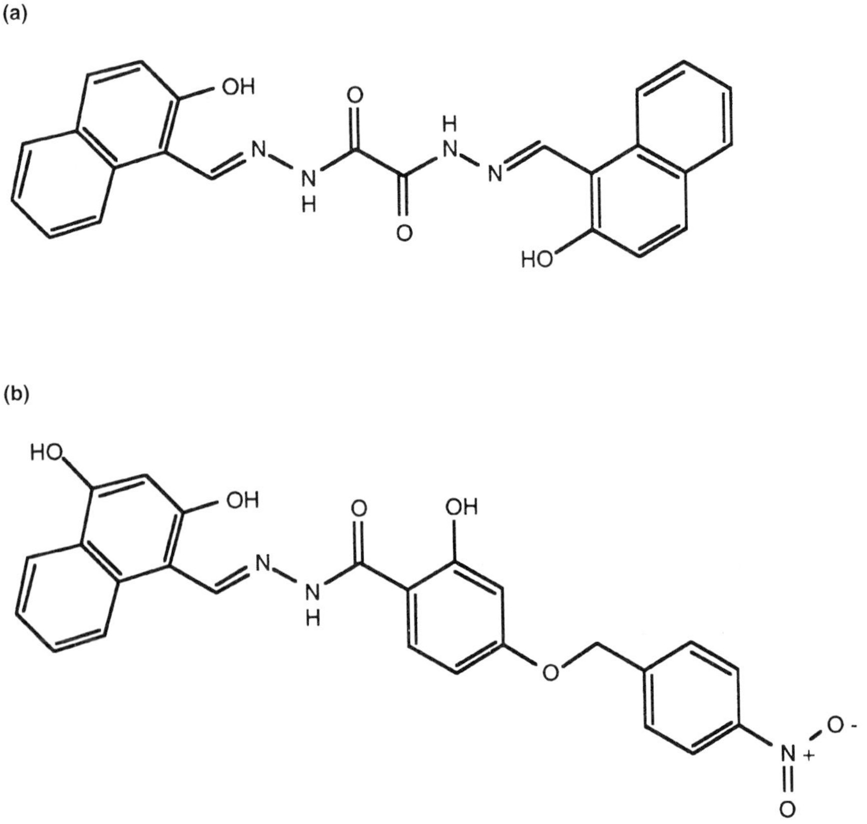

(a)

(b)

Figure 10 (a) The structure of an initial DOCK lead active in inhibiting a malarial protease (<10 μM) and in blocking parasite metabolism; (b) an analogue of the initial DOCK lead derived from examination of the DOCK binding model and active at 150 nM [70].

55,000 compounds in the Fine Chemicals Directory [3], and this subset was then used in a second DOCK calculation with a more detailed model of the proposed binding site and slightly different scoring parameters. Several hundred of the top-scoring molecules from the second DOCK run were examined graphically, and 43 molecules were selected for experimental testing. One of these compounds (Fig. 8a) inhibited the hemagglutinin conformational change reversibly and inhibited virus-mediated hemolysis [68]. This compound was too toxic for further antiviral testing, but a substructural analogue (see Fig. 8b) had similar activity in inhibiting the conformational change and showed antiviral activity in vitro [68].

Inhibitors of Parasitic Proteases

Homology models of a schistosomal serine protease and of a malarial cysteine protease were constructed using standard homology-modeling methods [69]. A DOCK search over the Available Chemicals Database [3] was performed against each of these proteases. For each protease, a set of 400 molecules were examined interactively, and the most promising were selected for testing. In each case, approximately 10% of the molecules chosen for testing were active at less than 100 μM. Two molecules were active at less than 10 μM against the schistosomal protease (Fig. 9). One molecule was active at less than 10 μM against the malarial protease (Fig. 10a). This compound was also tested for its ability to block the parasite metabolism and was active at a comparable concentration [69]. Further chemical modification around this compound was directed by the DOCK-generated binding model. This analogue design has resulted in a compound that is able to block the ability of the malaria parasites to infect or to mature in red blood cells at an IC_{50} of 150 nM [70] (see Fig. 10b). It is encouraging to note the success here, even with homology-modeled enzyme structures.

VI. DISCUSSION

Many tools, both commercial and academic, are now available to search databases of three-dimensional chemical structures. These methods fall into two general categories: 3D pharmacophore searching and searching versus a receptor site. The approaches are complementary and both have been successful in providing lead compounds with micromolar affinity. When knowledge of the receptor site is used in the discovery and design process, it is possible to check not only whether the prediction of activity is correct, but also whether the binding mode is predicted correctly. Examples of both correct- and incorrect-binding modes have been reported and, in one instance, the binding mode was influenced by the details of the crystallization. These results imply that the receptor-based methodology could be improved with better scoring functions and probably also by further conformation and orientation sampling. Occasionally, there may be several binding modes with similar energy that may be difficult to distinguish. In the absence of a receptor structure, it is more difficult to check whether a hit is interacting in a way consistent with the 3D pharmacophore hypothesis. In such situations, consistency of SAR between series may give some indication.

Most of the database search methods discussed here are designed to provide a list of hits that could be tested directly. Any of them may also provide new synthetic directions; for example, by suggesting a functional group replacement that had not been previously considered. The usefulness of a database search is to provide not only a hit list for screening, but also to provide the medicinal chemist with a variety of molecules that might inspire new synthetic directions.

ACKNOWLEDGMENTS

The author thanks Scott Dixon, Catherine Peishoff, and George Seibel for helpful comments on this manuscript.

REFERENCES

1. P. Gund, Pharmacophoric pattern searching and receptor mapping, *Ann. Rep. Med. Chem. 14*:288 (1979).
2. F. H. Allen, S. A. Bellard, M. D. Brice, B. A. Cartwright, A. Doubleday, H. Higgs, T. Hummelink, B. G. Hummelink-Peters, O. Kennard, W. D. S. Motherwell, J. R. Rodgers, and D. G. Watson, The Cambridge Crystallographic Data Centre: computer-based search, retrieval, analysis and display of information, *Acta Crystallogr. B35*:2331, (1979).
3. The Available Chemicals Database, Molecular Designs Limited Information Systems, Inc., 2132 Farallon Drive, San Leandro CA 94577.
4. Spresi Chemical Database, InfoChem GmbH, Grobenzell, Germany and Daylight Chemical Information Systems, Irvine CA.
5. The Chemical Abstracts Database, Chemical Abstracts Service, 2540 Olentangy River Rd., P.O. Box 3012, Columbus OH 43210.
6. G. W. A. Milne, J. A. Miller, et al., The NCI Drug Information System. Parts 1–6, *J. Chem. Inf. Comput. Sci. 26*:154 (1986).
7. The NCI Database in UNITY format, Tripos, Inc., 1699 S. Hanley Road, St. Louis MO 63144-2913.
8. G. W. A. Milne, M. C. Nicklaus, J. S. Driscoll, S. Want, and D. W. Zaharevitz, The NCI Drug Information System 3D database, *J. Chem. Inf. Comput. Sci 34*:1219 (1994).
9. The ACD-3D database, Molecular Designs Limited Information Systems, Inc., 2132 Farallon Drive, San Leandro CA 94577.
10. W. Fisanick, K. P. Cross, J. C. Forman, and A. Rusinko III, Experimental system for similarity and 3D searching of CAS Registry substances. 1. 3D substructure searching, *J. Chem. Inf. Comput. Sci. 33*:548 (1993).
11. A. Rusinko III, J. M. Skell, R. Balducci, C. M. McGarity, and R. S. Pearlman, CONCORD, University of Texas, Austin TX and Tripos Associates, St. Louis MO, 1988.

12. J. Gasteiger, C. Rudolph, and J. Sadowski, Automatic generation of 3D-atomic coordinates for organic molecules, *Tetrahedron Comput. Methodol.* *3*:537, (1990).

13. T. F. Havel, I. D. Kuntz, and G. M. Crippen, The theory and practice of distance geometry, *Bull. Math. Biol.* *45*:665 (1983).

14. D. Weininger, Rubicon, Daylight Chemical Information Systems, Irvine CA, 1995.

15. D. P. Dolata, A. R. Leach, and K. Prout, WIZARD: AI in conformational analysis, *J. Comput. Aided Mol. Design 1*:73 (1987).

16. A. R. Leach and K. Prout, Automated conformational analysis: directed conformational search using the A* algorithm, *J. Comput. Chem. 11*:1193 (1990).

17. W. T. Wipke and M. A. Hahn, Analogy and intelligence in model building, *Artif. Intell. Appl. Chem. 306*:136 (1986).

18. G. Klebe and T. Mietzner, A fast and efficient method to generate biologically relevant conformations, *J. Comput. Aided Mol. Design 8*:583 (1994).

19. E. V. Gordeeva, A. R. Katritzky, V. V. Shcherbukhin, and N. S. Zifirov, Rapid conversion of molecular graphs to three-dimensional representation using the MOLGEO program, *J. Chem. Inf. Comput. Sci. 33*:102 (1993).

20. G. M. Crippen, Distance geometry and conformational calculations, *Chemometrics Series* (D. Bawden, ed.), Research Studies Press (Wiley), New York, 1981.

21. J. Sadowski, J. Gasteiger, and G. Klebe, Comparison of automatic three-dimensional model builders using 639 X-ray structures, *J. Chem. Inf. Comput. Sci. 34*:1000 (1994).

22. S. K. Kearsley, D. J. Underwood, R. P. Sheridan, and M. D. Miller, Flexibases: a way to enhance the use of molecular docking methods, *J. Comput. Aided Mol. Design 8*:565 (1994).

23. A. Smellie, S. L. Teig, and P. Towbin, Poling: promoting conformational variation, *J. Comput. Chem. 16*:171 (1995).

24. E. J. Martin, J. M. Blaney, M. A. Siani, D. C. Spellmeyer, A. K. Wong, and W. H. Moos, Measuring diversity: experimental design of combinatorial libraries for drug discovery, *J. Med. Chem. 38*:1431 (1995).

25. N. E. Shemetulskis, J. B. Dunbar, Jr., B. W. Dunbar, D. W. Moreland, and C. Humblet, Enhancing the diversity of a corporate database using chemical database clustering and analysis, *J. Comput. Aided Mol. Design 9*:407 (1995).

26. S. M. Boyd, M. Beverley, L. Norskov, and R. E. Hubbard, Characterising the geometric diversity of functional groups in chemical databases, *J. Comput. Aided Mol. Design 9*:417 (1995).

27. S. E. Jakes and P. Willett, Pharmacophoric pattern matching in files of three-dimensional chemical structures: selection of interatomic distance screens, *J. Mol. Graphics 4*:12 (1986).

28. R. P. Sheridan, R. Nilakantan, A. Rusinko III, N. Bauman, K. S. Haraki, and R. Venkataraghavan, 3Dsearch: a system for three-dimensional substructure searching, *J. Chem. Inf. Comput. Sci. 29*:255 (1989).

29. J. H. Van Drie, D. Weininger, and Y. C. Martin, Aladdin: an integrated tool for computer-assisted molecular design and pharmacophore recognition from geometric, steric and substructure searching of three-dimensional molecular structures, *J. Comput. Aided Mol. Design 3*:225 (1989).

30. J. Greene, S. Kahn, H. Savoj, P. Sprague, and S. Teig, Chemical function queries for 3D database search, *J. Chem. Inf. Comput. Sci. 34*:1297 (1994).

31. P. A. Bartlett, G. T. Shea, S. J. Telfer, and S. Waterman, CAVEAT: a program to facilitate the structure-derived design of biologically active molecules, *Mol. Recog. Chem. Biol. Probl. 78*:182 (1989).

32. G. Lauri and P. A. Bartlett, CAVEAT: a program to facilitate the design of organic molecules, *J. Comput. Aided Mol. Design 8*:51 (1994).

33. F. H. Allen, J. E. Davies, J. J. Galloy, O. Johnson, O. Kennard, C. F. Macrae, E. M. Mitchell, G. F. Mitchell, J. M. Smith, and D. G. Watson, The development of versions 3 and 4 of the Cambridge Structural Database System, *J. Chem. Inf. Comput. Sci. 31*:187 (1991).

34. T. Hurst, Flexible 3D searching: the directed tweak technique, *J. Chem. Inf. Comput. Sci. 34*:190 (1994).

35. T. E. Mook, D. R. Henry, A. G. Ozkabak, and M. Alamgir, Conformational searching in ISIS/3D databases, *J. Chem. Inf. Comput. Sci. 34*:184 (1994).

36. N. W. Murrall and E. K. Davies, Conformational freedom in 3-D databases, *J. Chem. Inf. Comput. Sci. 30*:312 (1990).

37. D. E. Clark, P. Willett, and P. W. Kenny, Pharmacophoric pattern matching in files of three-dimensional chemical structures: implementation of flexible searching, *J. Mol. Graphics 11*:146 (1993).

38. D. E. Clark, G. Jones, P. Willett, P. W. Kenny, and R. C. Glen, Pharmacophoric pattern matching in files of three-dimensional chemical structures: comparison of conformational-searching algorithms for flexible searching, *J. Chem. Inf. Comput. Sci. 34*:197 (1994).

39. K. S. Haraki, R. P. Sheridan, R. Venkataraghavan, D. A. Dunn, and R. McCulloch, Looking for pharmacophores in 3-D databases: does conformational searching improve the yield of actives? *Tetrahedron Comput. Methodol. 3*:565 (1990).

40. I. D. Kuntz, J. M. Blaney, S. J. Oatley, R. Langridge, and T. E. Ferrin, A geometric approach to macromolecule–ligand interactions, *J. Mol. Biol. 161*: 269 (1982).

41. R. L. DesJarlais, R. P. Sheridan, G. L. Seibel, J. S. Dixon, I. D. Kuntz, and R. Vankataraghavan, Using shape complementarity as an initial screen in designing ligands for a receptor binding site of known three-dimensional structure, *J. Med. Chem. 31*:722 (1988).

42. B. K. Shoichet, D. L. Bodian, and I. D. Kuntz, Molecular docking using shape descriptors, *J. Comput. Chem. 13*:380 (1992).

43. E. C. Meng, B. K. Shoichet, and I. D. Kuntz, Automated docking with grid-based energy evaluation, *J. Comput. Chem. 13*:505 (1992).

44. E. C. Meng, I. D. Kuntz, D. J. Abrahan, and G. E. Kellogg, Evaluating docked complexes with the HINT exponential functional and empirical atomic hydrophobicities, *J. Comput. Aided Mol. Design 8*:299 (1994).
45. A. R. Leach and I. D. Kuntz, Conformational analysis of flexible ligands in macromolecular receptor sites, *J. Comput. Chem. 13*:730 (1992).
46. R. L. DesJarlais and J. S. Dixon, A shape- and chemistry-based docking method and its use in the design of HIV-1 protease inhibitors. *J. Comput. Aided Mol. Design 8*:231 (1994).
47. M. C. Lawrence and P. C. Davis, CLIX—a Search algorithm for finding novel ligands capable of binding proteins of known three-dimensional structure, *Proteins Struct. Funct. Genet. 12*:31 (1992).
48. S. Sudarasanam, G. D. Virca, C. J. March, and S. Srinivasan, An approach to computer-aided inhibitor design: application to cathepsin L, *J. Comput. Aided Design 6*:223 (1992).
49. R. L. DesJarlais, R. P. Sheridan, J. S. Dixon, I. D. Kuntz, and R. Venkataraghavan, Docking flexible ligands to macromolecular receptors by molecular shape, *J. Med. Chem. 29*:2149 (1986).
50. C. M. Oshiro, I. D. Kuntz, and J. S. Dixon, Flexible ligand docking using a genetic algorithm, *J. Comput. Aided Mol. Design 9*:113 (1995).
51. C. W. Crandell and D. H. Smith, Computer-assisted examination of compounds for common three-dimensional substructures, *J. Chem. Inf. Comput. Sci. 23*:186 (1983).
52. A. T. Brint and P. Willett, Identifying 3D maximal common substructures using transputer networks, *J. Mol. Graphics 5*:200 (1987).
53. A. T. Brint and P. Willett, Algorithms for the identification of three-dimensional maximal common substructures, *J. Chem. Inf. Comput. Sci. 27*: 152 (1987).
54. A. T. Brint and P. Willett, Upperbound procedures for the identification of similar three-dimensional chemical structures, *J. Comput. Aided Mol. Design 2*:311 (1988).
55. V. J. van Geerestein, N. C. Perry, P. D. J. Grootenhuis, and C. A. G. Haasnoot, 3D database searching on the basis of ligand shape using the SPERM prototype method, *Tetrahedron Comput. Methodol. 3*:595 (1990).
56. M. G. Bures, C. W. Hutchins, M. Maus, W. Kohlbrenner, S. Kadam, and J. W. Erickson, Using three-dimensional substructure searching to identify novel, non-peptidic inhibitors of HIV-1 protease, *Tetrahedron Comput. Methodol. 3*:673 (1990).
57. MedChem Database, Daylight Chemical Information Systems, Irvine CA.
58. J. Erickson, D. J. Neidhart, J. VanDrie, D. J. Kempf, X. C. Wang, D. W. Norbeck, J. J. Plattner, J. W. Rittenhouse, M. Turon, N. Wideburg, W. E. Kohlbrenner, R. Simmer, R. Helfrich, D. A. Paul, and M. Knigge, Design, activity, and 2.8 angstrom crystal structure of a C2 symmetric inhibitor complexed to HIV-1 protease, *Science 249*:527 (1990).
59. P. Y. S. Lam, P. K. Jadhav, C. J. Eyermann, C. N. Hodge, Y. Ru, L. T. Bacheler, J. L. Meek, M. J. Otto, M. M. Rayner, N. Wong, C.-H. Chang,

P. C. Weber, D. A. Jackson, T. R. Sharpe, and S. Erickson-Viitanen, Rational design of potent, bioavailable, nonpeptide cyclic ureas as HIV protease inhibitors, *Science 263*:380 (1994).

60. M. G. Bures, C. Black-Schaefer, and G. Gardner, The discovery of novel auxin transport inhibitors by molecular modeling and three-dimensional pattern analysis, *J. Comput. Aided Mol. Design 5*:323 (1991).

61. S. Wang, D. W. Zaharevitz, R. Sharma, V. E. Marquez, N. E. Lewin, L. Du, P. M. Blumberg, and G. W. A. Milne, The discovery of novel, structurally diverse protein kinase C agonists through computer 3D-database pharmacophore search. Molecular modeling studies, *J. Med. Chem. 37*:4479 (1994).

62. D. G. Alberg and S. L. Schreiber, Structure-based design of a cyclophilin–calcineurin bridging ligand, *Science 262*:248 (1993).

63. G. A. Weiss, E. J. Collins, D. N. Garboczi, D. C. Wiley, and S. L. Schreiber, A tricyclic ring system replaces the variable regions of peptides presented by three alleles of human MHC class I molecules, *Chem. Biol. 2*:401 (1995).

64. R. L. DesJarlais, G. L. Seibel, I. D. Kuntz, P. Oritiz de Montellano, P. S. Furth, J. C. Alvarez, D. L. DeCamp, L. M. Babe, and C. S. Craik, Structure-based design of non-peptide inhibitors specific for the human immunodeficiency virus-1 protease, *Proc. Natl. Acad. Sci. USA 87*:6644 (1990).

65. E. Rutenber, E. B. Fauman, R. J. Kennan, S. Fong, P. S. Furth, P. R. Ortiz de Montellano, E. Meng, I. D. Kuntz, D. L. DeCamp, R. Salto, J. R. Rose, C. S. Craik, and R. M. Stroud, Structure of a non-peptide inhibitor complexed with HIV-1 protease, *J. Biol. Chem. 268*:15343 (1993).

66. B. Chenera, R. L. DesJarlais, J. A. Finkelstein, D. S. Eggleston, T. D. Meek, T. A. Tomaszek, Jr., and G. B. Dreyer, Nonpeptide HIV protease inhibitors designed to replace a bound water, *Bioorg. Med. Chem. Lett. 3*:2717 (1993).

67. B. K. Shoichet, R. M. Stroud, D. V. Santi, I. D. Kuntz, and K. M. Perry, Structure-based discovery of inhibitors of thymidylate synthase, *Science 259*: 1445 (1993).

68. D. L. Bodian, R. B. Yamasaki, R. L. Buswell, J. F. Stearns, J. M. White, and I. D. Kuntz, Inhibition of the fusion-inducing conformational change of influenza hemagglutinin by benzoquinones and hydroquinones, *Biochemistry 32*: 2967 (1993).

69. C. S. Ring, E. Sun, J. H. McKerrow, G. K. Lee, P. J. Rosenthal, I. D. Kuntz, and F. E. Cohen, Structure-based inhibitor design by using protein models for the development of antiparasitic agents, *Proc. Natl. Acad. Sci. USA 90*:3583 (1993).

70. Z. Li, X. Chen, E. Davidson, O. Zwang, C. Mendis, C. S. Ring, W. R. Roush, G. Fegley, E. Sun, R. Li, P. J. Rosenthal, G. K. Lee, G. L. Kenyon, I. D. Kuntz, and F. E. Cohen, Anti-malarial drug development using models of enzyme structure, *Curr. Biol. 1*:31 (1994).

4

Three-Dimensional Quantitative Structure–Activity Relationship Analysis

A. J. Hopfinger
The University of Illinois at Chicago, Chicago, Illinois

John S. Tokarski
*The University of Illinois at Chicago, Chicago, Illinois, and
The Chem21 Group, Lake Forest, Illinois*

I. INTRODUCTION

Three-Dimensional Quantitative Structure–Activity Relationship (3D-QSAR) analysis is a sufficiently new area of computer-assisted molecular design (CAMD) that it lacks definition. Hence, this chapter begins with the construction of a tight definition of 3D-QSAR analysis and, in so doing, limits the types of CAMD approaches discussed. Many of the studies reported in the current comprehensive source on 3D-QSAR [1] do not fit the definition and are not included here.

Our definition of 3D-QSAR analysis composes two components arrived at by walking through the history of QSAR analysis. The first QSAR equations that took on a 3D flavor were those that included molecular property measures computed from 3D molecular modeling. In essence, the Hansch-type multiple linear regression (MLR) QSAR equations were supplemented with explicit 3D property measures. One of the first such QSARs incorporating molecular properties from explicit 3D computational chemistry methods, reported in 1974 [2], is the following:

$$\log(BA) = 11.070q_6 - 57.267q_7 - 3.447C_6^E + 31.115C_8^N + 10.456$$
$$N = 13 \qquad r = 0.967 \qquad s = 0.094 \qquad F = 28.88 \qquad (1)$$

where log(BA) is the insecticidal potency of a set $N = 13$ carbaryl derivatives for which q_6 and q_7 are the partial atomic charges on specific ring atoms, and the C_i^E and C_i^N are coefficients of the highest occupied and lowest empty molecular orbitals, respectively, for the ith atom. The q_i, C_i^E and C_i^N are taken from structure optimized CNDO/2 calculations. The correlation coefficient r, standard deviation of fit s, and significance descriptor F, are also listed.

Other statistical techniques, in addition to MLR analysis, have been used to develop functional relations between biological activity measures as dependent variables and 2D and 3D physicochemical molecular properties as independent variables. Overall, the first component in the definition of a 3D-QSAR is *an explicit computational relation relating biological activity to corresponding 2D and 3D molecular properties.* The second component to the 3D-QSAR definition is *a graphic representation of the 3D information packaged in the computational structure–activity relationship.*

Using this definition many approaches to receptor mapping and to pharmacophore design would not qualify as 3D-QSARs because explicit mathematical relationships of structure–activity are not generated, but are only graphically represented.

QSAR analysis, be it 2D or 3D, has almost exclusively been applied to structure–activity data sets for which molecular geometry of a common receptor is unknown. If the receptor geometry is known, intermolecular docking is usually performed to the exclusion of a QSAR analysis. Ligand–receptor binding modeling and QSAR analysis are almost viewed as incompatible with one another. Still, there is no reason physicochemical properties computed from ligand–receptor interaction modeling cannot be used in a 3D-QSAR. This was recognized more than 15 years ago and used to develop 3D-QSARs for anticancer anthracyclines intercalating into DNA [3]. A graphic representation of the ligand–receptor complex, and a MLR equation using the calculated binding energy as one of the independent variables, combine to satisfy our 3D-QSAR definition.

The inability to both accurately and completely compute ligand–receptor binding thermodynamics has prompted an increase in the use of QSAR techniques in intermolecular modeling. Hence, a formal distinction is made between a *receptor-independent 3D-QSAR* (RI 3D-QSAR), for which no receptor geometry is available and a *receptor-dependent 3D-QSAR* (RD 3D-QSAR), in which the receptor geometry is used in computing QSAR-independent variables.

2D-QSARs have been combined with graphic (nonthermodynamic) ligand–receptor docking [4] to demonstrate that the 2D-independent variables are consistent with plausible binding models. These are not receptor-dependent 2D-QSARs within the description of a RD 3D-QSAR given in the foregoing. The receptor geometry *is not used to compute* any independent variable in the MLR equation.

In principle, any type of dependent variable property measure, not just those within the class of biological activities, can be correlated to physicochemical features of the corresponding molecule. The label used for such a mapping is quantitative structure–property relationship (QSPR) [5]. Clearly, QSARs constitute a subset of the QSPRs. It is becoming increasingly common in the application of CAMD in materials and polymer science to develop QSPRs. QSPR equations to predict the glass transition temperature T_g, as a function of the molecular structure and properties of the polymer are particularly prevalent [5].

There also seems to be a growing interest in constructing 3D-QSPRs for properties such as $\log P$ and pk_a, which are often used as independent variables in QSARs [6a,b]. Ostensibly, these 3D-QSPRs are constructed to demonstrate a means of estimating physiochemical properties, such as pk_a, and not of biological activity.

3D-QSARs are developed for specific, highly anisotropic ligand–receptor interactions that correspond to in vitro biological assays. In the very limited applications of 3D-QSARs to in vivo data sets, the problem has usually been thought of in terms of a specific ligand–receptor interaction component (specific 3D descriptors) and a nonspecific transport, metabolism or other, component (general thermodynamic descriptors such as $\log P$). Overall, 3D-QSARs probe and extract information about a specific interaction involving the ligand, which almost always, also involves the ligand's receptor site. Thus, one useful way to compare and contrast 3D-QSAR methods is to identify what aspects of the general ligand–receptor-binding process are being considered in a particular 3D-QSAR formalism.

The binding free energy ΔG of a ligand L to a receptor R in a solvent medium M can be expressed as

$$\Delta G = G_{LR} - (G_L + G_R) = -kT \ln K \qquad (2)$$

where k is the gas constant, T is the temperature, and K is the binding constant. In terms of the applied ligand concentration C necessary to realize a particular bound concentration to a fixed quantity of R the general relation is usually valid,

$$-kT \ln K = a \log\left(\frac{1}{C}\right) + b \qquad (3)$$

or that

$$\log\left(\frac{1}{C}\right) = a'T \ln K + b' \tag{4}$$

Thus, for a fixed temperature T, $\log(1/C)$ and K are directly proportional to each other.

The free energy of the ligand–receptor complex G_{LR}, can be broken into its component terms,

$$G_{LR} = [G_{LR}(LL) + G_{LR}(RR) + G_{LR}(MM) + G_{LR}(LR)$$
$$+ G_{LR}(LM) + G_{LR}(RM)] \tag{5}$$

where $G_{LR}(XY)$ refers to the interaction between X and Y for the LR (bound, or complex) state. The variables X and Y can represnt both L, M, or R. Each of the terms in Eq. (5) can be further partitioned into enthalpy and entropy contributions. Because the work term $P\Delta V$ of binding is very small for small organic ligands binding to macromolecules at low combined solute (ligand and macromolecule) concentrations, the enthalpy terms, $H_{LR}(XY)$, can be represented by their internal energy $E_{LR}(XY)$ contributions and we have,

$$H_{LR} = E_{LR} = [E_{LR}(LL) + E_{LR}(RR) + E_{LR}(MM) + E_{LR}(LR)$$
$$+ E_{LR}(LM) + E_{LR}(RM)] \tag{6}$$

and for the entropy contributions $S_{LR}(XY)$, at some fixed temperature T,

$$S_{LR} = [S_{LR}(LL) + S_{LR}(RR) + S_{LR}(MM) + S_{LR}(LR)$$
$$+ S_{LR}(LM) + S_{LR}(RM)] \tag{7}$$

where in general

$$G_{LR} = H_{LR} - TS_{LR} \tag{8}$$

The corresponding unbound ligand G_L and receptor G_R free energies can be expressed in terms of their component XY interactions,

$$G_L = [G_L(LL) + G_L(LM) + G_L(MM)] \tag{9}$$

$$G_R = [G_R(RR) + G_R(RM) + G_R(MM)] \tag{10}$$

Each of the XY interaction free energy contributions in both Eqs. (9) and (10) can be broken down into their respective enthalpy and entropy contributions, as done for G_{LR}. Also, as done for G_{LR}, the enthalpy contributions $H_L(XY)$ and $H_R(XY)$ can be well-approximated by $E_L(XY)$ and $E_R(XY)$, respectively, for tight-binding at low L and R concentrations.

Overall, we can list the internal energy and entropy changes composing ΔG in Eq. (2) in terms of the XY interaction contributions. These contributions, and their representations, are given in Table 1 and provide a useful reference base to use in dissecting what aspects of ligand–receptor binding are considered in a particular 3D-QSAR approach.

An analysis of current 3D-QSAR approaches will reveal, perhaps not too surprisingly, that the intermolecular ligand–receptor binding interaction is the focus in developing these approaches. Solvent reorganization receives virtually no attention in any 3D-QSAR method. Entropy and the unbound states of L and R are also not considered in most 3D-QSARs. Still, emerging experimental studies of ligand–receptor binding suggest that each of the six classes of interactions in Table 1 can play a major role in the binding process, depending on the particular $LR(M)$ system [7].

II. RECEPTOR-INDEPENDENT 3D-QSAR ANALYSIS

A. Comparative Molecular Field Analysis

Introduction

To some 3D-QSAR analysis and *c*omparative *m*olecular *f*ield *a*nalysis (CoMFA) are one and the same [1,8]. CoMFA is by far the most often employed RI 3D-QSAR approach, reflecting a novel, conceptually satisfying scientific approach reduced to practice as a well-written and versatile software package. There are many reports in the literature of successful application of CoMFA that have not only led to predictive models within an analogue series of biologically active molecules [9], but also to insightful information on the general requirements for the expression of the activity.

Methodology and Implementation

One of us, AJH, remembers many stimulating discussions in the late 1970s with Dick Cramer, the inventor of the CoMFA approach, concerning how the shapes of molecules could be probed and represented, and how this data could be used to rationalize the biological behavior observed in the molecules. The conceptual frameworks of both CoMFA and molecular shape analysis (MSA; another 3D-QSAR approach described in this chapter) came partly from these discussions. A paraphrasing of Cramer's description of CoMFA is given here along with interjections on specific methodology changes, additions, and findings to the original method.

A QSAR study cannot be successful if the structural parameters do not actually relate to the differences in biological activity. A fresh approach to this question of structural parameterization was based on the combined beliefs that molecular shape somehow confers biological activity, and that ligand–receptor interaction seldom involves changes in covalent bonding.

Table 1 A Breakdown of the Interaction Terms, XY, for a $L + R \rightleftharpoons LR$ Binding Process in a Solvent Medium M at Low L and R Concentrations with the Concentration of Bound L Less Than R

Chemical unit (Z)	Type of interaction energy (XY)	Change in internal energy (symbols)	Change in entropy (symbols)
Ligand (L)	Intramolecular ligand conformational energy (LL)	$\Delta E_L(LL) = E_{LR}(LL) - E_L(LL)$	$\Delta S_L(LL) = S_{LR}(LL) - S_L(LL)$
Ligand (L)	Ligand solvation energy (LM)	$\Delta E_L(LM) = E_{LR}(LM) - E_L(LM)$	$\Delta S_L(LM) = S_{LR}(LM) - S_L(LM)$
Solvent medium (M)	Solvent reorganization energy (MM)	$\Delta E_M(MM) = E_{LR}(MM) - [E_L(MM) + E_R(MM)]$	$\Delta S_M(MM) = S_{LR}(MM) - [S_L(MM) + S_R(MM)]$
Receptor (R)	Intramolecular receptor conformational energy (RR)	$\Delta E_R(RR) = E_{LR}(RR) - E_R(RR)$	$\Delta S_R(RR) = S_{LR}(RR) - S_R(RR)$
Receptor (R)	Receptor solvation energy (RM)	$\Delta E_R(RM) = E_{LR}(RM) - E_R(RM)$	$\Delta S_R(RM) = S_{LR}(RM) - S_R(RM)$
Ligand–receptor (RL)	Intermolecular ligand–receptor energy (LR)	$\Delta E_{LR}(LR) = E_{LR}(LR)$	$\Delta S_{LR}(LR) = S_{LR}(LR)$

This philosophy is what most fundamentally distinguishes CoMFA from "classic QSAR." Quantum chemists have long been aware that potentials are an appropriate set of parameters to describe noncovalent intermolecular interactions. In pursuing CoMFA, it was believed that biological activity is especially sensitive to spatially localized differences in molecular field intensities. The concept of identifying those critical local differences by sampling field intensities on a Cartesian lattice came to Cramer immediately and naturally. However, several complications soon followed.

A major issue was the selection of force fields. It is notable that two intervening decades of intensive refinement have not yet required any nonbonded interaction fields other than electrostatic (usually coulombic) and steric (usually Lennard–Jones). These are the fields that seem to be universal in CoMFA, either directly as in the Tripos implementation, or indirectly, as in the Abbott/GRID implementation. It is likely that some form of a "hydrophobic field" will also prove quite important in CoMFA. There is also a need to develop a hydrogen-bond probe, because the combination of electrostatic and dispersion probes are not always adequate to portray ligand–receptor hydrogen-bonding. There are three major phases of CoMFA: setup, partial least-squares (PLS), and representation.

CoMFA setup. The overall CoMFA process is shown in Figure 1. The center of a CoMFA is a data table, shown in the middle of the figure. The first column was arbitrarily chosen to contain the biological activity or another experimentally determined property (the dependent variable). These are the values that can be predicted if the analysis succeeds. The remaining columns in the table are the structural parameters (the independent variables).

In CoMFA, each structural parameter column records the intensity of a particular type of interaction, at a particular point in space, with a probe atom of specified charge and steric properties for each of the compounds in the study. Thus, the cell pointed to by the arrow will record the net steric interaction energy of all the atoms in the particular molecule, aligned as shown, with a probe atom located at the lower left-hand corner of the Cartesian lattice. The electrostatic effect is also calculated and recorded in a different structural parameter column. The probe atom is then moved to another lattice intersection and the steric and electrostatic energies of interaction are recalculated and put into a different pair of columns. When all the lattice intersections have been traversed, filling out the first row of the data table, the next row of structural parameters is calculated by aligning the next compound within the lattice and repeating the probe atom traversal. When all compounds have been processed, each row of the resulting table will describe the fields exerted by a particular conformation of a molecule on any surrounding atoms.

Lattice

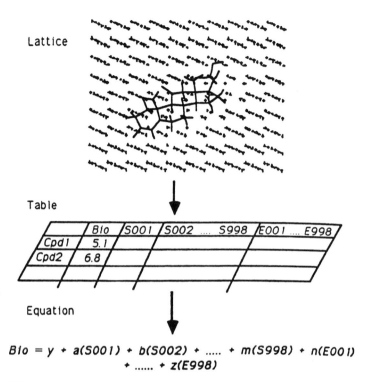

Table

Equation

$$Bio = y + a(S001) + b(S002) + \ldots + m(S998) + n(E001)$$
$$+ \ldots + z(E998)$$

Figure 1   A schematic illustration of the overall CoMFA process. (From Ref. 8.)

Partial least-squares and cross-validation in CoMFA.   A linear equation (the QSAR) is sought that relates biological activity to the intensity of the fields. The difficulty is to solve an equation having thousands of coefficients while supplying only a comparatively few biological measurements. Classic methods, such as MLR, that yield the unique solution are not applicable. CoMFA presents an enormously oversolved data set in that there are usually thousands of field measures over space to be mapped to a small number of biological measures, namely, one per compound. Partial least-squares (PLS) [10] provides an elegant filtering and weighting means of extracting the optimum solution to the oversolved data set generated by the field calculations in CoMFA.

Partial least-squares is an iterative procedure that applies two criteria to produce its solution. First, to extract a new component, the criterion is to maximize the degree of commonality between all of the structural parameter columns collectively and the experimental data. Second, in the evaluation phase of a PLS iteration, the criterion for acceptance of the principal component just generated is an improvement in the ability to predict, not to reproduce, the dependent variable.

The technique used in PLS to assess the predictive ability of a QSAR is cross-validation [11]. Cross-validation is based on the idea that the best way to assess predictive performance is to predict. When cross-validating, one pretends that one or more of the known experimental values is, in fact, unknown. The analysis being cross-validated is repeated, excluding the temporarily "unknown" compounds and then using the resulting equation to predict the experimental measurement of the omitted compound(s). The cross-validation cycle is repeated, until each compound has been excluded and predicted exactly once. The result of cross-validation is the sum of the squared prediction errors, sometimes called the predictive residual sum of squares (PRESS).

In PLS, the iterations continue until the PRESS converges. For evaluation of the overall analysis, the PRESS is commonly expressed as a cross-validated correlation coefficient r^2, or xv-r^2, value.

In CoMFA two r^2 values are encountered in addition to the xv-r^2 just discussed. The second r^2 is the classic, or conventional, r^2 and is a measure of how well a particular model reproduces or fits the input data. It is calculated in the same way as xv-r^2, except that PRESS is replaced by the sum of the squares of the differences between the least-squares fit and the experimental observations. In PLS both values are obtained, the xv-r^2 in the cross-validation step and the conventional r^2 in deriving the final best-fit model. The third r^2 value, the predictive r^2, arises after a QSAR has been used to predict the target property of structures not included in the training set.

There is one pitfall in using PLS. There is no guarantee that PLS will uncover every relation in the training set. The predictive r^2 value provides a bottom-line assessment of the analysis, including if a relevant relation has been identified by PLS.

Representation and Interpretation of a CoMFA Analysis

The goal of a QSAR study is to produce a linear equation, the QSAR itself. The thousands of terms in a CoMFA QSAR make it a particularly intractable expression for direct mathematical representation and exploration. However, as indicated in Figure 1, a CoMFA QSAR has the virtue that each numerical coefficient maps directly to a location in space. Thus, each lattice point has a QSAR coefficient. Hence, the CoMFA QSAR equation delineates volumes around lattice points for which QSAR coefficients show high associations between differences in field intensities and property values. Typically, there will be two contour levels displayed for each type of CoMFA field, highlighting the regions of greatest association: the most positive and the most negative. These contour maps are helpful in suggesting new compounds likely to have higher property values.

The CoMFA QSAR equation can also be used to predict property values, thereby providing a vehicle for ranking potential compounds for synthesis.

Some PLS equations have dominant independent variables in the components. In such situations, the dominant independent variables can be retained, while less significant independent variables are deleted, resulting in simplified corresponding MLR equations. The r^2 values of these MLR equations, provide a measure of how much "information" is lost in the simplification. If the information loss can be tolerated, the corresponding MLR equation can be explored in the same fashion as has become common for 2D-QSARs. The PLS to MLR simplification process is usually not possible for CoMFA QSAR equations. Even though only a few distinct volumes in space might define the essential mapping for the CoMFA QSAR, the number of lattice points (coefficients) needed to define the essential volume can be large.

CoMFA and Ligand–Receptor Binding

CoMFA is designed to characterize the ligand–receptor interaction (internal energy), $E_{LR}(LR)$, of Table 1. No other interaction or energy term in the ligand–receptor-binding process, as defined in Table 1, is explicitly considered in CoMFA. Moreover, CoMFA assumes the user provides (a) the "active" conformation of each ligand in the training set and (b) the relative-binding geometry (the alignment) of each ligand to the common receptor and, therefore, to one another as part of the input information for an analysis. There is no limitation in the iterative application of independent CoMFA studies on a common training set as a function of ligand conformation or relative alignment. In such an iterative process the r^2 could be optimized against conformation, alignment, or both. This approach does not appear to have been considered very frequently in training sets in which conformational flexibility or multiplicity of alignments is present. A partial attempt at optimizing against conformational flexibility is considered in the work of Nicklaus et al. [12], who developed an iterative procedure using CoMFA to identify the active conformation for a series of flexible protein–tyrosine kinase inhibitors.

From the foregoing discussion, CoMFA can be expected to perform best on sets of rigid analogues with well-defined alignment pharmacophores for which in vitro biological measures are available as independent variables. The in vitro activity requirement follows from the limitation of field-based molecular descriptors. These descriptors are designed to probe the receptor interaction. If in vivo activity is considered, and only field descriptors are used, there is likely to be questions of interpretation if any model (QSAR) is, in fact, realized.

Limitations

The alignment and active conformation problems span across all approaches to RI 3D-QSAR analysis. Hence, they are discussed where appropriate throughout this chapter, and only those issues characteristic of CoMFA are mentioned here.

Probes. Any chemical unit can be used as a field probe in a CoMFA analysis. Also, the number of field probes used to construct a 3D-QSAR is not limited. In practice, three (default) probes are usually employed: a steric probe, a positive-charge probe, and a negative-probe. The need for a hydrogen bond and "hydrophobic" probe has been recognized, and some models have been suggested [13]. Nevertheless, it is highly unlikely that any set of field probes will accurately reflect the composite field generated by the chemical units of the actual receptor. It is assumed that the selected set of field probes will at the least identify the major receptor field characteristics that differentiate the observed differences in biological activity for the training set of ligands.

There is no "recipe" for selecting the set of probes most useful in a CoMFA analysis. Rather, different sets need to be considered and evaluated in terms of the predictiveness of the resulting 3D-QSAR. Very few reported CoMFA analyses have considered how the choice of field probes impinges on the 3D-QSAR model. It is also important to remember that if nonspherically symmetric field probes, such as –OH and –COOH, are used, the orientational degrees of freedom must be explored for each translational state (grid point) considered.

Grid size. There are at least two considerations that arise under the heading of grid size. The first consideration is the resolution of the grid (i.e., the size of the cells). Current CoMFA studies seldom use grid resolutions less than 1 Å and, most often, 2 Å. The choice of grid resolution represents a compromise between computational practicality and detailing of the fields. If the grid resolution is too small, the number of field-points (cells) becomes too large to perform a timely analysis. Moreover, spatial information on field preference can be lost, through a "smearing-out" effect, if the cells become too small. Nevertheless, it should be kept in mind that grid cell resolution in the 1 to 2 Å range corresponds to, at best, differentiating single carbon–carbon bonds (1.54 Å) from one another.

One consequence of using relatively large grid resolutions is that different grid-based field representations will be generated as a function of the absolute spatial alignment. Cho and Tropsha noted this behavior in CoMFA analyses of three data sets [14]. These workers suggest that if the grid resolution is held fixed, the CoMFA analysis should be carried out as a function of absolute spatial alignment (alignment relative to the grid axes) to determine how sensitive the resultant 3D-QSAR models are to spatial alignment.

An alternative, and perhaps more general diagnostic evaluation of a CoMFA analysis, would be to explore the 3D-QSAR model as a function of grid resolution. The dependence of 3D-QSAR models on grid cell resolution does not appear to have been considered in most CoMFA studies.

Electrostatic potential function. The commercial version of CoMFA uses a $(\varepsilon r)^{-1}$ distance-dependent coulomb potential to evaluate electrostatic fields, where r is the probe–ligand atom distance and ε is the molecular dielectric. In the large majority of applications ε is set to the default value of unity. This form of the electrostatic probe potential function controls the magnitude of the field of a probe in space. Consequently, this function also controls the relative importance of the probe field potential to the fields of all other probes and, ultimately, the role of the field probe in the resultant 3D-QSAR.

It is highly unlikely that the electrostatic field in an anisotropic receptor site will orthotropically obey an $(r)^{-1}$ behavior. The electrostatic interaction behavior of atom-pair interactions of a solute in water (a polar environment much less complex than a receptor site) is better represented by a distance-dependent molecular dielectric, $\varepsilon = ar + b$, as first suggested by Hopfinger [15] and later used by Kollman et al. [16], than by $\varepsilon = 1$ (or any fixed scalar). Once again, little is reported in the literature concerning how different representations of the electrostatic field potential function might influence the resultant 3D-QSAR.

B. Molecular Shape Analysis

Introduction

A formalism that deals with the quantitative characterization, representation, and manipulation of molecular shape in the construction of a QSAR is *molecular shape analysis* (MSA) [17]. The derivation and application of MSA dates back to the late 1970s, when Hopfinger began to incorporate information from conformational energy calculations into QSARs [17]. In essence, there was an attempt to "marry" conformational analysis to Hansch analysis [18]. The common overlap steric volume (COSV) between a pair of superimposed molecules can be used as a global measure of molecular shape similarity in constructing QSARs [17,19–27]. Subsequently, the spatially integrated potential energy field was shown to be a complementary extension of COSV as a general QSAR shape descriptor [28,29].

In general, spatial similarity is often apparent for congeneric series that have limited flexibility. However, it can be difficult to see and determine molecular spatial similarity when the molecules in a series are flexible. One must consider the flexibility and associated internal energetics, the $\Delta E_L(LL)$ and $\Delta E_L(LM)$ of Table 1, of a molecule to properly define its complete molecular-shape profile. As a complication in considering the biologically relevant shape of a molecule, the intermolecular energetics on binding to a receptor, the $\Delta E_{LR}(LR)$ of Table 1, may stabilize conformations that are not the lowest-energy state in either vacuum or solution. Concerns about how to treat a series of flexible molecules impinge on drug design efforts to develop quantitative SAR models for activity.

Overall, the goals of MSA are (a) to identify the biologically relevant conformation without knowledge of the receptor geometry; then (b) in a quantitative fashion explain the activity of a series of analogues using only the structure–activity table.

Basic Operations of MSA

There are seven operations involved in the MSA formalism. The seven operations are listed in Figure 2 and are briefly described elsewhere [30,31].

Basic Operations to Investigate an SAR

1. Conformational Analysis

2. Hypothesize an "Active" Conformation

3. Select a Candidate Shape Reference Compound

4. Perform Pair-Wise Molecular Superpositions

5. Measure Molecular Shape

6. Determine Other Molecular Features

7. Construct a Trial QSAR

Use the Optimized QSAR for Ligand Design

Figure 2 The seven operations of MSA. (From Ref. 29.)

The final selection of the requirements for each operation (e.g., choice of the shape reference structure) is based on optimizing the 3D-QSAR in terms of its statistical significance. That is, the set of choices available for each operation is employed to generate trial 3D-QSARs. The 3D-QSAR that corresponds to the best-fit between observed activities and computed molecular features defines the specific requirements for each MSA operation.

Conformational analysis. The first operation in MSA is the conformational analysis of each of the compounds being investigated. A variety of approaches to perform conformational analyses have recently been reviewed [32a,b]. Development of unique strategies of conformational analysis employing sequential free and fixed valence geometry calculations to simultaneously optimize efficiency and reliability have been made. These strategies have been discussed previously [17,21,26,33].

The "active" conformation. The *active conformation* of a ligand is generally understood to be that ligand conformer state realized when the ligand is bound to the receptor. However, the active conformation, similar to any key physicochemical property of a bioactive compound in a QSAR, corresponds to the conformer state involved in the rate-limiting step controlling biological action. Most often this step is ligand–receptor binding, but might also be, for example, metabolic activation–deactivation, membrane transport, or generation of a transition state.

Because the MSA formalism is a RI-3D-QSAR technique, all information gleaned about the active conformation must come from the observed biological activities and corresponding intramolecular conformational properties computed for the ligands. The specification of an active ligand conformation permits a corresponding estimate of the change in intramolecular ligand energy on binding, $\Delta E_L(LL) = E_{LR}(LL) - E_L(LL)$ of Table 1. The $\Delta E_L(LL)$ can be used as a molecular feature in the construction of a 3D-QSAR.

The most successful strategy for identifying the active conformation of a set of ligand analogues, especially in vitro enzyme inhibitors, is the loss in biological activity–loss in conformational stability (LBA–LCS) model. The goal in the LBA–LCS model is to determine a low-energy (minimum) conformational state, common to active compounds, that is a high-energy, unstable state for inactive compounds. The premise implicitly made is that the loss in activity for the inactive analogues is a result of not being able to adopt the "active" conformation energetically available to the active compounds. Recently, Hopfinger and co-workers have developed a tensor-based representation of the general QSPR problem [34]. The general equation for a MSA 3D-QSPR relation is

Absolute

$$P_u = T_u \otimes [V_u(s,\alpha,B),F_u(p,r_{i,j,k},f,\alpha,B),H_u(h_p,\alpha,B),E_u(e_p,\alpha,B)] \tag{11}$$

Relative

$$P_{u,v} = T_{u,v} \otimes [V_{u,v}(s,\alpha,B),F_{u,v}(p,r_{i,j,k},f,\alpha,B),$$
$$H_{u,v}(h_p,\alpha,B),E_{u,v}(e_p,\alpha,B)] \tag{12}$$

where "Absolute" refers to models in which no reference state (structure) is used and "Relative" defines models based on some relative standard state, v. P is the dependent variable (activity) matrix, V, F, H, and E are four tensors which, respectively, incorporate the following information:

[V]: Intrinsic molecular shape (IMS) features that are usually highly dependent on conformation. The IMS features provide information on molecular shape within the steric contact surface of the molecule.

[F]: Molecular field (MF) features that are also highly dependent on conformation. The MF features provide information on molecular shape beyond the steric contact surface.

[H]: The remaining set of physicochemical features that are computed, such as lipophilicity, aqueous solubility, conformational entropy, and so forth, that may, or may not, exhibit dependence on conformation.

[E]: The set of experimental physicochemical features that have been measured for the compounds of interest. These features may, or may not, exhibit conformational dependence. Moreover, any conformational dependence may be realized only as a Boltzmann average for the feature, owing to the nature of the experimental measurement. Importantly one or more of these measured properties may, in fact, be used as the dependent variable endpoints in the construction of the QSPR.

Table 2 contains a set of definitions to facilitate the formulation of the MSA 3D-QSPR problem for a set of molecules, $\{M_u\}$. The quantity in brackets in Eqs. (11) and (12) is referred to as the **VFHE** composite tensor. A schematic illustration of Eq. (11) for which $E_{u,v}(e_p,\alpha,B)$ is "zero" is shown in Figure 3. In Eqs. (11) and (12) the T_u and $T_{u,v}$ are the transformation tensors that optimally map the **VFHE** tensor onto P_u and $P_{u,v}$, respectively. The determination of the transformation tensor is obviously the

Table 2 Definitions of Molecular Features and Entities Used to Construct the General MSA 3D-QSPR Formalism

Symbol	Definitions
u	Any compound in the trianing set, $\{M_u\}$
v	A reference compound
α	The set of conformations for the training set
β	The alignments for the training set
s	The set of intrinsic molecular shape features
p	The set of field probes
$r_{i,j,k}$	The spatial postitions at which the molecular field is evaluated
h_p	The set of nonmolecular shape and nonmolecular field features
e_p	The set of experimental measures
f	Field-related molecular features not derived from the p

Source: Ref. 34.

rate-limiting step in the practical application of the MSA 3D-QSPR tensor formalism. There are probably multiple ways of determining the transformation tensors, and one approach is given [34,35] and is applied to develop MSA 3D-QSARs for an analogue series of pyridobenzodiazepine inhibitors of muscarinic M_2 and M_3 receptors [35].

One useful feature of the MSA 3D-QSPR tensor formalism is that it overcomes the multiple alignment and active conformation problems by allowing as many trial choices as the user wishes. In the same spirit, the user can employ as many descriptors as wanted in the **VFHE** tensor. In the muscarinic 2 and 3 receptor inhibition study [35], as many as 359 conformations were considered for one of the 19 compounds in the training set, as three distinct alignments and 37 molecular descriptors were evaluated in the MSA 3D-QSAR tensor representation. For both the M_2 and M_3 receptor SAR, only two very similar 3D–QSARs were significant. Thus, the method was successful in making definitive conformational and alignment assignments as part of the 3D–QSAR model.

The shape reference structure. The current approach to identify the shape reference structure is to first place each compound in the data set in a possible active conformation. The selection of the possible active conformation is based on the information realized from one of the foregoing strategies for postulating active conformations. Each compound in each possible active conformation can be evaluated as the shape reference structure. The criterion for selecting the shape reference structure is to optimize the statistical significance of the corresponding 3D-QSAR. Another recent advancement in, and generalization of, MSA has been the construction of

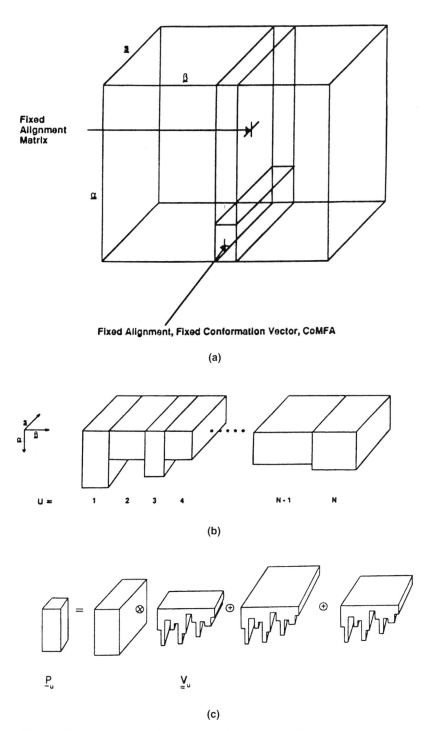

Figure 3 (a) A schematic representation of the IMS tensor for a single compound; (b) the complete IMS tensor for a set of N compounds presented in schematic form; (c) a schematic illustration of Eq. (11) in which the $\boldsymbol{E}_u$ tensor is zero. (From Ref. 34.)

candidate shape references from two, or more compounds, within, or outside, the training set [36]. These "mutant" shapes are generated by the common and difference volume combinations realized by multiple compound alignments or conformations. An example of a mutant reference shape generated in an MSA 3D-QSAR analysis of multiple analogue series of cholecystokinin A receptor antagonists is shown in Figure 4.

Molecular superposition (alignment). MSA requires that each compound in the data set, in each candidate active conformation, be compared with the shape reference. Such a comparison necessitates a pairwise molecular superposition, or alignment. The key is how to perform the alignment. The measure of molecular shape similarity is interdependent of the molecular alignment. Several pairwise molecular alignment criteria have been identified and used in applications [30,31]. The simultaneous evaluation of multiple alignments is intrinsic to the tensor representation of the general MSA 3D-QSAR [34] as described earlier.

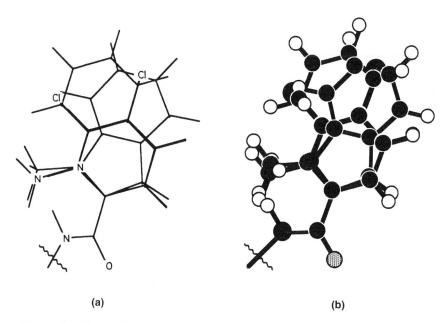

(a)   (b)

Figure 4 Shape reference "mutant" composed of the union of the van der Waals volume of the aligned and overlapped structures of four compounds in the training set. (a) stick; (b) ball and stick; and (c) space-fill representations of the mutant are shown. A common substructure to all four compounds is not shown. (From Ref. 36.)

Molecular shape measures. Several molecular shape similarity measures, $M(u,v)$, (u, test compound; v, reference) have been and are being proposed and explored. It is not meaningful to try to rank these $M(u,v)$ in terms of how "good" each is in general application. Rather, it appears that different $M(u,v)$ are application specific in terms of quality as a 3D-QSAR descriptor. Also, the $M(u,v)$ given here are far from a complete set.

Atom–pair-matching function

$$M_r(u,v) = \Sigma_i \, K_i r_{u,v}(i) \tag{13}$$

where the K_i are the user-selected "force constants" that provide the relative weight (importance) to minimizing the distance, $r_{u,v}(i)$, between the ith atom pair from u and v. Clearly, as $M_r(u,v) \rightarrow 0$, the alignment between u and v becomes better.

Atom–pair charge-matching function

$$M_c(u,v) = \Sigma_i \left(\frac{Q_u(i)Q_v(i)}{Q_T} \right) r_{u,v}(i) \tag{14}$$

$$\text{where } Q_T = \Sigma_i \, Q_u(i)Q_v(i) \tag{15}$$

is the product of the partial charges summed over all the atom pairs from u and v that are to be matched. The term $(Q_u(i)Q_v(i)/Q_T)$ takes the place of K_i in Eq. (13) and assumes the relative weighting factor for charge matching of atom pairs is proportional to the magnitudes of the charges of the atom pair. $Q_u(i)$ and $Q_v(i)$ are assumed to always have the same sign,

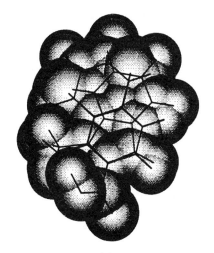

(c)

or they would not be matched. An investigator can modify the representation of the charge weighting term in Eq. (14) in any manner deemed appropriate.

Common overlap steric volume (COSV)

$$M_o(u,v) = V_u \cap V_v \tag{16}$$

where $V_u \cap V_v$ is the common overlap steric volume between the steric volumes of u, V_u, and the compound v, V_v. A complementary shape measure is the nonoverlap steric volume; that is the steric volume not shared by the molecules u and v.

Integrated spatial difference in field potential (ISDFP)

$$M_P(u,v) = (1/\Phi)[\int_\Phi [P_v(R,\Theta,\phi) - P_u(R,\Theta,\phi)]^2 d\Phi]^{1/2} \tag{17}$$

where $P_w(R,\Theta,\phi)$ is the potential field owing to compound w, as measured by probe p, at spherical coordinate postition (R,Θ,ϕ). Φ is the integraton volume considered in determining $M_p(u,v)$.

Weighted combination of COSV and ISDFP. The ISDFP and COSV are complementary in that overlap volume measures shape within the van der Waals surface formed by superposition of u and v, whereas ISDFP measures shape outside the van der Waals surface. Thus, it is useful to combine these two measures of shape similarity.

$$M_w(u,v) = \lambda[M_o(u,v)] + (1 - \lambda)M_p(u,v) \tag{18}$$

where λ is a weighting factor between the COSV and the ISDFP functions that is selected, as usual, to optimize the QSAR.

Time average COSV. The NMR studies of bound high-affinity ligands to receptor macromolecules indicate that the ligands can display considerable conformational freedom when bound [37]. Hence, a description of the active shape of a ligand may require a time-dependent component. One time-dependent molecular shape property is the time–average COSV defined as:

$$M_t(u,v) = (N)^{-1} \Sigma_i^N V_u(t_i) \cap V_v(t_i) \tag{19}$$

where $V_u(t_i)$ and $V_v(t_i)$ are the steric volumes of u and v at time t_i, and N is the number of time steps considered in a molecular dynamics (MD) trajectory of time length T. u and v are prohibited from straying away from their initial molecular alignment over time.

If the $M_t(u,v)$ values are subpartitioned over an (x, y, z)-grid, then a time-dependent MSA 3D-QSAR, which we also refer to as a 4D-QSAR, can be performed in a manner analogous to CoMFA. The individual grid cell $M_t(u,v)$ values, $[M_t(u,v)]_{x,y,z}$, replace the grid cell probe energies in the PLS data reduction.

An application of time-dependent MSA 3D-QSAR using $[M_t(u,v)]_{x,y,z}$ shape descriptors was performed for a set of 20 benzylpyrimidine inhibitors of dihydrofolate reductase [38]. A very significant MSA 3D-QSAR was found with the following statistical measures of fit, $N = 20$, $r^2 = 0.968$, and $xv–r^2 = 0.823$. The independent variables in the 3D-QSAR are the COSVs of a selected number of individual grid cells.

Figure 5 shows (a) the time-average probability of grid cell occupancy, $\langle P(v) \rangle_t$, for an active analogue, (b) the $\langle P(u) \rangle_t$ of an inactive analogue, and (c) the $M_t(u,v)$ for these two analogues. The grid cell index (x,y,z) is mapped onto the single scalar index, m^*, to permit a 2D representation. Figure 5c demonstrates that these two compounds each occupy different, as well as common, grid cells over time, with distinct probability of occupancy frequencies.

Combining $M(u,v)$ and $\Delta E_L(LL)$. Molecular-shape measures can be combined with $\Delta E_L(LL)$ outside a 3D-QSAR to define a distinct class of molecular-shape measures called the molecular commonality indices, $I_c(u,v,w)$,

$$I_c(u,v,w) = f_o[M(u,v)] - w\Delta E_u \tag{20}$$

where $\Delta e_u = \Delta E_L(LL)$ and w is either a user-selected weighting factor, or allowed to be determined in the 3D-QSAR-fitting process.

Determine other molecular features. Any property derived from the structure of a compound can be used as a nonshape feature in trial MSA 3D-QSARs. The descriptors of Hansch analysis, such as π, E_s, and σ [18], probably come first to mind. Reviews are available on nonshape molecular descriptors and the reader should consult these works [39,40]. Experience in developing MSA 3D-QSARs has led to beginning the analyses by selecting some thermodynamic descriptors and a few electronic descriptors, in conjunction with the COSV or other molecular shape measures. Such initial MSA 3D-QSARs contain thermodynamic, electronic, and molecular shape representations as activity correlates. These three general molecular property classes constitute the universe of possible sources of features that can govern biological activity. The remaining goal is identifying specific descriptors from the three classes that are unique to the data set being investigated.

Construction of trial MSA 3D–QSARs. The most often employed method to establish an MSA 3D-QSAR is MLR. However, other statistical methods can be used, and the reader is again referred to other reviews [41,42]. A unique aspect to MSA in generating a 3D-QSAR is that not only are all combinations of molecular descriptors sets considered in optimizing the statistical significance of the QSAR, but also the QSAR is optimized relative to steps 2–6 (see Fig. 2) of the MSA process. That is,

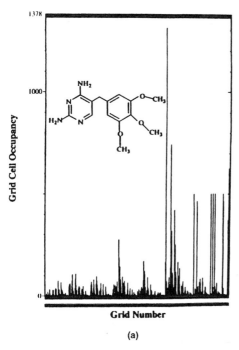

Grid Cell Occupancy

1.378

1000

0

Grid Number

(a)

Figure 5 The one-dimensional, m^*, plots of time-average grid cell occupancy: (a) an active analogue; (b) an inactive analogue; (c) the difference in cell occupancy, $M_t(u,v)$, for the active and inactive analogues. (From Ref. 38.)

the investigator cycles through steps 2–5 to optimize the molecular shape similarity or commonality contributions to the QSAR, and then mixes the shape terms with other descriptors in step 6 (see Fig. 2) to complete the statistical significance optimization process.

The evolutionary and feedback nature of the MSA formalism is ideal for the application of genetic algorithms (GA) [43] to optimize the 3D-QSARs. The genetic functions approximation (GFA), developed by Rogers [44], has been applied to some MSA 3D-QSAR problems with considerable success [45].

Representation and Interpretation of an MSA Analysis

A 3D-QSAR equation, or a set of equations, involving one or more molecular shape measures as independent variables, is available for the quantitative evaluation of the biological activity from a MSA. The molecular shape terms and, therefore, the 3D-QSAR equations, are measured relative to the reference structure of the MSA.

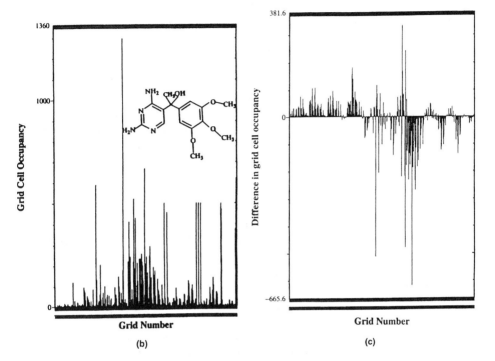

(b)

(c)

The graphic representation of an MSA is usually a picture of the most active compound in the training data set placed in the active conformation. Additional graphic representations can include the superposition of the 3D-QSAR descriptors, such as dipole moment, onto the molecular geometry of an analogue, alignment of one or more analogues onto the shape reference structure or most active analogue, or display of portions of one or more analogues to delineate the spatial nature of substructure 3D-QSAR features (regions of hydrophobicity, for example). Overall, once a significant MSA 3D-QSAR equation is realized, the investigator also knows the active molecular shape, alignment, and shape reference structure. The investigator can then package and graphically display this information.

C. 3D-QSARs from Molecular Similarity Matrices

Introduction

Richards and co-workers [46] have developed a 3D-QSAR approach based on comparing each molecule in a training set with every other. This is in contrast with the conventional working "rule" of relating activity of some test compound to its similarity to a *single* lead molecule. If there are N compounds in the training set being investigated, then a full pairwise compound shape similarity comparison leads to an N by N matrix in which each matrix entry is a measure of shape similarity between the corresponding pair of molecules.

Analysis of the full matrix implicitly introduces some of the location dependence of the steric and electrostatic parameters used within CoMFA methodology and has given excellent correlation with binding data for a steroid data set originally used in the evaluation and testing of CoMFA [46]. Good et al. [47] have extended the application of molecular similarity matrices to generate 3D-QSARs for other training sets and to explore different measures of shape similarity.

Methodology and Implementation

This approach, similar to CoMFA, assumes that the alignments and conformations used in an analysis are the "correct" ones. Conformational searching is not part of the procedure in the generation of structural properties of the similarity matrices. Presumably, different conformations could be tested by seeing which produces the best 3D-QSAR, as expressed from the similarity matrices.

The following indices have been used in the construction of the similarity matrices.

Carbo index. One of the most widely used expressions for the calculation of molecular similarity is the Carbo index [48,49]

$$R_{AB} = \frac{\int P_A P_B dv}{(\int P_A^2 dv)^{1/2}(\int P_B^2 dv)^{1/2}} \tag{21}$$

Molecular similarity R_{AB} is determined from the structural properties P_A and P_B of the two molecules being compared. The numerator measures property overlap, whereas the denominator normalizes the similarity result. As originally applied, electron density was used as the structural property P. More recently, electrostatic potential, electric field, and shape have been determined by application of modified versions of the ASP program [50].

Electrostatic potential for this and all other indices is evaluated at the intersections of a rectilinear grid constructed around the two molecules using point charge data. To avoid singularities at the atomic nuclei (where $1/r$ tends to infinity), evaluation is restricted to points outside the van der Waals volume of the molecules in the calculation. The resulting electrostatic values are then used to evaluate the indices numerically.

Meyer shape index. Meyer has proposed [51] a modified form of the Carbo equation to estimate molecular shape similarity. Similarity evaluations are the same as those applied to electrostatic potential and electric field calculations. For shape, every grid point is tested to see whether it falls inside the van der Waals surface of each molecule. The results are then applied to the following modified version of the Carbo index:

$$S_{AB} = \frac{B}{(T_A T_B)^{1/2}} \tag{22}$$

where B is the number of grid points falling inside both molecules, while T_A and T_B are the total number of grid points falling inside each individual molecule.

Hodgkin index. The Carbo index is sensitive to the shape of a property's distribution, rather than to its magnitude. To increase the sensitivity of the formula to a property's magnitude, the Hodgkin index [52] has been developed.

$$H_{AB} = \frac{2\int P_A P_B dv}{\int P_A^2 dv + \int P_B^2 dv} \tag{23}$$

Linear and exponential indices. The linear and exponential indices [53] evaluate electrostatic similarities at each individual grid point, the values are combined, and the total is divided by the number of grid points involved to determine the average similarity.

$$L_{AB} = \frac{\sum_{i=1}^{n}(1 - X)}{n} \qquad E_{AB} = \frac{\sum_{i=1}^{n}\exp^{-X}}{n} \tag{24}$$

where

$$X = \frac{|P_A - P_B|}{\max(|P_A|, |P_B|)} \tag{25}$$

$\max(|P_A|, |P_B|), (P_{max})$, is the larger electrostatic potential magnitude between P_A and P_B at the grid point where the similarity is being calculated. n is the number of grid points involved in the calculation.

Spearman rank correlation coefficient [54]. This statistical scalar has been used to measure the electrostatic potential similarity of two molecules over the intersections of an orthogonal grid, as used in CoMFA.

$$R_{AB} = 1 - \left(\frac{6\Sigma_{i=1}^{n} d_i^2}{n^3 - n} \right) \tag{26}$$

d_i is the difference in the electrostatic potential rank at point i of two structures, and n is the total number of grid points.

Statistical Analysis

The modified ASP programs construct a symmetric N by N data matrix. Column 1 and row 1 contain the similarities of structure 1 to all other compounds, column 2 and row 2 the same information for structure 2, ... This unmodified data matrix is analyzed using PLS (GOLPE program [55]) employing the leave-one-out cross-validation of all structures over X ($X > 10$) components. Matrices with more than Y ($Y > 30$) columns are reduced in size through D optimalization of their GAMMA values [55,56]. The D optimalization matrices, and all other matrices with fewer than Y components are then reduced using progressive-fixing exclusion. This procedure seeks to determine which variables aid correlation by the application of design matrices processed using fractional factorial design [57]. The resultant matrices are used to form a new cross-validated PLS model, and its variables are tested for predictiveness using GOLPE. Final models are tested by repeating the leave-one-out cross-validation analysis for up to three components.

D. Distance Geometry

Introduction

The use of interatomic distances as representations of shape has also shown success in 3D structure–activity modeling of molecules. Some workers have used the atomic coordinates of a pattern of atoms (thus distances) within a molecule to represent the key molecular shape attribute responsible for biological activity [58,59]. Another component in the evolution of using interatomic distances to represent molecular shape is the development and use of distance geometry [60].

Distance geometry permits not only the projection of important interatomic distances that relate to biological activity, but also to postulate critical intermolecular-binding distances that may be involved in the ligand–receptor interaction. The distance matrix, composed of the set of interatomic distances, is a convenient representation of molecular structure that is invariant to rotation and translation of the molecule, but that reflects changes in its internal degrees of freedom. The distance range matrix is an extension that has two values for each interatomic distance, representing the upper and lower limits, or range, allowed for a given interatomic distance owing to the conformational flexibility of the molecule.

Methodology and Implementation

Distance geometry, as the name implies, approaches geometric problems by focusing on the distances between points, rather than on coordinates or angles. In 3D-QSAR applications the points are atoms, and the geometric problems can include conformational analysis, molecular alignment, and ligand–receptor binding. Crippen and co-workers [60] have suggested that there are currently four methods of 3D-QSAR based on distance geometry [1]. An overview of each of these methods is given here.

Ensemble distance geometry. In this situation, a hypothesis is available about a possible common pharmacophore for a set of compounds (not necessarily analogues) that bind to the same, but unknown, receptor. Moreover, the groups in each molecule that correspond to the sites composing the common pharmacophore are identified. The goals of an analysis are to determine if the pharmacophore hypothesis is geometrically valid and, if it is, estimate the relative binding of the molecules to the receptor.

For a set of rigid molecules, the pharmacophore testing can be achieved by a best-fit alignment, depending solely on whole-molecule translations and rotations. However, the problem becomes appreciably more difficult for molecules that have conformational flexibility. Bond length and bond angle changes can usually be neglected relative to conformational flexibility because it is torsion angles that produce the major contributions to conformational (spatial) changes in a molecule.

Sheridan et al. [61] have formulated the fitting of flexible molecules to a common pharmacophore as a distance–geometry-embedding problem. The embedding problem consists of a set of upper and lower bounds on distance between some of the atoms of each molecule in a series. The absolute configuration of chiral centers, planarity of aromatic rings, or restrictions on torsion angles may also be provided. The solution is to find sets of atomic Cartesian coordinates for each molecule that satisfy the problem constraints.

Site pocket models. Site pocket models are another example of an applied distance geometry method [62]. The site model is composed of site points, or pockets, positioned in space such that a binding pocket is where a ligand could be located, and a nonbinding pocket represents the excluded volume of the receptor site. The objective in this approach is to find coordinates for the pockets and interaction parameters between pockets and ligand atoms, in an iterative fashion, such that the calculated binding affinity agrees with the observed values.

The method consists of evaluating the minimum and maximum distances between the ligand atoms for energetically allowed conformations. One then makes an initial hypothesis on the binding mode of the ligands at the binding site. The binding mode is defined as which atom of the ligand goes to which pocket. Because in the distance geometric representation atomic distances have ranges for flexible molecules, it is proposed that the active conformations be represented by a common distance range. The common distance range of user-selected superimposed atoms in the various ligands are evaluated and compared, which results in gradually decreasing the range and, thereby, contracting the possible conformational space for the series of ligands. Ultimately, embedding these distances (i.e., obtaining three-dimensional coordinates from interatomic distance ranges) will give the three-dimensional structure of the site pockets accommodating the ligand atoms. The site pockets are classified into different types to differentiate the nature or intensity of interaction. Assuming a linear function of the ligand–site pocket interactions, the binding energy can be calculated by the following general RI-3D-QSAR equation:

$$E_{\text{calc}} = -CE_c + \sum_{r=1}^{n_r} \sum_{o=1}^{n_o} \sum_{i=1}^{n_p} p_{a,i} \varepsilon_{r,i} \tag{27}$$

where E_c is the ligand conformational energy with some weight factor C, $p_{a,i}$ is the value of the ith physicochemical property attached to atom a, and $\varepsilon_{r,i}$ is the adjustable interaction energy parameter associated with the ith physicochemical property and the rth (binding) pocket, n_r is the number of site pockets, n_p is the number of physicochemical properties active in the site pocket, n_o is the number of ligand atoms occupying the site pocket. Typically, the physicochemical parameters include the atomic contribution to log$P$, the atomic contribution to molar refractivity, and atomic partial charge of each of the ligand atoms. Alternative binding modes, because of rigid rotations and translations and conformational flexibility, can also be evaluated, which results in reparameterizing the site pocket 3D-QSAR model. The optimal-binding mode is that which produces the most significant 3D-QSAR. The site pockets of a 3D-QSAR for a set of triazine inhibitors of dihydrofolate reductase [62] are shown in Figure 6.

REMOTEDISC. REMOTEDISC, a computer-aided receptor-modeling procedure [63] based on the site pocket model, addresses some of the problems inherent to the site pocket model. Ligand atoms that were positioned between pockets were ignored. If all possible atomic interactions are to be included in the model, more pockets of smaller spheres are required, but this increases the number of adjustable parameters to the detriment of the overall model. Another problem is the close coupling between hypothesized-binding modes and the resulting site geometry and energy parameters. The evaluation of alternative modes requires new ε values and,

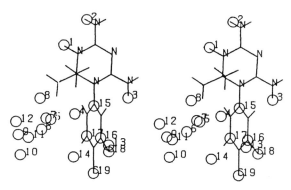

Figure 6 A stereographic representation of the distance geometry site pocket pharmacophore for a set of triazine inhibitors of dihydrofolate reductase. (From Ref. 62.)

possibly, also new site pocket coordinates. Because of the many geometrically feasible binding modes, convergence of the cycling process is questionable. These difficulties are resolved in REMOTEDISC by fixing the hypothesized-binding modes once and for all by a more rigorous conformational search and molecular superimposition procedure. Low-energy conformations of each ligand are found by a grid search, and a reference structure is chosen from this pool, using a priority function that takes into account experimental-binding energy and ligand internal energy. The reference structure is usually a strongly binding analogue. An optimal superimposition of the other ligands on the reference structure is realized by using physicochemical property matching. Once the ligands are superimposed, spherical site pockets are generated such that all atoms of all molecules are covered. However, to reduce the number of adjustable energy parameters, the pockets are classified as belonging to a limited number of types. The ε values depend on the type of pocket, instead of each pocket having its own unique set of energy parameters. REMOTEDISC results in identifying the dominant interactions for each site pocket by an examination of the relative importance of the various physicochemical properties taken as independent variables in the model.

Voronoi site modeling. One limiting feature of the site pocket method is its site definition—each pocket must be spherical and nonoverlapping—yielding a propagation of small pockets. Replacing the site pockets with Voronoi polyhedron regions as in the Voronoi site-modeling approach (VOROM method) [64] allows the user to minimize the number of regions needed to describe the binding site geometry. The method partitions space into distinct convex Voronoi regions. The sizes, shapes, and positions of these regions are determined by the coordinates of a single generating point, which ensures that each region, or Voronoi polyhedron, is just the set of points closer to its generating point than to any other generating point. To enhance algorithm efficiency, specified atomic groups of the ligands undergo molecular redefinition, or squashing, into single pseudoatoms, which retain the composite physicochemical properties of the component atoms. The new pseudoatoms are subsequently treated as actual atoms for the rest of the modeling sequence.

The conformational space (i.e., the shape) of the molecule remains the same for the condensed molecule because the interatomic distances of atoms and pseudoatoms still define the space-filling features of the molecule. Each molecule is subsequently broken down into convex sets of atoms. A convex set of atoms is any subset such that their convex frame contains only that subset. For a conformationally flexible molecule, different convex sets may be possible, depending on ligand conformation. The convex sets are then grouped into partitions. A *partition* of a molecule is defined to be a set of mutually exclusive and exhaustive convex sets. That is, each atom belongs to one and only one of the convex sets in the partition. The placement of the partitions among the binding regions is defined as the binding mode of the molecule. The number of regions in the site is user-defined and is kept at a minimum to maintain processing efficiency, but yet still be predictive. Usually, only a few regions are used to begin the process. The complexity of the site model is increased by adding more binding regions, and also different binding modes are employed until the experimental binding energy, which is represented as the upper and lower bounds of the observed binding energy, has been optimally predicted. The two bounds of the binding energy are introduced to take into account the experimental error involved in the measurement of these activity values. Increasing the experimental error bars leads to geometrically simpler models; however, one must be careful not to "oversimplify" the models to the point of losing too much structural detail in the Voronoi model.

To summarize, the result of distance-geometry approaches to developing RI 3D-QSARs, if successful, include a graphic 3D model of the binding site and the interaction energy parameters assigned to the different regions. In this way, it is possible to compute both intraligand and intermolecular ligand–receptor energy contributions to the overall binding process; that is, both $\Delta E_{L}(LL)$ and $\Delta E_{LR}(LR)$ of Table 1 can be estimated.

E. The Hypothetical Active-Site Lattice Model

The hypothetical active-site lattice approach (HASL) [65] is related to the CoMFA methodology and also to MSA. Whereas in CoMFA the field potentials of molecules at grid points outside the molecules are computed and analyzed, the HASL approach represents each of the shapes of the molecules as a collection of 3D grid points, which is termed the *molecular lattice*. The resolution of the HASL (i.e., the distance between the grid points) determines the number of lattice points that represent a molecule and also the resolution of the generated receptor map. User-defined conformations are selected to generate the HASL. Typically, conformations similar in shape are chosen. A reference compound is arbitrarily selected to begin the analysis. All grid points lying within the van der Waals radii of the atoms of the molecule are designated as "occupied" and constitute the molecular lattice. The electronic properties of the occupying atom(s) are represented discretely, such that the lattice points are labeled using a HASL type(s) ($+1$, 0, -1), according to the electron density of the atoms. This electronic property constitutes the fourth dimension of a molecular lattice, other properties being neglected.

A second molecule is next selected, its molecular lattice generated and compared with that of the reference molecule. The degree of correspondence between the two lattices is calculated according to a fitting function. To find the optimal alignment of the second molecule relative to the reference using the HASL, a systematic search procedure is performed that consists of a series of translational and rotational movements with a lattice generated at each step. After the best alignment of the two molecular lattices has been found, those lattice points of the fitted molecule that are not yet in common with the reference molecule are added to create a new larger reference lattice. This process is then repeated until all molecules in the training set are included and a reference lattice spanning the entire training set of compounds has been constructed. The HASL procedure is schematically illustrated in Figure 7 [66].

The two aims of the HASL approach are the prediction of activities of untested compounds, as well as the identification of substructures that most influence the observed activities. Initially, the observed biological activity measure of a molecule is uniformly divided among its lattice points. For lattice points that are common to several molecules, the partial activity contributions from the molecules are averaged. Starting with this "averaged" HASL the activity contributions of the individual active-site lattice points are adjusted by an iterative procedure to fit the observed activity data of the entire training set. This optimized, "iterated" HASL is then used as a calibrated template to predict the activities of untested com-

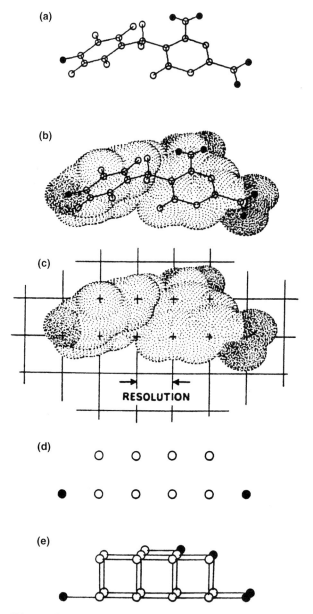

Figure 7 A schematic illustration of the HASL construction: (a) molecular structure in 3D space, containing different atoms (black and white); (b) superposition
of van der Waals molecular volume; (c) identification of molecular lattice points
imbedded within the molecular volume; (d) lattice points shown in two dimensions;
(e) a three- and four-dimensional view of these lattice points. (From Ref. 66.)

pounds. The activity of a particular molecule is predicted by summing all the partial activity values at points in common with the composite HASL. Examples of the use of this method to develop 3D-QSARs can be found [67,68]. HASL indirectly estimates differences in $\Delta E_{LR}(LR)$ of Table 1, based on user-chosen ligand conformations.

F. Genetically Evolved Receptor Models

Recently, Walters and Hinds have introduced "genetically evolved" receptor models (the GERM program) to establish 3D-QSARs [69]. The objective of this method is to produce atomic-level models of receptor sites based on a trial set of ligands. Receptor models are made by placing atoms at points in space in which they can simulate a receptor surface and interact with the ligands. Model aliphatic carbon atoms are distributed evenly over a sphere surrounding the training set of superimposed ligands, and their positions are adjusted to obtain maximal van der Waals attraction between the model carbon atoms and the ligand molecules. Once the positions of the carbons have been identified, they can be occupied by any of 14 atom types, including no atom at all. Because the receptor structure is unknown, the initial selection of the number of atoms, types of atoms, and their positions is random. New receptor models are evolved and evaluated using a GA method [43]. A conceptual illustration of a possible GERM is shown in Figure 8.

In a GA, the variables to be optimized are encoded as a sequence of bits in a linear string. Each variable is referred to as a gene, and the string containing all genes is designated as a chromosome. An initial population

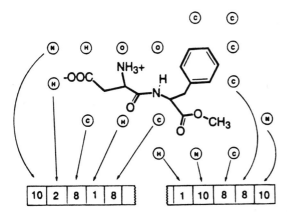

Figure 8 A conceptual representation of a GERM. (From Ref. 69.)

of chromosomes (strings) is generated, each chromosome in the population representing a different set of values for the variables. Each chromosome in the population is evaluated using a scoring scheme to measure how well it "solves" the problem under consideration. Chromosomes with good scores are preferentially selected for propagation of a new generation. Chromosomes with poor scores have a propensity to perish. The best-performing chromosome from one generation is frequently saved and survives unchanged into the next generation. A portion of the better chromosomes are copied directly into the next generation. Another portion of the better chromosomes also "mate" by a procedure called "crossover" to produce offspring, with a mixture of genes from both parents. In this procedure, a pair of chromosomes is lined up, a crossover point along the chromosome is selected, and portions of the bit string beyond the crossover point in each of the chromosomes are swapped. Occasionally, mutations are also produced by an alteration of single bits within the bit string. The population size of each generation remains constant. With succeeding generations, better-scoring chromosomes are formed. By continuing the parent solution–recombination process for several generations, the overall fitness of the population increases, resulting in natural selection and survival of the fittest: that is, a nonlinear optimization process is performed.

In the GERM scheme a chromosome consists of a list of atom types, "genes", (aliphatic H, hydrogen bonding H, aliphatic C, carbonyl C, hydroxyl O, and so forth), with each location in the chromosome corresponding to a specific location in space. A population is generated by randomly assigning an atom type code to every position of every individual chromosome. The "fitness" score for a given chromosome is produced by first calculating the sum of the intermolecular van der Waals and electrostatic energies between a chromosome (model) and each individual ligand. The criterion for measuring fitness is the correlation coefficient for the calculated energy versus activity. After a model has been evolved, it can be used to calculate bioactivities of other ligands when docked onto the model receptor. Intermolecular van der Waals and electrostatic energies are calculated between the model(s) and ligand, and the predicted bioactivity is interpolated from the calculated energy versus bioactivity correlation equation.

Walters and Hinds [69] have generated GERM models for a series of sweeteners, which show a high correlation between calculated intermolecular energy, $\Delta E_{LR}(LR)$ of Table 1, and bioactivity. These models also provide reasonable predictions of bioactivity for compounds that were not included in construction of the GERM.

There are several approximations and assumptions in this approach that have been recognized by these authors [69]. An active conformation and an alignment of each ligand in the receptor site are assumed. Furthermore, ligands and receptor models are treated as rigid entities. No intramolecular interactions are taken into account. The unbound state of the interacting ligand and receptor is not addressed. Finally, entropy and solvation terms are not included in the current energy-fitting function.

GERM models are not real receptors—they are composed of isolated atoms that are not coherent with protein structure. The models are collections of atom types and positions that distinguish relative potencies of bioactive compounds on the basis of calculating approximate intermolecular energies, $\Delta E_{LR}(LR)$. Nevertheless, evaluation of the best models may elucidate the pharmacophoric groups in a series of ligands.

G. Probing Rigid, High-Affinity Ligands

Milne and co-workers [70] have developed a model of the receptor site in the enzyme, protein kinase C (PKC), for which X-ray crystallographic data had not been reported at the time of their work. Their approach was to examine the interactions between probe molecules and crucial binding points of a rigid substrate having a high-binding affinity for the enzyme. This probe sampling analysis allowed construction of a receptor-site model by detailed examination of the hydrogen bond interactions between probe molecules and a receptor template.

Previous studies [71] have shown that the binding of phorbol esters to PKC essentially involves three of the phorbol atoms; namely, an oxygen of a carbonyl group and two hydroxyl groups. Hence, Milne et al. assumed a three-point pharmacophore in which there must be at least two hydrogen-bond donors and a hydrogen-bond acceptor. Thus, from the structure of phorbol, and the geometric characteristics of an optimum hydrogen bond, several possible structures for the receptor were postulated. The atoms of the receptor that are involved in hydrogen bonds with the crucial phorbol atoms were modeled by simple "probe" molecules. Methanol was used as the hydrogen bond donor and formaldehyde as a hydrogen bond acceptor at the binding site. Several orientations of these probe molecules are possible relative to the phorbol oxygens.

Evaluation of the three possible receptor models was accomplished by comparing the measured-binding affinities of several known PKC activators with the calculated-binding energies to see which of the models best reproduced the experimental data. Mapping of the pharmacophore derived from phorbol to the corresponding three-atom groups in various inhibitors was carried out by combined geometry and energy analyses. A measure of optimized geometric fit with the pharmacophore based on root mean square (RMS) values from the three-point fits was unable to distinguish between inhibitors with high-binding affinity and those of low affinity. The reason for this discrimination shortcoming, the authors propose, appears to be because superpositioning takes account of only the position of an atom, not its relative orientation to the rest of the ligand–receptor model system. Position alone is necessary, but in this example, an insufficient criterion for binding. Calculation of the explicit binding energies is necessary to solve this problem.

The binding energy (enthalpy) $E_{complex}$, between these PKC activator compounds and the three binding site models was calculated using the semiemperical quantum-mechanical method PM3 [73]. In the structure optimization process, the positions of the probe molecule atoms were kept fixed, and each of the ligands was allowed to move in space to find the position in which it could form the strongest interactions with the probe molecules. The energy of the ligand in the complex E_{ligand} was obtained by removing all the probe molecules from the complex and recalculating the energy of the system without geometry optimization. Similarly, after removal of the ligand from the complex and recalculation of the energy, without geometry optimization, the energy of formation of the model E_{model} was obtained. The binding energy $E_{binding}$ was then calculated using the following equation:

$$E_{binding} = E_{complex} - (E_{model} + E_{ligand}) \tag{28}$$

Equation (28) is an approximate representation of Eq. (6) and its terms are defined in Table 1.

One particular model was able to distinguish between two possible binding modes and gave binding energies better correlated to the experimental values than the other models. The major advantage of this model, compared with other previously proposed phamacophore models for PKC binding, is its ability to provide a quantitative evaluation of the strength of the hydrogen bonds that the ligand can form with the binding site in PKC. The model does break down for several compounds, and it was concluded that the differences in lipophilicity and flexibility among the ligands, which were not considered in the correlations, were largely responsible for the outlier behavior.

Protein kinase C is a lipid-soluble enzyme that interacts with ligands in the lipid phase. Thus, the free-energy change associated with the partitioning of a ligand between the aqueous and lipid phases and the free energy of the ligand's binding to PKC in the lipid phase both contribute to overall binding. Because it is difficult to calculate free energies in a lipid environment, the authors suggest that the difference in the binding affinities of two ligands can be estimated by computing the free-energy change in partitioning and adding the free-energy change on binding in the gas phase (i.e., the value obtained from the modeling experiment) for each ligand. The change in free energy during the partitioning process is related to the hydrophobicity of the ligand. If one assumes that the partitioning is a passive process, the efficiency with which a ligand transfers into a lipid phase is determined by the hydrophobicity of the ligand which, in turn, is a function of the aqueous solubility of the ligand. A quadratic correlation was found between ligand-binding affinity and aqueous solubility that accounts for, in some fashion, the free-energy change in partitioning. The free energy of binding can be further decomposed into enthalpy, which is estimated by the gas-phase enthalpy calculations, and entropy components. Entropy changes were restricted to those caused by immobilization of rotatable bonds of the ligand during its binding to the receptor, assuming that the transitional and rotational entropy losses are approximately the same for all ligands. A 3D-QSAR was obtained by MLR using the known K_i values as dependent variables:

$$2.303RT \log_{10}(K_i) = 6.62 + 1.505 \, \Delta H + 0.235 \, N_{rb} \tag{29}$$
$$+ 0.139 \, [\log(WS) + 2.832]^2$$

$$r^2 = 0.917; \quad SD = 0.64; \quad F(4,13) = 35.69$$

where ΔH is the binding energy calculated for the receptor model, N_{rb} is the number of rotatable bonds immobilized on binding, and $[\log(WS) + 2.832]^2$ is the contribution of the hydrophobicity represented by the water solubility WS of the ligand, as measured by the method developed by Klopman et al. [73]. Within the context of Table 1, Eq. (29) incorporates the $\Delta E_{LR}(LR)$ energy term and a representation of the change in conformational entropy and lipid solvation energy of the ligand.

H. Quantitative Binding Site Model, Compass

Jain et al. have developed an algorithm that analyzes structure–activity data to construct a "quantitative binding-site model." This algorithm, which the authors named Compass, is based on surface–only-type properties and predicts the bioactive conformation, alignment, and binding affinities of a series of ligands in an automated procedure [74,75]. Compass is allowed to choose from a pool of ligand conformations, found from a standard conformational search, that are within the program-defined cutoff of 5.0 kcal above the global energy minimum for each isomer. The conformations are placed in rough, initial orientations by an automated shape-based molecular alignment procedure. The alignment procedure relies on Compass's surface-based features, which include steric and hydrogen bond donor and acceptor features. These features are computed relative to a set of reference points uniformly placed on spheres, 6.0 and 9.0 Å in radius, centered at the origin of a Cartesian reference frame. The features are uniformly distributed in space. At each point, three distances are computed to the ligand: the distance to the van der Waals surface, the distance to the nearest potential hydrogen bond-donor, and the distance to the nearest potential hydrogen bond-acceptor. The hydrogen-bonding features have an associated directional component that is represented as a scalar strength between zero and 1. The direction strength captures the degree to which a vector going from the origin to the reference point is coincident with the direction of the hydrogen bond participant. This creates a single maximum for the possible interaction and eliminates degeneracies inherent in a pure distance feature. For uniformity, steric features have an associated constant strength of 1. The strengths are used to weigh the functions of the feature values.

The conformations of the ligands can be aligned to maximize their mutual similarity according to Compass's features. A specific conformation and orientation (i.e., alignment) is called a pose. A similarity measure m between some pose p and a reference pose r is defined as follows:

$$m(p,r) = \Sigma_i \left(\frac{e^{[-(f_i(p)-f_i(r))^2]/\sigma} s_i(p) s_i(r)}{\Sigma_j s_i(r)} \right) \quad (30)$$

A pose is specified by a conformation and six orientation parameters. The function, f_i, computes the ith feature value of a pose; the function s_i computes the strength of the feature. The exponential has a maximum when features from the poses correspond to one another, and it falls off toward zero as they diverge. The parameter σ controls the steepness of the decay. Maximizing m by varying the orientation parameters of p aligns the shape and polar functionality of p to that exhibited by the reference pose r. The strength term in the numerator enforces a matching directionality constraint on potential hydrogen bonds. The sum in the denominator normalizes each test ligand's similarity measure for the total strength of the reference pose, which may differ for different poses based on variations in hydrogen-bonding geometries relative to the feature reference points. The similarity function m is maximized using multiple initial starting alignments coupled with gradient descent on the derivative of m relative to the orientation parameters of p.

A procedure for developing an initial hypothesis of the bioactive conformations begins by selecting a set of poses (one per molecule) that maximize the joint similarity of all molecules to the most active ones, as defined by the binding data. Poses for ligands are selected in decreasing potency rank. Compass chooses conformations and alignments for each ligand by seeking bioactive poses of all active molecules that are similar to each other and are simultaneously different from the shapes that inactive molecules can adopt. For a molecule (m) each of its poses is compared with the poses of all other molecules using the similarity measure defined earlier, and the best matching pose for each is marked. The match scores are summed, weighted by the potency of the matched molecules, as measured by binding affinities. The pose of m that maximizes this sum is selected. The procedure continues until all molecules have a selected pose.

This initial hypothesis of a bioactive pose set is used for the first few iterations of neural network training. After this initial reliance on a fixed set of poses, the entire pool of possible poses is made available to the neural network model for the remaining training process. From these starting poses, an initial model of activity is constructed by training, with the shape and potential hydrogen-bonding features forming a particular pose as input, and experimentally observed activities as its desired output. Trial models are evaluated and refined using improved molecular poses, and the process iterates until it converges on a best pose for each molecule within the overall ligand–receptor model. New molecules are essentially "docked" into the resulting binding-site model using the analogous procedure to predict their affinities.

The flow diagram for the Compass procedure is shown in Figure 9. Because neural networks are used to create the model, a traditional QSAR equation is not produced. However, an analysis of this type does yield predicted activities and also other quantitative data (e.g., specific distance constraints from a proton donor to a ring), along with a qualitative visual model that shows favorable positions and relative contributions of steric and polar interactions. Compass makes indirect and relative predictions of combined $\Delta E_{LR}(LR)$ and $\Delta E_L(LL)$ internal energies as defined in Table 1.

Jain et al. performed a benchmark study of the Compass method [74] on a steroid-binding affinity prediction problem previously studied using CoMFA [8] and the molecular similarity matrix method [46]. A comparison of the predictive performance of the three methods, as measured by xv-r^2 values, revealed that Compass made better predictions than either CoMFA or the similarity matrix method for the set of ligands. The xv-r^2 values for the Compass, CoMFA, and molecular similarity method are 0.89, 0.69, and 0.53, respectively, for the CBG assay and 0.88, 0.44, and 0.74, respectively, for the TBG. Jain et al. also used Compass to construct a binding-site model of the $5HT_{1A}$ receptor from a training set of 20 compounds [75]. This 3D-QSAR model was able to predict the affinities, $-\log K_i$ values (with a mean predictive error of 0.55 log units relative to range of 3.52 for the actual values) and bioactive conformations of 35 new compounds.

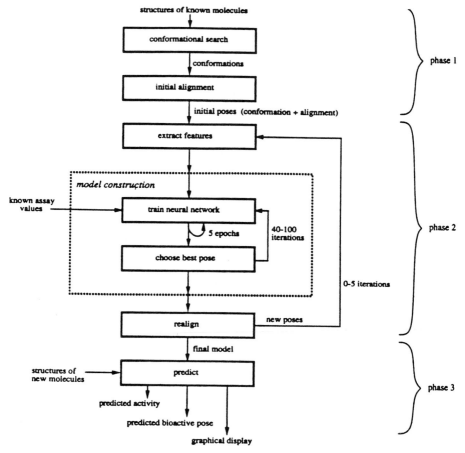

Figure 9   Flow diagram for the Compass procedure. (From Ref. 74.)

I.   3D-QSARs from GRID Probe Comparisons

Davis et al. used the GRID probe force field [76] to compute the interaction energy between a series of calcium channel agonists and an alkyl hydroxyl probe over a regular 3D grid around the target molecules to develop a 3D-QSAR [77]. The total energy of interaction, equal to the sum of electrostatic, steric, and hydrogen-bonding terms, at each grid point, along with CLOGP and CMR descriptors [78] for the ligands, were analyzed using PLS, as implemented inside the SIMCA multivariate analysis package [79]. A number of discrete regions in space are mapped out by positive- and negative-regression coefficient contours. A negative-regression coefficient/

PLS weight at a position in space indicates that as the interaction energy between the probe and the series of molecules becomes more negative, the ligands become more active. This could be due to a favorable electronic–hydrogen-bonding interaction with the receptor being identified, or to a less favorable steric interaction. Conversely, a positive-regression coefficient/PLS weight indicates that as the interaction energy across the set becomes more positive, the binding energy becomes higher. This higher-binding energy could be due to an unfavorable electrostatic interaction with the receptor, or to the identification of a region in space where it is favorable to place ligand steric bulk.

Part of this approach demonstrates how the interpretation of the resulting PLS model can be aided not only by examining the overall regression contour maps, but also by examining the individual PLS weighting maps. GRID points with high PLS weights are important in defining that component (i.e., are highly collinear with that component) and, therefore, contain similar information. Consequently, all mapped regions that weigh onto a single PLS component should have a single (common) statistical–physical interpretation. The authors also show that the quality of the model improves by removing redundant variables. The influence of variable scaling, especially when macroscopic descriptors (i.e., CLOGP and CMR) are evaluated along with the interaction energies as independent variables, have a significant affect on model predictivity.

J. Catalyst

Catalyst is a popular, turn-key commercial software package that establishes 3D-QSARs based on a training set of compounds and their activities against a common endpoint [80]. The compounds do not have to be highly homologous, although the 3D-QSAR models are usually most significant for analogue training sets. The turn-key aspect of the package refers to the user having to only sketch in the structures in the training set, input the corresponding activity measures, and provide some control data, such as the number of conformations to be sampled in the conformational search for the active conformation. Structure input and model building is quite easy; hence, many medicinal chemists find this package quite "user friendly." In addition, the 3D-QSAR is quite intuitive to the medicinal chemist. The graphic representation can be the most active compound in its active conformation with the 3D-pharmacophore found in the analysis superimposed on the compound. No QSAR equation is generated, but rather, the facility to rank the predicted activities of the training set of compounds, as well as any test compounds, based on the 3D-QSAR model. There is no explicit QSAR equation because the 3D-QSAR model is derived from weighted activity rules as well as from statistical fittings. The activity rules include matching hydrogen bond doner and acceptor bond vectors across the compounds and locating common spatial regions of hydrophobicity.

Catalyst does seem limited in some ways. The conformational search seems to be equally distributed, relative to flexible torsion angles, in terms of the number of conformations considered. No allowance is made for the fact that the torsion angles of a molecule do not have equal influence on its shape and conformation. The activity rules and their relative weighting of importance may be somewhat arbitrary and incomplete. The log$P$ and other whole-molecule physicochemical properties, for example, are not considered in 3D-QSAR model construction. The force field used in Catalyst has led to postulated active conformations that are quite high in energy (> 20 kcals mol higher than the global minimum) when evaluated by other force fields or by quantum mechanical methods.

Overall, Catalyst, similar to CoMFA, has proved to be a very popular and useful tool in molecular design. It has been particularly applied to test pharmacophore hypotheses as well as to generate activity hypotheses. Some workers have used Catalyst as a preprocessor to CoMFA for flexible molecules. Here the idea is to use Catalyst to provide the active conformations and alignments for CoMFA.

K.   Comparisons of Approaches and Validation

There is little in the way of comparisons of the various RI 3D-QSARs with one another for application to a common data set. Compass has been compared with both CoMFA and the molecular similarity matrix method and is discussed in the section on Compass. Moreover, very little has been done toward validation of RI 3D-QSAR methods. One straightforward validation process would be to consider a set of ligands for which the receptor-binding geometry is known as well as the binding constants of the ligands. The validation "measures" would be to see how much of the binding geometry and how accurately the binding constants can be predicted. In the spirit that validation should not focus on who is "right" and who is "wrong", but rather, when can a particular RI 3D-QSAR be expected to work, comparisons of methods should be undertaken. Crippen and co-workers have reported a comparison of some of their site pocket distance geometry models for dihydrofolate reductase inhibitors to the corresponding crystal complex geometries in their paper [1]. It would be highly informative if other 3D-QSAR methods were applied to the common data sets, and the results presented.

A set of 54 anticoccidial triazines [81] have been analyzed using (a) classic Hansch-type analysis [82], (b) CoMFA [83], (c) MSA [84], and (d) molecular similarity matrices [47]. The biological activity in this training set is log(1/MEC), where MEC is the lowest compound level, in parts per million, in feed preventing lesions in a test set of chicks prechallenged with oocysts of the coccidian parasite *Eimaria tenella*. That is, the test system is an in vivo model, and drug delivery factors, such as transport and metabolism, are inherent to the biological measures, as well as direct ligand–receptor binding. Thus, 3D-QSAR methods that address only direct ligand–receptor binding may be of limited applicability to this data set. Nevertheless, it is both interesting and insightful to compare and contrast the applications of the four foregoing 3D-QSAR methods. The RI 3D-QSARs from each of the four methods are given in Table 3.

The RI 3D-QSAR developed using molecular similarity matrices is the most significant model for all 54 analogues as measured by $xv\text{-}r^2$, whereas the MSA(2) model demonstrates how model quality is enhanced when outlier analysis is applied. Both the Hansch approach, using descriptors based on experimental measurements, and CoMFA, using only field descriptors, do not provide particulary good 3D-QSAR models.

A comparison of CoMFA (field only) and the CoMFA and Hansch models might indicate that the Hansch descriptors, in part, take into account in vivo factors on activity (transport as measured by log k'). However, the molecular similarity matrices approach presumably focuses only on ligand–receptor interactions, yet it is quite significant. In the MSA study, which included both in vivo and in vitro descriptors in model construction, V_{ov} (the COSV) and ΔD_x, a dipole moment component, were found in the optimum 3D-QSAR. These two descriptors most likely reflect direct ligand–receptor interactions. MSA also attempts to optimize the 3D-QSAR as a function of ligand conformation and alignment. The active conformation used in MSA is different from the conformation used in CoMFA. No assessment could be made for the conformations used in the molecular similarity matrices analysis. There is no way to estimate how the CoMFA and molecular similarity matrices models might be altered as a function of conformation. All methods appear to have used the common triazine ring as the alignment constraint.

The size of the training set ($N = 54$), coupled with the sizes of the various descriptor pools, leads to optimum model sizes (significant PLS components) of three independent variables. Whether a squared representation of a descriptor in combination with its linear value qualifies as two distinct terms might be debated.

Table 3 A Comparison of Various RI-3D-QSAR Models Developed for the Anticoccidal Triazine SAR Training Set

Method	N	Outliers	r^2	SD	xv-r^2	F	PLS components	Equation descriptors	Graphics	Active conformation	Alignment
Hansch	54	0	0.56	0.71	0.49	21.3	3	$(\log k')^2$, $\log k'^{a}$, δ_6^{b}	No	No	No
CoMFA (field only)	54	0	0.66	—[h]	0.47	—[h]	2	No[c]	Yes	—[d]	—[d]
CoMFA and Hansch	54	0	0.80	0.48	0.61	49.2	4	No	Yes	—[d]	—[d]
MSA(1)	54	0	0.70	0.59	0.64	28.7	3	$(V_{ov})^2$, $(V_{ov})^{e}$, ΔD_x^{f}	Yes	Yes	Yes
MSA(2)	51	3	0.83	0.46	0.81	36.0	3	$(V_{ov})^2$, (V_{ov}), ΔD_x^{f}	Yes	Yes	Yes
Molecular similarity matrices	54	0	—[h]	—[h]	0.73	—[h]	3	No[c]	No[g]	—[h]	—[h]

[a]Relative lipophilicity by HPLC [81].
[b]^{1}H-NMR chemical shift of position 6 of the triazine ring.
[c]Physicochemical descriptors not reported.
[d]A low-energy conformation selected and the largest common substructure chosen for alignment.
[e]COSV.
[f]Particular dipole-moment component.
[g]None given, but representations should be possible.
[h]Not reported.

III. RECEPTOR-DEPENDENT 3D-QSARS

A. Receptor-Dependent Molecular Shape Analysis

Hopfinger and colleagues [3] reported the first RD 3D-QSAR analysis, as defined in this review. A quantitative correlation of biological activities with calculated intermolecular binding energy and log$P$ is reported in their study. These authors modeled the intercalation of a series of doxorubicin-like anthracyclines (**I**) with a d(CpG) nucleotide dimer using a static intermolecular search and minimization technique [85]. A significant RD 3D-QSAR correlation equation,

$$\log\left(\frac{1}{C}\right) = 0.246[\log P] - 0.030[\log P]^2 - 0.423[IE \times 10] - 0.27$$

$$(31)$$

$$N = 29; \quad r = 0.901; \quad s = 0.289;$$

$$AE = \pm 11.9\%; \quad \log P_{opt} = 4.17$$

was constructed from this intermolecular modeling. The RD 3D-QSAR is dominated by [IE], the calculated global minimum intercalating binding energy of each analogue to the dinucleotide dimer. C is the concentration of anthracycline needed to increase the average life of a control group of cancer-infected mice, compared with a cancer-infected group not given therapy. AE is the average error of prediction; logP_{opt} corresponds to that value of log$P$ that maximizes its contribution to increasing log($1/C$). This RD3D-QSAR not only assigned a significant relation between measured anticancer activity and the specific intercalation binding energy of each

I

II

ligand, but it also supported a new (at the time) geometric mode of intercalator–DNA binding, which Hopfinger and Nakata had proposed [86], and that was subsequently supported by X-ray and NMR analyses [87,88]. 3D-QSARs relating cardiotoxicity of the set of anthracyclines to several physicochemical properties were also found. The two 3D-QSARs (anticancer and cardiotoxicity) were combined to develop a therapeutic index equation.

Hopfinger and Kawakami [89] employed MD simulations to determine the low-energy DNA intercalation thermodynamic properties for a set of 14 benzothiopyranindazole (BTPI) analogues (**II**). The calculated free-space binding (intercalation) energies by themselves, or in combination with ligand lipophilicity, which was found to be significant in the previously described RD 3D-QSAR [3], did not yield any significant RD 3D-QSAR model. However, the free-space binding energy combined with the aqueous desolvation energy of the intercalation complex led to highly significant RD 3D-QSAR. In this modeling scheme the aqueous desolvation energy, ΔE_d, is defined as

$$\Delta E_d = E_c - (E_l + E_r) \tag{32}$$

where E_c is the aqueous solvation energy of the lowest energy intercalation complex determined in the free-space MD simulation. E_l is the aqueous solvation energy of the isolated BTPI ligand in the conformation it adopts in the lowest-energy intercalation complex. Likewise, E_r is the aqueous solvation energy of the isolated $(G–C)_6$ duplex in the conformation it adopts in the lowest-energy MD intercalation complex. The desolvation energy is computed using a hydration shell model [15]. An example of an active [BTPI ligand–$(G–C)_6$] duplex is shown in Figure 10.

Drawbacks in this RD 3D-QSAR analysis include not considering the isolated ligand and receptor in their respective lowest-energy conforma-

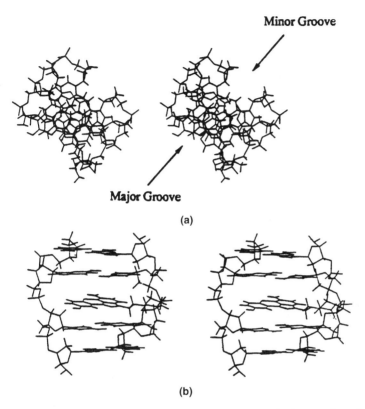

Figure 10 The "active" [BTPI ligand–(G–C)$_6$] duplex used to derive the RD 3D-QSAR, Eq. (31): (a) a top view; (b) a side view. (From Ref. 89.)

tions, and assuming the type of base pairs present in the active site. Nevertheless, this RD 3D-QSAR does consider all of the internal energy changes in Table 1, less, perhaps, solvent reorganization. No explicit entropy terms are considered, although the solvation energies used do include entropy in composite with internal energy.

B. A 3D-QSAR Based on the Intermolecular Contribution to Binding Energy

Holloway et al. [90] have established a high correlation between the intermolecular interaction energy calculated for HIV-1 protease inhibitor complexes and the observed in vitro enzyme inhibition, as measured by $-\log(IC_{50})$. A training set of 33 peptide mimetic analogue inhibitors, which differ in the P'_1 and P'_2 groups, was used to develop a regression equation that relates calculated interaction energies and $-\log(IC_{50})$ values.

Models of all inhibitors were built using the X-ray crystallographic structure of inhibitors of endothiapepsin and *Rhizopus* pepsin. The conformational flexibility of each inhibitor was "manipulated as necessary" to obtain a satisfactory fit in the X-ray crystal structure of the HIV-1 protease enzyme's active site. Inhibitor models (ligands in the enzyme's active site) were energy-minimized using the MM2X force field (developed at Merck Research Laboratories as an extension of the MM2 force field). The inhibitor was completely flexible, whereas the enzyme was completely static in the minimizations. If multiple conformational or orientational possibilities existed, the final inhibitor complex model was chosen on the basis of the lowest total energy (i.e., a balance between favorable intermolecular and intramolecular energies).

The calculated interaction energy E_{inter} is the intermolecular component of the total energy. In this study E_{inter} corresponds to the sum of the van der Waals (E_{vdw}) and electrostatic (E_{elec}) interactions between the inhibitor and the enzyme when the inhibitor is in an energy-minimized alignment and conformation in the rigid enzyme active site. The correlation between E_{inter} and $-\log(IC_{50})$ is premised on the authors' assumptions; (a) E_{inter} might be proportional to the enthalpy of binding (ΔH_{bind}), and (b) the entropy of binding (ΔS_{bind}) might be small or, more likely constant.

The RD 3D-QSAR equation derived using the L-689-502-inhibited X-ray crystal HIV-1 protease enzyme active site structure is

$$-\log(IC_{50}) = -0.16946(E_{inter}) - 15.707 \qquad (33)$$

$$N = 33; \qquad r = 0.885; \qquad xv\text{-}r^2 = 0.755$$

The RD 3D-QSAR equation was subsequently validated by successfully predicting the activity of proposed HIV-1 protease inhibitors in advance of synthesis as part of a structure-based design program.

The authors point out that their RD 3D-QSAR neglects some factors that can be key to binding, for example, (a) flexibility of the enzyme active site to accommodate different inhibitor structures; (b) the difference in enthalpic energy between the solution and bound conformations of the inhibitor and enzyme; and (c) the solvation–desolvation of the inhibitor and the enzyme, which may oppose or enhance the enzyme–inhibitor interaction. In terms of the energy contributions of Table 1, this study uses limited representations of $\Delta E_{LR}(LR)$ and $E_L(LL)$. The limitation comes from the rigid receptor constraint.

C. Comparative Binding Energy (COMBINE) Analysis

Ortiz et al. constructed RD 3D-QSARs [91] for a set of 26 inhibitors of human synovial fluid phospholipase A_2 (HSF-PLA$_2$) using a method they term comparative-binding energy (COMBINE) analysis which, as the name implies, is something of a receptor-dependent analogue method to CoMFA. For each ligand in the training set, intermolecular and intramolecular energies are calculated for the ligand–receptor complexes, the unbound ligands, and receptor, using the cff91 DISCOVER force field [92]. The goal of this aproach is to derive 3D-QSARs between experimental binding free energies (or biological activities) and a selected set of the energy terms found in Table 1. It is assumed for both the bound and the unbound species that one conformation can be chosen as representative of each respective ensemble. The conformational sampling of the reactants is limited to energy-minimized structures. Starting conformations and intermolecular alignments for each ligand were generated from related inhibitors cocrystallized with various sources of PLA$_2$ enzymes. To calculate the energy differences between bound and unbound states, the conformations of the free enzyme and the free inhibitors were modeled. The crystal structure of the free enzyme was optimized using the same protocol as that for the complexes. Conformations for the free inhibitors were determined by positioning each ligand in the local minimum nearest its conformation found in the complex and performing 1500 steps of conjugate gradient energy minimization.

The ligands are divided into fragments for the statistical analysis of the energy terms. All compounds are assigned the same number of fragments and "dummy" fragments are added to those inhibitors that lack a particular fragment. The fragments are chosen according to their spatial location in the protein-binding site, rather than by their chemical identity. The receptor is divided into regions (e.g., amino acid residues). The molecular mechanics force-field energy terms are divided into the intermolecular interaction energies between each fragment of the ligand and each region of the receptor, changes in the bonded (bond, angle, and torsion) and nonbonded (Leonard-Jones and electrostatic) energies of the ligand fragments on binding to the receptor, and the bonded and nonbonded energies of the receptor regions on binding of the ligand.

The total ligand–enzyme-binding energies correlate weakly with the experimental activities for the phospholipase training sets. However, when the PLS method, coupled to the GOLPE variable selection procedure [55], is applied to the components of the binding energies, a significant regression equation is obtained in which activity is correlated with the interaction energies of parts of the ligands and key regions of the enzyme. Wade and co-workers found that many of the energy terms included in the binding energy were not important in determining the differences in experimental activity because they were poorly correlated. One of the typical regression models derived by the COMBINE analysis contains 46 selected energy variables that seem to be responsible for most of the differences in inhibitory activity.

The COMBINE approach can be thought of as a receptor-dependent version of CoMFA, with the different regions of the receptor serving as probes for the elucidation of major interaction sites. This approach, contrary to CoMFA, does include intramolecular receptor and ligand energy contributions. The authors point out that the predictive ability of a COMBINE analysis may be enhanced by improvements in the description of the electrostatic energy term and the suitable representations of solvation and entropic effects. Approximate values of $\Delta E_{LR}(LR)$, $\Delta E_R(RR)$, $\Delta E_L(LL)$ (see Table 1) are currently considered in COMBINE.

D. De Novo Ligand Design Approaches

Several structure-based drug design methods, although not explicitly providing a 3D-QSAR equation or a procedure to compute the activity of ligands, still employ three-dimensional properties to rank potential drug candidates. These de novo ligand design algorithms are applicable when the structure of the receptor is available, and they generally involve predicting a ligand's complementarity to the receptor's active site by using a geometry or partial force–field-based scoring function. These methods are discussed elsewhere in this monograph.

IV. SUMMARY AND PERSPECTIVE

Current 3D-QSAR approaches focus on the characterization of the ligand–receptor interaction. This is true for both receptor-independent and receptor-dependent analyses. An implicit, or explicit, estimation of $\Delta E_{LR}(LR)$ of Table 1 is the primary objective. From a conceptual perspective, the ligand–receptor enthalpy interaction has become the dominant term in the binding. Hence, it is not surprising that QSAR models focus on the geometry and energetics of the ligand meeting the receptor. However, as stated by Eq. (2), and its constituent thermodynamic terms defined in Table 1, ligand–receptor binding involves many interactions besides $\Delta E_{LR}(LR)$. Available experimental data [7] suggests that every ligand–receptor system is unique relative to which binding interaction(s) may dominate the overall binding process. Thus, future method developments in 3D-QSAR analysis should explore ways to estimate and include all the thermodynamic terms in Table 1.

In particular, contributions from solvent (medium) and entropic changes realized in the binding process are largely ignored in current 3D-QSAR formalisms. A variety of solvation models are currently available, including hydration shell [15], solvent-exposed surface area [93], and explicit solvent molecule models [94]. These models can be used to estimate solvent effects on ligand–receptor binding. A major reason for not including solvation thermodynamics is the lack of reliability in making these calculations. This very real drawback cannot be ignored. However, it is still beneficial to see if the inclusion of solvation terms can enhance the quality and robustness of a 3D-QSAR.

A dramatic demonstration that entropy can play a major role in ligand–receptor binding can be gleaned from Table 4. The experimental measures of ΔH, ΔS, ΔG, and K_d are reported for a series of renin inhibitory peptides that were made and tested at Upjohn [95]. U-72407E has a much better ΔH of binding than U-72408E. Yet, both compounds have about the same ΔG and K_d measures; that is, they bind about the same to renin. The binding entropy ΔS of U-72407E is much larger than that of U-72408E, which negates the more favorable ΔH of binding of U-72407E.

Conformational entropy can be estimated from the conformational energy profile of a molecule by its partition function. Thus, in principle, the conformational entropy change after ligand–receptor binding can be computed. This translates into having an estimate of conformational entropy available in RD 3D-QSAR analyses. In practice, the estimates of entropy based on conformational or docking-space searching are only as good as the search. Most such searches are incomplete for flexible molecules.

An upper estimate of the unbound conformational entropy of both a ligand and a receptor can be made using torsion angle unit (TAU) theory [96]. These entropy estimates can, for example, be used as raw QSAR descriptors to rank and scale the relative flexibility of a set of ligands binding to a common receptor.

Some 3D-QSAR techniques or studies have considered the change in intramolecular stability $\Delta E_L(LL)$ in the overall binding process. The inclusion of $\Delta E_L(LL)$ in the development of a 3D-QSAR model appears to be largely dependent on the amount of effort given to hypothesizing an active

Table 4 Thermodynamic and Binding Parameters of Renin Inhibitory Peptides

Compound	K_d (μM)	ΔH^0 (kcal mol^{-1})	$-\Delta S^0$ (entropy units)	ΔG^0 (kcal mol^{-1})
[Leu-Val-OH]				
U-80215E	1	14.45	74.2	8.6
U-80631E	0.37	14.28	75.7	9.2
U-77646E	0.0054	28.75	131.1	11.2
U-77646E	0.013	20.33	105.5	12.4
[PheΨ[CH2NH]Phe]				
U-73777E	0.22	14.2	76.3	9.4
U-77451E	0.0025	26.7	125.3	12.2
U-71909E	0.029	13.7	78.4	10.6
[Statine]				
U-72407E	0.204	26.1	114.8	9.5
U-72408E	0.098	14.69	79.6	9.9
U-72409E	0.023	22.63	108.0	10.8
U-77455E	0.0017	21.3	108.9	12.4
[Phe-Phe]				
U-62168E	0.81	29.35	127.4	8.6
[LeuΨ[CH2NH]Val]				
U-76780E	0.008	33.56	144.3	11.3

Source: Ref. 95.

ligand conformation. We found [36] that $\Delta E_L(LL)$ is an essential descriptor for a RI 3D-QSAR model of a series of cholecystokinin A receptor antagonists.

The status of the calculation of binding constants is the topic of a very recent review [97]. Clearly, the ability to compute binding constants is intimately related to RD 3D-QSAR methodology. In fact, the limitations in being able to compute binding constants serves as a major impetus for developing RD 3D-QSARs. However, this review on binding constant calculations exposes what may be a fatal flaw in our attitude toward realizing reliable means of computing binding constants and, more generally, the thermodynamics of biomolecular processes.

This is an excellent review and perspective on protein–ligand binding. However, there are functional aspects to ligand–receptor binding not extensively covered in the perspective that include the following: (a) *Nonprotein receptor–ligand binding*: For example, the DNA intercalation binding process is less complex than protein–ligand binding relative to forcefield representation and geometric degrees of freedom. Several groups have recognized the advantages of modeling DNA intercalation binding and, in fact, some RD 3D-QSARs for intercalation processes are given in this chapter. (b) *Intermolecular modeling of synthetic polymers* [98]: Once again, interacting synthetic polymer systems are less complex than protein–ligand complexes. A considerable amount of information for estimating the complexing of synthetic polymers with one another has been generated. (c) *Statistical physics of ideal systems*: Theoretical physicists have explored the behavior of many types of interacting systems by both simulation and first-principles theory. Force fields have been developed that are accurate and provide understanding and insight on binding's free energy.

Overall, the idea of using simple model systems to probe how to calculate binding thermodynamics is not expressed in the review.

A case can be made that workers in biological applications of CAMD are "pigeon-holing" their approaches to methods development. It might be time for those CAMD scientists working in the biological sciences to look to other groups of workers, who, it can be argued, are better-trained to deal with the development of certain aspects of CAMD that are central to biological applications.

Perhaps, the most important point that can be made for validation of 3D-QSAR methods is that it should be done, and done extensively. There are an ever-increasing number of ligand–receptor systems for which an analogue series of ligands have had their respective affinities to the receptor measured, and the geometry of at least one analogue bound to the receptor is also known. Most often the measure of binding affinity is the ligand concentration necessary for a fixed biological response. However, there are also situations for which binding constants and even binding energies and entropies are available. Overall, these ligand–receptor systems constitute databases for the evaluation and the validation of both receptor-independent and receptor-dependent 3D-QSARs. It is important to remember that 3D-QSAR analysis involves not only achieving the "right" answer, but also "how much" of the right answer. A comparison of the experimental energetics and geometries of ligand–receptor systems to the corresponding calculated properties should answer the "How good?" and "How much?" validation questions. Moreover, these validation comparisons to multiple ligand–receptor databases should delineate the relative strengths of a given 3D-QSAR approach in general applications. Table 3 may illustrate a prototype example to validation and applicability.

To end on a positive note, evolutionary algorithms along with partial least-square techniques hold great promise for finding the optimal 3D-QSAR models in highly oversubscribed descriptor spaces. That is, the benefit of generating vast numbers of potential descriptors from three-dimensional computational chemistry calculations no longer becomes a liability in the statistical correlation phase of 3D-QSAR model development. CoMFA, molecular similarity matrix analysis, and the use of genetic algorithms in MSA [45] demonstrate the emerging potentials of the new statistical analysis tools.

REFERENCES

1. H. Kubinyi, ed., *3D-QSAR in Drug Design: Theory, Methods and Applications*, ESCOM Science, Leiden, 1993.
2. R. D. Cloney, I. J. King, V. M. Scherr, and A. J. Forgash, *Molecular and Quantum Pharmocology* (E. Bergmann and B. Pullman, eds.), D. Reidel Publishing, Dordrecht, 1974, p. 333.
3. A. J. Hopfinger, Y. Nakata, and N. Max, Quantitative structure–activity relationships of anthracycline antitumor activity and cardiac toxicity based upon intercalation calculations, *Intermolecular Forces* (B. Pullman, ed.), D. Reidel Publishing, Dordrecht, 1981, p. 431.
4. C. Dias Selassie and T. E. Klein, Building bridges: QSAR and molecular graphics, *3D-QSAR in Drug Design: Theory, Methods and Applications* (H. Kubinyi, ed.), ESCOM Science, Leiden, 1993, p. 257.
5. A. J. Hopfinger, M. G. Koehler, R. A. Pearlstein, and S. K. Tripathy, *J. Polym. Sci.* Part B: *Polym. Phys.* 26:2007 (1988).
6. (a) Y. C. Martin, C. T. Lin, and J. Wu, Application of CoMFA to D1 dopaminergic agonists: a case study, *3D-QSAR in Drug Design: Theory, Methods and Applications* (H. Kubinyi, ed.), ESCOM Science, Leiden, 1993, p. 643; (b) K. H. Kim and Y. C. Martin, Direct prediction of dissociation constants (pK_a's) of clonidine-like imidazolines, 2-substituted imidazoles, and 1-methyl-2-substituted-imidazoles from 3D structures using a comparative molecular field analysis (CoMFA) approach, *J. Med. Chem.* 34:2056 (1991).
7. M. C. Chervenak and E. J. Toone, A direct measure of the contribution of solvent reorganization to the enthalpy of ligand binding, *J. Am. Chem. Soc.* 116:10533 (1994).
8. R. D. Cramer, D. E. Patterson, and J. D. Bunce, Comparative molecular field analysis (CoMFA). 1. Effect of shape on binding of steroids to carrier proteins, *J. Am. Chem. Soc.* 110:5959 (1988).
9. U. Thibuat, Application of CoMFA and related 3D QSAR approaches, *3D-QSAR in Drug Design: Theory, Methods and Applications* (H. Kubinyi, ed.), ESCOM Science, Leiden, 1993, p. 661.
10. S. Wold, C. Albano, W. J. Dunn III, U. Edlund, K. Esbensen, P. Geladi, S. Hellberg, E. Johansson, W. Lindberg, and M. Sjöström, Multivariate data analysis in chemistry, *Chemometrics: Mathematics and Statistics in Chemistry* (B. R. Kowalski, ed.), D. Reidel, Dordrecht, 1987, p. 17.
11. R. D. Cramer III, J. D. Bunce, and D. E. Patterson, Crossvalidation, bookstrapping, and partial least squares compared with multiple regression in conventional QSAR studies, *Quant. Struct. Act. Relat.* 7:18 (1988).

12. M. C. Nicklaus, G. W. A. Milne, and T. R. Burke, QSAR of conformationally flexible molecules: comparative molecular field analysis of protein–tyrosine kinase inhibitors, *J. Comput. Aided Mol. Design 6*:487 (1992).

13. F. C. Wirecka, G. E. Kellogg, and D. J. Abraham, Allosteric modifiers of hemoglobin. 2. Crystallographically determined binding sites and hydrophobic binding/interaction analysis of novel hemoglobin oxygen effectors, *J. Med. Chem. 34*:758 (1991).

14. S. J. Cho and A. Tropsha, Cross-validated R^2-guided region selection for comparative molecular field analysis: a simple method to achieve consistent results, *J. Med. Chem. 38*:1060 (1995).

15. A. J. Hopfinger, *Conformational Properties of Macromolecules*, Academic Press, New York, 1973.

16. S. W. Weiner, P. A. Kollman, D. A. Case, U. C. Singh, C. Ghio, G. Alagona, S. Profeta, and P. Weiner, *J. Am. Chem. Soc. 106*:765 (1984).

17. A. J. Hopfinger, A QSAR investigation of dihydrofolate reductase inhibition by baker triazines based upon molecular shape analysis, *J. Am. Chem. Soc. 120*:7196 (1980).

18. S. H. Ungar, Whither QSAR? Wither QSAR?, *QSAR in Design of Bioactive Compounds* (K. Kuchar, ed.), J. R. Prous, Barcelona, 1984, p. 1.

19. A. J. Hopfinger, Inhibition of dihydrofolate reductase: structure activity correlations of 2,4-diamino 5-benzyl pyrimidines based upon molecular shape analysis, *J. Med. Chem. 24*:818 (1981).

20. A. J. Hopfinger, A general QSAR for dihydrofolate reductase inhibition by 2,4-diaminotriazines based upon molecular shape analysis, *Arch. Biochem. Biophys. 206*:153 (1981).

21. C. Battershell, d. Malhotra, and A. J. Hopfinger, Inhibition of dihydrofolate reductase: structure activity correlations of 2,4-diaminoquinazolines based upon molecular shape analysis, *J. Med. Chem. 24*:812 (1981).

22. A. J. Hopfinger and R. Potenzone, Jr., Ames test and antitumor activity of 1-(*X*-phenyl)-3,3-dialkyltriazenes, a quantitative structure–activity study based upon molecular shape analysis, *Mol. Pharm. 21*:187 (1982).

23. S. N. Mohammad, D. R. Bickers, and A. J. Hopfinger, Intrinsic mutagenicity of polycyclic aromatic hydrocarbons: a quantitative structure activity study based upon molecular shape analysis, *J. Theor. Biol. 102*:323 (1983).

24. M. Mabilia, R. A. Pearlstein, and A. J. Hopfinger, Molecular shape analysis using molecular graphics, *Molecular Graphics and Drug Design* (A. S. V. Burgen, G. C. K. Roberts, and M. S. Tute, eds.), Elsevier, Amsterdam, 1986, p. 158.

25. D. E. Walters and A. J. Hopfinger, Case studies of the application of molecular shape analysis to elucidate drug action, *J. Mol. Struct. (Theochem.) 134*:317 (1986).

26. R. L. Lopez de Compadre, R. A. Pearlstein, A. J. Hopfinger, and J. K. Seydel, A QSAR analysis of 4-aminodiphenylsulfone antibacterial agents using three-dimensional molecular modeling, *J. Med. Chem. 30*:900 (1987).

27. R. L. Lopez de Compadre, M. Koehler, S. Emery, A. J. Hopfinger, and J. K. Seydel, An extended QSAR analysis of some 4-aminodiphenylsulfone antibacterial agents using molecular modeling, *J. Quant. Struct. Act. Relat.* 6:111 (1987).

28. A. J. Hopfinger, Theory and application of molecular potential energy fields in molecular shape analysis: a QSAR study of 2,4-diamino-5-benzylpyrimidines as dihydrofolate reductase inhibitors, *J. Med. Chem.* 26:990 (1983).

29. A. J. Hopfinger, A QSAR study of the Ames mutagenicity of 1-(*X*-phenyl)-3,3-dialkyltriazenes using molecular potential energy fields and molecular shape analysis, *J. Quant. Struct. Act. Relat.* 3:1 (1984).

30. A. J. Hopfinger and B. J. Burke, Molecular shape analysis: a formalism to quantitatively establish spatial molecular similarity, *Concepts and Applications of Molecular Similarity* (M. A. Johnson and G. A. Maggiora, eds.), John Wiley & Sons, New York, 1990, p. 173.

31. B. J. Burke, Developments in molecular shape analysis to establish spatial molecular similarity among flexible molecules, Ph.D. Thesis, Department of Medicinal Chemistry and Pharmacognosy, University of Illinois at Chicago (1992).

32. (a) A. E. Howard and P. A. Kollman, An analysis of current methodologies for conformational searching of complex molecules, *J. Med. Chem.* 31:1669 (1988); (b) A. R. Leach, A survey of methods for searching the conformational space of small and medium-sized molecules, *Rev. Comput. Chem.* 2:1 (1991).

33. M. G. Koehler, K. L. Rowberg-Schaefer, and A. J. Hopfinger, A molecular shape analysis and quantitative structure–activity relationship investigation of some triazine–antifolate inhibitors of *Leishmania major* dihydrofolate reductase, *Arch. Biochem. Biophys.* 266:152 (1988).

34. A. J. Hopfinger, B. J. Burke, and W. J. Dunn III, A generalized formalism of three-dimensional quantitative structure–property relationship analysis for flexible molecules using tensor representation, *J. Med. Chem.* 37:3768 (1994).

35. B. J. Burker, W. J. Dunn III, and A. J. Hopfinger, Construction of a molecular shape analysis–dimensional quantitative structure–activity relationship for an analog series of pyridobenzodiazepinone inhibitors of muscarinic 2 and 3 receptors, *J. Med. Chem.* 37:3775 (1994).

36. J. S. Tokarski and A. J. Hopfinger, Three-dimensional molecular shape analysis–quantitative structure–activity relationship of a series of cholecystokinin-A receptor antagonists, *J. Med. Chem.* 37:3639 (1994).

37. M. S. Searle, M. J. Forster, B. Birdall, G. C. K. Roberts, J. Feeney, H. T. A. Cheung, I. Kompis, and A. J. Geddes, Dynamics of trimethoprim bound to dihydrofolate reductase, *Proc. Natl. Acad. Sci. USA* 85:3787 (1988).

38. W. J. Dunn III, A. J. Hopfinger, C. Catana, and C. Duraiswami, Solution of the conformation and alignment tensors for the binding of trimethoprim and its analogs to dihydrofolate reductase: 3D-quantitative structure-activity rela-

tionship study using molecular shape analysis, 3-way partial least squares regression, and 3-way factor analysis. *J. Med. Chem. 39*:4825 (1996).

39. R. Franke, *Theoretical Drug Design Methods*, Akademie-Verlag, Berlin (1984).

40. Y. C. Martin, A practitioner's perspective of the role of quantitative structure–activity analysis in medicinal chemistry, *J. Med. Chem. 24*:229 (1981).

41. P. P. Mager, *Multidimensional pharmacochemistry*, Academic Press, New York, 1984.

42. N. R. Draper and H. Smith, *Applied Regression Analysis*, John Wiley & Sons, New York, 1966.

43. J. Holland, *Adaptation in Artificial and Natural Systems*, University of Michigan Press, Ann Arbor MI, 1975.

44. D. Rogers, G/Splines: A hybrid of Freidman's multivariate adaptive regression splines (MARS) algorithm with Holland's genetic algorithm, *The Proceedings of the Fourth International Conference on Genetic Algorithms*, San Diego, July 1991.

45. D. Rogers and A. J. Hopfinger, Application of genetic function approximation to quantitative structure–activity relationships and quantitative structure–property relationships, *J. Med. Chem. 34*:854 (1994).

46. A. C. Good, S. So, and W. G. Richards, Structure–activity relationships from molecular similarity matrices, *J. Med. Chem. 36*:433 (1993).

47. A. C. Good, S. J. Peterson, and W. B. Richards, QSAR's from similarity matrices. Technique validation and application in the comparison of different similarity evaluation methods, *J. Med. Chem. 36*:2929 (1993).

48. R. Carbo, L. Leyda, and M. Arnau, How similar is a molecule to another? An electron density measure of similarity between two molecular structures, *Int. J. Quantum Chem. 17*:1185 (1980).

49. R. Carbo and B. Calabuig, Molecular similarity and quantum chemistry, *Concepts Applied Molecular Similarity* (M. A. Johnson and G. M. Maggiora, eds.), John Wiley & Sons, New York, 1990, p. 147.

50. Oxford Molecular Ltd., The Magdalen Centre, Oxford Science Park, Sanford on Thames, Oxford OX4 4GA, UK.

51. A. M. Meyer and W. G. Richards, Similarity of molecular shape, *J. Comput. Aid. Mol. Design 5*:426 (1991).

52. E. E. Hodgkin and W. G. Richards, Molecular similarity based on electrostatic potential and electric field, *Int. J. Quantum Chem. Quantum Biol. Symp. 14*: 105 (1987).

53. A. C. Good, The calculation of molecular similarity: alternative formulas, data manipulation and graphical display, *J. Mol. Graphics 10*:144 (1992).

54. M. Manaut, F. Sanz, J. Jose, and M. Milesi, Automatic search for maximum similarity between molecular electrostatic potential distributions, *J. Comput. Aid. Mol. Design 5*:371 (1991).

55. M. Baroni, G. Constantino, G. Cruciani, D. Riganelli, R. Valigi, and S. Clementi, GOLPE: an advanced chemometric tool for 3D-QSAR problems, *Quant. Struct. Act. Relat. 12*:9 (1993).

56. T. J. Mitchell, An algorithm for the construction of D-optimal experimental designs, *Technometrics 16*:203 (1974).

57. G. E. Box, W. G. Hunter, and J. S. Hunter, *Statistics for Experimenters*, John Wiley & Sons, New York, 1978, Chap. 12.

58. H. B. Weinstein, Z. Apfelderfer, S. Cohen, S. Maayani, and M. Sokolovsky, Molecular orbital studies on the conformation of pharmacological and medicinal compounds, *The Jerusalem Symposia on Quantum Chemistry and Biochemistry*, Vol. V: *Conformation of Biological Molecules and Polymers* (E. D. Bergmann and B. Pullman, eds.), Academic Press, New York, 1973, p. 531.

59. L. B. Kier, *Molecular Orbital Theory in Drug Research*, Academic Press, New York, 1971.

60. G. M. Crippen, Distance geometry analysis of the benzodiazepine binding site, *Mol. Pharm. 22*:11 (1982).

61. R. P. Sheridan, R. Nilakantan, J. S. Dixon, and R. Venkataraghavan, The ensemble approach to distance geometry: application to the nicotinic pharmacophore, *J. Med. Chem. 29*:899 (1986).

62. A. K. Ghose and G. M. Crippen, Use of physicochemical parameters in distance geometry and related three-dimensional quantitative structure–activity relationships: a demonstration using *Eschericha coli* dihydrofolate reductase inhibitors, *J. Med. Chem. 28*:333 (1985).

63. A. K. Ghose, G. M. Crippen, G. Revankar, P. McKernan, D. Smee, and R. Robins, Analysis of the in vitro activity of certain ribonucleosides against parainfluenza virus using a novel computer-aided molecular modeling procedure, *J. Med. Chem. 32*:746 (1989).

64. G. M. Crippen, Voronoi binding site models, *J. Comput. Chem. 8*:943 (1987).

65. A. M. Doweyko, The hypothetical active site lattice. An approach to modelling active sites from data on inhibitor molecules, *J. Med. Chem. 31*:1396 (1988).

66. A. M. Doweyko, New tool for the study of structure–activity relationships in three-dimensions, *Probing Bioactive Mechanisms* (P. Magee, D. R. Henry, and J. H. Block, eds.) *ACS Symp. Ser. 413*:82 (1989).

67. A. M. Doweyko and W. M. Mattes, An application of 3D-QSAR to the analysis of the sequence specificity of DNA alkylation by uracil mustard, *Biochemistry 31*:9388 (1992).

68. A. M. Doweyko, Three-dimensional pharmacophores from binding data, *J. Med. Chem. 37*:1769 (1994).

69. D. E. Walters and R. M. Hinds, Genetically evolved receptor models: a computational approach to construction of receptor models, *J. Med. Chem. 37*: 2527 (1994).

70. S. Wang, G. W. A. Milne, M. C. Nicklaus, V. E. Marquez, J. Lee, and P. M. Blumberg, Protein kinase C. Modeling of the binding site and prediction of binding constants, *J. Med. Chem. 37*:1326 (1994).

71. R. R. Rando and Y. Kishi, Structural basis of protein kinase C activation by diacylglycerols and tumor promoters, *Biochemistry 31*:2211 (1992).

72. J. J. P. Stewart, Optimization of parameters for semiemperical methods, *J. Comput. Chem. 10*:209 (1989).

73. G. Klopman, S. Wang, and D. M. Balthasar, Estimation of aqueous solubility of organic molecules by the group contribution approach. Application to the study of biodegradation, *J. Chem. Inf. Comput. Sci. 32*:474 (1992).

74. A. N. Jain, K. Koile, and D. Chapman, Compass: predicting biological activities for molecular surface properties. Performance comparisons on a steroid benchmark, *J. Med. Chem. 37*:2315 (1994).

75. A. N. Jain, N. L. Harris, and J. Y. Park, Quantitative binding site model generation: compass applied to multiple chemotypes targeting 5-HT_{1a} receptor, *J. Med. Chem. 38*:1295 (1995).

76. P. J. Goodford, A computational procedure for determining energetically favorable binding sites on biologically important macromolecules, *J. Med. Chem. 28*:849 (1985).

77. A. M. Davis, N. P. Gensmantel, E. Johansson, and D. P. Marriott, The use of the GRID program in the 3-D QSAR analysis of a series of calcium-channel agonists, *J. Med. Chem. 37*:963 (1994).

78. MEDCHEM, version 3.54; Daylight CIS: USA, 1993.

79. SIMCA 4.4; developed and distributed by Umetri AB, Umea, Sweden.

80. CATALYST, Biosyn/MSI, Inc., San Diego CA (1995).

81. M. W. Miller, U.S. Patent 3,905,971, Sept. 16, 1975.

82. J. W. McFarland, C. B. Cooper, and D. M. Newcomb, Linear discriminant and multiple regression analyses of anticoccidial triazines, *J. Med. Chem. 34*: 1908 (1991).

83. J. W. McFarland, Comparative molecular field analysis of anticoccidial triazines *J. Med. Chem. 35*:2543 (1992).

84. K.-B. Rhyu, H. C. Patel, and A. J. Hopfinger, A 3D-QSAR study of anticoccidial triazines using molecular shape analysis, *J. Chem. Inf. Comput. Sci. 35*: 771 (1995).

85. A. J. Hopfinger, M. G. Cardozo, and Y. Kawakami, Construction of quantitative structure–activity relationships (QSARs) from ligand–DNA molecular modeling studies, *Nucleic Acid Targeted Drug Design* (C. L. Propst and T. J. Perun, eds.), Marcel Dekker, New York, 1992, p. 151.

86. Y. Nakata and A. J. Hopfinger, *Biochem. Biophys. Res. Commun. 95*:583 (1980).

87. G. J. Quigley, A. H.-J. Wang, G. Ughetto, G. Van der Marel, J. H. Van Boom, and A. Rich, *Proc. Natl. Acad. Sci. USA 77*:7204 (1980).

88. (a) J. W. Lown, ed., *Anthracycline and Anthracenedione-Based Anticancer Agents*, Elsevier, Amsterdam, 1988; (b) L. P. G. Wakelin, *Med. Res. Rev. 6*: 275 (1986).

89. A. J. Hopfinger and Y. Kawakami, QSAR analysis of a set of benzothiopyranoindazole anti-cancer analogs based upon their DNA intercalation properties as determined by molecular dynamics simulation, *Anti-cancer Drug-Design* *7*:103 (1992).

90. M. K. Holloway, J. M. Wai, T. A. Halgren, P. M. D. Fitzgerald, J. P. Vacca, B. D. Dorsey, R. B. Levin, W. J. Thompson, L. J. Chen, S. J. DeSolms, N. Gaffin, A. K. Ghosh, E. A. Giuliani, S. L. Graham, J. P. Guare, R. W. Hungate, T. A. Lyle, W. M. Sanders, T. J. Tucker, M. Wiggins, C. M. Wiscount, O. W. Woltersdorf, S. D. Young, P. L. Darke, and J. A. Zugay, A priori prediction of activity for HIV-1 protease inhibitors employing energy minimization in the active site, *J. Med. Chem.* *38*:305 (1995).

91. A. R. Ortiz, M. T. Pisabarro, F. Gago, and R. C. Wade, Prediction of drug binding affinities by comparative binding energy analysis, *J. Med. Chem.* *38*: 2681 (1995).

92. J. R. Maples, U. Dinur, and A. T. Hagler, Derivation of force fields for molecular mechanics and dynamics from *ab initio* energy surfaces, *Proc. Natl. Acad. Sci. USA* *85*:5350 (1988).

93. D. Eisenberg and A. D. McLachlan, Solvation energy in protein folding and binding, *Nature* *319*:199 (1986).

94. G. Ciccotti and W. G. Hoover, eds., *Molecular Dynamics Simulation of Statistical Mechanical Systems*, North-Holland, Amsterdam, 1986.

95. D. E. Epps, J. Cheney, H. Schostarez, T. K. Sawyer, M. Prairie, W. C. Krueger, and F. Mandel, Thermodynamics of the interaction of inhibitors with the binding site of recombinant human renin, *J. Med. Chem.* *33*:2080 (1990).

96. M. G. Koehler and A. J. Hopfinger, Molecular modelling of polymers: 5. Inclusion of intermolecular energetics in estimating glass and crystal-melt transition temperatures, *Polymer* *30*:116 (1989).

97. Ajay and M. A. Murcko, Computational methods to predict binding free energy in ligand–receptor complexes, *J. Med. Chem.* *38*:4953 (1995).

98. Special issue on prediction of polymer form and properties, *J. Chem. Soc. Faraday Trans.* *91*:2355 (1995).

5

Computational Approaches to Chemical Libraries

David C. Spellmeyer, Jeffrey M. Blaney, and Eric Martin
Chiron Corporation, Emeryville, California

I. INTRODUCTION

A general rule of thumb in the pharmaceutical industry holds that one must screen 10,000 chemicals to find 1 that is a drug candidate. Although this is a large number of compounds, the chance of finding a drug—a compound approved by the US Food and Drug Administration (FDA) for a specific therapeutic use—is probably much lower. One source has said, "The odds of success are so low that oil wildcatters have a 'sure thing' by comparison" [1].

For decades, pharmaceutical companies have kept a permanent record of the compounds they have synthesized. These archives have often been screened as a method to improve their chances of discovering a novel, proprietary lead compound. Even though this often is an expensive and time-consuming proposition, several pharmaceuticals on the market today have derived from screening an in-house supply of compounds. Recently developed computational technologies, such as clustering [2], docking [3–5], and three-dimensional (3D) searching [6,7] have been applied to corporate databases as "filters" to lower the cost of screening and to improve the "hit" rate. This has been accompanied by advances in biological-screening technologies, which now make it possible to screen hundreds of thousands of compounds in a relatively short time period.

Companies are aware of the limitations inherent in their own archives. Often, no lead compounds are discovered after screening all the compounds in the archive. Therefore, it is often desirable to supplement the in-house database with compounds purchased from external sources [8]. The same computational selection tools used to filter databases are now being used to evaluate the "diversity" of a library and to fill "holes" in the corporate archives, or to substitute similar compounds that have been depleted over time.

This has become even more critical with the advent of combinatorial chemistry. Chemists are now able to synthesize thousands of compounds in weeks to months [9–12]. Combinatorial libraries require careful design before synthesis to ensure that the diversity of the corporate library is being expanded appropriately by new combinatorial syntheses. In fact, issues similar to the ranking or selection of compounds for screening are salient to library design of combinatorial experiments. Nearly every major pharmaceutical company has an active and growing combinatorial chemistry program that will provide more new compounds each year than are in the corporate archives today.

Innovative computational approaches are required to store and analyze the rapidly expanding amounts of chemical and biological data produced as a result of these advances. Recent reviews have covered the use of two-dimensional (2D) chemical databases [7,13,14]. Other chapters in this book present the generation and uses of 3D databases and pharmacophore mapping for drug discovery. Another chapter in this book describes the structure-based design approaches to "filtering" a chemical library. Therefore, this chapter will primarily address the use of chemical databases as a research tool for the experimental design of compound sets for screening. We will compare the approaches taken for the selective screening of corporate databases with combinatorial library design techniques. Finally, we will mention several uses of databases as tools for lead discovery, some of which touch on areas presented in much more detail in other chapters of this book.

II. BACKGROUND

In discussions that follow, we will refer to a *chemical library* as the physical collection of chemicals residing in bottles or tubes and sitting on a shelf. This is to be distinguished from the electronic compilation of the chemical structures of the physical collection, which we will refer to as a *database*.

Although many types of chemical libraries exist, it is often only the corporate library of individual compounds that is cataloged electronically. For instance, natural product libraries are the physical collection of the substances extracted from plant or marine extracts [15], from fermentation broths, or from biosynthetic manipulation of a species [16]. Because very few of these compounds have been identified, the vast majority of the chemical diversity in these types of libraries is unknown; hence, they are not cataloged, or are inadequately cataloged. Nonetheless, a significant amount of information does exist in corporate databases, and calculations can and have been quite successful in exploiting these databases for lead discovery and optimization.

The *corporate library* is the physical collection of all of the compounds that have been synthesized, characterized, and cataloged. In an effort to increase the structural diversity of the libraries and the chance that a hit will be discovered in broad screening, these libraries often include all the intended synthetic targets, plus the intermediates identified on the reaction sequence to a final product. Usually these materials have been purified and characterized before storage in the database. The size of corporate libraries varies, but is typically in the range of 50,000–500,000 compounds. Often, the number of readily available samples is lower than this as a result of sample depletion or degradation. Many of the compounds in a corporate library are closely related, the result of synthesizing hundreds to thousands of analogues in an active lead optimization program.

Unfortunately, the terminology in combinatorial chemistry is a bit less clear. A *combinatorial library* can refer to the physical collection of the vials containing the compounds that are thought to have been synthesized during a single combinatorial synthesis experiment. Likewise, the collection of several combinatorial libraries can also be termed a "library" in a manner akin to that just described.

A *corporate database* is an electronic representation of the compounds in the corporate library. Corporate databases typically include a two-dimensional structure of all of the compounds in the physical collection, the associated physical data on the compounds, and the biological data of the compounds. Over the last few decades, a variety of methods and tools have been developed to compile these libraries and databases. Bures et al. provide a good review of the representations and searching methods for 2D databases [7].

High-throughput screening of corporate archives has resulted in the discovery of potent lead compounds [17–19]. However, screening 500,000 individual compounds in a large number of assays can be expensive and time-consuming, and can lead to depletion of valuable chemical samples. Therefore, novel computational methods have been developed to decrease the number of compounds screened in broad-screening programs.

A common method is to "cluster" the corporate database to identify very similar compounds as a group [2]. Only one or two compounds from each of these clusters are then screened in the broad-screening program. This enhances the chances of finding an active compound by maximizing the diversity of the subset of compounds screened, while screening only a fraction of the number of compounds. The analysis required to cluster the corporate database can also be used to select compounds from external sources. One can augment the corporate database with compounds that contain features not present in the in-house collection.

Finally, the generation and storage of 3D coordinates for each of the compounds in the database has permitted 3D searching of corporate databases. One can rapidly search for the known pharmacophore of a receptor or enzyme, or even dock the 3D structures into the active site of a protein. The construction and application of 3D databases has been reviewed previously [7,20]. More recent work is covered in another chapter in this book.

Recent advances in combinatorial synthetic approaches facilitate the rapid extension of the corporate library. A wide variety of methods have been developed for combinatorial synthesis of chemical libraries. The development of these methods has been enhanced by the development of solid-phase chemistry techniques previously limited to peptide and oligo-nucleotide chemistries. Many types of reactions now are routinely carried out on the solid phase. Several excellent reviews include detailed descriptions of the benefits and disadvantages of many of these methods [9–12].

The choice of synthetic approaches to combinatorial chemistry is affected by the manner in which the compounds will be screened. One approach is to synthesize and screen compounds as combinatorial mixtures in which the compounds have been cleaved from a suitable resin and are free in solution. This method requires an iterative synthetic deconvolution scheme or an affinity selection process that can identify the compound with biological activity [21,22]. It assumes that one is able to successfully reproduce the chemistry used to generate the library. The tradeoff is that many thousands of compounds can be screened simultaneously. A second, closely related approach is to synthesize the combinatorial library as a mixture, and to screen those while they are still attached to the resin [23–26]. This approach requires a method to identify the resin particle that contains the active compound. This method does not require resynthesis. One must be concerned that the presence of the resin particle might result in a false-negative result. This can be avoided through the use of a partial-cleavage method [27]. A third approach is most similar to the traditional approach to medicinal chemistry. In this approach, one synthesizes and tests combinatorial libraries as individual compounds, either attached to or cleaved from the resin [10–12]. This approach saves the step of identification at the tradeoff of many thousands of additional biological screens.

Combinatorial chemical approaches offer advantages to the single-compound approach employed for years; however, there are some distinct difficulties inherent to this approach. Two examples are incomplete data and the vast amount of negative data obtained in a combinatorial experiment.

Often, a diversity experiment produces *incomplete data*. This can take several forms: In a mixture-based approach, there is no reliable analytical method to characterize an entire library. Thus, one is not absolutely certain that the compounds present in each mixture are actually the compounds that were intended owing to failure of reactions to reach completion or other causes. Also, the mixtures tested might not be equimolar, which could result in misleading data. In a single-compound parallel approach, there are likely insufficient analytical resources to characterize each compound. Thus, analysis can be performed on only a random sampling of the compounds synthesized. The synthesis of an active component of a library might fail and pass unnoticed in the analytical stage. Another example of incomplete data could be differential solubilities of related compounds: an active compound might not be soluble; hence, it would be missed.

The presence of *negative data*—compounds that show little or no activity on a biological target—is common to the industry. In combinatorial chemistry, the assumption can be made that if a mixture of compounds is inactive, then all of the compounds in that pool are inactive. Because libraries are frequently designed to have a modest hit rate, a tremendous amount of negative data is generated by combinatorial experiments. The challenge of how to exploit this data remains unsolved: inactive compounds provide information about the receptor and the subset of diversity space required to bind to the receptor, but this negative data is very indirect and much harder to use than positive data on active compounds. Imagine trying to describe a person's face well enough to pick it out of a crowd by what it does not look like, rather than by describing faces that are similar.

The goal of screening is to find one or more interesting active compounds with minimal time and effort. Automated high-throughput screening (HTS) and the screening of compound mixtures are two ways to increase the number of compounds screened. However, either of these methods increases the likelihood of screening errors. Errors take the form of either false-negative or false-positive results. In HTS of corporate archives, false-positive hits are a nuisance because they waste some time in follow-up experiments. False-negative hits, however, can be disastrous because the archive is a fixed resource. After screening the entire archive, if no leads have been found, the project is often finished and has failed. Thus, HTS programs are usually balanced to minimize the number of false-negative hits and to tolerate only a few false-positive ones. Because screening complex mixtures (more than 50 compounds) can increase the number of false-negative results, most companies choose to screen only very small mixtures (fewer than 50 compounds) or individual compounds.

However, screening combinatorial libraries differs from screening the individual compounds in a corporate archive because the chemical resource is no longer fixed: regardless of the synthetic approach, large numbers of new compounds can be produced, usually at higher and higher rates. Combinatorial libraries synthesized using a mixture approach offer an advantage over combinatorial libraries synthesized using an individual compound approach. First, mixtures greatly increase the number of available compounds, because the HTS hit rate is roughly proportional to the number of compounds screened; thus, synthesizing mixtures of 100 compounds allows one to make and screen 100 times more compounds. Even a 50% false-negative rate would still yield 50 times more leads. Although leads might be made and missed because of the false negative hits, that is more than compensated for by the large number of additional hits that otherwise would not have been made at all. With this many hits, the bottleneck to identification of an individual compound can be the synthetic deconvolution step. Thus, false-positives are now a greater problem than false-negatives. Short cuts, such as affinity selection, high-performance liquid chromatographic fractionation, or tagging methods, enable one to avoid spending significant amounts of time and resources on synthetic deconvolutions.

III. COMPUTATIONAL USES OF CORPORATE DATABASES IN LEAD DISCOVERY

A solely archival corporate database would be useless. One wishes to use the chemical structures and biological data to provide new active compounds faster than one would do by random choices. One can use computational methods to mine databases in a variety of ways. The result of such an endeavor is to synthesize and test novel compounds, either as individual compounds, or as a combinatorial library, or to prioritize the corporate archive for high-throughput screening. Regardless, there is a limit to the number of compounds one can make and test. Given this limited "budget," what does one choose? The choice of technique often depends on the nature of the target under study and the amount of information already known about that target.

Pharmaceutical research is driven by novel biological targets, about which little or nothing is known about the target or the ligands. In these situations, no structural information about the target is known, there are no ligands other than the endogenous ligand, and no correlation can be made with other systems in which more information is known. In this event, a broad-screening approach is desired in which one would minimize redundancy by choosing a diverse set of compounds for screening. In choosing the compounds from a corporate archive, one might use a clustering algorithm on the chemical structures and choose a member of each cluster for screening. In a combinatorial library, the library could be designed using an experimental design approach to choose the most diverse components. In either, one would ensure that as large a net had been cast as possible, and that the largest property space has been sampled for the given budget of molecules. This does not guarantee a lead, but does increase the chance of success.

A structure-based design approach is useful when a crystal structure of the target is known. Here, one can dock each member of a corporate database into the active site of a protein and rank-order the archive based on the goodness of the fit with the enzyme [5]. A combinatorial library design using a crystal structure could entail docking each potential reagent into the active site and biasing the library to those fragments [28]. Either way the likelihood for success is increased. There are now many examples of structure-based design of novel compounds, notably human immunodeficiency virus (HIV) protease inhibitors [29] and glycoprotein IIb/IIIa inhibitors [30,31].

One might know only a little about a specific target, but a great deal about a related biological target. It is possible to incorporate this information into the choice of molecules to screen. SmithKline Beecham's recent discovery of an endothelin receptor antagonist highlights the use of corporate databases in such an approach [19]. Little information about the endothelin receptors was known, other than that they are members of the 7-transmembrane–G protein-coupled receptor family. The vast amount of information available on ligands to other 7-transmembrane–G protein-coupled receptors (7TM/GPCRs) was used to hypothesize a pharmacophore for the endogenous peptide. The corporate database was scored based on similarity to ligands for the other 7TM/GPCRs and screened. This resulted in a lead compound with an affinity of about 1 μM, which was readily analogued to a compound with subnanomolar affinity.

A combinatorial library design might be biased toward pharmacophores from a known class of receptors. For example, workers from Chiron designed an *N*-substituted glycine combinatorial library that contained fragments known to be important to 7TM/GPCRs [22]. These workers chose to synthesize a small library (fewer than 5000 compounds) in which each compound contained at least one alcohol moiety and one aromatic moiety. Three alcohol fragments were chosen, two aliphatic and one aromatic. Four aromatic groups were chosen because they are important in central nervous system (CNS)-active compounds. The remaining library components were chosen to be as diverse as possible. They were able to identify ligands to two different receptors: CHIR-2279 binds to the α_1-adrenergic receptor with an affinity of 5 nM, and CHIR-4531 binds to the μ-opiate receptor with an affinity of 6 nM.

Finally, different computational approaches are taken when one is selecting compounds for screening and when one forms analogues from known hit compounds. When forming analogues, one can use the extensive quantitative structure–activity relation (QSAR) methods, developed over the last 30 years, to help guide the choice of compounds synthesized. Corporate databases can be screened for compounds that are similar to a known lead, thereby quickly gaining information about related compounds. Combinatorial approaches can also be used to form analogues. One could switch from the mixture approach to the single compound approach, in which each individual compound is chosen according to experimental design methods. One could also make mixtures of compounds with functionality similar to the hit compound(s). It is likely, however, that many of the pools will be active, and a rapid method of deconvolution or compound identification will be required.

We will discuss some of the underlying assumptions, techniques, and applications used in these examples.

A. What Does "Diverse" Mean?

We stated earlier that one wants diverse libraries for broad screening and similar compounds for lead optimization. Working definitions of these terms would be advantageous. Webster's dictionary defines *diverse* as "differing from one another" and *similar* as "having characteristics in common." The computational definition of *diverse* is a set of compounds that have properties that differ from one another. Conversely, a *similar* set of compounds would have properties that are very much alike. A set of diverse compounds would then be a set of compounds that are dissimilar to each other and to all other members of the set.

However, this leaves us with the problem of defining what similar means and how to define and determine the properties that we would use for our measure of similarity. As one might expect, a host of methods have been developed for defining molecular properties and similarity measures. Different properties may be relevant for different receptors. The notion of a universal set of properties or descriptors is undoubtedly naive.

B. Molecular Properties and Similarity Measures

One would like to define a similarity measure with these characteristics: (a) it should be easy to compute; (b) for a given biological target, it can produce high-similarity scores for compounds with comparable biological activity; and (c) it can produce low-similarity scores between compounds with differing biological activity.

Biological activity is impossible to calculate a priori, so we must assume that we can reconstruct the biological activity as a linear combination of some molecular properties. Thus, our similarity measure becomes a function of calculable molecular properties. We would like the similarity measure to include properties that are important for biological activity, such as molecular shape, molecular weight, or metabolic stability. Other properties, such as the geometric arrangement of the atoms in the molecules, the atom types, hydrogen-bonding capabilities, aromatic centers, lipophilic centers, electronic properties, and flexibility, should also be included. This is identical with the linear free-energy relation that is the underpinning of QSAR approaches. Unfortunately, many of these properties are difficult to define, let alone to calculate.

Oral bioavailability is one of the most desirable properties any pharmaceutically interesting molecule can possess. However, very few studies exist that give hard-and-fast rules about what makes a compound bioavailable. Many of the factors that affect bioavailability are unknown and are not calculable. For instance, formulation can have a profound effect on the bioavailability of a compound. Commonly, bioavailability is a complicated, unknown function of the lipophilicity, molecular weight, pK_a, shape, plus other descriptors.

The most common measure of lipophilicity, the estimated octanol/water partition coefficient ($\log K_{OW}$), can be calculated using a variety of programs, including CLOGP [32,33], LOGKOW [34], and HINT [35]. If these programs fail, an estimate can be made from the measured or calculated values for analogous compounds. Empirically, the correlation between the $\log P$ of compounds and their bioavailability suggests that compounds should not be too lipophilic and should not be too hydrophilic. A plot of the CLOGPs for the top 100 drugs in 1993 are shown in Figure 1.

Characterization of the molecular structure is calculated using topological indices, such as those as defined by Kier and Hall [36]. For example, in our library design approach, we perform principal components

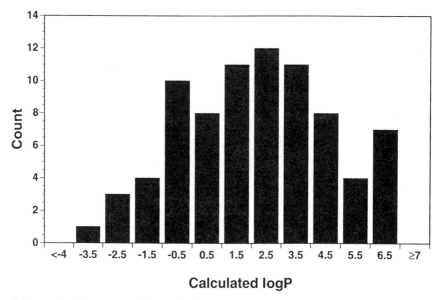

Figure 1 Histogram of the calculated logPs for the top-selling drugs in 1993.

analysis on a calculated set of a large number of descriptors. For each of our compounds, we calculate 70 connectivity indices, 7 shape indices, the ϕ-flexibility descriptor, molecular weight, and the numbers of elements, nonhydrogen atoms, and bonds [37]. However, many of these descriptors are closely related. for example, both the molecular weight and the number of bonds generally increase with an increase in the number of atoms. Therefore, these descriptors are reduced with principal components analysis to five or six principal components. These are latent properties that explain about 85–90% of the variance in the data. What results is a matrix in which the rows represent the compounds and the columns represent the principal components of these properties. The similarity between any two compounds A and B can then be defined as the distance between the two "property vectors" described by the PCA components for compounds A and B in this five- or six-dimensional space.

$$\text{Similarity} = [\Sigma_i(\mathbf{PC}_{iA} - \mathbf{PC}_{iB})^2]^{1/2} \tag{1}$$

These properties do not directly take into account the types of functionality present in the molecules. For example, one would like to have an idea of the types of molecular fragments that are present in the compounds of interest. A fragment-based "fingerprint" can be calculated for each compound. These fingerprints can then be compared with each other to define the similarity of the molecules. A Daylight fingerprint [38] is a binary string with 2048 bits, in which each bit indicates a presence or absence of a structural fragment. Two structures that are identical will have identical fingerprints. Two structures that are highly similar will have fingerprints that differ by only a few bits. This similarity is quantified using the Tanimoto coefficient (2), which compares the number of bits in common between the two fingerprints:

The Tanimoto coefficient is defined as:

$$Tc = N_{(A\&B)}/[N_A + N_B - N_{(A\&B)}] \tag{2}$$

where:

$N_{(A\&B)}$ = the number of bits in common between A and B
N_A = the number of bits in A
N_B = the number of bits in B

The Tanimoto similarity value is used in chemical problems because it is normalized for the complexity of the molecules. For example, the Tanimoto similarity between methylamine and methyl alcohol is less than the Tanimoto similarity between a benzodiazepine containing an amino group or a hydroxyl group. Figure 2 shows the level of differentiation that the Tanimoto similarity measure can produce. The top histogram shows the Tanimoto similarities of phenethylamine to all of the compounds (~19,000 compounds) in the Medchem94 database [38]. The second and third histograms show the similarities of captopril and ranitidine to the compounds in the Medchem94 database. Notice that there are few compounds with high similarity values (near 1.0) for all of the compounds, but that captopril and ranitidine have far fewer similar compounds than does phenethylamine, reflecting their more complex chemical structure. Note also that the vast majority of compounds are quite dissimilar (< 0.8) to each of these.

These descriptors might not account for the fact that atoms near the backbone systematically contribute to binding differently from those that are more remote. Thus, the chemical features of the structures can be further characterized with "receptor interaction" descriptors [37], which were developed to account explicitly for the directionality of the substituent relative to the backbone. Each atom in each potential substituent is characterized by six properties: the radius of the atom, whether the atom is acidic or basic, whether the atom is a hydrogen bond-acceptor or bond-donor, and whether or not the atom is aromatic. Within each potential substituent, all atoms in a given bond-count distance from the backbone constitute an *atom layer*. At each atom layer, the properties of the atoms that comprise that layer are summed, and each resulting atom layer is

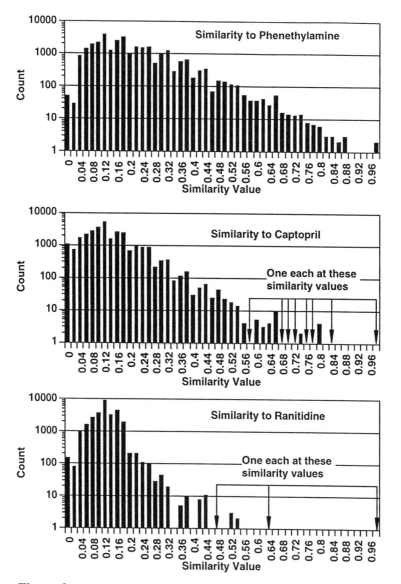

Figure 2 Histogram of the Tanimoto similarity values to selected compounds in the Pomona Medchem94 database.

H₃C—OH   H₃C—NH₂

Tanimoto Similarity = 0.22

Tanimoto Similarity = 0.97

{1}

stored into a table. To calculate similarity between pairs of substituents, the maximum and minimum values are determined for each corresponding pair of cells (columns) in their respective atom layer tables. The sum of the minima divided by the sum of the maxima yields the similarity between that pair of substituents. As with the chemical functionality descriptors, a dissimilarity matrix is computed, and multidimensional scaling (MDS), described in a later section, is applied. The atom layer similarities generally reduce to fewer dimensions than the chemical database fingerprints.

Figure 3 illustrates how each of the six atom properties are summed for all atoms within each layer (for up to 15 layers) to make a table of six columns (properties) by ten rows (layers). Other atomic properties, such as positive and negative partial charge, electrophilic and nucleophilic superdelocalizability, could also be added as columns to the tables. Interestingly, these descriptors allow for isosterism (e.g., that one acidic functionality can often substitute for another).

Other descriptors can also be used for clustering. Brown and coworkers [39,40] and Muskal [41] have used structural keys for clustering. These keys were developed for substructure searching, each representing an array of bits that signal the presence or absence of a specific fragment. Typically, fragments that are deemed important are cataloged in a fragment dictionary. Because one must avoid duplication of fragments and one must choose fragments that occur nearly equally, selecting which fragments to

Atom Layer Table for 1

Radius	Acid	Base	HBD	HBA	Ar
1	1.9	0	0	0	0	0
2	1.9	0	0	0	0	0
3	1.8	0	**0**	1	1	0
4	1.9	0	0	0	0	0
5	**3.5**	0	0	0	1	1
6	3.8	0	0	0	0	2
7	3.8	0	0	0	0	2
8	1.9	0	0	0	0	1
9	1.7	**1**	0	**0**	1	0
10	0	0	0	0	0	0

Atom Layer Table for 2

Radius	Acid	Base	HBD	HBA	Ar
1	1.9	0	0	0	0	0
2	1.9	0	0	0	0	0
3	1.8	0	**1**	**0**	**0**	0
4	1.9	0	0	0	0	0
5	**1.9**	0	0	0	**0**	1
6	3.8	0	0	0	0	2
7	3.8	0	0	0	0	2
8	1.9	0	0	0	0	1
9	1.7	**0**	0	**1**	1	0
10	0	0	0	0	0	0

$$\Sigma min / \Sigma max = 28.6/35.2 = \mathbf{0.81}$$

Figure 3   Receptor recognition similarity based on atom-layer tables.

include in the dictionary is difficult. Brown and co-workers mapped each of 153 fragments and the number of occurrences of the fragments into a 2048-bit word for their studies. The Tanimoto equation [see Eq. (2)] is used to calculate the similarities.

Brown and co-workers have also used 3D-substructural screens to create fingerprints that have some 3D characteristics [39,40]. Each of these fingerprints represents the geometric distances between several features in the range of 2–10 Å in 0.5-Å increments: oxygen, nitrogen, generic oxygen or nitrogen, aromatic ring centroids, carbonyl extensions, and normals to the plane of aromatic rings. A bit string of 336 bits was generated.

Fingerprints based on the pharmacophoric groups in a molecule have also been developed [39,40,42,43]. In these approaches, several pharmacophoric groups are defined. These are often defined as hydrogen bond-acceptors, donors, positive and negative charge, and aromatic centers. A fingerprint (or pharmacophore key) is generated by binning all of the distances between pharmacophoric groups in each molecule. These bins are biased so that the shorter, more common, distances are covered by more bins than are larger distances [42,43].

Chemical design encodes a fingerprint of three-point pharmacophores [43]. In this approach, diversity is quantified as the set of all possible three-point pharmacophores using four different pharmacophore types. There are

20 different pharmacophores using this approach, each comprises three atoms and three interatomic distances. Each pair of atoms in the pharmacophore can possibly lie from van der Waals (vdW) contact to about 15 Å apart. A total of 31 distance bins are used to catalog all of the possible pharmacophore space, ranging from vdW contact to 15 Å. The size of each 3D table of pharmacophores—called a *key*–generated is about 600 kilobytes (Kb). This can be prohibitive to store for each compound. Brown and co-workers have generated a fingerprint from this type of approach in which the keys are hashed into a 2048-bit word [39,40].

The computation of this key for rigid molecules is straightforward. However, most compounds have anywhere from a few to many rotatable bonds and low-energy conformations that must be considered when generating one of these keys. It is impossible to perform robust molecular mechanical energy calculations on an entire library of several hundred thousand compounds. Instead, a rule-based conformational analysis method is used to estimate the low-energy conformations for each molecule in the library [43]. The pharmacophores can then be tallied for all the acceptable conformations of all the molecules in the library.

Similarities defined with any (or all) of these property definitions can then be used for the selection or clustering of corporate databases.

C. Clustering Corporate Databases

The corporate archive is a limited resource and biological-screening efforts can be quite expensive. In choosing a set of compounds for biological screening, one would want to minimize the redundancy of the compounds selected for testing. Said differently, one would want to maximize the diversity of the compounds chosen. Corporate databases often contain several similar compounds. An obvious reason for this is that many similar analogues are synthesized, tested, and archived during the lead optimization phase of a therapeutic project. Over the years, several projects can lead to large numbers of similar compounds. One would want to select only a few of these closely related analogues for screening.

Methods of compiling lists of the compounds that are similar to each other is called *clustering*. A variety of methods for clustering chemical structures have been described [44]. Hierarchical methods of clustering are useful for smaller databases of fewer than 10^5 compounds, but scale poorly and are impractical for most larger corporate databases. A method of non-hierarchical clustering, the Jarvis–Patrick nearest-neighbor algorithm [45], has been most commonly applied to clustering of large databases because it does scale well and can be applied routinely to databases on the order of 10^5–10^6 compounds.

The Jarvis–Patrick method requires the calculation of all pair-wise similarities for the database. Storage of the entire list is computationally impractical. Instead, a list of the nearest neighbors is retained for each compound. Typically, only the 20 or so nearest neighbors of each compound are retained. The neighbor lists are rank-ordered based on the similarity measure. This calculation scales as the number of compounds squared and is the most time-limiting step in the calculation. However, it needs to be performed only once. The results can then be stored and used repeatedly. Clustering of the database is performed based on these lists of nearest neighbors. Two compounds are considered to be in the same cluster if they meet these two criteria: (a) they must both appear within each other's list of J nearest neighbors; and (b) they must share K of their J nearest neighbors. The Daylight Chemical Information System's implementation of the Jarvis–Patrick algorithm [46] uses a default in which a cluster is defined as having J = 14 and K = 8. This means that two compounds are in the same cluster if they share 8 of their 14 most similar compounds and that they are each within the set of 14 closest compounds to the other.

A single compound from each cluster can be selected as a representative of all members of the cluster. Typically, this is the member that is geometrically closest to the center of the cluster, and is often called the *centroid*, although it likely is not at the geometric center of the cluster. However, choosing one compound inherently means one is not selecting the remaining compounds. It is not unrealistic to believe that an active compound might be neglected in this method.

Often, about 10–30% of the database will contain compounds that do not cluster with any other compound in the database. These compounds are referred to as singletons and can be viewed as clusters of size 1. Because there are so many singletons, there is a tendency to want to group them together, either with each other, or with their nearest cluster. However, singletons represent unique or unusual compounds in the database, and might be quite useful in a broad-screening approach.

In addition, most pharmaceutical companies have archived compounds synthesized because they were thought to be therapeutically interesting. Thus, one is likely to find that many of the compounds in a database are closely related and that whole classes of compounds are not represented in a given database. Occasionally, this is desirable. For instance, one probably does not want transition-metal complexes in a pharmaceutical. However, it is entirely possible that the corporate database is not terribly diverse. In this situation, one would want to include compounds from chemical classes not represented in the database, either through the internal synthesis of these compounds or by the purchase of compounds from external sources. The clustering approach can be applied to solve this problem.

Shemetulskis and co-workers [8] have compared the Parke-Davis database (called CBI) with a set of compounds from Chemical Abstracts Services (CAST-3D) and with the collection of compounds available from Maybridge directly (MAY). The CBI database contains about 117,000 structures and MAY contains about 42,000 structures. The CAST-3D collection is a subset of the entire CAS database that was chosen (using clustering) as part of an effort to convert 2D to 3D coordinates. This list was pared down to remove metals and pure hydrocarbons, resulting in about 380,000 structures. The pair-list generation for the CAST-3D database required approximately 64 CPU days on a Silicon Graphics 4D/480 workstation. Clustering the composite whole of all of these databases was too computationally expensive. Therefore, Shemetulskis and co-workers subdivided the CBI and CAST-3D databases into subdatabases, with significantly fewer members, by choosing the centroids and singletons from a variety of clusterings employing different J and K values as described earlier. The resulting subdatabases were then clustered together and analyzed. They find that about 80% of the CAST-3D compounds are segregated into clusters that contain only CAS compounds. This would suggest that the chosen set of CAST-3D compounds are different from the in-house CBI compounds and might be valuable if purchased. In contrast, when the Maybridge database is clustered with the CBI compounds, only about 55% of the resulting clusters contain only Maybridge compounds. This suggests that there is overlap between the CBI and MAY. Nonetheless, significant additional diversity could be added to the CBI database through the purchase of about 55% of the Maybridge compounds or through the purchase of a significant portion of the CAST-3D database. Just as importantly, the MAY database represents a source of compounds that could replace dwindling supplies of the internal samples—a common consequence of random screening.

These workers carried out further analyses comparing the clustering results with a treatment employing the property descriptors CLOGP, CMR, and the calculated dipole moment. Both methods agree that there is more overlap between the CBI and the MAY databases than with CBI and the CAST-3D database.

Brown and co-workers [39,40] have compared several clustering methods using different chemical functionality descriptors to evaluate the ability of the methods to generate clusters containing similar biological activity (actives cluster with actives, inactives with inactives) in several biological screens, employing several fingerprinting methods, including structural keys, 3D keys, pharmacophore pairs, and 3D pharmacophores.

They evaluated the Jarvis–Patrick and three hierarchical clustering methods. In two of their clustering methods, the compounds were clustered using an agglomerative approach. In these methods, the similarities of all compounds in the data set are calculated, the two most similar compounds are then merged into a cluster [39,40]. The calculation then proceeds to merge either clusters of compounds until only one cluster remains. The remaining hierarchical clustering approach they employ is a divisive method. In this method, the dissimilarities of the compounds are compared. The two most dissimilar compounds are identified. All remaining compounds in the list are assigned to the least dissimilar of the two compounds. The largest-diameter cluster is then broken into two smaller clusters so that the largest remaining cluster has the smallest diameter. This continues for a total of $n - 1$ steps (where n is the number of compounds).

In this study, they found that the 2D structural descriptors are better at producing clusters of compounds with similar biological activity than are the 3D descriptors considered. They also found that the hierarchical clustering methods are able to separate the active and inactive compounds into clusters. In particular, the agglomerative methods perform better than the divisive method, and all perform better than the Jarvis–Patrick method. In three of four examples studied, the Jarvis–Patrick method performed substantially worse than the other methods [39,40]. This study highlights the risk in using the Jarvis–Patrick clustering method to select centroids for selective screening of a corporate database. Nonetheless, the Jarvis–Patrick method is the only method of the four that is applicable to the study of databases containing more than 100,000 structures.

D. Multidimensional Scaling

For experimental design of combinatorial libraries, we would like to have a euclidean description of the relations of the structure in the data set. Clustering methods do not provide this type of description.

For the topological descriptors, principal components analysis calculations will produce vectors of descriptors for each structure. These descriptors define a property space in which vectors that are spread far apart in space are diverse. We define similarity as the distance between the two property vectors. A matrix of similarities can then be easily generated by calculating all pair-wise distances for the compounds. This operation can be likened to determining the distances between all pairs of cities on a given map. Each city will have a specified coordinate on the map, and the distances can be directly calculated.

For fingerprints, however, we do not have these property vectors; we have only the binary data (the fingerprint), and the similarity matrix generated by calculating the Tanimoto similarity for all pairs of compounds. To use the information contained within the fingerprint similarity matrix, we must find a method to calculate property vectors that can reproduce the similarity matrix and also create a property space. In our city analogy, we would like to create an accurate map of the cities (assigning coordinates to each city) using only the intercity distances between all pairs of cities. A method called multidimensional scaling (MDS) allows us to derive individual property vectors that reproduce the Tanimoto similarities matrix (or a map from the intercity distances). MDS assigns coordinate vectors to each molecule in the minimum number of "dimensions" needed to reproduce the distances (i.e., similarities) within a specified error. Figure 4 shows the intercity "map" generated with MDS on the intercity distances shown in Table 1. Notice, the cities are fairly well placed relative to each other. A few minor displacements are seen, but the overall fit is quite good.

Multidimensional scaling produces a low-dimensional continuous space that reproduces the Tanimoto similarity matrix based on the binary fingerprints [37]. The results of this process can be used with statistical experimental design to select compounds that are either similar (small distances) or dissimilar (large distances) from each other. This presents an alternative to Jarvis–Patrick (J-P) clustering, which yields one set of compounds that are relatively near each other in space, with no direct measure of how "close" one set is relative to another. With the MDS method, we know the exact geometric relation between all the compounds in the data

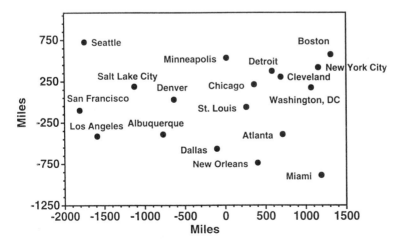

Figure 4   A map of US cities generated with multidimensional scaling.

Table 1 Intercity Distances Used to Calculate the Map Shown in Figure 4

	1	2	3	4	5	6	7	8	9	10	11	12	13	14	15	16	17	18
Albuquerque	0																	
Atlanta	1410	0																
Boston	2270	1115	0															
Chicago	1347	717	1013	0														
Cleveland	1627	780	667	345	0													
Dallas	654	788	1845	937	1185	0												
Denver	457	1425	2015	1026	1359	794	0											
Detroit	1569	743	714	288	173	1249	1285	0										
Los Angeles	804	2362	3028	2086	2388	1486	1062	2311	0									
Miami	2071	653	1541	1237	1274	1325	2065	1432	2785	0								
Minneapolis	1228	1131	1459	410	765	963	928	671	1993	1802	0							
New Orleans	1160	475	1619	926	1060	509	1344	1068	2009	857	1328	0						
New York City	2178	887	197	818	481	1620	1807	646	2797	1347	1234	1401	0					
St. Louis	1039	559	1196	302	578	629	879	543	1844	1197	609	677	1004	0				
Salt Lake City	625	1943	2405	1420	1753	1329	537	1656	703	2594	1321	1859	2214	1400	0			
San Francisco	1082	2482	3139	2151	2484	1734	1268	2390	384	3083	2052	2313	2945	2134	736	0		
Seattle	1443	2723	3126	2108	2463	2112	1314	2396	1143	3419	1661	2642	2924	2140	821	808	0	
Washington, DC	1892	634	471	712	375	1367	1705	525	2727	1070	1128	1149	235	835	2229	2960	2818	0

set. However, unlike J-P clustering, the MDS calculation can only be applied to data sets containing on the order of several thousand compounds, whereas J-P clustering can be readily applied to millions of compounds.

IV. COMBINATORIAL LIBRARY DESIGNS

A similar approach to that for clustering databases can be taken for library design. We catalogue the properties that we believe are important for biological activity, and perform calculations to decide which compounds to synthesize (as opposed to purchasing), based on these properties. Although the software and the molecular descriptors used in these methods are related, the size of the problems are dramatically different, leading to serious choices and compromises about the computational and synthetic approaches used for combinatorial library design. As an illustration, let us assume that we would like to create a combinatorial library that contains four positions of diversity and that the diversity at each of these positions arises from the inclusion of an amine in the synthesis. We can purchase well over 1000 amines. If it is possible to synthesize 20,000 compounds per week, the time it would take to synthesize the complete library containing all possible combinations of these amines would be about 1 million years. We must settle on making a fraction of the library that spans the diversity of the entire library.

One might argue that we should cluster the entire library, and select one member from each cluster for synthesis. Unfortunately, even this is computationally infeasible. To do would require the enumeration of the entire library and then to perform the clustering. In the foregoing example, if we could enumerate a compound and perform the nearest-neighbor's calculation on it in just 1 s, it would take about 31,000 years to calculate all the properties for all the molecules in the library. In fact, the practical upper limit for clustering is about 10^6 compounds. This same analysis holds for other design methods that require the enumeration of all members of the entire library.

Thus, there are difficult choices to be made to make the time required to perform the calculation manageable. One could reduce the size of the library under consideration to a more manageable size, say 10^6 or so. One could reduce the size of the calculation by eliminating members of the complete library a priori. Or, one could assume that the interactions between the points of diversity—or side chains—are going to be minimal, and perform intricate calculations on the side chains. Because there are approximately 1000 of these, the calculations can be quite rigorous and complex.

Figure 5 shows a schematic of the selection process involved in our
library design approach [37]. First, we select the data sets of the reagents
used in a combinatorial library (e.g., amines, alcohols, acids, or others).
For each of these sets, we calculate the topological indices, fingerprint
descriptors using MDS, and atom-layer descriptors, also using MDS. In
addition, we calculate the log$P$ of the structures. We then perform library
designs using a D-optimal design procedure that chooses a subset of structures from the larger set that are well spread out and nearly orthogonal in
property space (i.e., they are diverse). Often, there is some SAR or other
information that one would like to incorporate into the design. The D-
optimal algorithm can be used to "augment" the design by selecting additional structures that best complement those chosen structures, completing a design of a specified size, with maximum overall diversity.

It is often tempting to compare one library design with another, and
many often do. Often, significant differences in the basic assumptions or
compositions of each of the library design methods make direct comparisons of two designs impossible. To compare two library designs, one must
show that the descriptors developed in both methods can be used to predict
the other. Only then are comparisons between libraries valid.

A. Experimental Design

A common challenge in medicinal chemistry is to avoid the change-
one-single-thing (COST) approach to lead optimization [47,48]. In this
aesthetical-appealing approach, a molecule will be derivatized by holding
most of the molecule fixed and changing one and only one substituent.
Several molecules will be synthesized until the most active substituent is

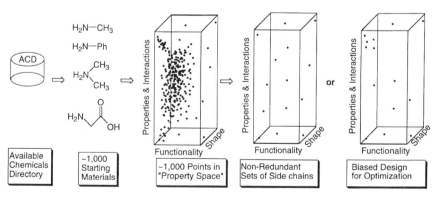

Figure 5 Schematic of selection of side chains for combinatorial library design.

found. A different substituent will then be altered until the most active substituent in that position is located. This iterative process, although simple, does not provide a good optimization protocol and usually does *not* even find a *local* minimum, let alone a global optimum. Often, the underlying response surfaces are highly complex and involve a large number of variables, which often interact with each other.

Statistical approaches to the design of experiments have several advantages to the COST approach. In these methods, many parameters (or substituents) are varied at the same time, covering as much of the response surface as possible during an experiment. Experimental design provides much better exploration of the property space, better results from fewer experiments, and the quality of the data becomes well-defined in the process. Though they have enjoyed success in other fields, experimental design approaches are relatively new to the pharmaceutical industry.

In combinatorial library design, we employ experimental design approaches both for diverse libraries used in broad screening and for lead optimization libraries. Doing so ensures that the libraries generated sample the biological response surface as efficiently as possible, given the limitations of the synthetic protocols.

It is possible to generate combinatorial libraries of the same size as a corporate library. However, it is unlikely that any one library design can span the same type of diversity as an entire corporate database. The compounds synthesized in a combinatorial experiment are closely related molecules; consequently, the overall diversity of the library is relatively small compared with a diverse corporate library. However, it is common to synthesize a large number of combinatorial libraries, each of which spans a different chemical space. Accordingly, one can design libraries that can and do span a large, diverse chemical space using different templates and different starting materials.

An example of this type of analysis is shown in Figure 6. Here, we use the chemical functionality fingerprints to estimate the total number of fragments that are present in a given library. We want to compare each library with the small molecules in the best-selling 100 drugs [49]. This is a diverse set of compounds and should give us an estimate of divers chemical functional groups. The two bottom bars represent the top 50 or top 100 best-selling small-molecule drugs. As you can see, a large number of functional groups (shown in solid bars as measured on the linear scale at the bottom of the graph) are present in these two data sets (number of compounds is shown in hashed bars, with a logarithmic scale at the top of the graph). The first three libraries are theoretical libraries of oligomers of nucleotides, saccharides, and peptides. Literally billions to trillions of compounds (hashed bars, top scale) can be synthesized, but the number of

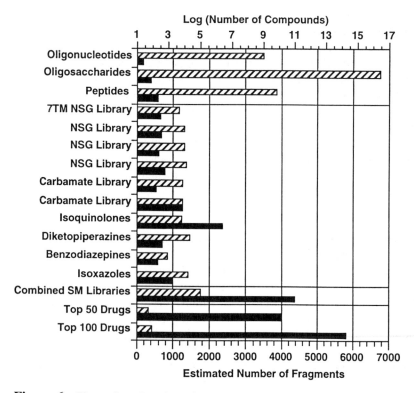

Figure 6 The variety (number of compounds) and the diversity (number of estimated fragments) in combinatorial libraries.

functional groups present in the libraries is small. The next library is our biased 7-*trans* membrane–G protein-coupled receptor biased NSG peptoid library [22]. Notice that with only about 5000 compounds, we produce more diversity than in several orders of magnitude more peptides. Several other libraries are presented, each with 10^3–10^4 compounds. Each displays more diversity than the peptides, but much less than the top drugs. Notice, however, that the combination of the ten nonpeptide libraries results in a total number of chemical fragments that is on the same order as the top 100 small-molecule drugs. Thus, we have generated libraries that are nearly orthogonal to each other and that do span a large diversity space.

B. Structure-Based Library Design

It has been suggested that combinatorial chemistry represents a step away from the structure-based paradigm that has become a standard in the search for new drugs. However, this is clearly not true. Combinatorial library design can incorporate structure-based drug design approaches. If the structure of a biological target is known, one can use structure-based design approaches to select or score the most likely scaffolds and substituents to use in a library. A library can then be designed to contain only the best fragments and scaffolds. This design can be supplemented with experimental design approaches to enhance the diversity (or similarity) of the design.

Martin et al. [50] have used a genetic algorithm (GA) to generate populations of mixed *N*-substituted glycine–peptide chimeric oligomers into a protein-active site. The ligands are docked into a homology model of a serine protease using distance geometry approaches and were optimized using the intermolecular energy from a force-field calculation as the scoring function for the GA. The optimization produced several families of structures that could then be used for the pharmacophoric hypothesis of a biased library design.

Sheridan et al. describe an approach similar to this in which they used a genetic algorithm to generate NSGs that maximized the value of a trend vector QSAR model based on small-molecule lead compounds [51]. This procedure identified several commonly seen side chains. These side chains could be used in a strongly biased combinatorial library design.

Martin et al. have also described a method to create fingerprints of side chains using 3D-docking calculations [50]. In this approach, the proposed side chains are docked into a small number of shapes arranged on a grid, starting with one sphere. If the structure does not fit into this shape, two-sphere shapes are tried. This continues until all of the shapes up to five spheres have been tried. This can be used to catalog the types and sizes of shapes that the structures fit into. These fingerprints are then treated with MDS and included in the library design approaches described in the foregoing section.

C. Library Design Using Three-Dimensional Pharmacophores

Chemical Design has described an alternative method to combinatorial library design. In their approach, one quantifies the diversity of the corporate database using the 3D pharmacophores described earlier [52,53]. The size of the pharmacophore key is prohibitively large to store for each molecule in even a modest library. Therefore, a common pharmacophore key for the entire library—or any subset of the library—is computed and stored. One then compares proposed compounds against the diversity of the corporate library. Any compound that contains no new pharmacophores is rejected as being already present in the database. Any compound with a new pharmacophore is included as one to be synthesized or purchased. The pharmacophore key can be visualized quite readily for small numbers of molecules.

In combinatorial library design, one can use this technique to select for synthesis only those compounds that exhibit most of the pharmacophores of the full combinatorial library. Molecules are eliminated by several criteria. First, all rigid compounds are eliminated because each would exhibit relatively few pharmacophores, and several would be required to cover the entire set of pharmacophores of the larger set. Second, molecules that are too flexible are eliminated because they require substantially more computational time to consider and analyze. Finally, a compound is eliminated if it exhibits a pharmacophore key that is not unique to those already included in the set selected for synthesis.

This requires the enumeration of all of the low-energy conformations of the set of compounds under consideration [43]. Although this is an acceptable task for sets of approximately 50,000 compounds or fewer, it is computationally unfeasible for millions to billions of compounds.

A similar approach can be used to select compounds to supplement the compounds already present in the corporate archives. Here, one would calculate the pharmacophore key of the corporate database. If one had enough disk storage, the pharmacophore key of each compound could be stored. The key of each commercially available compound could then be compared against the key or keys of the internal compounds. Only those compounds with a unique key would be purchased. If the compound supply has been depleted, one could search databases of commercially available compounds to find one that exhibits a pharmacophore key that is similar to the one that is being depleted.

REFERENCES

1. S. Shellenbarger, Lilly's new supercomputer spurs a race for hardware to quicken drug research, *Wall Street Journal*, August 14, 1990, p. 1.
2. P. Willett, *Similarity and Clustering in Chemical Information Systems*, John Wiley & Sons, New York, 1987, p. 54.
3. I. D. Kuntz, J. M. Blaney, S. J. Oatley, R. Langridge, and T. E. Ferrin, *J. Mol. Biol. 161*:269 (1982).
4. R. L. DesJarlais, R. P. Sheridan, J. S. Dixon, I. D. Kuntz, and R. Venkataraghavan, Docking flexible ligands to macromolecular receptors by molecular shape, *J. Med. Chem. 29*:2149 (1986).
5. J. M. Blaney and J. S. Dixon, A good ligand is hard to find: automated docking methods, *Perspect Drug Discov Design 1*:301 (1993).
6. Y. C. Martin, 3D database searching in drug design, *J. Med. Chem. 35*:2145 (1992).

7. M. G. Bures and Y. C. Martin, in *Topics in Stereochemistry*, Vol. 21 (E. L. Eliel and S. H. Wilen, eds.), John Wiley & Sons, New York, 1994, p. 467.
8. N. E. Shemetulskis, J. B. Dunbar, B. W. Dunbar, D. W. Moreland, and C. Humblet, Enhancing the diversity of a corporate database using chemical database clustering and analysis, *J. Comput. Aided Mol. Design 9*:407 (1995).
9. W. H. Moos, G. D. Green, and M. R. Pavia, Recent advances in the generation of molecular diversity, *Annu. Rep. Med. Chem. 28*:315 (1993).
10. M. A. Gallop, R. W. Barrett, W. J. Dower, S. P. Fodor, and E. M. Gordon, Applications of combinatorial technologies to drug discovery. 1. Background and peptide combinatorial libraries, *J. Med. Chem. 37*:1233 (1994).
11. E. M. Gordon, R. W. Barrett, W. J. Dower, S. P. Fodor, and M. A. Gallop, Applications of combinatorial technologies to drug discovery. 2. Combinatorial organic synthesis, library screening strategies, and future directions. *J. Med. Chem. 37*:1385 (1994).
12. N. K. Terrett, M. Gardner, D. W. Gordon, R. J. Kobylecki, and J. Steele, Combinatorial synthesis—the design of compound libraries and their application to drug discovery, *Tetrahedron 51*:8135 (1995).
13. Y. C. Martin, M. G. Bures, and P. Willet, in *Reviews in Computational Chemistry* (K. B. Lipkowitz and D. B. Boyd, eds.), VCH Publishers, New York, 1990.
14. C. Humblet and J. B. Dunbar, 3D database searching and docking strategies, *Annu. Rep. Med. Chem. 28*:275 (1993).
15. P. J. Hylands and L. J. Nisbet, The search for molecular diversity (I): natural products, *Annu. Rep. Med. Chem. 26*:259 (1991).
16. R. McDaniel, S. Ebert-Khosla, D. A. Hopwood, and C. Khosla, Rational design of aromatic polyketide natural products by recombinant assembly of enzymatic subunits, *Nature 375*:549 (1995).
17. R. M. Snider, J. W. Constantine, I. John, A. Lowe, K. P. Longo, W. S. Lebel, H. A. Woody, S. E. Drozda, M. C. Desai, F. J. Vinick, R. W. Spencer, and H.-J. Hess, A potent nonpeptide antagonist of the substance P (NK_1) receptor, *Science 251*:435 (1991).
18. M. Clozel, V. Breu, K. Burri, J.-M. Cassal, W. Fischli, G. A. Gray, G. Hirth, B.-M. Löffler, M. Müller, W. Neidhart, and H. Ramuz, Pathophysiological role of endothelin revealed by the first orally active endothelin receptor antagonist, *Nature 365*:759 (1993).
19. J. D. Elliot, M. A. Lago, R. D. Cousins, A. Gao, J. D. Leber, K. F. Erhard, P. Nambi, N. A. Elshourbagy, C. Kumar, J. A. Lee, J. W. Bean, C. W. DeBrosse, D. S. Eggleston, D. P. Brooks, G. Feuerstein, J. Robert, R. Ruffolo, J. Weinstock, J. G. Gleason, C. E. Peishoff, and E. H. Ohlstein, 1,3-Diarylindan-2-carboxylic acids, potent and selective non-peptide endothelin receptor antagonists, *J. Med. Chem. 37*:1553 (1994).
20. P. S. Charifson, A. R. Leach, and I. A. Rusinko, The generation and use of large 3D databases in drug discover, *Network Sci. 1*:(http://edisto.awod.com/netsci/Issues/Sept95) (1995).

21. R. N. Zuckermann, J. M. Kerr, M. A. Siani, and S. C. Banville, Design, construction and application of a fully automated equimolar peptide mixture synthesizer, *Int. J. Pept. Protein Res. 40*:497 (1992).

22. R. N. Zuckermann, E. J. Martin, D. C. Spellmeyer, G. B. Stauber, K. R. Shoemaker, J. M. Kerr, G. M. Figliozzi, M. A. Siani, R. J. Simon, S. C. Banville, E. G. Brown, L. Wang, and W. H. Moos, Discovery of nanomolar ligands for 7-transmembrane G-protein coupled receptors from a diverse (*N*-substituted)glycine peptoid library, *J. Med. Chem. 37*:2678 (1994).

23. S. Brenner and R. Lerner, Encoded combinatorial chemistry, *Proc. Natl. Acad. Sci. USA 89*:5381 (1992).

24. J. M. Kerr, S. C. Banville, and R. N. Zuckermann, Encoded combinatorial peptide libraries containing non-natural amino acids, *J. Am. Chem. Soc. 115*: 2529 (1993).

25. V. Nikolaiev, A. Stierandova, V. Krchnak, B. Seligmann, K. S. Lam, S. E. Salmon, and M. Lebl, Peptide-encoding for structure determination of non-sequenceable polymers within libraries synthesized and tested on solid-phase supports, *Pept. Res. 6*:161 (1993).

26. M. H. J. Ohlmeyer, R. N. Swanson, L. W. Dillard, J. C. Reader, G. Asouline, R. Kobayashi, M. Wigler, and W. C. Still, Complex synthetic chemical libraries indexed with molecular tags, *Proc. Natl. Acad. Sci. USA 90*:10922 (1993).

27. C. K. Jayawickreme, G. F. Graminski, J. M. Quillan, and M. R. Lerner, Creation and functional screening of a multi-use peptide library, *Proc. Natl. Acad. Sci. USA 91*:1614 (1994).

28. D. V. Vilet, M. H. Lambert, and F. K. Brown, Design of libraries based on the binding site: the merging of de novo design and combinatorial chemistry, Comp Division, 209th ACS National Meeting, Anaheim CA, American Chemical Society, 1995, 1, 034.

29. P. Y. S. Lam, P. K. Jadhav, C. J. Eyermann, C. N. Hodge, Y. Ru, L. T. Bacheler, J. L. Meek, M. J. Otto, M. M. Rayner, Y. N. Wong, C.-H. Chang, P. C. Weber, D. A. Jackson, T. R. Sharpe, and S. Erickson-Viitanen, Rational design of potent, bioavailable, nonpeptide cyclic ureas as HIV protease inhibitors, *Science 263*:380 (1994).

30. R. S. McDowell, T. R. Gadek, P. L. Barker, D. J. Burdick, K. S. Chan, C. L. Quan, N. Skelton, M. Struble, E. D. Thorsett, M. Ticshler, J. Y. K. Tom, T. R. Webb, and J. P. Burnier, From peptide to non-peptide. 1. The elucidation of a bioactive conformation of the arginine–glycine–aspartic acid recognition sequence, *J. Am. Chem. Soc. 116*:5069 (1994).

31. R. S. McDowell and D. R. Artis, Structure-based design from flexible ligands, *Annu. Rep. Med. Chem. 30*:265 (1995).

32. A. Leo, Calculating log P_{oct} from structures, *Chem. Rev. 93*:1281 (1993).

33. D. Weininger, CLOGP, 4.34 ed., Daylight Chemical Information Systems, Inc., Irvine, CA, 1994.

34. P. Howard and W. Meylan, LOGKOW, Syracuse Research Corp., Syracuse NY, 1993.

35. G. E. Kellogg, G. S. Joshi, and D. J. Abraham, *Med. Chem. Res. 1*:444 (1992).

36. L. H. Hall and L. B. Kier, in *Reviews in Computational Chemistry*, Vol. 2 (K. B. Kipkowitz and D. B. Boyd, eds.), VCH Publishers, New York, 1991, p. 367.
37. E. J. Martin, J. M. Blaney, M. A. Siani, D. C. Spellmeyer, A. K. Wong, and W. H. Moos, Measuring diversity: experimental design of combinatorial libraries for drug discovery, *J. Med. Chem 39*:1431 (1995).
38. D. Weininger, Thor, Daylight Chemical Information Systems, Irvine CA, 1993.
39. R. D. Brown, M. G. Bures, and Y. C. Martin, Similarity and cluster analysis applied to molecular diversity, Comp Division, 209th ACS National Meeting, Anaheim CA, American Chemical Society, 1994, 1, 003.
40. R. D. Brown and Y. C. Martin, Use of structure-activity data to compare structure-based clustering methods and descriptors for use in compound selection, Proceedings of the First Electronic Computational Chemistry Conference—CDROM (R. S. Rzepas, ed.), ARInternet: Landover MD, 1995.
41. S. M. Muskal, Enriching combinatorial libraries with features of known drugs, Comp Division, 209th ACS National Meeting, Anaheim CA, American Chemical Society, 1994, 1, 029.
42. R. P. Sheridan, R. Nilikantan, A. Rusinko, N. Bauman, K. Haraki, and R. Ventataraghavan, 3DSEARCH: a system for three-dimensional substructure searching, *J. Chem. Inf. Comput. Sci. 29*:255 (1989).
43. N. W. Murrall and E. K. Davies, Conformational freedom in 3D databases. 1. Techniques, *J. Chem. Inf. Comput. Sci. 30*:312 (1990).
44. J. M. Barnard and G. M. Downs, Clustering of chemical structures on the basis of 2-D similarity measures, *J. Chem. Inf. Comput. Sci. 32*:644 (1992).
45. R. A. Jarvis and E. A. Patrick, Clustering using a similarity measure based on shared near neighbors, *IEEE Trans. Comput.* C22:1025 (1973).
46. D. Weininger, Clustering package, Daylight Chemical Information Systems, Irvine CA, 1993.
47. S. Hellberg, M. Sjöström, B. Skagerberg, C. Wilkström, and S. Wold, On the design of multipositionally varied test series for quantitative structure–activity relationships, *Acta Pharm. Jugosl. 37*:53 (1987).
48. V. Austel, Experimental design in synthesis planning and structure–property correlations, *Methods Princ. Med. Chem. 2*:49 (1995).
49. The leading 100 drugs by worldwide sales, *Med. Ad. News*, May, 1994, p. 5.
50. E. J. Martin, J. M. Blaney, M. A. Siani, and D. C. Spellmeyer, Measuring diversity: experimental design of combinatorial libraries for drug discovery, Comp Division, 209th ACS National Meeting, Anaheim CA, American Chemical Society, 1995, 1, 032.
51. R. P. Sheridan and S. K. Kearsley, Using a genetic algorithm to suggest combinatorial libraries, *J. Chem. Inf. Comput. Sci. 35*:310 (1995).
52. Chem-X, Chemical Design, Ltd., Chipping Norton, UK, 1995.
53. K. Davies and C. Briant, Combinatorial chemistry library design using pharmacophore diversity, *Network Sci. 1*:(http://edisto.awod.com/netsci/Issues/July) (1995).

6

Receptor Preorganization for Activity and Its Role in Identifying Ligand-Binding Sites on Proteins

Brian K. Shoichet
Northwestern University Medical School,
Chicago, Illinois

I. INTRODUCTION

Imagine the ideal soluble protein, one optimized for its own stability in aqueous solution. This protein would bury most of its hydrophobic side chains from water and would expose most of its polar side chains to water. Those polar residues that were buried would interact with other polar groups of complementary functionality: positively charged residues with negatively charged residues, hydrogen bond donors with hydrogen bond acceptors. Residues would adopt low-energy conformations and everywhere would be well packed. This protein would maximize its complementarity to its water environment and to itself, within the constraints of chemical bonding. Such a protein would bind no ligand and have no function.

Now consider a functional protein, one that recognizes a ligand or catalyzes a reaction. These proteins are very different from our hypothetical stable protein. Rather than burying almost all of their hydrophobic residues, functional proteins often expose large patches of nonpolar surface to water. Rather than complementing every charged and polar residue with a residue

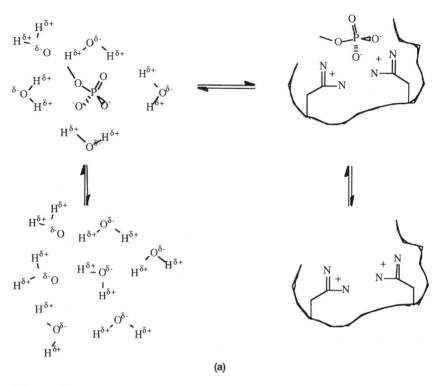

(a)

Figure 1 Preorganization of proteins to bind ligands: (a) Electrostatic aspects; (b) cavitation and hydrophobic aspects, water molecules are represented as *X*'s.

of opposite charge, functional proteins often cluster like charges in the same region of space. Some residues in functional proteins are found in high-energy conformations [1]. Although well-packed overall, functional proteins contain poorly packed regions. Such regions are typically at the active sites of functional proteins [2].

The features that distinguish functional proteins from our ideal stable protein are concentrated in the regions where ligands bind and reactions take place. Outside of these active sites, functional proteins adhere closely to the standards of the ideal protein. Their divergences from the ideal stable protein in the sites most connected with function are not accidental, but necessary. To achieve a stable, folded form, proteins must complement themselves: they must provide the keys to their own locks. In the area where a ligand is to bind such lock and key, self-complementarity must be absent; were it present the ligand would not bind. On binding to a protein,

(b)

ligands make the same sorts of complementary interactions that define the stable regions in proteins. To allow this to happen, the regions that will end up complementing the ligand, providing the lock to the ligand's key, must be preorganized to do so in the ligand's absence.

Several aspects of the preorganization of binding sites are illustrated in Figure 1. Water is a good solvent for the charged phosphate group (see Fig. 1a), its high dipole moment and small size allow it to respond to the introduction of such functionality by reorienting its dipoles to complement those of the ligand. Water is an excellent solvent for itself, and there is a cost to dissolving the phosphate. The dipoles of the water, to complement the charges of the ligand, must reorient into a high energy configuration relative to each other, compared with their configuration in the absence of the ligand. For water, there is a self-energy cost for solvating the phosphate. Conversely, the protein site (see Fig. 1a) pays no self-energy cost for interacting with the phosphate—its two arginines are preorganized into a high-energy configuration in the absence of the ligand. The protein prepaid the cost of attaining this high-energy configuration at the time of folding [3], it does not have to pay it again on ligand binding. For the hydrophobic ligand (see Fig. 1b), the cost to water on solvating the ligand is twofold—one of cavitation and one of hydrophobicity. Conversely, the apolar site into which the ligand binds is established in the absence of the ligand. The costs for displacing water molecules that fill the site in the apoprotein are balanced, at least partially, by the energy of liberating the waters from the confines of the apolar site. For at least one well-characterized site, there does not appear to be any water in the apoprotein, eliminating the cost for displacing bound waters on ligand binding [4] (see later discussion).

The preorganization of a protein to a high-energy conformation is the signature of a ligand-binding site. The greater the preorganization, the less it will resemble the hypothetical ideal stable protein, but the tighter a ligand of appropriate functionality will bind to it, all other effects being equal. In this chapter we will consider experimental and computational methods that seek to identify ligand-binding sites on proteins of known three-dimensional structure using this preorganization signature of potential-binding sites. These experimental and computational approaches can help us interpret protein structure for function and drug design.

II. PROTEIN–LIGAND INTERFACES

Protein–ligand interactions take several forms: ionic, ion–dipole, dipole–dipole, dipole–induced dipole, and instantaneous dipole-induced–dipole. Hydrogen-bonding is an important subcategory of polar interactions. Burial of nonpolar surface area has the added advantage of increasing the entrophy of the system through the hydrophobic effect [5]. We begin by considering examples of ligand–protein interfaces that highlight these interactions and the role of preorganization in determining the nature of the ligand site on the protein.

A canonical, simple-binding site is that created by Matthews and co-workers in T4 lysozyme [6] (Fig. 2). This site was made by substituting an alanine for leucine-99 (L99A), leaving a 150-$Å^3$ cavity in the center of the protein. This cavity is largely apolar; the only polar atoms in the site are main-chain nitrogens and oxygens, all of which form hydrogen bonds with other polar atoms, and one sulfur from a methionine in the site. Consequently, the ligands binding to this site are themselves largely apolar [4]: benzene, toluene, ethylbenzene, and other alkyl benzenes. As the ligands become larger and more hydrophobic, their binding energy increases. Benzene has a dissociation constant (K_d) of 100 μM from L99A, n-butyl benzene has a K_d of 20 μM. Ligands larger than n-butylbenzene have reduced

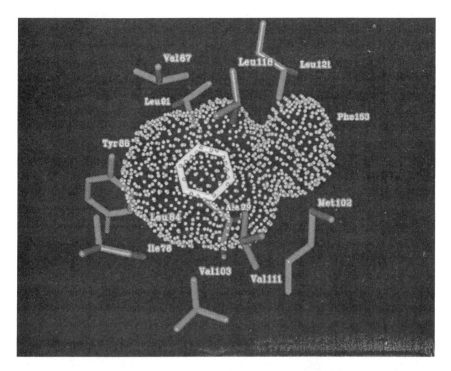

Figure 2 The cavity binding site of T4 lysozyme mutant L99A, shown with benzene bound. The residues that define the cavity are displayed, the molecular surface of the cavity is shown in dot format. Residues 84, 153, and 99 are labeled but are not displayed. (From Ref. 6.)

affinities. In the X-ray crystal structures of these complexes, the larger alkyl benzenes distorted the walls of the binding site, enlarging it. The site will tolerate some polar functional groups on the ligands; for instance, indole binds well. In the X-ray crystal structure of this complex determined by Morton et al. [4] the indole formed a nitrogen-to-sulfur hydrogen bond to Met-102. More polar residues, such as phenol, would not detectably bind to the mutant L99A lysozyme. The ligands that bound to the enzyme also stabilized it: the ligand–protein complexes were more stable to denaturation than the apoprotein.

This artificial-binding site illustrates several key features of preorganization in binding sites. The leucine-99 to alanine substitution that created the cavity reduces the complementarity of the protein for itself, reducing its stability. This reduction in self-complementarity sets up a potential complementarity for exogenous ligands that take the role formerly played by the leucine in the wild-type protein. On binding these ligands, the stability of the protein rises. Only ligands that can complement the chemistry of the cavity left by the mutation will bind: if the ligand is too polar, it will pay too high a cost for desolvation. Only ligands that are the right size will bind: if the ligand is too large it will not fit into the cavity. There is clearly some conformational play in the binding site, ligands that are larger than expected will be able to bind owing to conformational rearrangements of the site.

In contrast with the hydrophobic binding site of T4 lysozyme, the binding site in bacterial sulfate-binding protein (SBP) illustrates the sort of complementarity that can be achieved when polar interactions dominate (Fig.3) [7]. SBP binds to a sulfate ion through a network of hydrogen bonds. Somewhat surprisingly, most of these hydrogen bonds are with main-chain nitrogens. SBP is one of the purest examples of ligand com-

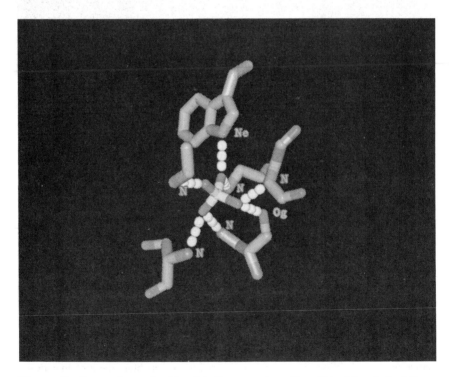

Figure 3 Interactions of sulfate-binding protein with sulfate. The dashed lines represent hydrogen bonds. (From Ref. 7.)

plementarity mediated through hydrogen-bond interactions. In aggregate, these interactions contribute approximately 10 kcal mol^{-1} to relative binding free energy of sulfate with SBP.

Proteins that recognize multifunctional ligands have multifunctional binding-sites. The folate-binding site of dihydrofolate reductase (DHFR) is a good example [8]. The highly polar pteridine rings of dihydrofolate or methotrexate—the substrate and a chemically related inhibitor—are complemented by hydrogen-bonding groups from the protein (Fig. 4). The apolar phenyl ring of the *p*-aminobenzoic acid group contacts residues Leu-27, Phe-30, Phe-49, Pro-50, and Leu-54. In the glutamylated "tail" region of methotrexate, the ligand carboxylates are complemented by charged protein residues. In the absence of the ligand, the structure of the binding site is largely, but not completely, maintained. In the apostructure, the

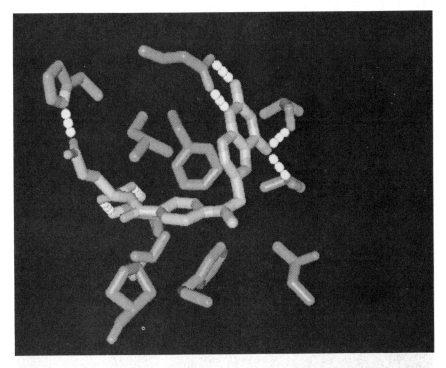

Figure 4 Methotrexate in complex with dihydrofolate reductase. The residues that interact with the phenyl ring of methotrexate are labeled. Hydrogen bonds are shown as dashed yellow lines; oxygens are red, nitrogens blue; the protein carbons are magenta, the methotrexate carbons are gray. See insert for color representation. (From Ref. 8.)

regions that will go on to bind to polar parts of the ligand are themselves polar. Residues with like charges and dipoles are concentrated in the same part of space, or are isolated in relatively hydrophobic grooves. In several instances, these polar residues make hydrogen bonds with water molecules that are displaced on binding to folate. In regions where the phenyl ring is to bind, an apolar surface area is exposed to solvent.

As the size of the ligand approaches that of the receptor, the complexity of the binding interface grows, and the distinction between ligand and receptor blurs. β-Lactamase–inhibitor protein (BLIP) buries 2600 Å^2 of surface area in its complex with TEM-1 β-lactamase [9]. In some regions of the interface BLIP introduces convex surface into a concave TEM-1 site, in other regions TEM-1 introduces convex features into concave sites of the inhibitor (Fig. 5). BLIP fits reading head-like loops into the active site of TEM-1. In this part of the interface we observe the

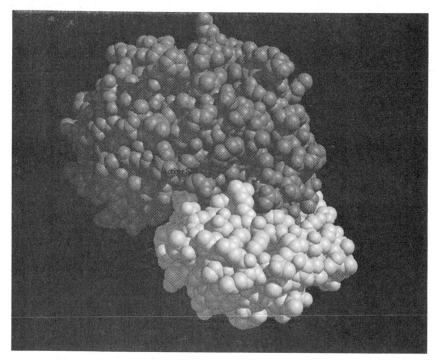

Figure 5   The hermaphrodite embrace of TEM-1 β-lactamase and BLIP. Each molecule has receptor-like and ligand-like qualities. The active site is marked. (From Ref. 9.)

greatest preorganization in the enzyme. In its unbound structure, the BLIP loops have high thermal factors and seem poorly localized [9]. In the absence of BLIP, the enzyme site preserves its coherence. In the region of the interface where TEM-1 is convex and BLIP is concave, it is the inhibitor that appears most preorganized for binding. In the absence of TEM-1, BLIP exposes a large number of hydrophobic amino acids to solvent, in a manner that is characteristic of many receptor sites.

Ligand preorganization may also play a role in small-molecule binding to proteins. Wiley and Rich [10] have argued that the exposure of high-energy surface area is a feature of many drugs. Drugs and drug candidates, such as clozapine and the DuPont–Merck human immunodeficiency virus HIV protease inhibitor (Fig. 6), are constrained by chemical bonding to expose the hydrophobic surface area to the solvent—the molecules cannot collapse upon themselves to reduce such surface area exposure. These molecules may be considered to be preorganized to adopt high energy conformations that are more likely to bind to receptors, relative to molecules

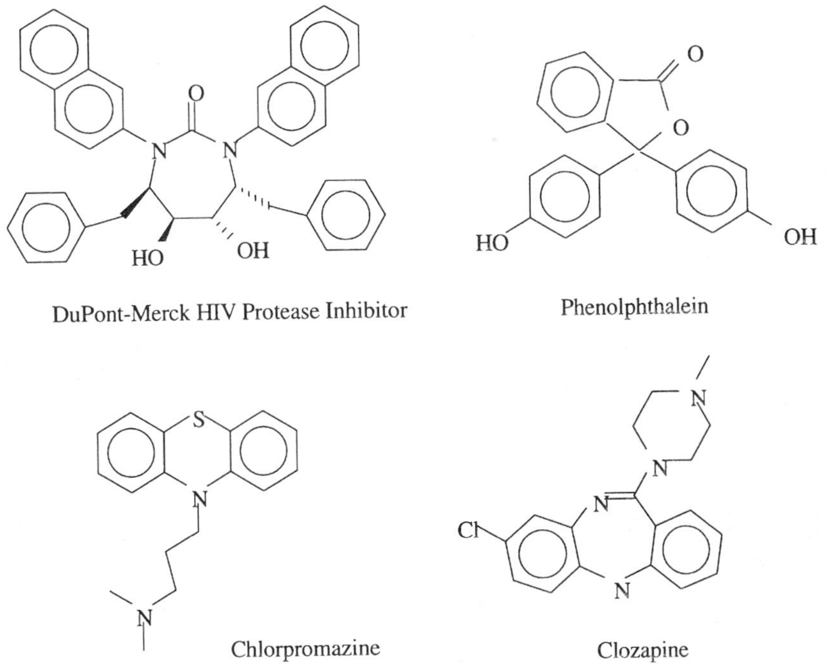

DuPont-Merck HIV Protease Inhibitor   Phenolphthalein

Chlorpromazine   Clozapine

Figure 6   Examples of inhibitors and drugs that are constrained to expose a large amount of hydrophobic surface area.

that are not so chemically constrained. Lam and colleagues recently invoked this notion of preorganization for binding [11] in their design of tight-binding inhibitors of HIV-1 protease [12]. One drawback of locating binding preorganization in small molecules is that they often cannot specify their interacting receptor to the same degree as the receptor can specify its ligand. Thus a ligand preorganized to expose a large amount of hydrophobic surface area may bind to several receptors, not just one. Ariens [13] has suggested that the lower specificity of antagonists, compared with their corresponding agonists, may reflect the greater hydrophobicity of the antagonists.

III. THE ROLE OF CONFORMATION CHANGE

On recognizing their ligands, some proteins undergo conformational change. Such change can take place on several scales [14]. Sometimes the conformational change is a matter of local accommodation, involving the rotation into different conformers of individual side chains. In response to binding phenolphthalein, for instance, the Arg-23 of thymidylate synthase changes its conformation to form a water-mediated hydrogen bond with a ligand carbonyl oxygen [15]. The rest of the binding site remains relatively fixed compared with the apostructure. This sort of local, residue-based change is also seen in TEM-1 β-lactamase in response to binding the BLIP protein. In TEM-1, Tyr-105 undergoes a 110° rotation in Chi 1, allowing the ligand to fit better into the binding site [9].

On a larger scale, elements of secondary structure can move together to either open or close a site in response to a ligand. On binding NAD-lactate, a ten-residue loop of lactate dehydrogenase rotates "down" on the ligand, closing off the active site. This loop movement allows ionic interactions between loop arginines and charged oxygens of the cofactor–substrate adduct. In the unliganded form of lactate dehydrogenase from dogfish muscle [16], this loop region is in an "open" conformation. This open conformation would not allow the favorable ionic interactions seen in the structure of the bound form (from pig muscle) [17]. The same sort of accommodation is seen with triose phosphate isomerase, for which a lid-like loop closes over the ligand, shielding it from solvent [18].

On a larger scale again, entire domains can change their relative positions in response to a ligand. In hexokinase [19] and maltodextrin-binding protein [20] such domain movements effectively bring two half-sites together—the full site exists only in the presence of the ligand. Calmodulin [21] has a characteristic dumbbell shape—two domains connected by a helix—in the absence of target-derived peptides. On binding to the targets, the central helix kinks in two, bringing the two domains together to form a single, globular domain, creating a new binding interface. At the far end of the spectrum, some DNA-binding proteins seem to exist only in a folded form in the presence of their cognate DNA [22].

Conformational change can take place on several levels of structural organization at the same time. Thymidylate synthase, on forming a ternary complex with dUMP and a folate-based inhibitor, shows a "segmental accommodation" [23], in which loops and helices move together to close down on the ligands. At the same time, individual residues, such as Arg-23, adopt different rotamers. Receptors can show different sorts of conformational change in response to different ligands: in binary complexes with dUMP or phenolphthalein analogs, segmental accommodation is not seen and the conformation of Arg-23 remains unchanged. In the complex between TEM-1 and penicillin G, unlike the BLIP–TEM-1 complex, Tyr-105 maintains the conformation observed in the apostructure.

Given these multiple levels of conformational change and their occasionally dramatic nature, it is appropriate to ask just how preorganized binding sites really are for their ligands. In transcription proteins such as MASH-1, the DNA-binding domain of which is unfolded in the absence of DNA [22] preorganization seems to lose all meaning. This is an unusual and perhaps extreme example, but even in the more common circumstances during which domain movement occurs, much of the binding site seems to exist only in the ligands presence. We must consider the possibility that a molten, highly flexible binding site is preferred to a more rigid, preorganized binding site.

Herschlag [24] and Fersht [25] have pointed out that when receptor flexibility is necessary for ligand binding, it will attenuate binding affinities relative to a situation for which flexibility is not required (i.e., if the protein is preorganized into its ligand-binding conformation in the absence of the ligand). Consider a receptor that can exist in two states, A and A* (Scheme 1). A is a lower-energy conformation of the receptor which binds the ligand poorly relative to A*, a higher energy conformation of the receptor. In the absence of the ligand (L), A will predominate in solution. In the presence of the ligand, A*L will predominate over AL. Now imagine the case where A* is the more stable state. A*L will again predominate—effectively A does not exist. The difference in binding affinities will be the difference in energies between A and A* (see $RT\ln K_{eq}$ in Scheme 1). By using this framework, we can understand the conformational changes observed on ligand binding as a preequilibrium to the optimal, preorganized state of the receptor. Conformational change thus *lowers* the binding affinity of the ligand to the receptor relative to the receptor's perfect, preorganized state.

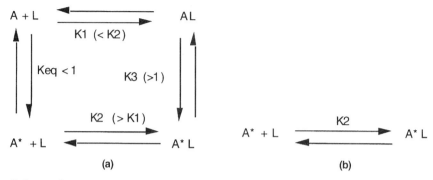

Scheme 1 The effect of conformational change on ligand binding: (a) Comparing the case for which receptor conformational change is necessary with the case (b) for which conformational change is not necessary for ligand binding. A ground state receptor conformation, A* high-energy conformation of receptor (in the absence of the ligand), L ligand.

Why then is conformational change so common? Several explanations have been suggested, we consider two here. First, the perfect preorganized state necessarily involves placing receptor functionality in high-energy configurations (the consequences of which are more fully discussed later). In the absence of the ligand, the overall folding energy of the protein might not be enough to stabilize the perfect preorganized state, leading to relaxation away from it. A second reason for conformational change is that this is often used as a signaling or regulatory event in the presence of multiple ligands. It is sometimes important, for instance, that a protein have an inactive conformation, and that it adopt its active conformation only under certain circumstances. This is true with maltodextrose-binding protein, for instance, which signals the presence of maltose to downstream targets by a considerable conformational change [20]. In general, an important feature of signal transduction cascades is that the kinases involved not be constituitively active, but only turn on under the proper circumstances, typically when they are themselves phosphorylated, methylated, or such by an upstream activator. In response to such chemical modification, the kinase will often change conformation, revealing a binding site that had previously been occupied by a self-inhibitory region. In these circumstances, conformational change reflects other constraints on the functioning of the enzyme and do not speak to the basis for receptor–ligand recognition, taken by themselves.

As a practical matter, conformational change muddies the notion of using preorganization as a guide to recognizing binding sites. The more dramatic the conformational change that a protein undergoes, the harder it will be to recognize what will ultimately be the binding site, in the absence of the ligand. In the limit, conformational change nullifies preorganization as a useful way of looking for binding sites. For most receptors, however, conformational change will be small enough that the preorganized-binding site can be recognized in the ligands absence. Going back to maltodextrin-binding protein, which undergoes significant domain movement on ligand binding, the binding site is largely established in the absence of the ligand, albeit as two halves, rather than a single site [20]. Conformational change is an important caveat to preorganization, and can reduce its usefulness, but it does not fundamentally affect the way we think of it, and we will not consider its role further here.

IV. SPECIFICITY OF BINDING SITES

The specificity of proteins in distinguishing among possible ligands and substrates is a fascinating feature of their action that has received much attention. Proteases such as trypsin and chymotrypsin, which have extensive sequence identity and superimposable main-chain folds, can distinguish with high specificities between peptides bearing charged or hydrophobic residues, respectively [26]. Trypsin has greater than 1 million-fold specificity for lysine-containing peptides over peptides with hydrophobic residues at the scissile bond, and chymotrypsin prefers aromatic hydrophobic amino acids over lysine residues at the siscile bond by up to 10 thousand-fold. Thymidylate synthase, which recognizes dUMP with micromolar K_m, discriminates against the highly similar dCMP with better than 300-fold specificity [27]. The bacterial sulfate-binding protein is highly specific for sulfate, preferring this anion to the isosteric phosphate by a factor of 100,000 [7]; conversely, the phosphate-binding protein prefers phosphate over sulfate to an equal degree [28].

Protein specificity may be considered an aspect of protein preorganization: proteins are preorganized to recognize a certain class of functional groups; not all functional groups will complement the binding site well. For instance, in trypsin, the specificity pocket is a deep depression in the surface of the enzyme, at the bottom of which lies an aspartate. This site is well suited to binding charged residues, such as lysine or arginine, but hydrophobic groups will be at a disadvantage, for they will bury the aspartate from water molecules, but will not interact well with it. In chymotrypsin, the pocket, although still deep, is now hydrophobic and is well suited to residues such as phenylalanine. Charged residues will be discriminated against, for on binding, they will bury a charged group without receiving any ionic compensation from the protein. The specificity of these two proteins depends on extensive interactions outside of the specificity pockets, not just the presence or absence of an aspartate [26]. Specificity is a fairly global feature of the structural and chemical organization of these binding sites.

This ability of enzymes and receptors to distinguish between substrates and agonists is the basis for the present view of their "exquisite specificity" [29]. In the last several years, results from several groups have suggested that the "tool and die-like" [30] specificity of a binding site for inhibitors or antagonists can be broader than has been previously supposed.

Investigators from several laboratories have shown that similar ligands can bind in different orientations in a given binding site, and the multiple-binding sites can exist on a given protein. In elastase, chemically similar peptide inhibitors bind in very different configurations to the enzyme (Fig. 7), even though the inhibitors are all potent (exhibiting K_i values of 2–12 nM) [31]. In rhinovirus coat protein, highly similar inhibitors of viral uncoating bound in two different orientations in the binding site (Fig. 8) [32]. As early as 1982, it was shown that pteridine analogues of folate bound to DHFR in different manners, making interactions with different residues within the same binding site [8]. In HIV-1 protease, nonpeptidic inhibitors bind to the enzyme in dramatically different configurations, depending on what seems to be an unimportant residue substitution at a position well-removed from the binding site [33]. Stout and co-workers have shown through mutagenesis, enzymology, and crystallographic studies that similar inhibitors of thymidylate synthase bind in very different orientations in the binding site [34]. In a fascinating study of the structural bases of antibody specificity, two different antibodies recognized the same hapten in very different manners using different residues [35]. This study generalizes an idea first introduced by Matthews, who suggested that the diversity of repressor structures and binding modes on DNA meant that there was no single "code" for recognition in these molecules [36].

In general, enzymes that recognize similar substrates can do so in different ways. Thus, dihydrofolate reductase binds to dihydrofolate in a manner different from the way thymidylate synthase binds methylene tetrahydrofolate, the mechanism and structure of zinc-type β-lactamases differs considerably from the serine-type β-lactamases [37], and so forth. There are examples for which enzymes, even when they are not evolutionarily related, *will* bind substrates using similar or identical sets of interactions; for example, the trypsin-like and subtilisin-like serine proteases. The point here is that similar substrates need not have similar enzymes or receptors—the structural and chemical codes for recognition are plastic.

Enzymes can sometimes recognize classes of inhibitors that are dissimilar to one another, and these will typically bind to different sites. Nu-

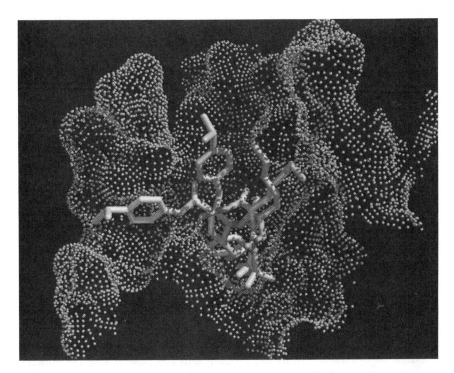

Figure 7 Similar inhibitors bind to elastase differently: The peptide trifluorace-tyl-L-lysyl-L-leucyl-p-isopropyanilide (carbons in gray) binds to elastase in a manner different from (molecular surface in red) the peptide trifluoroacetyl-L-lysl-L-phenylalanyl-p-isopropyanilide (carbons in orange). The trifluoromethyl and isopropylphenyl functionalities of each inhibitor are marked. Inhibitor nitrogens are blue, oxygens red, and fluorines magenta. See insert for color representation. (From Ref. 31.)

merous binding sites exist in hemoglobin for antisickling agents [38,39], the major histocompatibility complex (MHC)-II molecule has several different binding sites for different super antigen proteins [40]. In barnase, the substrate-analogue deoxydinucleotide d(GpC) bound to the enzyme in a site different from that expected for substrates [41]. In thymidylate synthase novel inhibitors bound to the enzyme differently from the substrates or inhibitors that resembled the substrates [15].

When first considered, the sometime low specificity of enzymes for inhibitors seems peculiar, given their high specificity for substrates. Why do enzymes not impose the same strict requirements for inhibitor complementarity as they do for substrates? Part of the answer may be that energy

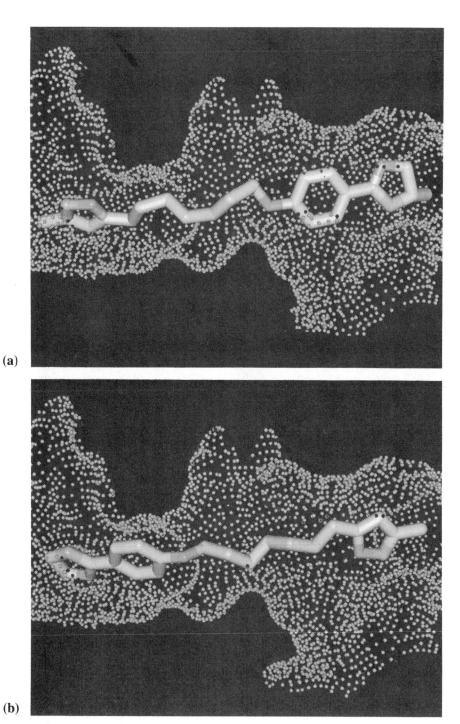

Figure 8 Similar antiviral compounds bind to rhinovirus coat protein in two different orientations: (a) Compound WIN I in the binding-site of rhinovirus coat protein; (b) compound WIN IV in the same site. Molecular surface of the binding site in dot format. (From Ref. 32.)

barriers for catalysis are so high [42] that constraints for recognizing the transition state have few tolerances. Enzymes probably do recognize a variety of substrates and transition states, but the rates of catalysis for most of them will be slow enough that they are not seen to turnover in the typical experiment. Mutant enzymes with reduced activity might show reduced specificity for the natural substrate. Recent results in T4 lysozyme for which a mutant enzyme proceeds through a different mechanism, recognizing a different stereoisomer along the reaction path [43], are consistent with this view. Sometimes enzymes will have evolved to distinguish between similar biological molecules that are present in their cellular environments. A constraint in the evolution of thymidylate synthase, for instance, may well have been that it distinguishes between dUMP and dCMP. For nonsubstrate-like inhibitors, to which organisms have not been exposed over evolutionary time, such a specificity pressure would not be present. Less teleologically and more biophysically, the novel inhibitors often take advantage of interactions outside the substrate recognition residues. Binding sites are typically considerably larger than the substrates they recognize, and inhibitors can often take advantage of residues the ligands do not use. The purpose of these additional residues is often unclear: as far as the catalytic or ligand response cycle is concerned, they may have roles in the trajectory of the ligands or products on or off the binding site, or they may have structural roles. The noncatalytic binding of nucleotides to barnase and phosphorylase has been explained as representative of pre- or post-catalytic-binding modes [41,44]. Different transition-state analogues of β-lactamases bind in different modes to the enzymes [45–47]. The different geometries may represent different high-energy intermediates along the catalytic pathway. These nonsubstrate sites and modes may have no functional "purpose"; they may be "happy monsters" that have arisen over the evolution of the enzyme and are a secondary phenomenon of the construction of the active site cavity.

If preorganization of the binding site is the signature of ligand binding, it clearly does not uniquely specify what ligand should bind, especially when the ligand is an inhibitor. The existence of one chemical class of ligand does not preclude the binding of very different classes; the existence of one binding site does not preclude the existence of other binding sites. Whatever the reason for the multiplicity of sites and modes, their discovery has renewed interest in methods to discover possible binding sites and possible ligands for them from first principles of structure and chemistry. We now turn to consider experimental and computational methods for identifying where ligands can bind to protein surfaces, and what ligands can bind at these sites.

V.   EXPERIMENTAL METHODS FOR IDENTIFYING BINDING SITES

We will consider two approaches to identifying binding sites. The first targets the receptor using site-directed mutagenesis, attempting to discover through perturbation of receptor properties signatures for functional regions. The second method uses X-ray crystallography directly to probe for different areas on the protein to which ligand functional groups might bind.

A.   Protein Mutagenesis and Stability Studies of Proteins

We have suggested that the ability of proteins to bind to their ligands is because of the preorganization of the protein-binding sites in high-energy conformations (see Fig. 1). This preorganization makes the proteins better solvents for the ligand than its alternative solvent, water. The high energy of binding sites should destabilize the ligand-free protein relative to some mutant protein that does not have the binding site.

The hypothesis that there is a balance between stability and function can be stated as: *protein residues that contribute to catalysis or ligand binding are not optimal for protein stability.* This function–stability hypothesis predicts that it usually should be possible to replace residues known to be important for function, reducing protein activity, but concomitantly, increasing the stability of the folded protein.

To test this hypothesis directly, we made substitutions in the active site of T4 lysozyme [43], an enzyme well characterized for the effects of mutation on structure and stability [48]. Five residues were replaced; the roles of these residues in chemical catalysis or ligand binding had been established previously by enzymatic or structural studies. These included two residues implicated in chemical catalysis, Gln-11 and asp-20 [49], as well as three others thought to have a role in substrate binding, gly-30, ser-117, and asn-132. We measured the thermodynamic stability and kinetic activity of the mutant lysozymes. To determine the structural consequences of the substitutions, we determined X-ray crystallographic structures for several of these proteins.

Our results in T4 lysozyme support the stability–activity hypothesis. At all five sites we were able to make substitutions that decreased the activity, but increased the stability of T4 lysozyme (Fig. 9). Many of these substitutions stabilize T4 lysozyme considerably more than any previously characterized point mutations in this enzyme; however, not all substitutions stabilized the protein. This is not inconsistent with the stability–function hypothesis, which predicts that some substitutions at functional residues should stabilize a protein, but not all substitutions will necessarily do so.

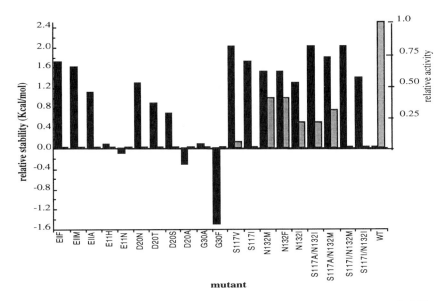

Figure 9 Comparison of the stability and activity of mutant lysozymes: Stability changes relative to the native protein are solid (left-hand scale), activity changes versus the native protein are dotted(right-hand scale).

For those mutants that are stabilized, the increase in stability appears to have a similar origin: the native protein is preorganized to complement the ligand or the transition state, whereas the substituted residues complement their local protein environment. Because this local environment is the substrate-binding site, the increased stability of the mutants comes at the expense of catalytic activity. The improved complementarity of the substituted residues for the their local environment can arise from improved electrostatic, van der Waals, or hydrophobic interactions, or through a reduction of strain present in the native protein (Warshel and co-workers have described a theoretical basis for the relation between stability and the electrostatic component of preorganization in active sites; see [3]). A detailed description of the trade-off between activity and stability among these residues has been presented [43].

The relation between protein stability and function should be a general phenomenon. Results from several other proteins support this view [43]. I draw attention to the work of Srere and co-workers on citrate synthase [50] and the work of Fersht and co-workers on barnase [51] and barstar [52], who explained their results in terms similar to the stability–function trade-off we have described here, focusing on electrostatic aspects of this hypothesis. In Cro, repressor stability has been significantly improved by substitutions of DNA-binding residues, at the cost of reduced operator affinity [53]. These residues occur in convex regions of the protein's surface, suggesting that the interplay between stability and function is not limited to the concave environments typical of enzyme active sites. The finding that most main-chain conformational strain occurs in the functional regions of proteins [1], and the view of enzymes as having an "entatic state" [54], are also consistent with the hypothesis.

Several caveats to the stability–function hypothesis must be mentioned. We do not mean to suggest that every substitution of a functional residue will improve stability—some residues will complement the site better than others, some will complement the site worse than the native residue. An appropriate analogy is that of a ligand binding to an active site. A particular active site will bind some ligands better than others, some ligands will not bind detectably. The hypothesis also makes no claims about how optimized a particular protein is for function or stability. It might be possible to improve the stability and the activity of a protein with the same substitution (in practice single substitutions that improve the activity of a protein have been rare).

If it is true, as I have argued here, that binding sites destabilize a protein, it also should be true that the ability to stabilize a protein by residue substitution indicates that a binding site exist. Imagine the following experiment: substitutions are made in various interesting grooves or ridges seen in the surface of a protein of determined three-dimensional structure. Some of the substitutions significantly stabilize the protein, which would suggest that a binding site exists for a ligand, although not which ligand. Significant stabilization is open to interpretation. Substitutions on the surface of a protein are typically thought to be stability neutral. Any substitution that increases the stability of the protein more than 500 calories might be considered to be significant. When reversible thermal denaturations are not possible, a change of 2° in the T_m would be significant. Until now only the positive control of this experiment has been conducted—only known binding sites, such as T4 lysozyme or barnase, have been mutated. Experiments that use the method to predict new binding sites are only just beginning.

B. Crystallographic Methods to Determine Binding Sites

In principle, it should be possible to take any given ligand or functional group, add it to a protein (either before or after crystallization) and determine where it goes using X-ray techniques. Indeed, this is probably the most common method currently used for finding and mapping binding sites. Once one has determined the structure of a receptor–ligand complex one can often tell a great deal about what is important for ligand binding, and where on the protein one should design against for new ligand functionality. The more extensive the protein–ligand interface, the more information one will have from such a structure. An interesting recent example is the structure of TEM-1 β-lactamase, a key enzyme for bacterial resistance to penicillin antibiotics and, hence, a drug target, in complex with β-lactamase inhibitor protein (BLIP; see Fig. 5). It has been suggested that the BLIP protein, although not itself being useful as a drug against β-lactamases, can be used as a guide to design smaller peptide- or nonpeptide-based inhibitors [9].

It is not always possible to determine a protein–ligand complex structure with the appropriate ligand. Often the compound of interest will be insoluble under the conditions during which the protein crystallizes, sometimes the protein crystals will deform and crack when the ligand is added, rendering them useless for structure determination. Sometimes it is unclear what the "appropriate" ligand should be. Ideally, one would like to be able to map out all possible-binding sites for a potential ligand—this will help define what the potential ligand will be. Naturally, this cannot be done with any one, particular ligand. Although an X-ray crystal structure can be rich in information, it says little about the energetics of the interactions seen between the ligand and the protein—it is often difficult to know which interactions are important and which are not.

To overcome these problems, several investigators have turned to small, highly soluble ligands as representative functional groups and determined where they bind to the protein at high concentration. These small ligands are probes for where particular functional groups might bind to the protein. Fitzpatrick and co-workers have immersed protein crystals into organic solvents, either neat or as aqueous mixtures, and then determined the three-dimensional structures by X-ray crystallography [55]. Crystals of subtilisin, grown from aqueous mother liquor, were transferred into each of acetonitrile, acetic acid, and ethanol, among others. The new solvent was allowed to diffuse through the crystals, which were then re-transferred into fresh solvent several more times. Occasionally it was necessary to chemically cross-link the crystals to maintain their structural integrity. The resulting structures have several intriguing features (Fig. 10). Overall, the protein is not affected much by the change from water buffer to the organic solvent. This is explained by the retention by the crystal of most of its water of hydration on being immersed in the organic solvent. Most of the water molecules bound to the protein in aqueous buffer are also found when the mother liquor is exchanged for the organic solvent. Some few solvent molecules are also seen in the structure—typically these have dis-

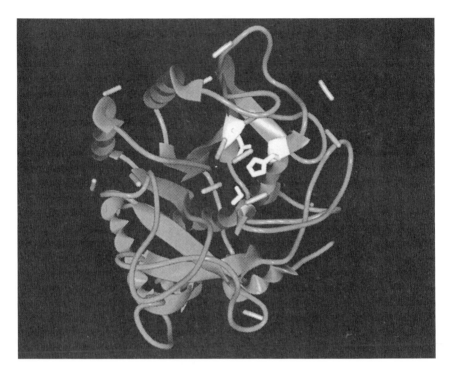

Figure 10   Acetonitrile (gray with blue tips) binding to subtilisin (red): The catalytic triad of subtilisin is in green. See insert for color representation. (From Ref. 55.)

placed water molecules that formerly occupied particular sites. Different solvents bind at different sites on the protein surface.

These results are explained by particular and, arguably, general features of the surface of subtilisin. Different parts of the surface of the enzyme will be better setup to accommodate different functional groups. Acetonitrile molecules bind at sites different from those of methanol molecules. Effectively, the protein is being probed for places where different functional groups might bind. One might imagine a ligand that is built up from a composite picture of where the different functional groups bind. This would have natural applications to ligand and drug design. An advantage of this method is that it is relatively unbiased for what ligand to design, but nevertheless, suggests specific functionalities to include. It is also agnostic in which site to design for—the locations of the solvent molecules on the protein are the only guide. Indeed, the organic solvent molecules, although binding predominantly in the active site, also bind in other regions of the protein [55].

Several other groups have investigated the binding of small molecules to proteins by X-ray crystallography. Urea binds to specific sites on DHFR (H. P. Yennawar and C. K. Farber, unpublished; protein data bank structure 1DDR). Again, the structure of the enzyme remains essentially unchanged. Similar work has been conducted against hen egg white lysozyme, using ligands such as ethanol [56], bromoethanol [57], dimethyl sulfoxide [58], and urea [59].

C. NMR Methods to Determine Binding Sites

Fesik and co-workers have recently published a method, SAR by NMR, that experimentally probes for binding sites for molecular fragments using NMR [78]. A library of small molecule ligands is screened against an enzyme or receptor, looking for those that bind. Affinity as well as structural conformation and orientation are determined by NMR. As with the crystallographic methods, different fragments are observed to bind in different sites. Because the authors chose larger molecular fragments they found ones with higher affinity than those used in the crystallographic experiments. This, and their knowledge of the ligand orientations on the protein, allowed them to link fragments together synthetically, to arrive at a compound with an affinity of 49 nM for the receptor. More recently still, NMR has been used to observe the binding of small molecules such as DMSO, methanol, and acetonitrile tolysozyme [79].

The use of small ligands as probes for binding sites has many attractive features, as we have discussed. For technical reasons relating to the stability of the crystal, this method will not be useful for every protein, or every functional group. This criticism may also be applied to the mutagenesis–stability approach. Some proteins are poorly behaved in temperature studies, and many proteins are difficult to reversibly denature by temperature. Although the both methods return trustworthy, often surprising, information about binding sites on proteins, both require considerable effort. We now turn to consider computational methods for interpreting structure for function. These methods require no experimentation, at least at the beginning, and are relatively inexpensive to use. They do not directly measure binding or binding sites; therefore, the information that they return is less trustworthy than the experimental methods. Similar to the experimental methods, they can return surprising insights into possible binding sites and functions for proteins. Similar to the experimental methods, they recognize preorganization for binding present in the structure of the protein.

VI. COMPUTATIONAL METHODS FOR IDENTIFYING BINDING SITES

The computational methods preceded the experimental methods in considering preorganization to be a signature of ligand binding. With the possible exception of inorganic biochemists such Williams [54], computational biochemists such as Warshel were first to advertise the role of preorganization in biological recognition [3,60].

A. Graphical Methods

Probably the most widely used computational methods in day-to-day work are those involving molecular graphics. The advent of high-resolution graphics devices and high-speed workstations has, in principle, allowed every computational chemist to have a graphics workstation on his or her desk. The programs are widely used for interactive identification of binding sites, investigation of binding interactions, design of new molecules, and so forth. One of the great strengths of these methods is that they allow for, in fact depend on, the knowledge of the scientist. Because they are so influenced by the user, it is difficult to attribute general principles to their operation; we will not consider them further here. It is appropriate only to mention several of the techniques that have had the most influence. These include the molecular surface technique (MS program) [61], first suggested by Richards [62]; the GRASP program [63]; the UCSF graphics package Midas-Plus [64]; the ribbons algorithm [65]; the crystallographic modeling package O [66]; the integrated simulations program MacroModel [67] and the several commercial packages including SYBYL (Tripos Associates) and Insight (Biosym). The preceding list is not meant to be exhaustive.

B. GRID

Among the first methods to probe for binding sites using biological structure and computational simulation was the GRID program introduced by Goodford [68]. The program calculates a three-dimensional lattice that encloses the active site of the protein. The molecular potential of the protein is evaluated on the basis of a potential function that includes Lennard–Jones, electrostatic, and hydrogen bond terms. A probe functional group is placed at every lattice point. Functional groups such as amines, hydroxyls, and methyls are among those commonly used as probes. The functional group has particular atomic properties, such as charge, van der Waals characteristics, and so forth, that when mapped onto a particular grid point allow an interaction energy (E_{int}) to be calculated:

$E_{\text{int},xyz)} = \sum \mathbf{PA}$ $\mathbf{P} = potential,$ $\mathbf{A} = probe\ atom$

Grid points that give favorable interaction energies with particular functional groups identify regions where such functional groups, if placed in the binding site, would complement it. In this manner, a topographic map of the binding site can be constructed for different functionalities.

GRID has been used extensively by pharmaceutical chemists for inhibitor design and elaboration. Perhaps the best example of its use is the design of a new inhibitor of neuraminidase [69]. Here, GRID identified a high concentration of negative potential adjacent to the sialic acid-binding site, predicting that a charged amino group would interact well with two glutamate residues. Synthesis of analogues of sialic acid that included amino or guanidinyl groups led to compounds with high-binding affinity for the enzyme. X-ray crystallographic analysis demonstrated that the analogues were taking advantage of the new site in the expected manner.

C. Spheres

Another widely used method [70] is the shape complementarity method first introduced by Kuntz [71]. Spheres are calculated to complement local areas of curvature in the molecular surface of a protein. Where such curvature exists, the possibility exists that a ligand atom could fit into it, as a ball into a socket. The location of the spheres thus defines pseudo-atom positions where a ligand atom might fit to complement a groove or pit in the protein's surface. The spheres can be given chemical characteristics according to what functional groups are around them, thereby expanding the information from simply geometric potential to chemical potential as well [72].

D. HSITE

A favored feature of protein–ligand interactions is the hydrogen bond. Danziger and Dean [72] introduced the program HSITE to identify regions on a receptor surface that are set up to donate or accept hydrogen bonds to a potential ligand. By using distance and angle criteria, potential hydrogen bond donors and acceptors are located on the protein. Such donors and acceptors that are not themselves complemented by groups on the protein are free to interact with the ligand. In regions where such groups are concentrated, three-dimensional lattices are calculated. At each lattice point the ability of a ligand atom to either accept or donate a hydrogen is evaluated. In this way HSITE calculates a map that describes potential hydrogen-bonding regions on the protein.

E. X-SITE

Molecular databases such as the Protein Databank Bank (PDB) [74] are rich sources of information for molecular interactions and binding sites. Laskowski and colleagues have considered interactions within proteins represented in the PDB to map out preferred interaction types and geometries for given probe atoms [75]. With a subset of well-resolved, unrelated proteins, the preferred environments for 26 probe atoms, all of which occur in proteins, are mapped spatially. The preferred environments are computed based on which three-atom fragments surround a given probe most often in the data set.

With these preferred environments in hand, the surface of a particular protein may be searched for binding sites. Any given patch of surface will have a particular distribution of functionality, which is analyzed in terms of three-atom fragments. The different atoms that make up the 26 probes have different likelihoods of being found close to different fragments, and the surface patches, therefore, can be judged as being more or less likely to complement a particular probe atom. Rather than attempt to give an energy score to these preferences, the authors highlight the surface regions that are within the top 10% for complementing any particular probe. The method was tested on several complexes of known three-dimensional structure and was able to accurately reproduce the location of many of the ligand atoms.

F. MCSS

Perhaps the computational method that most closely corresponds to an experimental method is the MCSS program introduced by Karplus and colleagues [76]. The method begins with an empty binding site in a protein of known structure. Overlapping, noninteracting molecular fragments are distributed throughout the volume of this site. The molecules are given kinetic energy, and they proceed to explore the binding site of the protein according to the CHARMM potential function [77]. Sites that interact favorably with the probes will be more populated during the course of this trajectory then unfavorable sites. By using multiple fragments and multiple trajectories the favored configurations of various fragment molecules can be calculated within the site of the protein. This is the computer version of the protein crystal–solvent experiments undertaken by Ringe [55] and others. As in the experimental version, different fragments will find different protein sites. A composite image of a potential ligand can, in principle, be stitched together from the different fragments.

VII. INTEGRATING THEORY AND EXPERIMENT

The computational and experimental methods for discovering binding sites are undergirded by the same principle: protein-binding sites are preorganized to accommodate a ligand even in the absence of that ligand. In the apoprotein, this preorganization leads to a network of unsatisfied protein functionality that in structural parts of the protein would be interacting with other residues. The computational methods that we have considered recognize these areas of uncompensated functionality either chemically (e.g., GRID, HSITE, X-SITE), or geometrically (Spheres), or by exploring the energy surface of the protein (MCSS). The experimental methods seek these areas of uncompensated functionality by finding either protein groups, through site-directed mutagenesis and stability measurements, or ligand groups, by exposing the crystals to high concentrations of small molecules that can fill these sites.

The experimental methods find true-binding sites. Their drawback is that they cannot be used on every interesting target. Some crystals will not tolerate high concentrations of urea, formic acid, and so forth. Neither can rigorous stability measurements be performed on every protein. Both experimental methods can also be quite time-consuming. Conversely, the computational methods, in principle, can be applied to any protein of known or modeled three-dimensional structure. Their drawback is that they have never been tested fully: Their reliability is unknown. Until recently, direct tests of these methods have been difficult. With the advent of the new mutagenesis and crystallographic methods of probing for binding sites, direct testing of the computational methods may soon be possible.

Until such time, structure-based identification of binding sites will have a strong qualitative component to it. I hope that I have convinced the reader that even at a qualitative level, binding sites stand out in protein structures. The preorganization of protein structures for function creates regions of unsatisfied potential that signal the existence of a binding site. At least some of these signals should be easily recognized within the structure of your favorite protein.

REFERENCES

1. O. Herzberg and J. Moult, Analysis of the steric strain in the polypeptide backbone of protein molecules, *Proteins 11*:223–229 (1991).
2. F. M. Richards, The interpretation of protein structures: Total volume, group volume distributions and packing density, *J. Mol. Biol. 82*:1–14 (1974).
3. A. Warshel, F. Sussman, and J.-K. Hwang, Evaluation of catalytic free energies in genetically modified proteins, *J. Mol. Biol. 201*:139–159 (1988).

4. A. Morton and B. W. Matthews, Specificity of ligand binding in a buried nonpolar cavity of T4 lysozyme: Linkage of dynamics and structural plasticity, *Biochemistry 34*:8576–8588 (1995).

5. Y. Nozaki and C. Tanford, The solubility of amino acids and two glycine peptides in aqueous ethanol and dioxane solutions. Establishment of a hydrophobicity scale, *J. Biol. Chem. 246*:2211–2217 (1971).

6. A. E. Eriksson, W. A. Baase, J. A. Wosniak, and B. W. Matthews, A cavity-containing mutant of T4 lysozyme is stabilized by buried benzene, *Nature 355*:371–373 (1992).

7. B. L. Jacobson and F. A. Quiocho, Sulfate-binding protein dislikes protonated oxyacids; a molecular explanation, *J. Mol. Biol. 204*:783–787 (1988).

8. J. T. Bolin, D. J. Filman, D. A. Matthews, R. C. Hamlin, and J. Kraut, Crystal structures of *E. coli* and *L. casei* DHFR refined to 1.7 Angstrom resolution. 1. General features and binding of methotrexate, *J. Biol. Chem. 257*: 13650–13662 (1982).

9. N. C. J. Strynadka, et al. Molecular docking programs successfully predict the binding of a beta-lactamase inhibitory protein to TEM-1 beta-lactamase, *Nature Struct. Biol. 3*:233–239 (1996).

10. R. A. Wiley and D. H. Rich, Peptidomimetics derived from natural products, *Med. Res. Rev. 13*:328–384 (1993).

11. D. J. Cram, The design of molecular hosts, guests and their complexes, *Science 240*:760–767 (1988).

12. P. Y. S. Lam, et al. Rational design of potent, bioavailable, nonpeptide cyclic ureas as HIV protease inhibitors, *Science 263*:380–384 (1994).

13. E. J. Ariens, in *Drug Design* Vol. 1 (E. J. Ariens, ed.), Academic Press, New York, 1971, p. 177.

14. R. Huber and W. S. Bennett, Functional significance of flexibility in proteins, *Biopolymers 22*:261–279 (1983).

15. B. K. Shoichet, K. M. Perry, D. V. Santi, R. M. Stroud, and I. D. Kuntz, Structure-based discovery of inhibitors of thymidylate synthase, *Science 259*: 1445–1450 (1993).

16. C. Abad-Zapatero, J. P. Griffith, J. L. Sussman, and M. G. Rossmann, Refined crystal structure of dogfish M4 apo-lactate dehydrogenase, *J. Mol. Biol. 198*: 445–467 (1987).

17. C. R. Dunn, H. M. Wilks, D. J. Halsall, T. Atkinson, A. R. Clarke, H. Muirhead, and J. Holbrook, Design and synthesis of new enzymes based on the lacate dehydrogenase framework, *Philos. Trans. R. Soc. B. 332*:177–184 (1991).

18. T. Alber, W. A. Gilbert, D. R. Ponzi, and G. A. Petsko, The role of mobility in the substrate binding and catalytic machinery of enzymes, *Ciba Found. Symp. 93*:4–24 (1983).

19. W. S. Bennett and T. A. Steitz, Structure of a complex between yeast hexokinase A and glucose. II. Detailed comparisons of conformation and active site configuration with the native hexokinase B monomer and dimer, *J. Mol. Biol. 140*:211–230 (1980).

20. A. J. Sharff, L. E. Rodseth, J. C. Spurlino, and F. A. Quiocho, Crystallographic evidence of a large ligand-induced hinge–twist motion between the two domains of the maltodextrin binding protein involved in active transport and chemotaxis, *Biochemistry 31*:10657 (1992).

21. W. E. Meador, A. R. Means, and F. A. Quiocho, Modulation of calmodulin plasticity in molecular recognition on the basis of X-ray structures, *Science 262*:1718–1721 (1993).

22. D. Meierhan, C. el-Ariss, M. Neuenschwander, M. Sieber, J. F. Stackhouse, and R. K. Allemann, DNA binding specificity of the basic-helix–loop–helix protein MASH-1, *Biochemistry 34*:11026–11036 (1995).

23. W. R. Montfort, K. M. Perry, E. B. Fauman, J. S. Finer-Moore, G. F. Maley, L. Hardy, F. Maley, and R. M. Stroud, Structure, multiple site binding, and segmental accommodation in thymidylate synthase on binding dUMP and an anti-folate, *Biochemistry 29*:6964–6976 (1990).

24. D. Herschlag, The role of induced fit and conformational changes of enzymes in specificity and catalysis, *Biorg. Chem. 16*:62–96 (1988).

25. A. Fersht, *Enzyme Structure and Mechanism*, W. H. Freeman & Co., New York, 1985.

26. L. Hedstrom, L. Szilagyi, and W. J. Rutter, Converting trypsin to chymotrypsin: The role of surface loops, *Science 255*:1249–1253 (1992).

27. L. Liu and D. V. Santi, Exclusion of 2'-deoxycytidine 5'-monophosphate by asparagine 229 of thymidylate synthase, *Biochemistry 32*:9263–9267 (1993).

28. H. Luecke and F. A. Quiocho, High specificity of a phosphate transport protein determined by hydrogen bonds, *Nature 347*:402–406 (1990).

29. N. Kasinos, G. A. Lilley, N. Subbarao, and I. Haneef, A robust and efficient automated docking algorithm for molecular recognition, *Protein Eng. 5*:69–75 (1992).

30. L. Pauling and M. Delbruck, The nature of the intermolecular forces operative in biological processes, *Science 92*:77–79 (1940).

31. C. Mattos, B. Rasmussen, X. Ding, G. A. Petsko, and D. Ringe, Analogous inhibitors of elastase do not always bind analogously, *Nature Struct. Biol. 1*: 55–58 (1994).

32. J. Badger, I. Minor, M. J. Kremer, M. A. Oliveira, T. J. Smith, and J. P. Griffith, *Proc. Natl. Acad. Sci. USA 85*:3304–3308 (1988).

33. E. Rutenber, et al. Structure of a non-peptide inhibitor complexed with HIV-1 protease, *J. Biol. Chem. 268*:15343–15346 (1993).

34. T. Stout, D. Tondi, D. Barlocco, M. Rinaldi, R. M. Stroud, B. K. Shoichet, and M. P. Costi, Structure-based design of specific inhibitors of thymidylate synthase from bacteria (in preparation, 1997).

35. R. L. Malby, W. R. Tulip, V. R. Harley, J. L. McKimm-Breschkin, W. G. Laver, R. G. Webster, and P. M. Colman, The structure of a complex between the NC10 antibody and influenza virus neuraminidase and comparison with the overlapping binding site of the NC41 antibody, *Structure 2*:733–746 (1994).

36. B. W. Matthews, Protein-DNA interaction. No code for recognition, *Nature* *335*:294–295 (1988).

37. A. Carfi, S. Pares, E. Euee, M. Galleni, C. Duez, J. M. Frere, and O. Dideberg, The 3-D structure of a zinc metallo-β-lactamase from *Bacillus cereus* reveals a new type of protein fold, *EMBO J. 14*:4914–4921 (1995).

38. A. A. Mehanna and D. J. Abraham, Comparison of crystal and solution hemoglobin binding of selected antigelling agents and allosteric modifiers, *Biochemistry 29*:3944–3952 (1990).

39. M. F. Perutz, G. Fermi, D. J. Abraham, C. Poyart, and E. Bursaux, *J. Am. Chem. Soc. 108*:1064–1078 (1985).

40. T. S. Jardetzky, J. H. Brown, J. C. Gorga, L. J. Stern, R. G. Urban, and D. C. Wiley, *Nature 368*:711–718 (1994).

41. S. Baudet and J. Janin, Crystal structure of a barnase–d(GpC) complex at 1.9 A resolution, *J. Mol. Biol. 219*:123–132 (1991).

42. A. Radzicka and R, Wolfenden, A proficient enzyme, *Science 267*:90–93 (1995).

43. B. K. Shoichet, W. A. Baase, R. Kuroki, and B. W. Matthews, A relationship between protein stability and protein function, *Proc. Natl. Acad. Sci. USA 92*: 452–456 (1995).

44. S. M. Sprang, N. B. Madsen, and S. G. Withers, Multiple phosphate positions in the catalytic site of glycogen phosphorylase: Structure of the pyridoxal-5′-pyrophosphate coenzyme–substrate analog, *Protein Sci. 1*:1100–1111 (1992).

45. K. Usher, L. Blaszczak, B. K. Shoichet, and J. R. Remington, (in preparation, 1997).

46. C. C. Chen, J. Rahil, R. F. Pratt, and O. Herzberg, Structure of a phosphonate-inhibited beta-lactamase. An analog of the tetrahedral transition state/intermediate of beta-lactam hydrolysis, *J. Mol. Biol. 234*:165–178 (1993).

47. E. Lobkovsky, E. M. Bilings, P. C. Moews, J. Rahil, R. F. Pratt, and J. R. Knox, Crystallographic structure of a phosphonate derivative of the *Enterobacter cloacae* P99 cephalosporinase: Mechanistic interpretation of a β-lactamase transition-state analog. *Biochemistry 33*:6762–6772 (1994).

48. B. W. Matthews, Structural and genetic analysis of protein stability, *Annu. Rev. Biochem. 62*:139–160 (1993).

49. R. Kuroki, L. Weaver, and B. W. Matthews, A covalent enzyme–substrate intermediate with saccharide distortion in a mutant of T4 lysozyme, *Science 262*:2030–2033 (1993).

50. W. Zhi, P. A. Srere, and C. T. Evans, *Biochemistry 30*:9281–9286 (1991).

51. E. M. Meiering, L. Serrano, and A. R. Fersht, *J. Mol. Biol. 225*:585–589 (1992).

52. B. Schreiber, A. M. Buckle, and A. R. Fersht, Stability and function: two constraints in the evolution of barstar and other proteins, *Structure 2*:945–951 (1994).

53. A. A. Pakula and R. T. Sauer, Amino acid substitutions that increase the thermal stability of the lambda Cro protein, *Proteins 5*:202–210 (1989).

54. R. J. Williams, The entatic state. *Cold Spring Harbor Symp. Quant. Biol. 36*: 53–62 (1972).

55. P. A. Fitzpatrick, A. C. U. Steinmetz, D. Ringe, and A. M. Klibanov, Enzyme crystal structure in a neat organic solvent, *Proc. Natl. Acad. Sci. USA 90*: 8653–8657 (1993).

56. M. S. Lehmann, S. A. Mason, and G. J. McIntyre, Study of ethanol–lysozyme interactions using neutron diffraction, *Biochemistry 23*:5862–5869 (1985).

57. A. Yonath, A. Podjarny, B. Honig, W. Traub, A. Sielecki, O. Herzberg, and J. Moult, Binding of dimethyl sulfoxide to lysozyme in crystals, studied with neutron diffraction, *Biophys. Struct. Mech. 4*:27–36 (1977).

58. M. S. Lehmann and R. R. D. Stansfield, Binding of dimethyl sulfoxide to lysozyme in crystals, studied with neutron diffraction, *Biochemistry 28*: 7028–7033 (1989).

59. A. C. W. Pike, and K. R. Acharya, A structural basis for the interaction of urea with lysozyme, *Protein Sci. 3*:706–710 (1994).

60. A. Warshel, Energetics of enzyme catalysis, *Proc. Natl. Acad. Sci. USA 75*: 5250–5254 (1978).

61. M. L. Connolly, Solvent-accessible surfaces of proteins and nucleic acids, *Science 221*:709–713 (1983).

62. F. M. Richards, Areas, volumes, packing, and protein structure, *Annu. Rev. Biophys. Bioeng. 6*:151–176 (1977).

63. A. Nicholls, K. A. Sharp, and B. Honig, Protein folding and association: Insights from the interfacial and thermodynamic properties of hydrocarbons, *Proteins 11*:281–296 (1991).

64. T. E. Ferrin, C. C. Huang, L. E. Jarvis, and R. Langridge, The MIDAS display system, *J. Mol. Graph. 6*:13–27 (1988).

65. M. Carson and C. E. Bugg, Algorithm for ribbon models of proteins, *J. Mol. Graph. 4*:121–122 (1986).

66. T. A. Jones, J. Y. Zou, S. W. Cowan, and M. Kjeldgaard, Improved methods for binding protein models in electron density maps and the location of errors in thes models. *Acta Crystallogr. A47*:110–119 (1991).

67. F. Mohamadi, N. G. J. Richards, W. C. Guida, R. Liskamp, M. Lipton, C. Caufield, G. Chang, T. Hendrickson, and W. C. Still, Macromodel, *J. Compt. Chem. 11*:440–467 (1990).

68. P. J. Goodford, A computational procedure for determining energetically favored binding sites on biologically important macromolecules, *J. Med. Chem. 28*:849–857 (1985).

69. M. V. Itzstein, et al., Rational design of potent sialidase-based inhibitors of influenza virus replication, *Nature 363*:418–423 (1993).

70. I. D. Kuntz, Structure-based strategies for drug design and discovery, *Science 257*:1078–1082 (1992).

71. I. D. Kuntz, J. M. Blaney, S. J. Oatley, R. Langridge, and T. E. Ferrin, A geometric approach to macromolecule–ligand interactions, *J. Mol. Biol. 161*: 269–288 (1982).

72. B. K. Shoichet and I. D. Kuntz, Matching chemistry and shape in molecular docking, *Protein Eng.* 6:723–732 (1993).
73. D. J. Danziger and P. M. Dean, Automated site-directed drug design: The prediction and observation of ligand point positions at hydrogen-bonding regions on protein surfaces. *Proc. R. Soc. Lond. Ser. B 236*:115–124 (1989).
74. F. C. Bernstein, T. F. Koetzle, G. J. B. Williams, E. F. Meyer, Jr., M. D. Brice, J. R. Rodgers, O. Kennard, T. Shimanouchi, and M. Tasumi, The Protein Data Bank: A computer-based archival file for macromolecular structure, *J. Mol. Biol. 112*:535–542 (1977).
75. R. A. Laskowski, J. M. Thornton, C. Humblet, and J. Singh, X-SITE: Use of empirically derived atomic packing preferences to identify favourable interaction regions in the binding sites of proteins, *J. Mol. Biol. 259*:175–201 (1996).
76. A. Miranker and M. Karplus, Functionality maps of binding sites: A multicopy simultaneous search method, *Proteins 11*:29–34 (1991).
77. B. R. Brooks, R. E. Bruccoleri, B. D. Olafson, D. J. States, S. Swaminathan, and M. Karplus, CHARMM: A program for macromolecular energy, minimization, and dynamics calculations, *J. Comput. Chem. 4*:187–217 (1983).
78. S. B. Shuker, P. J. Hajduk, R. P. Meadows and S. W. Fesik, Discovering high affinity ligands for proteins: SAR by NMR, *Science 274*:1531–1534 (1996).
79. E. Liepinsh and G. Otting, Organic solvents identify specific ligand binding sites on protein surfaces, *Nature Biotechnology 15*:264–268 (1997).

7

Comparative Protein Modeling

Manuel C. Peitsch
Glaxo Wellcome Research and Development R.A., Geneva, Switzerland

I. INTRODUCTION

Insights into the three-dimensional (3D) structure of a protein are of great assistance when planning experiments aimed at understanding protein function and during the process of drug design. Although protein structure elucidation techniques have made tremendous steps forward in the last years, they are often hampered by difficulties in obtaining sufficient protein, diffracting crystals, and many other aspects. The rate of sequence determination is roughly 50-fold higher than the rate of structure elucidation. The gap between known 3D structures and available amino acid sequences is growing rapidly. In fact the Swiss-Prot database [Bairoch and Boeckmann, 1992] contains more than 43,000 sequences, whereas the Brookhaven Protein Data Bank (PDB) [Bernstein et al., 1977] contains 3000 entries, approximately 1000 of which are distinct proteins. In this context, it is not surprising that predictive methods to derive the 3D structure of a protein are rapidly gaining interest.

Accurate and reliable protein–ligand interaction studies require high-resolution structures that can be obtained only by experimental means. Such structures, however, are generally unavailable during the early stages of a drug design project, and the identification of functional residues is usually derived from "blind," site-directed mutagenesis experiments and, to a lesser extent, by structure–activity relations based on assaying small molecules and peptides. The design of these mutagenesis experiments, however, could be rationalized to a much higher degree by the use of "low-resolution" protein models. Theoretical protein-modeling methods can frequently yield such low-resolution models that bear valuable information about the spatial arrangement of essential residues.

The 3D structure of a protein is determined not only by its amino acid sequence, but also by the molecular environment present at the time of folding. The rules underlying this process are largely unknown, and this hinders the prediction of a protein's 3D structure solely from its amino acid sequence (modeling de novo) and in the absence of a structural template. Attempts to predict the 3D structure of proteins de novo generally start with the prediction of their secondary structure using a palette of well-known techniques, which are based on the statistical distribution of amino acids in known 3D structures [Chou and Fasman, 1974; Garnier et al., 1978]. and the fine analysis of multiple sequence alignments [Benner, 1992]. Despite all the progress made in this field, the accuracy of secondary structure prediction remains less than (60–70%), which does not allow tertiary structure modeling with an acceptable level of reliability. The most recent advances [Srinivasan and Rose, 1995] in the prediction of protein structure from its amino acid sequence alone is based on the generation of a large number of random conformations selected by simplified force fields. This novel approach will provide a more reliable prediction method (up to 90%) for secondary and supersecondary structures, because it seems to work best for stretches of 50 residues. Along a similar line, a novel rule-based method was developed to predict the tertiary structure of G protein-coupled receptors [Herzyk and Hubbard, 1995]. The method is based on the assumption that it is possible to generate models of the transmembrane regions of these receptors using (a) nonstructural experimental data (i.e., mutagenesis and ligand binding) available for at least one member of a particular receptor subfamily; (b) the multiple sequences alignment of all known members of this subfamily; and (c) the 2D projection map available for bovine rhodopsin [Schertler et al., 1993]. The methodology also requires the clear definition of the sequence of the transmembrane regions. This is normally achieved by combining the helix assignments determined by Baldwin [1993], with those obtained from the multiple sequence alignments using programs such as TMAP [Persson and Argos, 1994] and TopPred [von Heijne, 1992]. These data are then translated into various distance and torsion restraints and an associated penalty function. Monte Carlo-simulated annealing [Kirkpatrick et al., 1983] is then used to globally optimize the penalty function and produce an optimal model.

Comparative protein modeling, on the other hand, first attempts to relate an amino acid sequence to a structural family and, then, generates atomic coordinates based on selected structural templates [Browne et al.,

1969; Greer, 1981; Blundell et al., 1987; Greer, 1991]. Here we will focus on comparative protein modeling, which is the most reliable method to date.

II. COMPARATIVE PROTEIN MODELING METHODS

Proteins from different sources with diverse biological functions can have similar sequences, and it is generally accepted that high-sequence similarity is reflected by distinct structural similarity. Indeed, the relative mean square deviation (rmsd) of the C-α atoms for protein cores sharing 50% residue identity is expected to be approximately 1 Å [Chothia and Lesk, 1986]. This has served as the premise for the development of comparative protein-modeling methods (also called knowledge-based protein modeling), by which a model for a new (target) sequence is extrapolated from the known 3D structure of related family members (templates) [Browne et al., 1969; Greer, 1981, 1991; Blundell et al., 1987].

Today, more than 50% of the newly solved protein structures appear to be related to known folding motifs [Blundell and Doolittle, 1992]. This is consistent with the idea that only a limited number of protein folds exist. The maximum number of these protein families has been estimated to be approximately 1000 [Chothia, 1992], and the number of families with distinct topologies to be approximately 500–700 [Blundell and Johnson, 1993]. According to Orengo and colleagues [Orengo et al., 1993], the PDB presently contains 150 nonhomologous folds, meaning that they do not share a common evolutionary origin. As time passes, an ever-increasing number of structural folds will be known, which should allow the identification of modeling templates for an ever-growing number of amino acid sequences. One may now find a suitable-modeling template for over 8000 sequences from the Swiss-Prot database, based on sequence similarity searches using such tools as BLAST [Altschul et al., 1990].

A. Template Identificatoin and Multiple Sequence Alignment

The first step in comparative model building is the identification of at least one suitable template structure. The most straightforward method of accomplishing this consists of scanning a database of protein sequences derived from the PDB database entries with the target sequence using algorithms such as BLAST [Altschul et al., 1990] and FastA [Pearson and Lipman, 1988]. If the degree of identity between the potential template and the target is greater than 30%, a model of the target sequence can be built with reasonable accuracy. However, if the degree of identity is too low to identify an unequivocal modeling template, then "threading" can be applied to search for the most suitale protein fold corresponding to the target sequence [Finkelstein and Reva, 1991; Jones et al., 1992; Bryant and Lawrence, 1993; Sippl and Weitckus, 1992]. Threading, or "inverse folding" addresses the question: "What known protein fold corresponds best to my sequence?" These methods evaluate the sequence-to-structure compatibility using an empirical Boltzman-like potential derived from a table of observed residue contacts in known protein folds.

In a second step, one has to generate a multiple alignment of the target and the template sequences. In some instances, a multiple sequence alignment that includes all known members of a protein family, can help identify common conserved sequence regions and allow a more accurate alignment of the target sequence with the selected templates. This alignment is essentially a description of the spatial correspondence between target and template residues. If several template structures are used, their sequences must be aligned by using structure, rather than sequence, similarity criteria. Thus, the proper boundaries between common secondary structural elements and loops can be clearly defined.

B. Coordinate Generation

Model coordinate building can now begin. Initially, an average framework for the target sequence will be calculated, based on the multiple sequence alignment described in the foregoing. The spatial location for as many atoms of the target as possible will be derived from the postions of the corresponding atoms in the template structures. The coordinates will be calculated as a weight-averaged postion, based on the corresponding atoms available from the templates. Each template will contribute to the average to an extent determined by its local degree of sequence similarity to the target [Peitsch, 1995, 1996]. Because the selected templates do not contain structural information about nonconserved loops and many of the side chains, these must be rebuilt in consecutive steps.

Rebuilding nonconserved loops is often performed using a "spare parts" algorithm as described by Jones and Thirup [1986; Greer, 1990]. Although most of the known 3D structures available share no sequence or structural similarity with the target and templates, there might be similarities in the loop regions, which can be inserted in the protein model. Each loop is defined by its length and the geometry of its "stems"; namely, the coordinates of the α-carbon (C-α) atom of the four residues preceding and following the loop. The fragments that correspond to the loop definition are extracted from the PDB entries if the rmsd computed for their stems is lower than a specified cutoff value. Furthermore, only fragments that do not overlap with neighboring parts of the structure are considered possible candidates. The accepted spare parts are sorted according to their rmsd and their degree of sequence similarity with the target. The best-fitting fragment is then added to the model.

Because the spare parts algorithm does not always lead to convincing solutions, especially for longer loops (more than eight residues), one might have to complement this approach with methods using conformational space-searching techniques. Loops modeled with these methods are filtered according to criteria such as the surface exposure of hydrophobic moieties and relative conformational energies [Bruccoleri et al., 1988].

Under certain circumstances, one might have to rebuild the main-chain atoms in some regions of a model. This is best performed by a method showing some similarity with the loop-construction process just described. Indeed, pentapeptides derived from the backbone structures of the high-resolution structures (less than 1.9-Å resolution) from the PDB are used as spare parts. These pentapeptides are fitted to five consecutive C-α atoms, and the main-chain carbonyl and nitrogens are derived from the best-fitting elements [Peitsch, 1996].

In the final step of coordinate generation, it is necessary to know the geometry of fully defined side chains, and to build those that are incomplete or lacking. This can be achieved by using libraries of allowed side-chain rotamers. Such tables are deduced from the highest-resolution structures from the PDB, and each rotamer is ranked according to its frequency of occurrence [Ponder and Richards, 1987]. More sophisticated tables provide the distribution of the side-chain rotamers based on backbone conformations (helix, sheet, turn, and coil). Whereas optimization of the fully defined side-chain geometries is performed by replacing each one by its best-fitting rotamer, the partially defined and missing residues are built by searching for a combination of side-chain conformations that minimizes the steric overlaps in the model structure.

C. Model Optimization

At this point, all atoms of a protein model have spatial coordinates. To optimize the stereochemistry of the model, and to minimize unfavorable nonbonded contacts, force-field calculations, such as energy minimization and molecular dynamics, can be applied. As a general rule, such computations should be kept to a minimum, because extensive force-field computations generally cause models to drift away from an experimental control structure. For instance, the approximate treatment of electrostatic interactions by conventional force fields can induce artificial structural effects and, thereby, lead to excessive structural deviations relative to the template structure.

III. MODEL EVALUATION

The technical aspects of comparative protein modeling described in the foregoing imply that the accuracy of a model is essentially limited by the deviation of the templates relative to the experimental control structure. It is unlikely that a theoretical protein model can be more accurate than average crystallographic precision, or the difference between a nuclear magnetic resonance (NMR) solution structure and the crystal structure of the same protein [Harrison et al., 1995]. As a consequence, the C-α atoms of protein models sharing 35–50% sequence identity with their templates, will generally deviate by 1.0–1.5 Å from their experimental counterparts. These values are expected because comparison of identical proteins for which the structure was elucidated independently, or in different crystal forms, deviate by 0.16–0.79 Å for the backbone atoms of the core [Chothia and Lesk, 1996]. Furthermore, two NMR and two crystal structures of interleukin-4 showed rmsd of 1.15–1.53 Å on C-α atoms [Smith et al., 1994]. These values reflect experimental errors as well as the influence of the molecular environment on protein structure.

Nonconserved loops and side chains are expected to be the least reliable portions of a protein model. Indeed, nonconserved loops often deviate markedly from control crystal structures. This phenomenon reflects the limitations of the loop-rebuilding methods (see foregoing). Frequently, however, these loops also correspond to the most flexible parts of the protein, as evidenced by their high crystallographic temperature factors and multiple solutions in NMR experiments. One reason for the inaccuracy of loop-rebuilding methods is that even short loops can potentially adopt a very large number of conformations that cannot be generated and ranked efficiently by computational methods (a peptide of ten residues, considering only four allowed-angle combinations, could potenitally adopt 105,107 conformations). A second reason is that loops are also often subject to unpredictable intermolecular contacts in the crystal lattice that will favor a group of conformations over all others. The conformations of the same loops in a solution structure might be very different.

The core residues, which are the least variable in any given protein family, are usually in essentially the same orientation as in experimental control structures, whereas far larger deviations are observed for surface amino acids. This is expected because the core residues are generally well conserved, and the rotamers of their side chains are constrained by neighboring residues. In contrast, the more variable surface amino acids will tend to show more deviations because there are few steric constraints imposed on them.

Some structural aspects of a protein model can be verified using methods based on the inverse-folding approach. Two of them—namely, the 3D-profile-based [Bowie, et al., 1991] verification method [Lüthy et al, 1992] and ProsaII [Sippl, 1993], are widely used. The 3D profile of a protein structure is calculated by adding the probability of occurrence for each residue in its 3D context [Lüthy et al., 1992]. Each of the 20 amino acids has a certain probability to be located in one of 18 environmental classes (defined by criteria such as solvent-accessible surface, buried polar and exposed nonpolar area, and secondary structure) as defined by Eisenberg and colleagues. In contrast, ProsaII [Sippl, 1993] relies on empirical pseudoconformational energy potentials derived from the pairwise interactions observed in well-defined protein structures. These terms are summed over all residues in a model and result in a more (more negative) or less (more postitive) favorable energy.

Both methods can detect a global sequence to structure incompatibility and errors corresponding to topological differences between the template and target. They also allow the detection of more localized errors, such as β-strands that are "out of register" or buried charged residues. These methods, however, are unable to detect the more subtle structural inconsistencies often localized in nonconserved loops, and cannot provide an assessment of the correctness of their geometry.

The stereochemistry of a model can be properly assessed by computing the backbone and torsion angles, and by measuring the accuracy of each bond length and angle using such programs as PROCHECK [Laskowski et al., 1993]. These tests, however, are of no value in determining the correctness of a protein model. Indeed, miss-traced protein chains in crystal structure can have acceptable crystallographic R factors and pass all stereochemical tests such as PROCHECK, and still be completely wrong. In turn, a protein model with a few residues in the disallowed region of the Ramachandran plot and inaccurate bond lengths, can still be of value to design mutagenesis experiments.

The accuracy of the model determines the extent to which it can be used. Low-resolution models, those derived from templates sharing less than 70% residue identity with the target, are helpful to rationalize site-directed mutagenesis experiments aimed at the identification of residue essential for a given molecular recognition and binding process. On the other hand, models based on more closely related templates may be useful during a compound optimization process. For example, models of closely related species variants of an enzyme may allow the optimization of drug specificity.

IV. COMPUTERS

With the rapid development of computer hardware and networks, displaying molecular structures and protein modeling are both becoming available to an ever-growing number of scientists. Besides the well-established commercial software packages (Biosym/MSI, Tripos, OML), which generally require powerful computer hardware, several systems that allow protein modeling (see the following) and molecular visualization on personal computer are emerging [Richardson and Richardson, 1993; Sayle, 1993; Peitsch, 1995, 1996]. Such tools enable experimentalists to perform simple protein-modeling tasks, and to visualize molecular structures without heavy investments. As time passes, these software packages will become increasingly powerful, and they should become a fundamental component of modern biomedical research.

V. AUTOMATED PROTEIN MODELING BY SWISS-MODEL

The bringing of protein-modeling capabilities to the scientists' desktop is essential for the broad application of these methods in molecular biology and drug design. Because protein modeling requires a fair amount of computing time, these tasks are best performed on powerful servers with inexpensive client software at the user's end. Swiss-Model [Peitsch, 1995, 1996] was designed to address this growing need. Hereafter is a description of this system, that can be reached on the Internet through the Worldwide Web.

A. The Search for Related Proteins

To determine if a modeling request can be carried out, Swiss-Model compares the target sequence with all proteinaceous chains of the Brookhaven Protein Data Bank, using both FastA [Pearson and Lipman, 1988] and BLAST [Altschul et al., 1990]. Sequences with a FastA score 10.0 standard deviations above the mean of the random scores and a Poisson unlikelihood probability $P(N)$ of 10–5 (BLAST) will be considered for model building. The choice of template structures is further restricted to those that share at least 35% residue identity with 40% of the target sequence. All requests that do not comply with these criteria end at this stage, and the user is notified by E-mail.

B. Generation of a Multiple Sequence Alignment

The target sequence is added to a structurally corrected multiple sequence alignment generated from the 3D structures of the selected templates, using the best-scoring regions of sequence similarity obtained by the SIM algorithm [Huang and Miller, 1991]. Residues that are not appropriate for model building (e.g., those located in nonconserved loops) will be ignored during the initial framework-building process. Thus, the core and the loops common to both the target and the templates will be built using the supplied structural information. The coordinates of the model are then generated by the automated protein-modeling tool ProMod, using the methods described in the foregoing [Peitsch, 1995, 1996].

C. Further Refinement

Idealization of bond geometry and removal of unfavorable nonbonded contacts are automatically performed by energy minimization with CHARMM [Brooks et al., 1983], using the PARAM22 parameter set and a cutoff distance for interactions of 8 Å. The refinement of the primary model generated by ProMod is accomplished by 50 steps of steepest descent, followed by 200 steps of conjugate gradient energy minimization.

D. 3D Profile Calculation

Swiss-Model provides a quality assessment of the generated protein models. ProMod and ProsaII [Sippl, 1993] are used to compute the 3D profile [Lüthy et al., 1992] and the sequence-to-structure fitness of the model. The results of these computations are returned to the user in ready-to-print ProstScript files.

E. Model Confidence Factors

Molecular models usually contain a mixture of regions that are well defined by the used template structures and other areas that require complete rebuilding. To distinguish between these regions, we need to define confidence factors. Clearly, there will be a higher degree of confidence in regions similar to several closely overlapping template structures, than for others that are based on only one-template structure. Even the latter regions are still better defined than loops built using segments from unrelated structures. ProMod, therefore, computes a model confidence factor (termed the C-factor) during framework building. This data is stored in the crystallographic temperature factor (B-factor) fields in the coordinate files sent by Swiss-Model. As with B-factors, low C-factors indicate low structural variability of the given residues and high confidence. A high degree of flexibility and dispersion is reflected by a high C-factor. Most molecular visualization programs have functions that will color atoms according to these values, providing the user with a graphic interpretation of structural variability. The similarities between target and template sequences are not considered, because the expected deviation of the model based on this criterion can be deduced from the work of Chothia and Lesk [1986]. A maximal C-factor (lowest confidence) is automatically assigned to all non-conserved loops and side chains.

F. The Worldwide Web Interface

URL: http://expasy.hcuge.ch/swissmod/SWISS-MODEL.html

The Swiss-Model server is reachable on the Worldwide Web (WWW) and requests can be submitted through easy-to-fill forms using WWW-browsers such as NCSA-Mosaic or Netscape. All results are returned to the user by E-mail. Swiss-Model also provides links to other servers relevant to protein structure as well as detailed help in hypertext format. Because protein modeling is heavily dependent on the alignment between target and template sequences, Swiss-Model provides two distinct modes of function accessible through two separate forms:

The First Approach Mode. This mode allows the user to submit a sequence or its Swiss-Prot identification code. In this mode, Swiss-Model will go through the complete procedure described in the foregoing. The first approach mode also allows the user to define a choice of preselected template structures, thereby overruling the automated selection procedure.

The Optimize Mode. This mode allows the user to recompile a model by submitting altered sequence alignments and ProMod command files. The sequence alignment procedure, which is fully automatic in the first approach mode, may yield nonoptimal alignments and, consequently, lead to erroneous models. The automated alignment of moderately similar sequences is often imprecise, and the boundaries of nonconserved loops are frequently ill-defined and misaligned. These regions of the sequence alignments, therefore, must be corrected by hand to overcome these weaknesses. The optimize mode allows the user to perform such corrections and to request the remodeling of the sequence by submitting a supplied sequence alignment. This is best done by altering the sequence alignment file sent back by Swiss-Model after a first approach mode request. Usually, it is not necessary to further optimize a model after the first approach mode if none of the insertions or deletions were made in secondary structure elements, such as helices and strands. Also a model that yields acceptable 3D profile and ProasII plots (sequence-to-structure fitness) does not need to be further optimized.

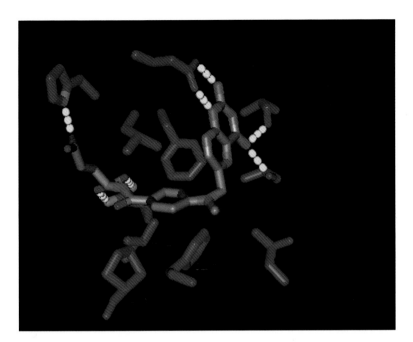

Figure 6.4 Methotrexate in complex with dihydrofolate reductase: The residues that interact with the phenyl ring or methotrexate are labeled. Hydrogen bonds are shown as dashed yellow lines, oxygens are red, nitrogens blue, protein carbons are magenta, and the methotrexate carbons are gray.

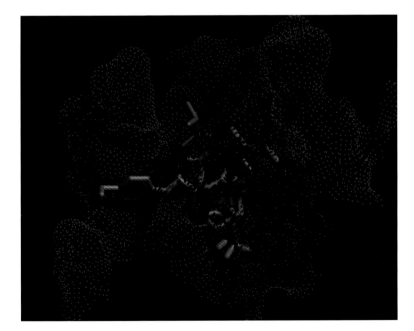

Figure 6.7 Maltodextrin-binding protein in the presence (orange) and absence (green) of *d*-maltose (gray and red): The two globular domains of the protein undergo a rigid-body "hinge-bending" rotation of 35° on binding maltose.

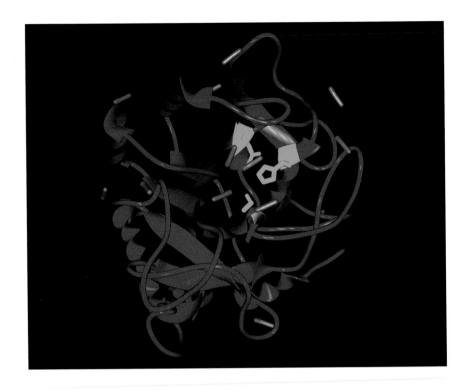

Figure 10 Acetonitrile (gray with blue tips) binding to subtilisin (red): The catalytic triad of subtilisin is in green.

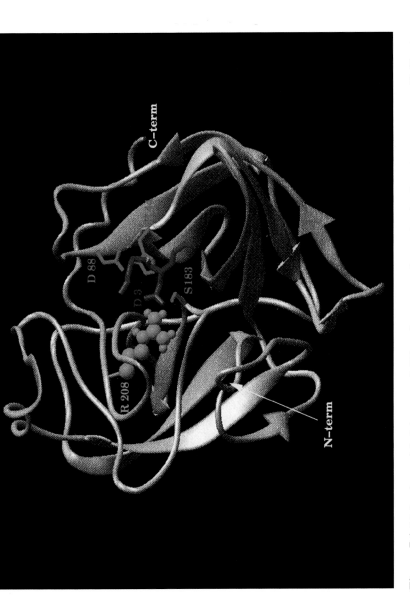

Figure 7.1 Molecular model of the cytotoxic T-lymphocyte granule associated serine esterase granzyme B. The structure of granzyme B is shown as a gray ribbon, while the peptide substrate Ala-Ala-Asp-Gly is depicted by red sticks. The side chain of the substrate aspartate points into the S1 pocket which is partially filled by Arg 208 (blue space-filling). The residues of the catalytic triad (His 44, Asp 88, and Ser 183) are shown in green.

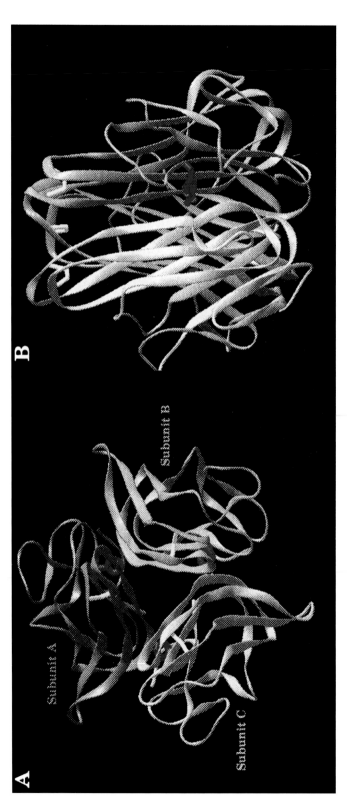

Figure 7.2 Top (A) and side (B) view of the molecular model of the trimeric Fas ligand. The three subunits are depicted in different colors, while the cystein-bonds are shown in yellow. The Phe 273, which is mutated in *gld* mice and causes a lymphoproliferative disease, is shown in magenta.

VI. EXAMPLES

A. The Substrate Specificity of Granzyme B

The results and interpretation of this example can be obtained through the automated protein-modeling server Swiss-Model.

Cytotoxic T lymphocyte-mediated killing is central to the immunological defense against tumors, viral infections, and transplanted tissue [Lowin et al., 1995]. Activated cytotoxic T lymphocytes possess dense cytoplasmic granules that contain various proteins that take part in the "lethal hit" delivery. Besides perforin, which is responsible for the lesions often associated with target cell lysis, several serine proteases (mouse granzymes A–G; human granzyme A, B, and H) were discovered within these granules [Lowin et al., 1995]. Only the substrate specificities of granzymye A and D were readily apparent because they are trypsin-like.

To determine the substrate specificity of mouse and human granzyme B, molecular models of both serine esterases were built [Murphy et al., 1988; Peitsch and Tschopp, 1994; Lowin et al., 1995]. The model structures were constructed using comparative protein-modeling methods described in this chapter. The selected structural templates were the experimentally elucidated structures of mast cell protease II, α-chymotrypsin, and trypsin. All templates share between 35 and 40% residue identity with granzyme B. One could use several more templates, for the structures of pancreaticlastase, leukocyte elastase, thrombin, kallikrein, and tonin are also known. Models generated with six or more templates do not, however, yield better results and do not differ markedly from the model obtained with the four aforelisted structures. Also, none of the nonconserved loops of granzyme B were conserved in them. These structures can thus be considered superfluous and are not necessary to obtain a model of granzyme B. Analysis of the amino acid sequences revealed an arginine in position +25 (human Arg-208) relative to the active site serine. In the model structure (Fig. 1 see insert), the side chain of Arg-208 is oriented toward the active site, and partially fills the binding pocket. Granzyme B was thus predicted to cleave substrates with negatively charged side chains. Furthermore, the model indicated that granzyme B should prefer aspartic over glutamic acid, because aspartic acid has a shorter side chain. These predictions were later supported by experimental evidence demonstrating that granzyme B cleaves synthetic peptide substrates preferentially after aspartic acid and more weakly after glutamic acid [Poe et al., 1991; Odake et al., 1991].

B. Analyzing the Interaction Between FAS and Its Ligand

The results and interpretation of this example cannot be obtained through the automated protein-modeling server Swiss-Model, because the degree of sequence similarity between target and template structures is low.

The Fas ligand (FasL) is a member of a type II membrane protein superfamily consisting of tumor necrosis factor (TNF-α and TNF-β; lymphotoxin-α), lymphotoxin-β, CD27L, CD30L, CD40L, and 4-1BB. The Fas receptor (Fas) is a member of the TNF-receptor family, which comprises receptors for the foregoing ligands. Despite the diversity of the biological activities elicited by these ligands, most of the ligands induce cellular differentiation or proliferation with two exceptions. The FasL, and under some circumstances TNF, are responsible for rapid induction of apoptosis in receptor-bearing cells [see references in: Singer et al., 1994; Golstein, 1995; Peitsch and Tschopp, 1995; Hahne et al., 1995].

Comparative protein modeling of the Fas ligand and the other members of that superfamily (based on the TNF-α and TNF-β crystal structures) is a typical example of how low-resolution models can serve as a basis for the rational planification of site-directed mutagenesis experiments [Peitsch and Tschopp, 1995]. Given the protein model, one can define potential sites for receptor–ligand interaction and design appropriate experiments to identify the key residues. In addition, these models can help understand the structural consequences of naturally occurring mutants as shown for CD40L [summary in Callard et al., 1993] and FasL [Hahne et al., 1995] (Fig. 2 see insert).

REFERENCES

Altschul, S. F., W. Gish, W. Miller, E. W. Myers, and D. J. Lipman, Basic local alignment search tool, *J. Mol. Biol. 215*:403–410 (1990).

Bairoch, A. and B. Boeckmann, The SWISS-PROT protein sequence data bank, *Nucleic Acids Res. 20*:2019–2022 (1992).

Baldwin, J. M. The probable arrangement of the helices in G protein-coupled receptors, *EMBO J. 12*:1693–1703 (1993).

Benner, S. A. Predicting de novo the folded structure of proteins, *Curr. Opin. Struct. Biol. 2*:402–412 (1992).

Bernstein, F. C., T. F. Koetzle, G. J. B. Williams, E. F. Meyer, M. D. Brice, J. R. Rodgers, O. Kennard, T. Shimanovichi, and M. Tasumi, The Protein Data Bank: A computer-based archival file for macromolecular structures, *J. Mol. Biol. 112*:535–542 (1997).

Blundell, T. L. and R. F. Doolittle, Sequence and topology—an inverse approach to the old folding problem, *Curr. Opin. Struct. Biol. 2*:381–383 (1992).

Blundell, T. L. and M. S. Johnson, Catching a common fold, *Protein Sci. 2*:877–883 (1993).

Blundell, T. L., B. L. Sibanda, M. J. Sternberg, and J. M. Thornton, Knowledge-based prediction of protein structures and the design of novel molecules, *Nature 326*:347–352 (1987).

Bowie, J. U., R. Luethy, and D. Eisenberg, A method to identify protein sequences that fold into a known three-dimensional structure, *Science 235*:164–170 (1991).

Brooks, B. R., R. E. Bruccoleri, B. D. Olafson, D. J. States, S. Swaminathan, and M. Karplus, CHARMM: A program for macromolecular energy, minimization and dynamics calculation, *J. Comput. Chem. 4*:187–217 (1983).

Browne, W. J., A. C. T. North, d. C. Philipps, K. Brew, T. C. Vanaman, and R. L. Hill, A possible three-dimensional structure of bovine alpha-lactalbumin based on that of hen's egg white lysozyme, *J. Mol. Biol. 42*:65–86 (1969).

Bruccoleri, R. E., E. Haber, and J. Novotny, Prediction of the folding of short polypeptide segments by uniform conformational sampling, *Biopolymers 26*: 137–168 (1988).

Bryant, S. H. and C. E. Lawrence, An empirical energy function for threading protein sequences through the folding motif, *Proteins Struct. Funct. Genet. 16*:92–112 (1993).

Callard, R. E., R. J. Armitage, W. C. Fanslow, and M. K. Spriggs, CD40 ligand and its role in X-linked hyper-IgM syndrome, *Immunol. Today 14*:559–564 (1993).

Chothia, C., One thousand families for the molecular biologist, *Nature 357*:543–544 (1992).

Chothia, C. and A. M. Lesk, The relation between the divergence of sequence and structure in proteins, *EMBO J. 5*:823–826 (1986).

Chou, P. Y. and G. D. Fasman, Prediction of protein conformation, *Biochemistry 13*:222–245 (1974).

Finkelstein, A. V. and B. A. Reva, A search for the most stable fold of proteins, *Nature 351*:497–499 (1991).

Garnier J., D. J. Osguthorpe, and B. Robson, Analysis of the accuracy and implications of simple methods for predicting the secondary structure of globular proteins, *J. Mol. Biol. 120*:97–120 (1978).

Golstein, P., Fas-based T cell-mediated cytotoxicity, *Curr. Top. Microbiol. Immunol. 198*:25–37 (1995).

Greer J., Comparative model building of mammalian serine proteases, *J. Mol. Biol. 153*:1027–1042 (1981).

Greer, J., Comparative modelling methods: Application to the family of mammalian serine proteases, *Proteins Struct. Funct. Genet. 7*:317–334 (1990).

Greer, J. Comparative modelling of homologous proteins, *Methods Enzymol. 202*: 239–252 (1991).

Hahne, M., M. C. Peitsch, M. Irmler, M. Schröter, B. Lowin, R. Rousseau, C. Bron, T. Renno, L. French, and J. Tschopp, Characterisation of the non-functional Fas ligand of *gld* mice, *Int. Immunol 7*:1381–1386 (1995).

Harrison, R. W., D. Chatterjee, and T. Weber, Analysis of six protein structures predicted by comparative modeling techniques, *Proteins Struct. Funct. Genet.* *23*:463–471 (1995).

Herzyk, P. and R. E. Hubbard, An automated method for modelling seven-helix transmembrane receptors from experimental data, *Biophys. J. 69*:2419–2442 (1995).

Huang, X. and M. Miller, A time-efficient, linear-space local similarity algorithm, *Adv. Appl. Math. 12*:337–357 (1991).

Jones, D. T. and S. Thirup, Using known substructures in protein model building and crystallography, *EMBO J. 5*:819–822 (1986).

Jones, D. T., W. R. Taylor, and J. M. Thornton, A new approach to protein fold recognition. *Nature 358*:86–89 (1992).

Kirkpatrick, S., C. D. Gellat, and M. P. Vecchi, *Science 220*:671–680 (1983).

Laskowski, R. A., M. W. MacArthur, D. S. Moss, and J. M. Thornton, PROCHECK: A program to check the stereochemical quality of protein structures, *J. Appl. Crystalogr. 26*:283–291 (1993).

Lüthy, R., J. U. Bowie, and D. Eisenberg, Assessment of protein models wth three-dimensional profiles, *Nature 356*:83–85 (1992).

Lowin, B., M. C. Peitsch, and J. Tschopp, Perforin and granzymes: Crucial effector molecules in cytolytic T lymphocyte and natural killer cell-mediated cyto-toxicity, *Curr. Top. Microbiol. Immunol. 198*:1–24 (1995).

Murphy, M. E., J. Moult, R. C. Bleackley, H. Gershenfeld, I. L. Weissman, and M. N. James, Comparative molecular model building of two serine protein-ases from cytotoxic T lymphocytes, *Proteins Struct. Funct. Genet. 4*:190–204 (1988).

Odake S., C.-M. Kam, L. Narasimhan, M. Poe, J. T. Blake, O. Krähenbühl, J. Tschopp, and J. C. Powers, Human and murine cytotoxic T lymphocyte serine proteases: Subsite mapping with peptide thioester substrates and inhibition of enzyme activity and cytolysis by isocoumarins, *Biochemistry 30*:2217–2227 (1991).

Orengo, C. A., T. P. Flores, W. R. Taylor, and J. M. Thornton, Identification and classification of protein fold families, *Protein Eng. 6*:485–500 (1993).

Pearson, W. R. and D. J. Lipman, Improved tools for biological sequence compar-ison, *Proc. Natl. Acad. Sci. USA 85*:2444–2448 (1988).

Peitsch, M. C., ProMod and Swiss-Model: Internet-based tools for automated com-parative protein modelling, *Biochem. Soc. Trans. 24*:274–279 (1996).

Peitsch, M. C., Protein modelling by E-mail, *Biotechnology 13*:658–660 (1995).

Peitsch, M. C., and J. Tschopp, Granzyme B, *Methods Enzymol. 244*:80–87 (1994).

Peitsch, M. C. and J. Tschopp, Comparative molecular modelling of the Fas-ligand and other members of the TNF family, *Mol. Immunol. 32*:761–772 (1995).

Persson, B. and P. Argos, Prediction of transmembrane segments in proteins util-ising multiple sequence alignments, *J. Mol. Biol. 237*:182–192 (1994).

Poe, M., J. T. Blake, D. A. Boulton, M. Gammon, N. H. Sigal, J. K. Wu, and H. J. Zweerink, Human cytotoxic lymphocyte granzyme B. Its purification from granules and the characterization of substrate and inhibitor specificity, *J. Biol. Chem. 266*:98–103 (1991).

Ponder, J. W. and F. M. Richards, Tertiary templates for proteins. Use of packing criteria in the enumeration of allowed sequences for different structural classes, *J. Mol. Biol. 193*:775 (1987).

Richardson, D. C. and J. S. Richardson, The kinemage: A tool for scientific communication, *Protein Sci. 1*:3–9 (1992).

Sayle, R. A. and E. J. Milner-White, Biomolecular graphics for all, *Trends Biochem. Sci. 20*:374–376 (1995).

Schertler, G. F. X., C. Villa, and R. Henderson, Projection structure of rhodopsin, *Nature 362*:770–772 (1993).

Singer, G. G., A. C. Carrera, A. Marshak-Rothstein, C. Martinez, and A. K. Abbas, Apoptosis, Fas and systemic autoimmunity: The MRL-lpr/lpr model, *Curr. Opin. Immunol. 6*:913–920 (1994).

Sippl, M. J. and S. Weitckus, Detection of native-like models for amino acid sequences of unknown three-dimensional structure in a data base of known protein conformations, *Proteins Struct. Funct. Genet. 13*:258–271 (1992).

Sippl, M. J. Recognition of errors in three-dimensional structures of proteins, *Proteins Struct. Funct. Genet. 17*:355–362 (1993).

Smith, L. J., C. Redfield, R. A. G. Smith, C. M. Bobson, G. M. Clove, A. M. Gronenborn, M. R. Walter, T. L. Naganbushan, and A. Wlodawer, Comparison of four independently determined structures of human recombinant interleukin-4, *Nature Struct. Biol. 1*:301–310 (1994).

Srinivasan, R. and G. D. Rose, LINUS: A hierarchic procedure to predict the fold of a protein, *Proteins Struct. Funct. Genet. 22*:81–99 (1995).

von Heijne, G., Membrane protein structure prediction. Hydrophobicity analysis and the positive-inside rule, *J. Mol. Biol. 225*:487–494 (1992).

8

Docking Conformationally Flexible Molecules into Protein Binding Sites

Millard H. Lambert

Glaxo Wellcome Inc., Reserach Triangle Park, North Carolina

I. INTRODUCTION

Advances in molecular biology, protein expression and purification, X-ray crystallography, and nuclear magnetic resonance (NMR) spectroscopy have recently led to high-resolution structures for numerous important proteins. In principle, it should be possible to design highly potent ligands quickly, directly, and routinely from the structures of the target proteins. Although this ultimate goal of structure-based drug design is far from reality, structure-based methods have played an important role in many recent drug discovery projects [1–5; see Chap. 1].

Structure-based drug discovery necessarily depends on experimental methods for obtaining purified protein, for synthesizing and testing compounds, and for solving the structures, as well as theoretical methods for designing new compounds. Although there is always room for improvement, the current experimental methods are generally adequate; the principal obstacle to structure-based design is the theoretical methodology. The minimal theoretical methodology required for structure-based drug design includes molecular-docking calculations, binding energy estimation, and molecular design. Docking calculations are needed to predict how new, hypothetical compounds will bind to the protein. Methods for estimating the binding energy are needed to identify the best of the candidate compounds. Molecular design techniques would then be used in an iterative cycle with docking methods and binding energy estimation to find synthetically accessible compounds that optimize the binding affinity. An ideal theoretical toolkit would also include methods for building protein models by homology, as well as methods for predicting bioavailability and pharmacokinetics.

This chapter reviews the methods used in docking small flexible molecules into protein-binding sites, emphasizing the methods appropriate for lead optimization in drug discovery projects. This includes a brief discussion of previously unpublished algorithms used in the MVP program at Glaxo Wellcome [6]. Elsewhere in this volume [see Chap. 3] DesJarlais reviews the application of molecular-docking calculations to lead discovery by database screening. Ajay et al. [see Chap. 10] review the estimation of binding energies, and Murcko [see Chap. 9] reviews molecular design. Other reviews of the protein–ligand docking problem [7,8] as well as brief reviews of molecular docking [4,9,10] are also recommended. The protein–protein docking problem generally involves more drastic approximations and, thus, different algorithms; this area has been reviewed [11]. Also, a recent protein–protein docking "challenge" compares six different methods [12]. Much of the methodology for protein–ligand docking calculations has been inherited from earlier work in small-molecule conformational searching and macromolecular energy calculations. A very clear survey of conformational searching is available [13], as well as a thorough review of energy calculations in protein modeling [14].

II. ENERGY IN MOLECULAR DOCKING CALCULATIONS

The stable structures of a small molecule correspond to minima on the multidimensional energy surface, with alternative conformations populated according to their free energies. The free energy of a particular conformation is equal to the solvated free energy at the minimum, with a small correction for the configurational entropy about the minimum [15]. Anfinsen's renaturation experiments [16] showed that this basic principle of statistical physics also applies to proteins [17]. Thus, although there are specific proteins that become trapped in a local minimum because of barriers to folding or covalent modification, most proteins probably fold to the conformation of minimum free energy [17]. The same argument should apply to reversibly binding ligands; therefore, it seems reasonable to assume that small molecule ligands adopt the binding mode of lowest free energy within the protein binding site. This very reasonable assumption is the ultimate basis for the use of energy in molecular-docking calculations.

A. Energy Calculations in Binding Energy Estimation

Energy minimization is routinely used to optimize geometries within the binding site and to select the best structure from a set of possible structures. The calculated energies can also be used to estimate the binding energy. The estimation of binding energies is reviewed in Chapter 10. However, because docking methods are heavily dependent on methods for estimating the energy, we cover some of the basic principles here.

The free energy of binding is the change in free energy that occurs on binding,

$$\Delta G_{binding} = G_{complex} - G_{separated} \tag{1}$$

where $G_{complex}$ and $G_{separated}$ are the free energies of the complexed and noninteracting protein and ligand, respectively. Ideally, these free energies are calculated by integrating over all possible configurations of the protein, ligand, solvent system, for example:

$$G_{complex} = -kT \log \left(\int \cdots \int_{complex} e^{-E/kT} \, dq_1 \cdots dq_n \right) \tag{2}$$

where T is the temperature, k is the Boltzmann constant, $q_1 \ldots q_n$ are the coordinates, and the integral is restricted to configurations of the complexed or separated forms [18]. Unfortunately, there are astronomical numbers of accessible configurations for protein–ligand systems, and it is impossible to compute these integrals directly. Free energy perturbation methods allow direct calculation of certain differences in free energies [19]. However, free energy perturbation still requires relatively large amounts of computer time, provides very limited conformational searching, and remains technically difficult. Consequently, most docking studies use approximate methods.

One common approximation is to represent solvation by an empirical model. In one approach, the solvent molecules are replaced with a dielectric medium, and then, the electrostatic effects of solvation are modeled by solving the Poisson–Boltzmann equation [20–22]. The application of sophisticated electrostatic computations to binding energy estimation [23–25] and molecular docking calculations [26,27] is in its infancy, and remains technically difficult, but already appears promising. Another approach represents the effects of solvation according to the solvent-exposed surface areas of the atoms [28–31], or the occupied volumes around the atoms [32]. These approaches cannot handle electrostatics accurately, but at least, can direct polar groups to the solvent and lipophilic groups to the interior.

Several recently developed methods [33], including the MVP procedure [6], attempt to estimate the free energies by summing over discrete minimized structures,

$$G = -kT \log \left(\sum_{\text{minima}} e^{-E/kT} \right) \tag{3}$$

Here, G_{complex} and $G_{\text{separated}}$ are obtained separately by summing over minimized structures of the complexed and separated forms, respectively. In general, this requires an explicit conformational search of the noninteracting protein and ligand, as well as the complex. The energies involved should include some representation for solvation, as discussed in the foregoing. The entropy about each minimum can be estimated from the second-derivative matrix [34] or from the number of initial structures associated with the minimum [33]. Other procedures neglect the configurational entropy and estimate the binding energy directly from the best structures of the complexed and separated forms.

In these approaches, the free energy of binding $\Delta G_{\text{binding}}$ is calculated as the difference of two nearly equal numbers, G_{complex} and $G_{\text{separated}}$. Small errors in either of the two energies can lead to relatively large errors in the calculated binding energy. Also, this approach requires explicit consideration of both the complexed and the uncomplexed forms. Thus, many procedures attempt to estimate the binding energy directly from the energy of the complex. In general, there is no reason to expect the total energy of the complex to be related to the binding energy. However, the interaction energy between the protein and the ligand does often show a good correlation with binding energy, at least within a series of related molecules [35]. This approach clearly neglects terms that are frequently important; however, the interaction–energy approach is the most practical with commonly available software.

Note that errors may arise from poor models for solvation and electrostatics, poorly parameterized molecular mechanics force fields, inaccurate representations for atomic charge distributions, and neglect of configurational entropy. Errors may also arise from incomplete conformational searching, incomplete energy minimization, or even mistyped atoms or incorrect ionization and tautomer forms. Drug design depends on the differences in binding energies of different inhibitors, and these calculated $\Delta\Delta G$ values can accumulate certain errors even more readily than the individual $\Delta G_{\text{binding}}$ values.

B. Empirically Corrected Energy Calculations in Binding Energy Estimation

Recognizing the errors that usually occur in molecular mechanics energy calculations, some authors have sought to rescale components of the energy to correct for physical deficiencies in the models, or to minimize the "noise" and maximize the "signal." For example, Aqvist et al. [36] compute the components of the interaction energy from molecular dynamics simulations, rescale the electrostatic component according to linear response theory, and then rescale the van der Waals component to fit experimental-binding energies. The COMBINE procedure [37] treats the van der Waals and coulombic interactions between each residue in the protein–ligand complex as separate variables in a large regression analysis. Approximately 50 of these variables are selected and are then rescaled, as necessary, to fit experimental-binding energies, yielding a semiempirical model for binding energies.

C. Empirical Approaches to Binding Energy Estimation

Although detailed energy calculations appear to be the most general approach to binding energy prediction, accurate calculations are still technically difficult, and incomplete or sloppy energy calculations are probably worse than useless. For many applications, it is better to use empirical approaches that are easier to apply and less subject to computational error. For example, the early work by Kuntz' group emphasized molecular shape, because shape complementarity is certainly essential and can be computed easily and accurately [38–40]. More recently, Kuntz has added chemical information [41,42], molecular mechanics energies [43], and empirical hydrophobicities [44]. Bohm has developed a scoring function that takes account of hydrogen bonds, ionic interactions, lipophilic contact surface, and the number of rotatable bonds [45]. The parameters in the scoring function were adjusted to reproduce known binding constants for 45 protein–ligand complexes with high-resolution structures. Several other scoring functions focus primarily or exclusively on buried and exposed hydrophobic and hydrophilic surfaces [46,47]. Wallqvist et al. [48] have extended this approach by parameterizing a buried surface model that includes interactions between buried atoms.

Some of the empirical scoring functions have been remarkably accurate in test cases with rigid ligands. However, all of the current empirical scoring functions omit certain interactions that are sometimes important. For example, most of the scoring functions omit the internal energy of the ligand. Although this is appropriate when the ligand is held fixed, it would allow unreasonable ligand conformations if the ligand is subjected to conformational searching.

III. DOCKING BY ENERGY MINIMIZATION

Energy minimization is an important technique in molecular-docking calculations. The utility and limitations of energy minimization were illustrated in early calculations where several substrates were docked into chymotrypsin [49,50]. In peptides, chymotrypsin hydrolyzes the amide bond on the C-terminal side of lipophilic side chains. N-Acetyl-phenylalanine amide was used as a model substrate in the foregoing study. Chymotrypsin hydrolyzes the C-terminal amide in this molecule, to release N-acetylphenylalanine and ammonia. Mechanical models were built for chymotrypsin and the substrate molecule to help define starting points for energy minimization and to help visualize the minimized structures. Energy contour maps and minimization were used to identify the minimum energy conformations of the model substrate in isolation [49]. Then, to define possible binding sites, the acetyl-phenylalanine amide molecule was minimized from ten different starting orientations, all located about 12 Å outside the active site. In these energy minimization calculations, the substrate molecule slides down the energy gradient toward the protein. In general, the ligand could "catch" on some protruding group near the binding site. However, the active site in chymotrypsin is largely exposed, and in this example, the substrate molecules dropped into the binding site without encountering any obstacles. The ten different minimized structures clustered into four different overlapping binding sites, one of which corresponded to the specificity pocket identified in an earlier X-ray crystallographic study [51]. Interestingly, this "correct" binding mode did not have the lowest energy at this stage of the calculation. This reflects the incomplete sampling of the large number of minima within each binding mode.

Additional calculations were carried out to examine the four possible binding sites in greater detail [50]. Starting positions and orientations were obtained with the mechanical models by manipulating the substrate within each of the four binding positions. A total of 74 minimizations were carried out for the acetyl-phenylalanine amide, giving a number of refined geometries with lower energies than that obtained previously. The authors noted that the energies before minimization failed to predict the geometry correctly, owing to steric repulsions in the hand-built structures. However, these steric overlaps were successfully relaxed in the minimization, and the binding mode with the lowest minimized energy was very similar to that revealed in the X-ray crystallographic study [51]. Similar calculations were carried out for three other substrates (acetyl-tyrosine, acetyltryptophan, and formyl-tyrosine), giving plausible geometries in all cases. However, the calculated binding energies did not correlate well with the experimental K_M values, a deviation the authors attributed primarily to solvation.

This work of Platzer and colleagues is perhaps the very first docking study that used energy calculations to predict geometry and binding affinity; it is perhaps also the very first docking calculation where the authors attribute the disagreement with experiment to solvation. The study clearly illustrates the usefulness of energy minimization, and shows that it is easier to predict the geometry than the binding energy. However, some of the techniques would not be used in the same way today. For example, although mechanical models may still provide the best intuitive "feel" for a binding site, the computer graphics representations available today are almost as intuitive, and far easier to build and manipulate. Also, there are now much faster ways to discover binding sites on the surface of a protein. Nonetheless, energy minimization remains essential to refine the geometries (and corresponding energies) of structures initially obtained by other methods.

IV. INTERACTIVE MOLECULAR GRAPHICS

Molecular graphics is an essential tool in studies of protein–ligand interactions, and should not be neglected in large-scale docking studies [52,53]. Molecular graphics is used to examine experimentally determined structures of protein–ligand complexes and to build new, modified compounds within an active site. Interactive molecular graphics programs generally allow the user to rotate and translate the ligand within the active site and to rotate selected torsions within the ligand. With sufficient patience and manual dexterity, it is possible to dock a flexible molecule into a protein-binding site. Some of the graphics programs include interfaces to energy minimization programs, allowing the hand-built structures to be optimized. Alternative conformations may then be explored by the extremely tedious iterative procedure where successive energy-minimized structures are manipulated and then reminimized. One difficulty with this approach is that the internal coordinate manipulations required to obtain desired structures are not intuitively obvious; time is often wasted searching for the right set of rotatable bonds. The Sculpt program [54] allows a user to pick an atom with the mouse, and then manipulate it directly, while continually maintaining reasonable bond lengths, bond angles, and torsions with a Lagrange multiplier procedure. Sculpt simulates the physical behavior of the protein, propagating deformations through the model in a realistic manner, and keeping the model in a conformation that locally minimizes the energy.

This should make human intuition much more effective in interactive molecular docking exercises.

Interactive docking exercises become very tedious when more than a few molecules must be considered. An alternative approach uses automated docking procedures to generate plausible bound structures in advance. A representative selection of these structures is then examined with molecular graphics programs. For example, alternative binding modes of a single ligand may be stored as successive frames in a molecular dynamics trajectory file, and then visualized with a molecular dynamics animation facility [55]. As the user scrolls forward or backward through the set of structures, the animation facility displays and continuously updates the energy, together with the geometry and hydrogen bond monitors. It is often useful to display the molecular surface within the active site [56], colored according to electrostatic potential [22]. As discussed earlier, the methods for estimating binding energies are not yet very accurate. With a good graphic representation, a chemist can apply his or her knowledge of the structure–activity relation and of the shortcomings of binding energy estimation procedures, to identify the most plausible binding modes more accurately.

V. DOCKING BY SUPERIMPOSITION

Users of molecular graphics packages commonly "dock" new ligands into binding sites by superimposing selected atoms from the ligand onto corresponding atoms from another ligand already positioned in the site. This usually works well if the new ligand is very similar to the reference ligand. Alternatively, one can use atoms from unrelated ligands, crystallographic water molecules, or even energetically favorable positions in space [57] as "target points" for the superimposition. Alternative positions and orientations within the active site may be explored by selecting different sets of atoms or target points and repeating the superimposition.

The original DOCK program [38] automated this technique by running thousands of superimpositions, and scoring the resulting trial structures according to shape complementarity. The target points for the superimposition operations are called "spheres" in DOCK terminology, and may be selected from a crystal structure, or they may be constructed directly from the molecular surface. Although a proper rotation is fully determined by superimposition of three noncolinear points, DOCK required superimposition of at least four ligand atoms onto four target points. If there are m heavy atoms in the ligand, and n target points or spheres in the binding site, then there are m times n different ways to match the first atom with the first target point. After the first pair has been matched, there are $(m - 1)(n - 1)$ remaining ways of making the second pair, and $(m - 2)(n - 2)$ ways of making the third pair, and so on. Small-molecule ligands typically have 10–20 heavy atoms, and the binding site is typically represented by 20–60 target points, so that the total number of four-pair matchings is in the billions. However, the vast majority of these matchings are geometrically impossible. For example, if the first and second atoms are 3 Å apart, then they cannot simultaneously be matched with target points that are 15 Å apart. The original DOCK program used distance tolerances of 1–2 Å to restrict the matching algorithm to geometrically plausible pairings [38]. The iteration through potentially matchable target points can be accelerated with "distance binning," where target points are grouped according to their distance from the first target point [49]. Kuntz and co-workers have explored heuristic-matching algorithms that preferentially select more distant atoms [40] and have extended the matching algorithm to include chemical information [41,42]. Their "Directed DOCK" superimposition procedure uses shape complementarity as well as hydrogen bonding to find positions and orientations [41]. The procedure uses two types of target points: one type corresponding to the conventional "sphere centers," and the other type corresponding to the specific positions that a ligand atom would occupy if it made an idealized hydrogen bond with the protein. The Directed DOCK matching algorithm then pairs ligand atoms with conventional sphere center target points (as in the original DOCK program), and it also pairs ligand heteroatoms with corresponding hydrogen-bonding target points.

The original DOCK scoring function relied on shape complementarity [38]. A force-field scoring function has been added, with interaction energies computed in advance at points on a grid [43]. Because small displacements of the ligand can dramatically reduce van der Waals overlap energies, the Kuntz group has added rigid-body energy minimization for use with the force-field scoring [58]. An alternative scoring function, based on hydrophobicity, has also been developed and incorporated [44].

Different versions of the DOCK program have been used successfully to screen chemical databases for small molecule ligands [4,59–64] and to dock protein ligands into protein binding sites [65]. The experimental structures have not always agreed with the predicted structures [62,66], but improved compounds have, nonetheless, been obtained from these leads [62,66]. A more complete description of the methodology and its applications is given in Chapter 3.

Several other research groups have developed programs that use the general DOCK superimposition method. CLIX positions ligands with a two-point superimposition, followed by a rotation around the resulting axis, with an optional displacement to relieve clashes, if necessary [67]. FLOG includes an efficient matching algorithm, a heavy-atom grid-based force-field scoring function, and a simplex rigid-body minimizer [68]. LUDI was originally developed for de novo design [69], but includes facilities for rigid-body docking by superimposition [70]. Targeted-DOCK allows ligand atoms and spheres to be prioritized and reweighted [71].

The original DOCK paper [38] observed that a good geometric fit is obtained when the molecular surfaces of the ligand and receptor come into contact over a large region. Thus, ideally, the ligand should be docked into the binding site by superimposing points from the molecular surfaces, instead of atoms and sphere centers. However, even at low dot densities, there are many more surface points than atoms, so that vastly more surface point matchings are possible. This fact led Kuntz and co-workers to use the more approximate atom and sphere centers approach. Recently, however, several groups have developed algorithms for the more demanding surface-fitting problem. Bacon and Moult [72] trace a spiral path over the molecular surface within the binding site, starting from some selected point deep in the active site, and then trace a similar spiral path over the surface of the ligand. The spiral paths effectively organize the surface points into a linear sequence, so that corresponding points on the protein and ligand surfaces can be identified and then superimposed. Alternative ligand orientations can be generated by tracing alternative spiral paths. Nussinov and co-workers represent the molecular surface by an extremely sparse set of "critical" surface points [73]. Geometric-hashing schemes based on distances [74] or Cartesian coordinates [75] are then used to rapidly identify matchable surface points. These hashing algorithms are an extension of the distance "binning" used in DOCK, and are similar to methods for object identification in computer vision [74]. With careful selection of surface points and with geometric hashing, the surface point approach appears to be competitive with the 2.0 version of DOCK [75].

VI. DOCKING FLEXIBLE MOLECULES BY SUPERIMPOSITION

The superimposition paradigm works extremely well with rigid molecules, but is less well-suited for those that are conformationally flexible. One approach is to generate multiple conformations for the molecule in advance and then dock each conformation into the binding site independently [68,76,77]. The Merck group uses distance geometry to generate up to 300 alternative conformations for each molecule, and they then use pairwise root-mean-square (rms) deviations to select a set of up to 25 dissimilar conformers for inclusion in the database [76]. With this approach, FLOG has successfully identified highly flexible inhibitors of the human immunodeficiency virus (HIV) protease from a multiconformer database [78]. The Glaxo Wellcome group uses a similar approach, except that the structures obtained with distance geometry are refined by molecular mechanics energy minimization [77]. Searches through the resulting database with the DOCK program successfully identified micromolar inhibitors of collagenase and cyclin-dependent kinase 2 [77].

DesJarlais et al. [39] developed an alternative approach that divides the conformationally flexible molecule into rigid fragments, each of which is independently docked into the protein binding site. The high-scoring fragment positions and orientations are recombined with energy minimization to obtain the docked ligand. Although the original approach is limited to relatively rigid molecules, the general idea is very powerful, and leads to a family of de novo design programs, as discussed in the following.

Leach and Kuntz dock a single rigid "anchor" fragment into the binding site and then use systematic conformational searching to find low-energy conformations for the flexible substituents [41]. Candidate positions and orientations for the anchor fragment are obtained with the Directed DOCK algorithm (see previous section). These positions and orientations are screened according to score, and are then clustered to eliminate redundant starting geometries. The flexible substituents are then reattached to the anchor fragment, in each of its clustered positions, and the rotatable bonds are searched with a systematic conformational search procedure to find low-energy binding modes for the complete molecule (the systematic conformational search is described later in Sec. XVI). Leach and Kuntz illustrate the method by docking methotrexate into dihydrofolate reductase (DHFR). The pteridine ring system is the largest rigid substructure; thus, it was chosen as the anchor fragment. Directed DOCK generated 1530 alternative positions and orientations for the anchor fragment. Screening by hydrogen bonding, shape complementarity score, and coulombic energy reduced this to 60 positions and orientations. Cluster analysis then identified 16 representative positions and orientations. The flexible substituent was attached to the anchor fragment in each of these 16 positions, and the 11 rotatable bonds were searched, yielding a total of 6795 alternative structures for the full methotrexate molecule in the binding site. Twenty of these were selected by further screening and clustering for refinement by energy minimization. The structure with the best energy was very similar to the X-ray crystallographic structure, with an rms deviation of 0.9 Å.

The Leach and Kuntz procedure [41] is heavily dependent on the rigidity of the anchor fragment. However, some molecules, such as peptides, may not contain any suitable rigid substructure. Itai and co-workers have developed an alternative procedure, called ADAM, that adjusts the conformation of the anchor fragment to better fit the target points before superimposing it into the active site [79–81]. Whereas Leach and Kuntz apply distance screens to eliminate poor matchings, ADAM uses energy minimization to find a ligand conformation with a better fit. This adjusted conformation is then superimposed into the active site. Side chains are added to the anchor fragment and subjected to systematic search, and then the fully-built ligand is refined by energy minimization. The ADAM procedure focuses on hydrogen-bonding interactions instead of shape complementarity. Alternative approaches that use metric matrix embedding to fit flexible ligands onto target points are described in Sec. XIV.A.

VII. SELECTING REPRESENTATIVE CONFORMATIONS

Multiconformer databases [68,77] attempt to represent the flexibility of a molecule with a few, selected conformations. The speed of database searches clearly depends on the number of structures; hence, it is generally important to select the conformers carefully. The same problem arises in conventional conformational search and analysis calculations, for which it is often necessary to select representative conformations for more detailed analysis. For example, a conformational search might yield thousands of candidate conformations, of which a few hundred might be selected for energy minimization, detailed solvation calculations, or graphic analysis.

Cluster analysis is often used to select representative structures. Note however, that most methods of cluster analysis are designed to discover the natural grouping of a multivariate data set [82]. This is appropriate for the analysis of experimental [83] or computed [84] conformations, or to help understand the range of structures explored in a molecular dynamics trajectory [84–86]. However, the goal in selecting representative conformations is to sample a range of important conformations. Very often, most of the conformations fall into several large clusters, with the remaining conformations scattered around the edges of the primary clusters. Cluster analysis methods always select a single structure from each cluster, and this approach can oversample the outliers and undersample the range of conformations within the larger clusters. This problem is particularly serious with the commonly used single-linkage method, because it often finds very large, elongated clusters [82].

Smellie and co-workers avoid the problems of cluster analysis by selecting sets of conformations that cover the widest range of conformational space [87,88]. More recently, these researchers have developed "poling," an approach in which the potential energy surface is modified to penalize the conformational space around conformers already included in the representative set [89]. With this approach, a conformational search is biased toward different conformations. Leach uses the A* algorithm to directly identify a sequence of most different conformations, where the conformational similarity is measured by the rms deviation of the torsional angles [90]. This again avoids the need to carry out a complete conformational search.

The MVP program uses a "filtering" algorithm to select a representative set of low-energy structures [6]. In this approach, the conformations are sorted by energy, and then considered one at a time, starting with the lowest energy structure. The first structure is always selected, and then subsequent structures are selected if the rms deviation from the prior structures is greater than a specified tolerance. The rms deviations may be calculated with or without optimal superimposition [91,92], as appropriate for conformational search and molecular docking calculations, respectively. The effect is to filter out structures with rms deviation less than the tolerance, preferentially retaining the lowest energy structures. The MVP program applies this filtering procedure on every cycle of growth in a buildup calculation, as discussed later. This gives a representative set of low-energy structures, without actually searching the complete conformational space.

VIII. METHODS FOR LINKING FRAGMENTS AND CLOSING LOOPS

As discussed earlier DesJarlais et al. [39] break flexible molecules into rigid fragments, dock the fragments into the binding site independently, and then recombine the fragments with energy minimization. As originally described, this approach seems limited to the very few molecules that can be broken into two or three rigid fragments. However, the method can be extended to a wider range of molecules by allowing conformationally flexible linker segments. The general problem is to find linker conformations that connect the prepositioned fragments without distorting the bond lengths bond angles.

This flexible linker problem is closely related to the conformational analysis of cyclic molecules and also to the prediction of protein loop conformations in homology modeling. In each case, an arbitrary choice of the torsional angles would give a grossly distorted structure, leaving the fragments unconnected, the ring open, or the loop unclosed. However, several specific strategies have been developed to ensure ring closure in conformational search calculations. Go and Scheraga [93] showed that exact ring closure constrains six torsional angles in a molecule represented with rigid bond lengths and bond angles, and they derived a series of equations to compute these six torsional angles. Bruccoleri and Karplus [94] modified the Go and Scheraga approach by allowing variations in bond angles. This modified loop closure algorithm is included in the CONGEN program [95].

The random tweak procedure [96] uses a Lagrange multiplier method to enforce the ring closure constraint with minimal conformational perturbation. Zheng et al. [97,98] use bond length scaling and energy minimization to effect ring closure. Several procedures "grow" molecules one bond at a time into alternative conformations. During this process, the two growing "arms" must remain close enough together to allow the remaining unbuilt bonds to close the ring. This provides a constraint that can be applied to the partially built structures [99,100] or to the range of torsions considered in the next cycle of growth [101]. Corner-flapping [102] and torsion-flexing [103] movements can be used to throw linkers, loops, and cycles into new conformations, without severely distorting the covalent geometry.

DeLisi and co-workers have developed fragment linking methods to dock flexible peptides into the class-I MHC receptors [104,105]. X-ray crystal structures show that the nine-residue peptides bind the MHC receptors in an extended conformation, with the charged N- and C-termini fitting into well-defined pockets. These workers take advantage of this feature by initially docking the N- and C-terminal residues of the peptide into the corresponding pockets, and then using a loop closure algorithm [95,97] to find a peptide conformation that connects the N- and C-terminal residues.

The fragment-linking idea is useful in molecular docking calculations, but probably much more important for de novo design. The typical approach is to dock a wide range of groups into the binding site, and then to seek linkers that connect two or three of these groups into synthetically accessible molecules [69,106–111]. This area is reviewed elsewhere [112].

IX. MOLECULAR DYNAMICS

One could imagine a molecular dynamics calculation that simulated the motion of a drug-like molecule as it diffuses into the active site of the protein, exploring alternative conformations and binding modes, and eventually choosing one particular binding mode. Dynamics could account for solvation as well as flexibility in both the protein and the ligand in a natural and accurate manner. Unfortunately, a true simulation of the docking process is not yet possible. Molecular dynamics simulations of protein–ligand complexes immersed in aqueous solvent are limited to about 10 ns with present-day computers. Drug-like molecules generally require microseconds or longer to find a stable binding mode within a protein binding site [113], and this time scale will probably remain beyond the reach of routine molecular dynamics calculations for many years.

A recent simulation of the streptavidin–biotin complex [114] illustrates the strengths and weaknesses of molecular dynamics. The dynamics calculation simulated an earlier experiment in which atomic force microscopy (AFM) was used to pull the biotin molecule out of its binding site in streptavidin [115,116]. The force required to rupture the complex was measured from the deflection of the AFM cantilever arm as 250 pico Newtons. Translated into more familiar units, this is a force of 3.6 kcal/mol Å, comparable with the maximum force of a single hydrogen bond in vacuum. The covalent connection between the biotin and the cantilever arm was simulated by a harmonic restraint between the linker atom in biotin and a point in space. The motion of the cantilever arm was simulated by moving this point with specified velocity out of the binding site. In the original experiment, the AFM cantilever tip was moved slowly, so that the unbinding process required milliseconds. Because this time scale is not feasible for dynamics calculations, the "virtual" cantilever tip was moved about 1 million times faster, rupturing the complex on a nanosecond time scale. Simulations were then repeated with a range of different velocities on this general time scale. The calculated rupture force increased with rupture velocity, but extrapolation back to the experimental velocity gave good agreement with the AFM rupture force. This shows that molecular dynamics can simulate an "undocking" process. Note, however, that the calculation depended on having a strong restraining force to pull the molecules apart on the nanosecond time scale. No corresponding restraints would be available in ordinary docking calculations unless the bound structure is already known.

Nevertheless, modified molecular dynamics algorithms and protocols can sometimes be useful in generating alternative orientations and conformations in docking calculations. The SHAKE algorithm is commonly used in Cartesian coordinate simulations to hold bond lengths fixed, allowing a slightly longer time step [117]. Internal coordinate dynamics calculations with fixed bond lengths and bond angles could allow significantly longer time steps [118]. High-temperature dynamics can be used to increase the breadth of the search [119].

A related approach simulates different types of motion at different temperatures [120]. For example, the translational motion of the ligand may be simulated at high temperature, while internal motion is simulated at room temperature, and the motion of the receptor is simulated at lower temperatures, giving an exploratory search that visits many possible binding modes [120]. The local elevation method helps broaden the search by penalizing structures that have already been visited [121]. The mixed Monte Carlo stochastic dynamics method carries out alternating cycles of Monte Carlo and molecular dynamics, using the Monte Carlo cycles to jump over barriers, and using the molecular dynamics cycles to explore neighboring low-energy structures [122]. Restraints could be used in any of these approaches to focus the search on structures of interest. "Snapshots" from the trajectories would then be refined by energy minimization [123].

One feature of dynamics is that it generates a continuous sequence of physically realizable structures. This can be a disadvantage, because there may be high-energy barriers between different binding modes of interest. In a dynamics simulation, the ligand might have to disengage from the protein to explore alternative binding modes, and this motion might require large amounts of computer time, or be prevented by restraints. A second disadvantage of dynamics, and particularly high-temperature methods, is that computer time is consumed manipulating or refining structures with distorted bond lengths and bond angles. Although distorted structures do occur on femtosecond time scales, chemical intuition and most analysis procedures are oriented toward undistorted, time-averaged structures. Most of the other methods described in this review save computer time be retaining reasonable bond lengths and bond angles throughout the calculation.

X. MULTIPLE COPY SIMULTANEOUS SIMULATION

One very simple docking procedure would place the ligand in a random position, orientation, and conformation within the protein binding site, and then use energy minimization or molecular dynamics to refine the interaction with the protein. In the simplest form of Monte Carlo minimization, this random placement and optimization could be repeated many times to yield a set of low-energy binding modes. This "memoryless" approach differs from the conventional metropolis approach [124] in that successive structures are completely independent and unrelated. The procedure samples uniformly through the allowed region, instead of following a trajectory that might be confined to one low-energy region.

The sequential Monte Carlo minimization approach can be used to characterize the binding site and the range of positions and orientations available to a small ligand molecule. However, the sequential approach is not very efficient with larger, flexible ligands because so much computer time is wasted on minimizations that are trapped in high-energy configurations and because many of the successful minimizations converge to the same local minima. The multiple copy simultaneous search (MCSS) method [125] generates 1000–5000 starting positions for the ligand, and then minimizes all the structures simultaneously, allowing each copy of the ligand to interact with the field of the protein, but not with the other copies of the ligand. The simultaneous simulation procedure saves computer time by suspending the minimizations periodically (e.g., every 1000 steps) to identify redundant minimizations that are converging to the same minimum.

Note that when the protein is held fixed, as in the original application to molecular docking [125], the simultaneous minimizations do not communicate except at the redundancy checking steps. Thus, when the protein is held fixed, one may use sequential, partial minimizations, with periodic redundancy checking, to achieve the same effect. The MVP program [6] uses a sequential filtering minimization procedure, described in Section XVII.E of this review, to refine large numbers of structures efficiently.

When the protein is allowed to move, the simultaneous simulation method makes it possible to generate many ligand trajectories in the presence of a single protein trajectory [104,126]. The computational efficiency is improved because the internal energy of the protein is calculated only once per step for the whole ensemble of ligands [104,126]. Protein flexibility in multiple copy, simultaneous minimization may also be effective in smoothing the energy surface to give enhanced sampling efficiency [127]. A further smoothing of the potential energy surface may be obtained when the solvent molecules are explicitly included in the simulation.

B. Metropolis Monte Carlo

The independent-sampling Monte Carlo minimization methods do not learn from experience and, thus, cannot focus on low-energy structures discovered during the sampling. By contrast, metropolis Monte Carlo procedures generate a sequence of structures that can first locate and then explore low-energy regions of the conformational space [124]. Metropolis Monte Carlo is similar to molecular dynamics in this respect. The approaches are also similar in that both can have difficulty climbing over barriers and both can get "stuck" in particular regions of the conformational space.

A metropolis Monte Carlo procedure starts by calculating the energy of the initial structure. The procedure then applies a small movement to the molecular system, and calculates the new energy. If the movement decreases the energy, then the new structure is automatically accepted. If the energy increases, then the structure is accepted with probability $e^{-\Delta E/kT}$, where ΔE is the (positive) change in energy, k is the Boltzmann constant in appropriate units, and T is the temperature chosen for the calculation; this rule is commonly called the *metropolis criterion* for acceptance. The original paper proved that a sequence of structures generated according to this procedure would eventually populate the available states according to the Boltzmann distribution, thereby simulating a thermodynamic system [124]. This proof is the basis for the use of metropolis Monte Carlo in free energy calculations [128].

The efficiency of a metropolis Monte Carlo procedure depends on the "moves" allowed. Liquid argon can be handled efficiently with Cartesian coordinate movements, where a single randomly selected atom is given a small displacement in a random direction. More complex liquids, such as water, can be modeled accurately with rigid liquid molecules subject to small translational and rotational movements [128]. However, rotation and translation of a large, rigid ligand within a binding site usually leads to collisions with the protein. Consequently, rigid body metropolis should be much less efficient than the DOCK superimposition approach in rigid body docking. Nevertheless, rigid body metropolis can be effective when highly focused searching is needed, or when distance constraints are available [129]. Conformationally flexible molecules present a more difficult challenge. Simple displacements of individual atoms or functional groups lead to grossly distorted geometries and collisions with neighbors. Goodsell and Olson [130] use torsional rotations, together with rigid body rotations and translations, to dock flexible molecules into rigid protein binding sites. On each step, a small random variation is applied to each degree of freedom, and the energy of the new structure is evaluated by interpolation from grid points. The temperature is gradually reduced from an extremely high initial value ($kT = 100$ kcal mol^{-1}) to a final value near room temperature. This simulated annealing temperature-reduction protocol [131] allows the ligand to explore a range of binding modes before "annealing" into a particular low-energy mode. This approach has been used in several studies [132–135].

The simple simulated annealing protocol generates only one refined structure in each simulation. Goodsell and Olson [130] carried out several separate simulations to find alternative binding modes. Hart and Read used a larger number of randomly generated starting positions in their multiple-start Monte Carlo (MSMC) procedure [136]. Flexible ligands were represented by independent rigid fragments, assuming that low-energy fragments could be reassembled into useful ligands. Each run starts from a randomly generated initial position and orientation within a cube centered on the binding site. The first part of each Monte Carlo run uses the distance to the protein surface as part of the energy function, effectively "floating" ligand fragments from partially buried random starting points to the protein surface. The remainder of the Monte Carlo run uses a conventional grid-based energy function, with the metropolis criterion applied at progressively lower temperatures.

XII. MONTE CARLO MINIMIZATION

Torsional coordinate movements preserve bond lengths and angles, but can still lead to collisions, particularly in a tightly packed protein binding site. Li and Scheraga introduced a Monte Carlo minimization procedure that refines the perturbed structure by energy minimization before applying the metropolis criterion [137]. The energy minimization is not a random movement, and its inclusion in the procedure effectively disrupts the Boltzmann distribution. However, the goal in conformational search calculations is not to simulate a thermodynamic ensemble, but rather, to search the relevant conformational space rapidly. The minimization step can dramatically improve the effectiveness of the search in tightly packed geometries by making small conformational adjustments to obtain low-energy structures. Li and Scheraga originally applied the Monte Carlo minimization approach to a linear peptide chain in free space [137]. Several other groups have now adapted the approach for molecular docking calculations [138–140].

One problem with conventional metropolis Monte Carlo is that its "memory" retains only a single structure. The MCMM procedure of Still and colleagues [138] retains a number of structures through the calculation, any of which could be selected for random variation and energy minimization. Various structure selection strategies have been investigated. Energy-based selection strategies tend to search some low-energy regions effectively while neglecting other low-energy regions. A usage-directed strategy that selected the least-used low-energy structure gave a more uniform search of the range of low-energy structures [138]. The random variation step in MCMM permits various "move" operations, including random variation of one or more torsional angles, random displacement of atoms, and random rotation or translation of the molecule as a rigid unit for molecular docking calculations. MCMM also includes torsional flexing [103] and special checks for ring closure, both before and after energy minimization. The MCMM procedure has been incorporated into the MacroModel BATCHMIN program [141,142] and used extensively in molecular docking calculations [143].

The ICM procedure of Abagyan et al. [140] uses internal coordinates for energy minimization as well as for its Monte Carlo move operations. The principal rationale for the use of internal coordinates in refinement is the reduction in the number of minima. Abagyan et al. [140] support this idea by subjecting distorted structures of a 29-residue protein to energy minimization in internal coordinates and in Cartesian coordinates. The internal coordinate energy minimizations were able to recover the original, undistorted structure even for relatively large distortions, whereas Cartesian coordinate minimizations were almost always trapped in other local minima [140]. Molecular docking calculations are carried out in ICM with a Brownian Monte Carlo minimization procedure that scales random rotations according to the radius of gyration or the moment of inertia tensor, so that molecular rotations and translations give atomic displacements of similar size. The procedure has been applied successfully in several test cases [140,144].

XIII. GENETIC ALGORITHMS

Genetic algorithms and evolutionary programming have recently been used in flexible-docking calculations [145–150], as well as a variety of other problems in molecular structure [151]. These approaches are loosely based on ideas from genetics and natural selection, in which a population of individuals evolves over many generations under some selective pressure [152].

In a simulation, each individual has a single "chromosome," represented as a string of integers, often ones and zeros. A "fitness function" translates the chromosome into a number, effectively evaluating the "fitness" of the individual. On each generation, some (or most) of the less-fit individuals are "killed," or eliminated from the population. Pairs of surviving individuals are "mated," leading to children with chromosomes derived from the parents by mutation and recombination. In point mutations, a randomly selected integer in the chromosome is incremented by a random amount. In the recombination or "crossover" events, randomly selected homologous segments of the parent chromosomes are interchanged. Children may also be obtained directly from a single parent with one or more point mutations. In addition, one or more of the best individuals may be passed unchanged into the next generation. The process is iterated over many generations, leading to a population with increasingly fit individuals.

In the application to the molecular-docking problem, the chromosome encodes the position, orientation, and conformation of the ligand. The conformation is represented by a list of torsional angles, each stored as an integer or in a "gray-coded" binary format. The position and orientation are typically represented by a translation vector and Euler angles. However, alternative representations are possible, and Oshiro and co-authors obtain the position and orientation by superimposing selected ligand atoms onto corresponding target points or spheres in the binding site [147]. In this approach, the chromosome includes the superimposition lists instead of the explicit translation vector and Euler angles. A similar approach [146] involves superimposition of hydrogen-bonding groups.

The ideal fitness function is the total energy of the protein–ligand system, but approximations must be used in practice. The Agouron procedure [150] uses a simplified united atom empirical interaction potential. Jones and associates [146] use quantum mechanically parameterized hydrogen bond energies as the primary term in the fitness function, while the UCSF procedures [147,148] calculate interaction energies by interpolation on a precomputed grid. The Sandia procedure [145] uses a full molecular mechanics force field, and optionally, a solvation model [153] based on approximate surface areas [154]. The Agouron procedure uses the simplest energy term, and runs the fastest, docking typical ligands in approximately 10 min. The Sandia procedure uses the most comprehensive energy function, requiring 10–100 h for a complete docking calculation. However, the extra computer time does seem to buy more accurate estimates of the binding energy [153]. Individuals with low energy are considered to be the most fit, and these are selected most frequently to generate children for the next generation.

The chromosomes may be subject to mutation and recombination in the reproduction process. Mutations randomly perturb the x, y, and z translations, the three Euler angles, and the torsional angles. Recombination events transfer coordinates between chromosomes. Very often, a recombination event will transfer a contiguous set of coordinates corresponding to a low-energy substructure within the ligand, effectively transplanting the low-energy substructure from one copy of the ligand to another. Thus, recombination provides a mechanism for distributing favorable combinations of coordinates throughout the whole population. Most of the procedures use both mutation and recombination to generate structural variation. However, the mutation rate is typically much lower than the recombination rate; hence, most of the orientational and conformational variation probably arises from recombination. The Agouron evolutionary programming procedure [150] is an exception in that it relies entirely on "asexual" reproduction, in which children are generated directly from a single parent without recombination. In this procedure, structural variation is obtained by mutating all of the coordinates by a small, random amount, instead of mutating a small number of randomly selected coordinates.

Several of these procedures include interesting deviations from the basic genetic algorithm strategy. The Sandia procedure [145] uses a "growth" algorithm that starts by docking a pivot atom and its immediate substituents into the active site. This will be discussed in Section XVII.C. The Agouron procedure [150] smooths the energy landscape by softening the pair interaction potential for the first few generations. This allows the ligand to penetrate the protein core during the early stages of the simulation, exploring structures that would otherwise be blocked by high-energy barriers. Subsequent hardening of the interaction potential "funnels" the ligand into energetically favorable binding modes.

It is useful to compare the genetic algorithm approaches with earlier methods. Leaving the exotic vocabulary aside, most of the steps and operations in a genetic algorithm have counterparts in conventional Monte Carlo approaches. For example, probabilistic selection according to fitness corresponds to acceptance or rejection under the metropolis criterion. Mutations correspond exactly to the random variation operations in conventional Monte Carlo approaches. However, recombination is apparently a novel operation, with no obvious counterpart in the previous molecular docking Monte Carlo literature; the closest analog may be the use of rotamer libraries in side-chain conformational searching [155]. The experience with genetic algorithms suggests that recombination is useful in certain problems, and that it would make sense to implement recombination operations in conventional Monte Carlo programs. Another important feature of genetic algorithms is the explicit use of a population of individuals with different orientations and conformations. The best of the Monte Carlo procedures [138] also have this feature, allowing any of the retained structures to be selected for subsequent steps. However, a considerable amount of work is still carried out with less-efficient metropolis procedures that retain only a single structure. Thus, although some of the differences are purely semantic, the genetic algorithm approach has inspired some important contributions, and includes some of the best algorithms available.

XIV. THEORY OF DISTANCE GEOMETRY

Distance geometry is a branch of mathematics that uses the distances between points as the principal representation in geometric problems [156]. In chemical structure problems, distance geometry provides a general method for converting interatomic distance information into three-dimensional coordinates. The approach has been used extensively to generate molecular structures from NMR data, for NOESY cross-peaks can be translated into distance constraints [157]. Several excellent reviews are available. In particular, Blaney and Dixon [158] describe the application to flexible docking. Other reviews emphasize the mathematical theory [159], or application to conformational searching [13,160], receptor modeling [161], or NMR [162–164]. Crippen [165] and Crippen and Havel [166] have written books on distance geometry and its applications.

The first practical, numerically stable distance geometry procedure was developed by Crippen and co-workers [159,167,168]. To explain the procedure, which is called metric matrix embedding, we consider a system with n atoms, and initially assume that all $n(n - 1)/2$ interatomic distances d_{ij} are known. The objective is to calculate the vectors x_i from the center of mass to the ith atom, for each of the n atoms. We will assume that the x_i lie in a d dimensional space, where d is usually 3, but could be greater than 3. Crippen and Havel [168] showed that, for each atom, the distance d_{io} from the center of mass may be calculated as

$$d_{io} = \frac{1}{n} \sum_{j=1}^{n} d_{ij}^2 - \frac{1}{n^2} \sum_{j=2}^{n} \sum_{k=1}^{j-1} d_{jk}^2 \tag{4}$$

For any two atoms i and j, the three distances d_{io}, d_{jo}, and d_{ij} define a triangle where the distances d_{io} and d_{jo} from the center of mass correspond to the vectors x_i and x_j, respectively. The law of cosines can be rearranged to calculate the dot product of these two vectors,

$$x_i \cdot x_j = \frac{d_{io}^2 + d_{jo}^2 - d_{ij}^2}{2} \tag{5}$$

These dot products may be collected into the n by n "metric" matrix $\mathbf{G}$, with elements $g_{ij} = x_i \cdot x_j$. Similarly, the row vectors x_i may be collected in the same order into an n by d coordinate matrix $\mathbf{X}$. The relation may then be written in matrix notation as

$$\mathbf{G} = \mathbf{X}\mathbf{X}^T \tag{6}$$

Since the metric matrix $\mathbf{G}$ is symmetric, it can be diagonalized to give

$$\mathbf{G} = \mathbf{U}\mathbf{D}\mathbf{U}^T \tag{7}$$

where $\mathbf{D}$ is the diagonal matrix of eigenvalues and $\mathbf{U}$ is the corresponding matrix of eigenvectors. The coordinate matrix can be identified from this expression as $\mathbf{X} = \mathbf{U}\mathbf{D}^{1/2}$, and the coordinates may be calculated as

$$x_{ij} = \lambda_j^{1/2} u_{ij} \tag{8}$$

If the original distances d_{ij} were computed from a real molecule in three-dimensional space, then the first three eigenvalues λ_1, λ_2, and λ_3 will be positive, and the rest will be zero. In this case, the calculated coordinates x_{ij} will have nonzero components only for $j = 1$, 2, and 3, and will thus lie in a three-dimensional space. In general, however, one can choose interatomic distances that cannot be embedded into a three-dimensional space. The metric matrix-embedding procedure indicates this situation by returning more than three nonzero eigenvalues. When this occurs, the best three-dimensional approximation to the desired structure is obtained by using the three largest eigenvalues, essentially projecting the structure onto its three longest principal axes. Leach [13] and Blaney and Dixon [158] give some simple numerical examples, and also discuss the similarity to principal component analysis.

The foregoing derivation assumed that all $n(n - 1)/2$ interatomic distances were known exactly. In actual practice, very few distances are known accurately. Some of the distances may be determined directly from the covalent structure of the molecule. For example, chemical bonds constrain the bonded atoms very tightly, and the corresponding 1–2 distances may be taken as the ideal bond lengths. Similarly, the 1–3 distances may be calculated from ideal bond angles. However, 1–4 distances depend on the intervening torsional angle, giving the longest possible distance in the *trans* (or *anti*) conformation, and the shortest possible distance in the *cis* (or *syn*) conformation. Atoms separated by more than three bonds are subject to even greater uncertainty. However, one can generally assume that these atoms will be no farther apart than the sum of the intervening bond lengths, and will come no closer than the sum of their van der Waals radii. Experimental information from NOESY spectra, fluorescence phototransfer, or chemical cross-linking experiments may be available to tighten these limits. For example, an NOE cross-peak might indicate an interproton distance of 2–5 Å.

Distance geometry programs generally retain upper and lower bounds on each of the $n(n - 1)/2$ distances. The upper and lower bounds initially obtained from the covalent connectivity and experimental information are usually not as tight as possible. To see this, consider an NOE between an amide proton (HN) in one residue and a C-α proton (HA) from another residue. The NOE might lead to an explicit 5.0 Å upper limit on the interproton distance. However, because the H–N and H–C bond lengths are known to be 1.0 and 1.1 Å, respectively, this NOE also implies that the amide nitrogen is within 6.0 Å of the HA atom, and that the C-α is within 6.1 Å of the HN atom. Implied limits of this type can be deduced by "triangle inequality bounds smoothing," in which triplets of atoms are examined to make the bounds as tight as possible. Distance geometry programs normally include efficient algorithms [159,169] that iterate through triplets of atoms to eliminate this triangle inequality slack from the distance bounds. Distances in three-dimensional spaces must also satisfy a tetrangle inequality, as well as higher-order relations. An algorithm for "tetrangle inequality smoothing" has been developed, but is apparently too slow for practical use [170].

The metric matrix-embedding procedure requires a full set of $n(n - 1)/2$ distances. A few of these distances may be determined exactly, but most of the distances are merely constrained to some interval. To run the embedding procedure, these unknown distances are selected randomly from the allowed intervals. It might seem absurd to select distances at random, but it is roughly consistent with the spirit of Monte Carlo, where torsions are varied at random. Thus, after distances are selected, the embedding procedure is used to generate a three-dimensional structure, which may then be refined by conventional energy-based methods. The overall randomize, embed, refine sequence is repeated many times in exactly the same manner as in Monte Carlo minimization calculations.

Some problems can arise when the random distances are selected independently [171]. To see this, consider an *n*-octane molecule with carbons numbered 1 through 8. Certain distances are fixed from the covalent connectivity, e.g., $d_{78} = 1.5$ Å, and $d_{68} = 2.5$ Å. The other distances must be selected randomly. The random selection procedure could easily choose $d_{17} = 3.0$ Å and then choose $d_{18} = 8.0$ Å, because both of these values lie within the respective allowed ranges. However, the simultaneous choice of 3 and 8 Å leads to an impossible structure, because C-7 and C-8 are bonded and thus 1.5 Å apart. The metric matrix-embedding procedure can still force these structures into three dimensions with distortions that are eventually removed by energy refinement. However, the inconsistent distances do alter the sampling properties of the distance geometry procedure, so that some regions of the conformational space are grossly undersampled [172,173]. This problem can be corrected by using triangle bounds smoothing to update the upper and lower bounds after each random distance was selected. Havel showed that this "metrization" process dramatically improved the sampling properties [173]. Subsequently, Kuszewski et al. argued that a much faster "partial metrization" algorithm samples the conformational space almost as well [174].

A. Docking with Distance Geometry

Blaney and Dixon [158] illustrate the use of distance geometry by docking an ester-containing substrate molecule into the active site of chymotrypsin. The protein was represented by 55 atoms from the active site, plus a single dummy atom near the center of a hydrophobic pocket. These atoms were held rigid by setting the upper and lower distance bounds equal to the actual distances from the X-ray crystal structure. The upper and lower bounds for the substrate were determined from the covalent connectivity, effectively allowing all rotatable bonds to vary. To prevent interpenetration, lower bounds for the protein–substrate distances were taken from the sum of the van der Waals radii. Then, a phenyl ring in the substrate was constrained to lie within 2 Å of the dummy atom in the hydrophobic pocket. In this example, the catalytic mechanism required the ester group to fit between the catalytic residues Ser-195 and His-57, and the oxyanion hole. This requirement was translated into five additional distance constraints.

The remaining distances were then chosen randomly in the usual randomize, embed, refine sequence, leading to several very similar bound structures. This example is unusual in that so many good constraints were available, permitting essentially just one bound structure.

Blaney used a similar approach in earlier calculations where an ester-containing phospholipid molecule was docked into the active site of phospholipase A_2, again using constraints derived from the catalytic mechanism [175]. The binding modes shown in the stereo figures [175] appear to be very similar to that of an amide inhibitor in a subsequent X-ray study [176]. This predicted structure was the starting point for design of nonphospholipid inhibitors. Distance geometry was used to dock these designed compounds into the active site, this time without mechanism-based constraints. The overall process led to compounds with relatively good in vitro activity [175].

Specific distance constraints between the ligand and the protein can focus the search dramatically. Crippen and co-workers [166,177,178] made tentative matches between selected atoms in the ligand and selected atoms in the receptor. Their procedures add artificial constraints between the matched atoms, and use metric matrix embedding to generate a three-dimensional structure. The constrain, embed, refine sequence is then repeated with different matchings of ligand and receptor atoms to search the full range of positions, orientations, and conformations. In one variation [178], the matchings are confined to hydrogen-bonding groups, whereas the embed includes all of the heavy atoms from the surface of the active site. Another variation [166] uses dummy atoms to represent the volume available in the active site cavity, and a few (purely repulsive) atoms to represent the surface of the protein. The dummy atoms, called site points in Crippen's nomenclature, are similar to the target points, or spheres, used by DOCK [38] and the other superimposition procedures. But when DOCK uses a rigid body superimposition to fit the ligand onto the spheres, the distance geometry procedures use the metric matrix-embedding procedure to carry out a flexible superimposition.

The rigid body and distance geometry superimposition approaches both iterate over many different atom matchings to search the range of possible positions and orientations. Note, however, that additional levels of iteration are required in the distance geometry procedures to search the range of possible conformations. This additional level of searching can be achieved by matching larger numbers of atoms. Thus, a rigid (proper) rotation can be specified by matching three ligand atoms with three receptor atoms. Matching a fourth ligand atom with some atom in the receptor would probably then require an adjustment to the conformation. Matching that fourth ligand atom to a different receptor atom would force a different conformation. By matching larger numbers of atoms at a time, the distance geometry procedures can drive a search through the conformational space of the ligand. Crippen and co-workers [166,177,178] have developed relatively efficient algorithms that use the available upper and lower distance bounds to search the space of geometrically feasible matchings.

XV. SYSTEMATIC SEARCH ALGORITHMS

All of the methods described in the foregoing carry out an irregular search of the conformational and orientational space. The sampling of the space is generally not uniform and may be quite spotty. This is clear in molecular dynamics, where a simulated structure will remain near the starting structure until, by chance, it finds a valley through the surrounding barriers. Monte Carlo procedures and genetic algorithms can make larger jumps through the space, but still sample very unevenly. Even when the sampling is more uniform, it remains random. For example, the metric matrix-embedding procedure drives its search by choosing distances randomly between ι pper and lower bounds. Random searches are necessarily hit or miss; they cannot guarantee that the global minimum has been located. One can obtain statistical evidence for comprehensiveness by running the procedure to saturation. But it is clearly inefficient to rediscover the same structures many times. Constraints can focus the search on a particular region, but do not overcome the fundamentally capricious nature of these methods.

Systematic approaches offer some hope of overcoming these problems. Systematic searches have been used extensively in small-molecule conformational analysis for many years. The simplest approach is a grid search, where each rotatable bond is rotated from $-180°$ to $+180°$, typically in steps of $20°-60°$. With a step size of $30°$, there are 12 rotameric states for each rotatable bond. The procedure generates all combinations of rotameric states. For a molecule with two rotatable bonds, the grid search procedure generates 12×12 structures, corresponding to 144 points on a two-dimensional grid. The number of structures required increases geometrically with the number of rotatable bonds. Thus, a molecule with ten rotatable bonds would require generation of $12^{10} = 62$ billion conformations. Accurate estimation of the energy requires energy minimization, and if each minimization consumed 1 s, then the complete calculation would require almost 2000 years.

Docking calculations require an additional search over ranges of x, y, and z, and over the full range of rotations corresponding to the three Euler angles. The most direct approach would position a ligand on successive grid points within the binding site, rotating the ligand to sample the space of orientations. Pincus and co-workers used this general approach in a very early study where a flexible disaccharide was docked into the active site of lysozyme [179,180]. A coordinate system was defined with the z-axis directed along the length of the active site cleft. Translations along the z-axis, and rotations about the z-axis, were sampled uniformly over the full range, with step sizes of 3 A and 30°. Because the cleft is quite narrow, the x and y translations were sampled over a very limited range, and the x and y rotations were confined to a 45° cone. Grid searches of the six coordinates were carried out for each of three low-energy conformations of the disaccharide molecule. Thirteen structures had energies within 5 kcal of the best structure, and were refined by energy minimization. The best of the minimized structures occupied the sites expected experimentally [180].

Leach used a similar systematic search to position the ligand in his recent DEE/A* calculations [181]. The anchor fragment was positioned at successive points on a grid, and then rotated into 22 different orientations. Each orientation was checked for overlap with the protein backbone. Calculations with trypsin and the rigid ligand benzamidine used a grid spacing of 1.0 A, and identified a total of 4465 nonoverlapping positions and orientations. Calculations with the antibody McPC 603 and the flexible ligand phosphocholine involved seven precomputed conformations of the ligand with a grid spacing of 1.5 A, and identified a total of 13,478 nonoverlapping positions, orientations, and conformations. The DEE/A* algorithm was then used to adjust the protein side-chain conformations for each of the ligand positions and orientations, as discussed in the following.

Note that it is geometrically impossible to sample the space of orientations uniformly, except for special low-resolution samplings corresponding to the symmetry operations of the dodecahedron and icosahedron [182]. In their soft-docking algorithm, Jiang and Kim introduce a formula to calculate the angle between two rotation operations [183]. This allows a procedure to generate rotation matrices randomly or from evenly spaced Euler angles, rejecting the rotation matrices that come within some cutoff angle of a previously used rotation. More recently, Harrison and co-workers generated random rotation matrices from random unit quarternions [184]. The resulting collection of rotations is not perfectly uniform, but at least has a constant-sampling density.

Jiang and Kim [183] represent the protein and the ligand with filled or empty cubes in a three-dimensional lattice, essentially "digitizing" the two molecules. The lattice representation for the ligand is recomputed for each new orientation of the ligand. Ligand positions are then obtained by seeking translations that superimpose surface cubes from the ligand onto surface cubes from the protein; this avoids the need to iterate explicitly over x, y, and z. Vakser and co-workers [185] have developed a similar approach in which the object function measuring the protein–ligand fit is cast in the form of a spatial correlation function. Optimal ligand translation vectors then correspond to peaks in the correlation function. This correlation function can be calculated rapidly from the spatial Fourier transforms of the protein and ligand lattices. More recently, good results have been obtained with partial [186] and very low resolution [187] lattice representations. This approach has been extended by using Fourier–Green functions to rapidly calculate a molecular mechanics interaction energy [184]. This approach was used to predict binding geometries and energies for a series of trypsin inhibitors [188]. An alternative digitization approach is employed, in which the binding surfaces of two proteins are represented by their distances outward from sectioning planes [189]. Here, the docking calculation requires iteration over the separation and orientational angles, as well as different sectioning planes. In principle, ligand flexibility could be handled in any of these procedures by repeating the entire analysis for successive ligand conformations. However, this would not be particularly efficient, and all of the studies described in the foregoing were carried out with rigid ligands.

XVI. TREE SEARCHES

The basic grid search algorithm can be improved dramatically in conformational analysis by using a *tree* data structure to organize the calculations. The tree in Figure 1 represents a grid search of a molecule with three rotatable bonds, using a step size of 120°. This molecule might be hexane, aspirin, or any other molecule that has exactly three rotatable bonds (terminal methyl groups are normally not included in the search). The three nodes in the first level of the tree correspond to the *gauche-minus* ($-60°$), *gauche-plus* ($+60°$), and *trans* (180°) conformations of the first rotatable bond. The nodes in the second level then correspond to conformations of the second bond. For example, the three nodes below the *trans* node correspond to the three conformations where the first bond is *trans* and the second bond is g^-, g^+, and t. Similarly, nodes in lower levels correspond to bonds farther out in the molecule.

A grid search can be carried out by traversing the tree, rotating the first bond for nodes on the first level, the second bond for nodes on the second level, and so on, and then rotating the final bond, and running an energy minimization, for each node on the terminal level. The efficiency of the tree search procedure depends on the order in which the bonds are

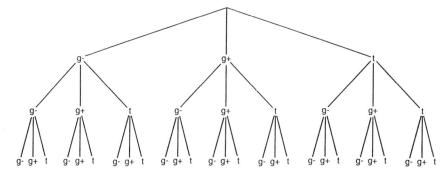

Figure 1   Tree representation of a conformational search of a molecule with three rotatable bonds, assuming a step size of 120°. The *gauche-minus, gauche-plus,* and *trans* conformational states are indicated by g^-, g^+, and t. There are a total of 27 possible conformations, $g^- g^- g^-, \ldots, ttt$.

rotated. The MVP program [6] generates an ordering of the rotatable bonds by starting from some "root" atom, and working outward through the covalent structure of the molecule. Lipton and Still use a similar approach, starting from one end of the molecule [99]. During the search, the rotations are always applied to the atoms on the outward side of the bond, leaving the atoms on the inward side fixed. With this arrangement, the root atom and its immediate substituents are fixed in space through the entire calculation. Additional atoms become fixed in space as the search process moves downward through the search tree. Note that the sequence with which atoms become fixed in space is identical with the growth process that occurs in MVP buildup calculations, discussed in Section XVII.E.

Now suppose that the first and second torsions are given values that turn the molecule back on itself, so that atoms overlap. To take a well-known example from the conformational analysis of alkanes, consecutive g^+/g^- bonds bring the 1–5 atoms close together in a "*syn*-pentane" conformation. The *syn*-pentane contact is relatively soft, but hard overlaps can occur with other combinations of torsions in large molecules. The tree data structure is useful here because it explicitly connects related conformations. Thus, if an overlap occurs at a particular node in the tree, then it also occurs in all conformations below that node. These daughter nodes may be eliminated, or "pruned," from the search tree, avoiding the need to generate and minimize the corresponding conformations. This early overlap checking and pruning can improve the efficiency of small-molecule conformational searching significantly. More dramatic improvements can be obtained within protein binding sites because the geometry is so tightly constrained.

Distance constraints are easily incorporated into this approach. If a constraint is violated at a particular node, then the daughter nodes may be immediately eliminated. Similar methods can be used to handle cyclic molecules [99]. A specific ring-closure bond is selected and temporarily broken to allow free rotation within the ring. The ideal bond length is then represented as a distance constraint that is applied at the search tree node corresponding to ring closure. Conformations that leave the ring open are thus detected and eliminated. As discussed earlier, the tree search process applies rotations, and thus defines atomic positions sequentially, along the two "arms" of a ring. These arms must remain close enough together to allow the remaining undefined bonds to close the ring. The efficiency of the process can thus be improved by checking these partially defined ring structures, rejecting those conformations that could not be closed by the remaining bonds [99,100].

Marshall and co-workers [190,191] have developed a similar systematic search procedure that achieves an additional speedup by analyzing distance constraints into ranges of allowed and disallowed torsions. This procedure is used extensively in pharmacophore modeling, where one assumes that different active molecules assume conformations that present key functional groups to the receptor with a common geometry. Marshall's search procedure can carry out searches on a series of active molecules, expressing the results from each search in turn as distance constraints that are applied to subsequent molecules in the series [191]. This "active analog approach" may also be useful in molecular docking calculations, where one could assume that corresponding atoms from different ligands make the same interactions with the protein.

Leach and Kuntz have developed a procedure that docks a single, rigid anchor fragment into the binding site and then uses systematic conformational searching to fit the flexible substituents into the binding site [41]. Their Directed dock procedure for positioning the anchor fragment was discussed earlier in this review (see Sec. V). Their systematic conformational search uses the tree data structure, with several novel features. Ring conformations are searched by iterating over prestored fragment conformations (discussed in the following). Acyclic bonds are initially searched with very large stepsizes. These crude initial conformations are then adjusted to relieve steric problems and to improve hydrogen bond interactions. This algorithm uses artificial intelligence techniques to identify appropriate conformational adjustments [192]. In certain cases, the adjusting algorithm should be functionally similar to partial energy minimization. However, in certain cases, the adjusting algorithm could find two distinct structures that relieve the strain, or that make interactions, in two different ways. By contrast, minimization could never find more than one such structure. The algorithm has been applied in various docking problems; calculations where methotrexate was docked into dihydrofolate reductase are described in Section VI.

XVII. CONFORMER BUILDUP APPROACHES

Conventional tree searches can handle molecules with up to about ten rotatable bonds, although additional degrees of freedom can be handled when the geometry is constrained. Scheraga and co-workers have introduced several approaches that can handle much larger molecules. The most generally applicable of these is the buildup, where alternative conformations are "built-up" by combining precomputed low-energy conformations of different submolecules. The application to peptides is particularly convenient, because peptides can easily be divided into smaller subpeptides or individual amino acids. To simulate the environment in the fully built peptide, the subpeptides and amino acids are represented with N-acetyl and N'-methyl amide end groups. Exhaustive conformational search calculations were used to identify the low-energy minima for each of the 20 naturally occurring amino acids [193,194], as well as the 400 possible dipeptides [K. D. Gibson and H. A. Scheraga, unpublished data]. For example, with an energy cutoff of 5 kcal, the analysis located 7 conformations of alanine, 18 conformations of phenylalanine, and 103 conformations of glutamine. Lysine and arginine are significantly more flexible, with 178 and 210 conformations, respectively, below 3 kcal. Glycine is a special case, represented by the 12 minima occurring in the X-Gly and Gly-X dipeptides [195].

We will illustrate the buildup procedure by describing calculations on met-enkephalin [196], a pentapeptide with the amino acid sequence Tyr-Gly-Gly-Phe-Met. In the single residue analysis discussed earlier, these amino acids have 30, 12, 12, 18, and 87 minima below 5 kcal, respectively. Candidate conformations for the pentapeptide could be obtained by forming all combinations of the single-residue conformations. This simple approach would lead to $30 \cdot 12 \cdot 12 \cdot 18 \cdot 87 = 6.8$ million pentapeptide conformations. The buildup procedure uses the energies of partially constructed peptides to focus the search on the most likely conformations, avoiding the need to minimize all 7 million structures. We will initially describe a simplified buildup approach [197] instead of the more complex strategy actually followed by Vasquez and Scheraga. In the simplified approach of Gibson and Scheraga, the first cycle of growth starts at the N-terminus, with the 30 alternative tyrosine conformations. In the second cycle of growth, these 30 conformations are combined with each of the 12 glycine conformations to give $30 \cdot 12 = 360$ candidate conformations for the Tyr-Gly dipeptide. Each of these is refined by energy minimization, and high-energy structures are eliminated. The minimization sometimes brings distinct starting structures to the same minimum, in which case the redundant structures are also eliminated. The 5 kcal cutoff and redundancy checking often eliminate about three-fourths of the conformations, which would then leave about 100 conformations. In the third cycle of growth, these 100 retained Tyr-Gly conformations are combined with the 12 conformations for the second glycine, and the resulting 1200 Tyr-Gly-Gly conformations are refined by energy minimization. Elimination of high-energy and redundant structures might then leave about 300 structures for the tripeptide. In the fourth cycle of growth, these 300 Tyr-Gly-Gly structures are combined with the 18 phenylalanine structures to give 5400 Tyr-Gly-Gly-Phe structures, of which perhaps 1000 would be retained. Finally, in the fifth cycle of growth, the addition of the 87 alternative methionine structures would give 87,000 candidate structures. A final round of energy minimization would then be used to refine the structures for the fully built pentapeptide.

The number of structures under the 5 kcal cutoff increases geometrically with each new residue. This is exactly what one should expect for conformational search problems. Consider the situation with a grid search: assuming that the amide bonds are held fixed, met-enkephalin has 18 rotatable bonds. If the torsions are searched with a step size of 30°, requiring 12 grid points per bond, then the complete search would involve $12^{18} = 2.7 \times 10^{19}$ conformations. A tree search would allow recognition and elimination of some sterically impossible structures. However, in this case, there are no external constraints, so the improvement would not be particularly dramatic. The conformational search problem increases combinatorially with the number of rotatable bonds. This is true for any systematic search technique. The advantage of the buildup procedure is that the search is more focused, and the combinatorial explosion is better controlled.

A. Alternative Buildup Strategies

Several variations on this theme have been explored. In their original calculations on enkephalin, Vasquez and Scheraga [196] built up two overlapping tripeptides (Tyr-Gly-Gly and Gly-Phe-Met), instead of simply working from one end of the molecule. This symmetric buildup strategy brings the Gly-Phe, Phe-Met, and Gly-Phe-Met interactions into the calculation at an earlier stage, eliminating some additional conformations earlier in the process. In general, the efficiency is also improved by building the most constrained fragments first. DeLisi and co-workers have used ideas from dynamic programming to apply smaller cutoffs to different subsets of conformations [198,199]. The A* algorithm modifies the buildup approach by estimating the energy of the best fully built structure that could result from each partially built structure [200]. This is discussed in greater detail later.

The buildup procedure can also be applied in a more abstract manner. Lambert and Scheraga [201] divide the conformational space of an amino acid into four regions, α, ϵ, α^*, and ϵ^*. The single-residue classifications correspond loosely to right-handed α-helical conformation, the conventional extended conformation, and the mirror images of these two conformations, respectively. Within this system, tripeptide segments can be classified into $4 \cdot 4 \cdot 4 = 64$ possible conformations. For example, the $\alpha\alpha\alpha$ state describes a tripeptide in which all three residues adopt the α-conformation, as typically observed in α-helices. The $\epsilon\epsilon\epsilon$ state describes three residues in the ϵ-conformation, as typically observed in β-sheets. The $\epsilon\alpha^*\alpha^*$ state describes the type-I' turn conformation often seen in β-hairpins [202]. Many of the other known structural motifs also correspond to distinct tripeptide conformation states in this representation. We then carried out an analysis of tripeptide conformations in the protein data bank to derive parameters for estimating the probability that a tripeptide adopts each of these conformational states. The conformation of an entire protein chain may be represented by listing the conformational states of each of the residues [203]. A chain with n-residues could adopt any of 4^n alternative conformations in this representation. The probabilities of each of these chain conformations may be estimated from the calculated probabilities of the overlapping tripeptides. An important advantage of the overlapping tripeptides is that nearest-neighbor interactions are incorporated, so that the cooperativity of α-helix and β-strand formation is modeled more accurately. Large amounts of computer time would be required to compute all 4^n chain conformation probabilities. Consequently, we used a probability-directed buildup procedure to generate the 1,000–10,000 most-probable chain conformations. The approach is similar to that of Gibson and Scheraga [197], except that the buildup is directed by calculated probabilities instead of energies. We generated three-dimensional structures from the most probable chain conformations using an importance-sampling minimization procedure that took advantage of the known distribution of conformers within each tripeptide conformational state [204]. The over-all *p*robability-directed *i*mportance-*s*ampling *m*inimization (PRISM) procedure was successful in calculating a structure for a 36-residue peptide in relatively good agreement with a prior X-ray crystal structure [204]. However, the empirical parameters are restricted to peptides and protein segments with the 20 naturally occurring amino acids.

B. Docking Peptides with the Buildup Approach

Pincus and associates used a buildup approach in very early calculations where various oligosaccharides were docked into lysozyme [180]. Grid searches and energy minimization were used to dock alternative conformations of a disaccharide into the active site cleft. Several trisaccharide structures were obtained by attaching an additional monosaccharide unit in various different conformations [179] to either end of the docked disaccharide. The alternative trisaccharide structures were refined by energy minimization, and then used in an additional cycle of buildup to obtain tetrasaccharides. A subsequent study extended the buildup calculation to pentasaccharides and hexasaccharides [205].

The GROW program [206] automated this approach to docking. In its original form, the program was restricted to peptides. An amino acid library was generated by running 5000 cycles of Monte Carlo minimization [141,142] on each of the 20 standard amino acids, represented as N-acetyl-N'-methylamides. The conformations were generated with partial minimization, so that the library includes slightly distorted structures around each of the local minima. Redundant conformations were eliminated, leaving, for example, 53 structures for proline, 171 for alanine, and 4987 for arginine. Assembly of the peptide begins from an anchoring amide bond unit prepositioned in the binding site. The GROW procedure attaches the first amino acid to this anchor unit by superimposing its N-terminal amide onto the corresponding atoms of the anchor amide. Alternatively, growth can proceed in the opposite direction by superimposing the C-terminal amide. The GROW procedure iterates over 300–1000 randomly selected amino acid conformations from the library, estimating the interaction with the protein, and saving the 10–100 conformations that give the best energy. The energies are estimated with the AMBER force field [142], together with a solvation model [28] based on approximate surface areas [154]. The procedure is then repeated for the second residue, the third residue, and so on, until peptide assembly is complete. Aside from the degree of automation, the principal difference between the GROW procedure and Scheraga's buildup procedure is that Scheraga's procedure uses energy minimization to refine the intermediate, partially built structures. In a docking calculation, these minimizations allow the partially built structures to relax more precisely into the binding site cavity. Moon and Howe compensate for this, to some extent, by using a much larger library of slightly distorted amino acid conformations. However, the lack of energy minimization does make the GROW procedure very sensitive to the initial position and orientation of the anchor unit. In its "unrestricted" mode, the GROW procedure iterates over alternative amino acids at each stage of the buildup. In this mode, GROW acts as a de novo design program, searching for the best amino acid sequence as well as the best conformation. The GROW program has been used extensively in studies of peptide-like ligands bound to the HIV protease [207]. The predicted structure of one such peptide is in partial agreement with the subsequently published crystal structure [208].

C. Docking General Organic Molecules with the Buildup Approach

Although most of the published work has been done with peptides, carbohydrates, and nucleic acids, buildup approaches are not restricted to polymeric molecules. A recent version of the GROW procedure can use several nonamide linkers to combine molecular fragments [209]. The molecular fragments are obtained by searching the Cambridge Crystallographic Database [210] for molecules with the specific linkers. The LUDI program [69], can run several types of calculations. In one mode of operation [211], LUDI can position library fragments to make bonds to specified positions on an anchor fragment, without restriction to amides or other special bond types. This is an advantage, because it permits construction of a wider range of molecules. However, it is also a disadvantage because LUDI can easily construct molecules that would be difficult or impossible to synthesize. The LUDI program iterates through the fragment library, tentatively adding each fragment successively to each allowed bonding position on the anchor and then estimating the binding energy using an empirical scoring function [45]. The original LUDI fragment library included more than 500 molecules. However, LUDI is intended more for do novo design than for conformational searching, and most of the molecular fragments are present as a single conformation, or as a very small number of conformations. Extended multiconformer fragment libraries would be needed to carry out extensive conformational searches. Also, like the GROW program, LUDI does not carry out energy minimization.

A number of other de novo design programs use the same general fragment assembly approach as GROW and LUDI. Whereas GROW and LUDI assemble molecules from relatively large fragments, GroupBuild [112], Sprout [212], and the Chemical Genesis algorithm [213] use small fragments, and Legend [214] and GrowMol [215] build molecules from individual atoms. Addition of an atom or fragment generally creates a new torsion, which is then searched with a coarse step size, or given a random torsional angle. Currently, however, none of these programs would carry out an extensive conformational search for any particular molecule. The Chemical Genesis algorithm uses energy minimization during the fragment assembly and recombination processes, and GrowMol uses energy minimization as part of the scoring process. However, the other programs never use gradient minimization. These simple approaches are appropriate at the current level of de novo design, because the principal goal is to generate ideas for possible synthesis. However, future progress will probably depend on more accurate estimation of binding energies and this, in turn, will depend on more extensive conformational searching and energy minimization.

Most of the de novo design programs are limited to relatively simple bonding operations. Additional fragment-linking operations, such as ring fusions and spiro joins, may be needed to construct certain molecules. Leach and co-workers have implemented a range of fragment-joining operations [216] in their WIZARD and COBRA programs [13,217]. These programs use a fragment-assembly process to search the conformational space of a small molecule in isolation. Flexible fragments are represented in the library by multiple conformers, and distance geometry can be used to generate conformations for groups that are not already included in the library [218]. For each new molecule, the programs start by identifying the conformational units corresponding to groups in the library [219,220]. The conformational unit with the largest number of connections is designated as the "crucial unit," and is taken as the root of a search tree [221]. A conformation of the molecule is constructed by joining alternative conformations of the library fragments onto the crucial unit. To search the entire conformational space, the program generates all possible combinations of library fragment conformations. Alternatively, the A* algorithm, discussed in the following section, can be used to focus on the low-energy structures [200]. Leach and Kuntz used some of these ideas to handle ring structures in their tree–search docking algorithm [41]. However, most of these refinements to the fragment assembly approach have not yet been applied to molecular docking calculations.

Judson and co-workers use a "growing" algorithm in their genetic algorithm docking procedure [145]. This algorithm avoids the complexity of fragment-linking operations by simply excluding unbuilt atoms from the molecular mechanics energy calculations. However, the genetic algorithm still uses the full chromosome, and rotational, translational, and torsional movements are applied to the entire molecule, including the unbuilt part. In the early stages of the simulation, the energy calculations are restricted to the "pivot" atom and its immediate substituents, allowing it to find a range of low-energy positions and orientations in the active site. Then, as the genetic algorithm simulation progresses, additional layers of atoms are included in the molecular mechanics energy. The genetic algorithm simulation is continued for several generations after the entire molecule has been included in the energy calculations. This approach is not limited by the availability of pregenerated conformers in a fragment library. However, the approach does sacrifice some of the efficiencies normally obtained with pregenerated conformers.

D. The A* Algorithm and Dead-End Elimination

Leach has adapted the general A* algorithm [222] from artificial intelligence to a wide range of problems in conformational analysis [90,181, 200,223]. His application of the A* algorithm is similar to the buildup approach in that it uses the energies of partially built structures to direct the conformational search. However, whereas the traditional buildup approach uses the partially built energies directly, the A* algorithm attempts to estimate the energy of the fully built structure that would result from each partially built structure. To use the nomenclature from artificial intelligence, each partially built structure is scored by an evaluation function

$$f* = g* + h*, \tag{9}$$

where $g*$ is the calculated energy of the partially built structure, and $h*$ is the estimated energy change upon completing the structure. In small-molecule conformational analysis, the energy required to complete the structure may be estimated as the sum of the best energies of the remaining, unbuilt fragments [200]. For example, if the unbuilt part consists of a cyclohexane ring on a five-carbon linker, then $h*$ may be estimated as the energy of the cyclohexane ring in the chair conformation, plus the energy of the linker in the all-*trans* conformation.

In principle, the $f*$ evaluation function makes it possible to compare the energies of conformers at different stages of construction. To take peptide conformational analysis as an example, the $f*$ function would bring the energies of dipeptides, tripeptides and tetrapeptides to the same scale. The A* algorithm uses this information to concentrate on the best structures. For example, if a particular tripeptide conformation gives a good score, then the A* algorithm will build it to the tetrapeptide stage immediately, without also building the other tripeptide conformations. If the tetrapeptide energy looks good, as judged by the $f*$ evaluation function, then the A* algorithm will then build it on to the pentapeptide stage. However, if the tetrapeptide energy turns out to be worse than expected, then the A* algorithm can backtrack to some other tripeptide conformation. By contrast, the conventional buildup approach would build all the selected tetrapeptides at once, and the then build all the selected pentapeptides at once. When the completion energy h^* is estimated accurately, the A* algorithm should be more efficient than the conventional buildup algorithm, because it does not need to build as many suboptimal conformers.

The A* algorithm can be applied to side chain conformational searching [181] if the side chains are restricted to discrete rotameric states [154]. Here, g^* is the sum of the previously built side chain energies, and h^* is the sum of the best possible energies for each of remaining unbuilt side chains. If n' of the n side chains have been built, then

$$g^* = \sum_{i=1}^{n'} E_{ir}^1 + \sum_{i=1}^{n'} \sum_{j=1}^{i-1} E_{irjs}^2 \qquad (10)$$

where r and s refer to the actual rotameric states of the ith and jth side chains, E_{ir}^1 is the internal and backbone interaction energy for the ith side chain in the rth rotameric state, and E_{irjs}^2 is the interaction between the ith and jth side chains in the rth and sth rotameric states, respectively. The completion energy is taken as

$$h^* = \sum_{i=n'+1}^{n} E_i^{min} \qquad (11)$$

where for each unbuilt side chain E_i^{min} is taken as the minimum energy over the full range of rotameric states:

$$E_i^{min} = \min_r \left(E_{ir}^1 + \sum_{i=1}^{n'} E_{irjs}^2 + \sum_{i=n'+1}^{n} \min_s(E_{irjs}^2) \right) \qquad (12)$$

To facilitate calculation of these energies, Leach precomputes all of the E_{ir}^1 and E_{irjs}^2. Now, the A* algorithm could be used to directly search the full set of side chain rotamers. However, Desmet et al. showed that a simple rule, called the "dead-end elimination theorem," could be used to eliminate certain high-energy rotameric states from a conformational search [224]. Expressed mathematically, the theorem eliminates rotamer r of residue i if there is some other low-energy rotamer s such that

$$E_{ir}^1 + \sum_{j \neq i} \min_t (E_{irjt}^2) > E_{is}^1 + \sum_{j \neq i} \max_t(E_{isjt}^2). \qquad (13)$$

Expressed somewhat less precisely in words, the theorem eliminates rotamer r if its *best* possible energy is still *worse* than the *worst* possible energy of some other rotamer s [225]. They also set forth a similar rule for pairs of rotamers [224]. In their first study, the single and pairwise dead-end elimination rules were applied iteratively to the side-chain rotamers in insulin to eliminate most of the possible rotamers. The few remaining rotameric states were searched with a modified buildup procedure, leading to a final low-energy structure that predicted 72% of the side chains correctly. Their second study corrected an error in the pair rule and then showed how the modified rule could be applied to the insulin problem.

In his DEE/A* procedure, Leach applies a modified (single) dead-end elimination rule to eliminate side chain rotamers that would lead to a structure more than 5 kcal above the global minimum, and then uses the A* algorithm to search through the remaining rotamers. The combination is remarkably efficient, and allows the complete side chain search to be repeated for a large number of different ligand positions and orientations [181]. Calculations were carried out with trypsin and the antibody McPC 603, using benzamidine and phosphocholine, respectively, as the ligands. Leach selected 61 and 42 side chains for searching in trypsin and McPC 603, respectively. The complete side chain search required approximately 25 s for each orientation of benzamidine in trypsin, and 60 s for each orientation (and all seven conformations) of phosphocholine in McPC 603. Similar calculations were carried out on trypsin and McPC 603 without the ligand. Surprisingly, these calculations indicated that there are more low-energy side chain conformations in the complexes than in the apo-proteins.

The DEE/A* algorithm appears to be an important advance for side-chain conformational searching. The principal disadvantage of the approach is its restriction to discrete rotameric states. The current implementations [181,224,225] do not relax overlaps with the protein backbone or between pairs of side chains. Long experience has shown that unrelaxed structures often have very high energies owing to small overlaps, and the DEE/A* algorithm depends on these energies to select between alternative conformations. Interestingly, a recent study by Vasquez suggests that the restriction to rotameric states is appropriate for the combinatorial search, but that subsequent minimization could improve the accuracy [226]. Note also that the ligand positions and orientations were obtained by a grid search, as discussed earlier in this review, and the ligand conformations were obtained from a separate conformational search of the ligand in isolation [181]. It will be interesting to see whether dead-end elimination and the A* algorithm can be adapted to handle these ligand degrees of freedoms efficiently.

E.   The MVP Buildup Algorithm

The MVP program [6] uses a modified buildup algorithm in both docking and conformational search calculations. In a simple conformational search calculation, the algorithm starts by identifying a root atom and all the rotatable bonds. The rigid group containing the root atom is always included in the molecular mechanics energy calculations (this corresponds to the anchor fragment in the docking calculations). The first cycle of growth "activates" the first rotatable bond outward from the root atom, and brings the atoms immediately dependent on this rotatable bond into the energy calculations. To take a specific example, activation of the side chain CA–CB bond in lysine would bring the CG, HB1, and HB2 atoms into the energy calculations. Atoms farther out in the side chain depend on additional rotatable bonds, and are not included in the energy calculations until their parent bonds have been activated. After the dependent atoms have been included, the MVP program rotates the bond from $-180°$ to $+180°$, calculating the energy in steps of $3°$. This rotation traces out an energy profile, and the MVP program retains the conformations corresponding to the minima along the profile. For example, in the lysine side chain or in straight-chain alkanes, the profile has minima at approximately $-60°$, $+60°$, and $180°$, corresponding to the g^-, g^+, and t conformations. These retained structures are then refined by torsional coordinate energy minimization.

The second cycle of growth activates the second rotatable bond. In a protein calculation, this second bond could be the CB–CG bond in the lysine residue, or some other backbone or side chain rotatable bond. Alternatively, in an n-alkane, this would be the next bond in the molecule. The atoms immediately dependent on the bond are brought into the energy calculations, and then the bond is rotated from $-180°$ to $+180°$ to obtain the torsional energy profile. The torsional profile is calculated separately for each of the three structures retained in the previous cycle of growth, because the different conformations of that bond can perturb the torsional profile of the new bond. However, we will restrict our discussion here to the "idealized" alkane, in which the profile would again have minima at exactly $-60°$, $+60°$, and $180°$. This idealized alkane would thus have nine conformations overall, g^-g^-, . . . , tt (a real alkane will have additional structures owing to splitting of the g^-g^+ and g^+g^- conformations). All nine of these would be refined by torsional coordinate energy minimization. The third cycle of growth would activate a third rotatable bond, which would be rotated from $-180°$ to $+180°$ for each of the retained structures, giving 27 new conformations for refinement by torsional coordinate minimization.

In idealized alkanes, successive cycles of the growth process lead to 3, 9, 27, 81, 243, 729, . . . , retained structures. In practice, the MVP program places a limit on the number of structures retained. This is similar to the approach used in our earlier PRISM buildup [203], but differs from Scheraga's original approach, where all structures within a specified energy cutoff were retained. Typically, the limit in MVP calculations is 200 structures (although much larger limits are sometimes used). In the simple alkane example discussed in the forgoing, the limit would be applied after obtaining 243 structures in the fifth cycle. In this example, the MVP-filtering process is used to select 200 representative low-energy conformations from the full set of 243 structures. The filtering algorithm does not simply select the 200 conformations with the lowest energy, but rather, selects a set of significantly different low-energy conformations that "cover" a large volume of the conformational space; this is discussed in Section VII of this review. The 200 selected representative structures would be retained for the sixth cycle. Then, in an idealized alkane, rotation of the sixth rotatable bond would give $3 \times 200 = 600$ new structures, which would again be filtered into a representative set of 200 structures for the next cycle. The process continues, generating several hundred new structures for each rotatable bond, and then filtering back into a representative set of 200 starting structures for energy minimization and the next cycle of growth.

The basic algorithm is modified slightly for cyclic molecules. The current ring closure algorithm carries out a two-dimensional grid search of the last two rotatable bonds in the ring. The algorithm then uses torsional coordinate energy minimization to refine all the minima from the two-dimensional grid, as well as a representative set of low-energy flanking structures. The algorithm can rapidly recover all envelope and twist–chair conformations of cyclopentane, and all chair and twist–boat conformations of cyclohexane [227]. The algorithm is much less efficient for macrocycles, but can still generate good, low-energy structures. The efficiency can be improved dramatically by manually applying distance constraints to keep the growing arms of the partially-built ring close enough together to allow the remaining unbuilt bonds to close the ring.

Docking calculations use exactly the same buildup approach, except that the program must find initial positions and orientations for the rigid anchor unit. The MVP program currently includes algorithms based on superimposition and Monte Carlo minimization. The superimposition approach is similar to the Directed DOCK algorithm [41] discussed earlier, except that the MVP procedure refines each anchor position by rigid body energy minimization. This approach is very fast, but requires prior specification of a set of target points in the binding site. The Monte Carlo minimization approach applies random rotations and translations to the anchor unit, and then carries out partial rigid body energy minimization, using the metropolis criterion to accept or reject the new structure. This approach is similar to the procedure of Still and co-workers discussed earlier [138], except that MVP treats the anchor as a rigid body in the minimization. Monte Carlo minimization can generate good-quality, low-energy binding modes for the anchor unit. However, the user must specify distance constraints between the anchor unit and the protein to prevent the anchor unit from popping out of the binding site. MVP will typically retain 200 different positions and orientations for the anchor unit with either approach. When the first rotatable bond is activated, MVP will calculate the torsional profile separately for each of these anchor positions and orientations. If the torsional profiles have more than three minima each, then the first cycle of growth will give approximately $3 \times 200 = 600$ alternative structures for the partially grown molecule. These structures are refined by internal coordinate minimization, and then filtered to select 200 representative structures. The growth process in a docking calculation is thus virtually identical to the process in a conventional conformational search calculation.

Internal coordinate energy minimization is applied to all partially built structures after each cycle of growth. In a docking calculation, this internal coordinate minimization includes the rotational and translational coordinates of the anchor unit, as well as the torsional coordinates corresponding to the rotatable bonds. This allows the molecule to relax into its binding site as the growth process continues, and makes the overall process much less sensitive to the initial position and orientation of the anchor unit. When growth is complete, the MVP program switches to Cartesian coordinate energy minimization to allow a more complete relaxation. Energy minimization is much slower in Cartesian coordinates than in torsional coordinates, so the MVP program uses a filtering minimization protocol to focus on the best structures. The typical filtering minimization protocol consists of three successive rounds of partial energy minimization, with redundancy checking between rounds. The first round of minimization refines all 200 structures to an rms gradient of 2.0 kcal A^{-1}. Structures within the same energy basin will tend to minimize to the same point. The MVP program applies the filtering procedure just discussed to recognize these and other redundant structures, selecting a set of 100 representative structures from the full set of 200. The second round of minimization refines these 100 structures to an rms gradient of 0.5 kcal A^{-1}. The filtering algorithm is applied again to select 50 representative structures. Then, the third and final round of minimization refines these 50 structures to an rms gradient of 0.1 kcal A^{-1}. These 50 representative structures would be used in the estimates of the free energy, or written out to a file for graphic examination. The filtering minimization protocol can usually identify the best structures much faster than complete minimization of all 200 structures.

The MVP program uses the Biosym CVFF [228] and CFF91 [229] force fields to compute the molecular mechanics energies and forces. Currently, MVP computes the conventional and anharmonic terms, but not the cross terms. Solvation is normally represented by a solvation shell model similar to those described by Scheraga [28–30]. MVP uses an analytical algorithm to compute the solvent accessible surface areas [230], as well as the gradient of the surface area with respect to atomic coordinates [231]. This allows the MVP program to include the solvation forces in energy minimization and molecular dynamics calculations. The analytical surface algorithm is extremely fast, and will be described elsewhere [232]. The MVP solvation model separates the solvation energy into hydrophobic and electrostatic terms, and then scales the electrostatic term according to the dielectric constant chosen for the molecular mechanics calculations. Alternatively, MVP can obtain a more accurate estimate of the electrostatic term by submitting the coordinates to the DelPhi program for electrostatic calculations [22].

The MVP program uses approximations to the energies during the buildup, and then shifts toward more accurate energies when the buildup is complete. For example, solvation energies are estimated from approximate solvent-accessible surface areas [154,233] during the buildup, and then from exact analytical surface areas at the end of the calculation [232]. Also, solvation energies are normally not included in the torsional coordinate minimizations during the buildup, but may be included in the final minimizations. Similarly, van der Waals and coulombic interactions are typically calculated with a 6 Å cutoff during the buildup, and then recalculated with a 100 Å cutoff at the end of the calculation. The protein is normally held fixed, but selected atoms or residues may be allowed to relax in the energy minimizations, and selected side chains may be included in the buildup conformational search. The final binding energies are calculated from Eqs. (1) and (3) in the binding energy estimation section of this review.

XVIII.   THE MVP PROGRAM

Structure-based drug design projects generally require a wide range of different calculations, usually carried out with several different semicompatible programs. Available molecular modeling software is remarkably diverse, not just in the methods used, but also in the scripting languages, file formats, and even the interpretations given to fields in the standard file formats. We have tried to solve some of these problems by bringing a wide range of different methods into the MVP program with a common scripting language. Inevitably, this creates some new problems, but development of new methods is accelerated by the availability of extensive subroutine libraries using the same core data structures.

The current MVP program includes facilities for amino acid sequence analysis, protein homology modeling, and a range of molecular mechanics calculations. The Evans and Sutherland molecular graphics interface in the original Cornell version has been deleted in the current Glaxo Wellcome version. The current version includes facilities for structural analysis [234], secondary structure prediction [201,203], and multiple sequence alignment based on primary, secondary [235], and tertiary structure. Alignments can be annotated and colorized according to the three-dimensional structure or other available information. MVP uses the sequence alignments for homology modeling [236] and superimposition [237]. MVP uses molecular mechanics calculations in protein ligand docking (as discussed earlier), as well as homology modeling [236] and small molecule conformational searching. MVP can use a relaxation matrix analysis to obtain structures from NMR data [238]. MVP has special facilities to automatically determine atom types, charges and ionization states at specified pH, as well as facilities to carry out simple chemical reactions on specified molecules. These automation facilities were used in recent calculations where thousands of compounds were constructed from starting "materials" in chemical databases, and then docked into protein binding sites [239; P. S. Charifson and M. H. Lambert, unpublished data].

XIX. CONCLUSION

Flexible-docking algorithms are now widely recognized as an essential tool for structure-based drug design. Earlier work focused on the rigid docking problem, and a number of programs have been used to efficiently dock rigid molecules into protein binding sites. However, most molecules of interest in drug discovery are conformationally flexible, and these flexible molecules present a much more difficult challenge. This review shows that substantial progress has been made, particularly over the last 3 years. Current methods involve a surprisingly wide range of different techniques, including molecular dynamics, metropolis Monte Carlo, Monte Carlo minimization, genetic algorithms, distance geometry, tree searching, buildup approaches, and rigid-body methods with multiconformer databases.

It is tempting to try to compare the different methods. However, most of the methods are evolving quite rapidly, and the programs involved would probably be obsolete before the comparison appeared in print. Consequently, this review focuses on the basic methods and algorithms. A thorough understanding of the algorithms is probably the best guide in selecting or developing methods for new problems and for interpreting the results.

Binding energy estimation remains a serious problem, even when the geometries are known accurately. It is sobering to note that the binding energies obtained in many contemporary studies are only slightly better than those obtained 25 years ago [50]. However, except for free energy perturbation, all current approaches still neglect one or more important terms in the free energy expressions. Our hope is that a proper consideration of the complete problem will give improved estimates of the binding energy. Meanwhile, current methods can often be applied within a series of related compounds, and empirical approaches continue to improve rapidly.

ACKNOWLEDGMENTS

I thank Max Vasquez for reading the manuscript and making numerous suggestions. I thank Paul Charifson, Max Vasquez, Roger Williams, Ken Gibson, Jim Veal, Lee Kuyper, Steve Jordan, Tai-he Xia, Jean-Yves Trosset, Andrew Leach, Frank Brown, Peter Jeffs, Mike Cory, Ray Unwalla, Tom Darden, Steve Freer, Harold Scheraga, and Tack Kuntz for helpful discussions of the docking problem, binding energy estimation, and structure-based design.

REFERENCES

1. R. C. Jackson, Update on computer-aided drug design, *Curr. Opin. Biotechnol.* 6:646–651 (1995).
2. C. L. M. J. Verlinde and W. G. J. Hol, Structure-based drug design: Progress, results and challenges, *Structure* 2:577–587 (1994).
3. W. C. Guida, Software for structure-based drug design, *Curr. Opin. Struct. Biol.* 4:777–781 (1994).
4. I. D. Kuntz, Structure-based strategies for drug design and discovery, *Science* 257:1078–1082 (1992).
5. M. A. Navia and M. A. Murcko, Use of structural information in drug design, *Curr. Opin. Struct. Biol.* 2:202–210 (1992).
6. M. H. Lambert and H. A. Scheraga, Molecular viewing program. A general program for molecular mechanics calculations developed at Cornell University and Glaxo Wellcome.
7. R. Rosenfeld, S. Vajda, and C. DeLisi, Flexible docking and design, *Annu. Rev. Biophys. Biomol. Struct.* 24:677–700 (1995).
8. J. M. Blaney and J. S. Dixon, A good ligand is hard to find: Automated docking methods, *Perspect. Drug Discovery Design* 1:301–319 (1993).

9. T. P. Lybrand, Ligand-protein docking and rational drug design, *Curr. Opin. Struct. Biol.* 5:224–228 (1995).

10. G. Jones and P. Willett, Docking small-molecule ligands into active sites, *Curr. Opin. Biotechnol.* 6:652–656 (1995).

11. J. Cherfils and J. Janin, Protein docking algorithms: Simulating molecular recognition, *Curr. Opin. Struct. Biol.* 3:265–269 (1993).

12. N. C. J. Strynadka, M. Eisenstein, E. Katchalski-Katzir, B. K. Shoichet, I. D. Kuntz, R. Abagyan, M. Abagyan, M. Totrov, J. Janin, J. Cerfils, F. Zimmerman, A. Olson, B. Duncan, M. Rao, R. Jackson, M. Sternberg, and M. N. G. James, Molecular docking programs successfully predict the binding of a β-lactamase inhibitory protein to TEM-1 β-lactamase, *Nature Struct. Biol.* 3:233–239 (1996).

13. A. R. Leach, A survey of methods for searching the conformational space of small and medium-sized molecules, *Reviews in Computational Chemistry*, Vol. 2 (K. B. Lipkowitz and D. B. Boyd, eds.), VCH Publishers, New York, 1991, pp. 1–55.

14. M. Vasquez, G. Nemethy, and H. A. Scheraga, Conformational energy calculations on polypeptides and proteins, *Chem. Rev.* 94:2183–2239 (1994).

15. K. D. Gibson and H. A. Scheraga, The multiple-minima problem in protein folding, *Structure*, Vol. 1, *From Proteins to Ribosomes* (R. H. Sarma and M. H. Sarma, eds.), Adenine Press, 1988, pp. 67–94.

16. C. B. Anfinsen, Principles that govern the folding of protein chains, *Science* 181:223–230 (1973).

17. C. B. Anfinsen and H. A. Scheraga, Experimental and theoretical aspects of protein folding, *Adv. Protein Chem.* 29:205–300 (1975).

18. In the approximation of classic statistical mechanics, the constant temperature, constant volume free energy A actually involves an additional integral over conjugate momenta, a factor involving Planck's constant, and factors of $N!$ for each class of identical particles. However, the momentum integral can be separated and represented as a constant factor, and then all of the factors cancel out in any subsequent calculations of free energy differences. The constant temperature, constant pressure free energy G takes the integrand as $e^{-(E+pV)/kT}$, and requires one additional integral over volumes. However, the pV term is essentially negligible in condensed phases at ordinary pressures, and the volume integral is dominated by the contribution at the optimal volume. Thus, the simplified expression may be used for binding energy estimation. See D. A. McQuarrie, *Statistical Mechanics,* Harper & Row, New York, 1976.

19. P. Kollman, Free energy calculations: Applications to chemical and biochemical phenomena, *Chem. Rev.* 93:2395–2417 (1993).

20. A. Warshel and J. Aqvist, Electrostatic energy and macromolecular function, *Annu. Rev. Biophys. Biophys. Chem.* 20:267–298 (1991).

21. M. K. Gilson, Theory of electrostatic interactions in macromolecules, *Curr. Opin. Struct. Biol.* 5:216–223 (1995).

22. B. Honig and A. Nicholls, Classical electrostatics in biology and chemistry, *Science 268*:1144–1149 (1995).
23. J. Shen and F. A. Quiocho, Calculation of binding energy differences for receptor–ligand systems using the Poisson–Boltzmann method, *J. Comput. Chem. 16*:445–448 (1995).
24. J. Shen and J. Wendoloski, Binding of phosphorus-containing inhibitors to thermolysin studied by the Poisson–Boltzmann method, *Protein Sci. 4*: 373–381 (1995).
25. T. Zhang and D. E. Koshland, Jr., Computational method for relative binding energies of enzyme–substrate complexes, *Protein Sci. 5*:348–356 (1996).
26. M. Zacharias, B. A. Luty, M. E. Davis, and J. A. McCammon, Combined conformational search and finite-difference Poisson–Boltzmann approach for flexible docking, *J. Mol. Biol. 238*:455–465 (1994).
27. R. M. Jackson and M. J. E. Sternberg, A continuum model for protein–protein interactions: Application to the docking problem, *J. Mol. Biol. 250*: 258–275 (1995).
28. T. Ooi, M. Oobatake, G. Nemethy, and H. A. Scheraga, Accessible surface areas as a measure of the thermodynamic parameters of hydration of peptides, *Proc. Natl. Acad. Sci. USA 84*:3086–3090 (1987).
29. J. Vila, R. L. Williams, M. Vasquez, and H. A. Scheraga, Empirical solvation models can be used to differentiate native from near-native conformations of bovine pancreatic trypsin inhibitor, *Proteins Struct. Funct. Genet. 10*:199–218 (1991).
30. R. L. Williams, J. Vila, G. Perrot, and H. A. Scheraga, Empirical models in the context of conformational energy searches: Application to bovine pancreatic trypsin inhibitor, *Proteins Struct. Funct. Genet. 14*:110–119 (1992).
31. L. Wesson and D. Eisenberg, Atomic solvation parameters applied to molecular dynamics of proteins in solution, *Protein Sci. 1*:227–235 (1992).
32. P. F. W. Stouten, C. Frommel, H. Nakamura, and C. Sander, An effective solvation term based on atomic occupancies for use in protein simulations. *Mol. Simulat. 10*:97–120 (1993).
33. J. Wang, Z. Szewczuk, S. Y. Yue, U. Tsuda, Y. Konishi, and E. O. Purisima, Calculation of relative binding free energies and configurational entropies: A structural and thermodynamic analysis of the nature of non-polar binding of thrombin inhibitors based on hirudin, *J. Mol. Biol. 253*:473–492 (1995).
34. A. T. Hagler, P. S. Stern, R. Sharon, J. M. Becker, and F. Naider, Computer simulation of the conformational properties of oligopeptides. comparison of theoretical methods and analysis of experimental results, *J. Am. Chem. Soc. 101*:6842–6852 (1979).
35. M. K. Holloway, J. M. Wai, T. A. Halgren, P. M. D. Fitzgerald, J. P. Vacca, B. D. Dorsey, R. B. Levin, W. J. Thompson, L. J. Chen, S. J. deSolms, N. Gaffin, A. K. Ghosh, E. A. Giuliani, S. L. Graham, J. P. Guare, R. W. Hungate, T. A. Lyle, W. M. Sanders, T. J. Tucker, M. Wiggins, C. M. Wiscount, O. W. Woltersdorf, S. D. Young, P. L. Darke, and J. A. Zugay, A

Priori prediction of activity for HIV-1 protease inhibitors employing energy minimization in the active site, *J. Med. Chem. 38*:305–317 (1995).

36. J. Aqvist, C. Medina, and J.-E. Samuelsson, A new method for predicting binding affinity in computer-aided drug design, *Protein Eng. 7*:385–391 (1994).

37. A. R. Ortiz, M. T. Pisabarro, F. Gago, and R. C. Wade, Prediction of drug binding affinities by comparative binding energy analysis, *J. Med. Chem. 38*: 2681–2691 (1995).

38. I. D. Kuntz, J. M. Blaney, S. J. Oatley, R. Langridge, and T. E. Ferrin, A geometric approach to macromolecule–ligand interactions. *J. Mol. Biol. 161*: 269–288 (1982).

39. R. L. DesJarlais, R. P. Sheridan, J. S. Dixon, I. D. Kuntz, and R. Venkataraghavan, Docking flexible ligands to macromolecular receptors by molecular shape, *J. Med. Chem. 29*:2149–2153 (1986).

40. B. K. Shoichet, D. I. Bodian, and I. D. Kuntz, Molecular docking using shape descriptors, *J. Comput. Chem. 13*:380–397 (1992).

41. A. R. Leach and I. D. Kuntz, Conformational analysis of flexible ligands in macromolecular receptor sites, *J. Comput. Chem. 13*:730–748 (1992).

42. B. K. Shoichet and I. D. Kuntz, Matching chemistry and shape in molecular docking, *Protein Eng. 6*:723–732 (1993).

43. E. C. Meng, B. K. Shoichet, and I. D. Kuntz, Automated docking with grid-based energy evaluation, *J. Comput. Chem. 13*:505–524 (1992).

44. E. C. Meng, I. D. Kuntz, D. J. Abraham, and G. E. Kellogg, Evaluating docked complexes with the HINT exponential function and empirical atomic hydrophobicities, *J. Comput. Aided Mol. Design 8*:299–306 (1994).

45. H.-J. Bohm, The development of a simple empirical scoring function to estimate the binding constant for a protein–ligand complex of known three-dimensional structure, *J. Comput. Aided Mol. Design 8*:243–256 (1994).

46. N. Horton and M. Lewis, Calculation of the free energy of association for protein complexes, *Protein Sci 1*:169–181 (1992).

47. V. Nauchitel, M. C. Villaverde, and F. Sussman, Solvent accessibility as a predictive tool for the free energy of inhibitor binding to the HIV-1 protease, *Protein Sci. 4*:1356–1364 (1995).

48. A. Wallqvist, R. L. Jernigan, and D. G. Covell, A preference-based free-energy parameterization of enzyme-inhibitor binding. Applications to HIV-1 protease inhibitor design, *Protein Sci. 4*:1881–1903 (1995).

49. K. E. B. Platzer, F. A. Momany, and H. A. Scheraga, Conformational energy calculations of enzyme–substrate interactions. 1. Computation of preferred conformations of some substrates of α-chymotrypsin, *Int. J. Protein Pept. Res. 4*:187–200 (1972).

50. K. E. B. Platzer, F. A. Momany, and H. A. Scheraga, Conformational energy calculations of enzyme–substrate interactions. 2. Computation of the binding energy for substrates in the active site of α-chymotrypsin, *Int. J. Protein Pept. Res. 4*:201–219 (1972).

51. T. A. Steitz, R. Henderson, and D. M. Blow, Structure of crystalline α-chymotrypsin. III. Crystallographic studies of substrates and inhibitors bound to the active site of α-chymotrypsin, *J. Mol. Biol.* 46:337–342 (1969).

52. W. C. Ripka and J. M. Blaney, Computer graphics and molecular modeling in the analysis of synthetic targets, *Topics in Stereochemistry*, Vol. 20 (E. L. Eliel and S. H. Wilen, ed., Wiley, New York, 1991, pp. 1–85.

53. A. J. Olson and G. M. Morris, Seeing our way to drug design, *Perspect. Drug Discov. Design 1*:329–344 (1993).

54. M. C. Surles, J. S. Richardson, D. C. Richardson, and F. P. Brooks, Jr., Sculpting proteins interactively: Continual energy minimization in a graphical modeling system, *Protein Sci. 3*:198–210 (1994).

55. Biosym Technologies, San Diego. *Insight II Reference Guide*, 1990.

56. M. L. Connolly, Solvent-accessible surfaces of proteins and nucleic acids, *Science 221*:709–713 (1983).

57. P. J. Goodford, A computational procedure for determining energetically favorable binding sites on biologically important macromolecules, *J. Med. Chem. 28*:849–857 (1985).

58. E. C. Meng, D. A. Gschwend, J. M. Blaney, and I. D. Kuntz, Orientational sampling and rigid-body minimization in molecular docking, *Proteins Struct. Funct. Genet. 17*:266–278 (1993).

59. R. L. DesJarlais, R. P. Sheridan, G. L. Seibel, J. S. Dixon, I. D. Kuntz, and R. Venkataraghavan, Using shape complementarity as an initial screen in designing ligands for a receptor binding site of known three-dimensional structure, *J. Med. Chem. 31*:722–729 (1988).

60. R. L. DesJarlais, G. L. Seibel, I. D. Kuntz, P. S. Furth, J. C. Alvarez, P. R. Ortiz de Montellano, D. L. DeCamp, L. M. Babe, and C. S. Craik, Structure-based design of nonpeptide inhibitors specific for the human immunodeficiency virus 1 protease, *Proc. Natl. Acad. Sci. USA 87*:6644–6648 (1990).

61. K. D. Stewart, T. A. Fairley, J. A. Bentley, C. W. Andrews, and M. Cory, Automated 3D docking: Inhibitors of α-chymotrypsin, *Med. Chem. Res. 1*: 439–443 (1992).

62. B. K. Shoichet, R. M. Stroud, D. V. Santi, I. D. Kuntz, and K. M. Perry, Structure-based discovery of inhibitors of thymidylate synthase, *Science 259*: 1445–1450 (1993).

63. C. S. Ring, E. Sun, J. H. McKerrow, G. K. Lee, P. J. Rosenthal, I. D. Kuntz, and F. E. Cohen, Structure-based inhibitor design by using protein models for the development of antiparasitic agents, *Proc. Natl. Acad. Sci. USA 90*: 3583–3587 (1993).

64. D. L. Bodian, R. B. Yamasaki, R. L. Buswell, J. F. Stearns, J. M. White, and I. D. Kuntz, Inhibition of the fusion-inducing conformational change of influenza hemagglutinin by benzoquinones and hydroquinones, *Biochemistry 32*:2967–2978 (1993).

65. B. K. Shoichet and I. D. Kuntz, Protein docking and complementarity, *J. Mol. Biol. 221*:327–346 (1991).

66. E. Rutenber, E. B. Fauman, R. J. Keenan, S. Fong, P. S. Furth, P. R. Ortiz de Montellano, E. Meng, I. D. Kuntz, D. L. DeChamp, R. Aslto, J. R. Rose, C. S. Craik, and R. M. Stroud, Structure of a non-peptide inhibitor complexed with HIV-1 protease, *J. Biol. Chem. 268*:15343–15346 (1993).
67. M. C. Lawrence and P. C. Davis, CLIX: A search algorithm for finding novel ligands capable of binding proteins of known three-dimensional structure, *Proteins Struct. Funct. Genet. 12*:31–41 (1992).
68. M. D. Miller, S. K. Kearsley, D. J. Underwood, and R. P. Sheridan, FLOG: A system to select "quasi-flexible" ligands complementary to a receptor of known three-dimensional structure, *J. Comput. Aided Mol. Design 8*: 153–174 (1994).
69. H.-J. Bohm, The computer program LUDI: A new method for the de novo design of enzyme inhibitors, *J. Comput. Aided Mol. Design 6*:61–78 (1992).
70. H.-J. Bohm, On the use of LUDI to search the Fine Chemicals Directory for ligands of proteins of known three-dimensional structure, *J. Comput. Aided Mol. Design 8*:623–632 (1994).
71. R. L. DesJarlais and J. S. Dixon, A shape- and chemistry-based docking method and its use in the design of HIV-1 protease inhibitors, *J. Comput. Aided Mol. Design 8*:231–242 (1994).
72. D. J. Bacon and J. Moult, Docking by least-squares fitting of molecular surface patterns, *J. Mol. Biol. 225*:849–858 (1992).
73. S. L. Lin, R. Nussinov, D. Fischer, and H. L. Wolfson, Molecular surface representation by sparse critical points, *Proteins Struct. Funct. Genet. 18*: 94–101 (1994).
74. R. Norel, D. Fischer, H. L. Wolfson, and R. Nussinov, Molecular surface recognition by a computer vision-based technique, *Protein Eng. 7*:39–46 (1994).
75. D. Fischer, S. L. Lin, H. L. Wolfson, and R. Nussinov, A geometry-based suite of molecular docking process, *J. Mol. Biol. 248*:459–477 (1995).
76. S. K. Kearsley, D. J. Underwood, R. P. Sheridan, and M. D. Miller, Flexibases: A way to enhance the use of molecular docking methods, *J. Comput. Aided Mol. Design 8*:565–582 (1994).
77. P. S. Charifson, A. R. Leach, and A. Rusinko III, The generation and use of large 3D databases in drug discovery, *Network Sci. 1* (Sept. 1995).
78. M. D. Miller, R. P. Sheridan, S. K. Kearsley, and D. J. Underwood, Advances in automated docking applied to human immunodeficiency virus type 1 protease, *Methods Enzymol. 241*:354–370 (1994).
79. M. Yamada and A. Itai, Development of an efficient automated docking method, *Chem. Pharm. Bull. 41*:1200–1202 (1993).
80. M. Yamada and A. Itai, Application and evaluation of the automated docking method, *Chem. Pharm. Bull. 41*:1203–1205 (1993).
81. M. Y. Mizutani, N. Tomioka, and A. Itai, Rational automatic search method for stable docking models of protein and ligand, *J. Mol. Biol. 243*:310–326 (1994).
82. J. A. Hartigan, *Clustering Algorithms*, Wiley, New York, 1975.

83. P. Murray-Rust and J. Rafferty, Computer analysis of molecular geometry, part VI: Classification of differences in conformation, *J. Mol. Graph. 3*: 50–59 (1985).

84. P. S. Shenkin and D. Q. McDonald, Cluster analysis of molecular conformations, *J. Comput. Chem. 15*:899–916 (1994).

85. M. E. Karpen, D. J. Tobias, and C. L. Brooks III, Statistical clustering techniques for the analysis of long molecular dynamics trajectories, *Biochemistry 32*:412–420 (1993).

86. J. M. Troyer and F. E. Cohen, Protein conformational landscapes: Energy minimization and clustering of a long molecular dynamics trajectory, *Proteins Struct. Funct. Genet. 23*:97–110 (1995).

87. A. Smellie, S. D. Kahn, and S. L. Teig, Analysis of conformational coverage. 1. Validation and estimation of coverage, *J. Chem. Inf. Comput. Sci. 35*: 285–294 (1995).

88. A. Smellie, S. D. Kahn, and S. L. Teig, Analysis of conformational coverage. 2. Applications of conformational models, *J. Chem. Inf. Comput. Sci. 35*: 295–304 (1995).

89. A. Smellie, S. L. Teig, and P. Towbin, Poling: Promoting conformational variation, *J. Comput. Chem. 16*:171–187 (1995).

90. A. R. Leach, An algorithm to directly identify a molecule's "most different" conformations, *J. Chem. Inf. Comput. Sci. 34*:661–670 (1994).

91. W. Kabsch, A solution for the best rotation to relate two sets of vectors, *Acta Crystallogr. A32*:922–923 (1976).

92. W. Kabsch, A discussion of the solution for the best rotation to relate two sets of vectors, *Acta Crystallogr. A34*:827–828 (1978).

93. N. Go and H. A. Scheraga, Ring closure and local conformational deformations of chain molecules, *Macromolecules 3*:178–187 (1970).

94. R. E. Bruccoleri and M. Karplus, Chain closure with bond angle variations, *Macromolecules 18*:2767–2773 (1985).

95. R. E. Bruccoleri and M. Karplus, Prediction of the folding of short polypeptide segments by uniform conformational sampling, *Biopolymers 26*: 136–168 (1987).

96. P. S. Shenkin, D. L. Yarmush, R. M. Fine, H. Wang, and C. Levinthal, Predicting antibody hypervariable loop conformations. I. Ensembles of random conformations for ringlike structures, *Biopolymers 26*:2053–2085 (1987).

97. Q. Zheng, R. Rosenfeld, S. Vajda, and C. DeLisi, Loop closure via bond scaling and relaxation, *J. Comput. Chem. 14*:556–565 (1993).

98. Q. Zheng, R. Rosenfeld, S. Vajda, and C. DeLisi, Determining protein loop conformation using scaling–relaxation techniques, *Protein Sci. 2*:1242–1248 (1993).

99. M. Lipton and W. C. Still, The multiple minimum problem in molecular modeling. Tree searching internal coordinate space, *J. Comput. Chem. 9*: 343–355 (1988).

100. G. M. Smith and D. F. Veber, Computer-aided, systematic search of peptide conformations constrained by NMR data, *Biochem. Biophys. Res. Commun.* *134*:907 (1986).

101. N. Weinberg and S. Wolfe, A comprehensive approach to the conformational analysis of cyclic compounds, *J. Am. Chem. Soc.* *116*:9860–9868 (1994).

102. H. Goto and E. Osawa, Corner flapping: A simple and fast algorithm for exhaustive generation of ring conformations, *J. Am. Chem. Soc.* *111*: 8950–8951 (1989).

103. I. Kolossvary and W. C. Guida, Torsional flexing: Conformational searching of cyclic molecules in biased internal coordinate space, *J. Comput. Chem.* *14*:691–698 (1993).

104. R. Rosenfeld, Q. Zheng, S. Vajda, and C. DeLisi, Computing the structure of bound peptides: Application to antigen recognition by class I MHCs, *J. Mol. Biol.* *234*:515–521 (1993).

105. U. Sezerman, S. Vajda, J. Cornette, and C. DeLisi, Toward computational determination of peptide-receptor structure, *Protein Sci.* 2:1827–1843 (1994).

106. R. A. Lewis, D. C. Roe, C. Huang, T. E. Ferrin, R. Langridge, and I. D. Kuntz, Automated site-directed drug design using molecular lattices, *J. Mol. Graph.* *10*:66–78 (1992).

107. A. Caflisch, A. Miranker, and M. Karplus, Multiple copy simultaneous search and construction of ligands in binding sites: Application to inhibitors of HIV-1 aspartic protease, *J. Med. Chem.* *36*:2142–2167 (1993).

108. M. B. Eisen, D. C. Wiley, M. Karplus, and R. E. Hubbard, HOOK: A program for finding novel molecular architectures that satisfy the chemical and steric requirements of a macromolecule binding site, *Proteins Struct. Funct. Genet.* *19*:199–221 (1994).

109. G. Lauri and P. A. Bartlett, CAVEAT: A program to facilitate the design of organic molecules, *J. Comput. Aided Mol. Design* 8:51–66 (1994).

110. A. R. Leach and S. R. Kilvington, Automated molecular design: A new fragment-joining algorithm, *J. Comput. Aided Mol. Design* 8:283–298 (1994).

111. A. R. Leach and R. A. Lewis, A ring-bracing approach to computer-assisted ligand design, *J. Comput. Chem.* *15*:233–240 (1994).

112. S. H. Rotstein and M. A. Murcko, GroupBuild: A fragment-based method for de novo drug design, *J. Med. Chem.* *36*:1700–1710 (1993).

113. G. G. Hammes, *Enzyme Catalysis and Regulation*, Academic Press, New York, 1982.

114. H. Grubmuller, B. Heymann, and P. Tavan, Ligand binding: Molecular mechanics calculation of the streptavidin–biotin rupture force, *Science 271*: 997–999 (1996).

115. E. L. Florin, V. T. Moy, and H. E. Gaub, Adhesion forces between individual ligand–receptor pairs, *Science 264*:415–417 (1994).

116. V. T. Moy, E. L. Florin, and H. E. Gaub, Intermolecular forces and energies between ligands and receptors, *Science 266*:257–259 (1994).

117. J. P. Ryckaert, G. Ciccotti, and H. J. C. Berendsen, Numerical integration of the Cartesian equations of motion of a system with constraints: Molecular dynamics of n-alkanes, *J. Comput. Phys. 23*:327–341 (1977).
118. K. D. Gibson and H. A. Scheraga, Variable step molecular dynamics: An exploratory technique for peptides with fixed geometry, *J. Comput. Chem. 11*:468–486 (1990).
119. R. E. Bruccoleri and M. Karplus, Conformational sampling using high-temperature molecular dynamics, *Biopolymers 29*:1847–1862 (1990).
120. A. Di Nola, D. Roccatano, and H. J. C. Berendsen, Molecular dynamics simulation of the docking of substrates to proteins, *Proteins Struct. Funct. Genet. 19*:174–182 (1994).
121. T. Huber, A. E. Torda, and W. F. van Gunsteren, Local elevation: A method for improving the searching properties of molecular dynamics simulation, *J. Comput. Aided Mol. Design 8*:695–708 (1994).
122. F. Guarnieri and W. C. Still, A rapidly convergent simulation method: Mixed Monte Carlo/stochastic dynamics, *J. Comput. Chem. 15*:1302–1310 (1994).
123. Biosym Technologies, *Discover Reference Guide,* San Diego, 1993.
124. N. Metropolis, A. W. Rosenbluth, M. N. Rosenbluth, A. H. Teller, and E. Teller, Equation of state calculations by fast computing machines, *J. Chem. Phys. 21*:1087 (1953).
125. A. Miranker and M. Karplus, Functionality maps of binding sites: A multiple copy simultaneous search method, *Proteins Struct. Funct. Genet. 11*:29–34 (1991).
126. R. Elber and M. Karplus, Enhanced sampling in molecular dynamics: Use of the time-dependent Hartree approximation for a simulation of carbon monoxide diffusion through myoglobin, *J. Am. Chem. Soc. 112*:9161–9175 (1990).
127. Q. Zheng and D. J. Kyle, Multiple copy sampling: Rigid versus flexible protein, *Proteins Struct. Funct. Genet. 19*:324–329 (1994).
128. W. L. Jorgensen and C. Ravimohan, Monte Carlo simulation of differences in free energies of hydration, *J. Chem. Phys. 83*:3050–3054 (1985).
129. S.-Y. Yue, Distance-constrained molecular docking by simulated annealing, *Protein Eng. 4*:177–184 (1990).
130. D. S. Goodsell and A. J. Olson, Automated docking of substrates to proteins by simulated annealing, *Proteins Struct. Funct. Genet. 8*:195–202 (1990).
131. S. Kirkpatrick, D. D. Gelatt, Jr., and M. P. Vecchi, Optimization by simulated annealing, *Science 220*:671–680 (1983).
132. D. S. Goodsell, H. Laubel, C. D. Stout, and A. J. Olson, Automated docking in crystallography: Analysis of the substrates of aconitase, *Proteins Struct. Funct. Genet. 17*:1–10 (1993).
133. B. L. Stoddard and D. E. Koshland, Jr., Prediction of the structure of a receptor–protein complex using a binary docking method, *Nature 358*: 774–776 (1992).

134. B. L. Stoddard and D. E. Koshland, Jr., Molecular recognition analyzed by docking simulations: The aspartate receptor and isocitrate dehydrogenase from *Escherichia coli, Proc. Natl. Acad. Sci. USA 90*:1146–1153 (1993).

135. A. R. Friedman, V. A. Roberts, and J. A. Tainer, Predicting molecular interactions and inducible complementarity: Fragment docking of Fab–peptide complexes, *Proteins Struct. Funct. Genet. 20*:15–24 (1994).

136. T. N. Hart and R. J. Read, A multiple-start Monte Carlo docking method, *Proteins Struct. Funct. Genet. 13*:206–222 (1992).

137. Z. Li and H. A. Scheraga, Monte-Carlo minimization approach to the multiple-minima problem in protein folding, *Proc. Natl. Acad. Sci. USA 80*:6611 (1983).

138. G. Chang, W. C. Guida, and W. C. Still, An internal coordinate Monte Carlo method for searching conformational space, *J. Am. Chem. Soc. 111*: 4379–4386 (1989).

139. A. Caflisch, P. Niederer, and M. Anliker, Monte Carlo docking of oligopeptides to proteins, *Proteins Struct. Funct. Genet. 13*:223–230 (1992).

140. R. Abagyan, M. Totrov, and D. Kuznetsov, ICM-A new method for protein modeling and design: Applications to docking and structure prediction from the distorted native conformation, *J. Comput. Chem. 15*:488–506 (1994).

141. F. Mohamadi, N. G. J. Richards, W. C. Guida, R. Liskamp, M. Lipton, C. Caufield, G. Chang, T. Hendrickson, and W. C. Still, MacroModel—an integrated software system for modeling organic and bioorganic molecules using molecular mechanics, *J. Comput. Chem. 11*:440–467 (1990).

142. W. C. Still, *Batchmin User Manual Version 4.0.* Department of Chemistry, Columbia University, New York, 1993.

143. W. C. Guida, R. S. Bohacek, and M. D. Erion, Probing the conformational space available to inhibitors in the thermolysin active site using Monte Carlo/energy minimization techniques, *J. Comput. Chem. 13*:214–228 (1992).

144. M. Totrov and R. Abagyan, Detailed ab initio prediction of lysozyme–antibody complex with 1.6 Å accuracy, *Struct. Biol. 1*:259–263 (1994).

145. R. S. Judson, E. P. Jaeger, and A. M. Treasurywala, A genetic algorithm based method for docking flexible molecules, *J. Mol. Struct. 308*:191–206 (1994).

146. G. Jones, P. Willett, and R. C. Glen, Molecular recognition of receptor sites using a genetic algorithm with a description of desolvation, *J. Mol. Biol. 245*:43–53 (1995).

147. C. M. Oshiro, I. D. Kuntz, and J. S. Dixon, Flexible ligand docking using a genetic algorithm, *J. Comput. Aided Mol. Design 9*:113–130 (1995).

148. K. P. Clark and Ajay, Flexible ligand docking without parameter adjustment across four ligand–receptor complexes, *J. Comput. Chem. 16*:1210–1226 (1995).

149. R. P. Meadows and P. J. Hajduk, A genetic algorithm-based protocol for docking ensembles of small ligands using experimental restraints, *J. Biomol. NMR 5*:41–47 (1995).

150. D. K. Gehlhaar, G. M. Verkhivker, P. A. Rejto, C. J. Sherman, D. B. Fogel, L. J. Fogel, and S. T. Freer, Molecular recognition of the inhibitor AG-1343 by HIV-1 protease: Conformationally flexible docking by evolutionary programming, *Chem. Biol.* 2:317–324 (1995).

151. P. Willett, Genetic algorithms in molecular recognition and design, *Trends Biotechnol.* 13:516–521 (1995).

152. S. Forrest, Genetic algorithms: Principles of natural selection applied to computation, *Science 261*:872–878 (1993).

153. R. S. Judson, Y. T. Tan, E. Mori, C. Melius, E. P. Jaeger, A. M. Treasurywala, and A. Mathiowetz, Docking flexible molecules: A case study of three proteins, *J. Comput. Chem.* 16:1405–1419 (1995).

154. W. Hasel, T. F. Hendrickson, and W. C. Still, A rapid approximation to the solvent accessible surface areas of atoms, *Tetrahedron Comput Methodol. 1*: 103–116 (1988).

155. J. W. Ponder and F. M. Richards, Tertiary templates for proteins. Use of packing criteria in the enumeration of allowed sequences for different structural classes, *J. Mol. Biol.* 193:775–791 (1987).

156. L. M. Blumenthal, *Theory and Applications of Distance Geometry,* Chelsea Publishing, Bronx NY, 1970.

157. K. Wuthrich, Protein structure determination by nuclear magnetic resonance spectroscopy, *Science 243*:45 (1989).

158. J. M. Blaney and J. S. Dixon, Distance geometry in molecular modeling, *Rev. Comput. Chem.* 5:299–335 (1994).

159. T. F. Havel, I. D. Kuntz, and G. M. Crippen, The theory and practice of distance geometry, *Bull. Math. Biol.* 45:665–720 (1983).

160. D. B. Boyd, Aspects of molecular modeling, *Rev. Comput. Chem. 1*:321–354 (1990).

161. J. M. Blaney and J. S. Dixon, Receptor modeling by distance geometry, *Annu. Rep. Med. Chem.* 26:281–285 (1991).

162. W. Braun, Distance geometry and related methods for protein structure determination from NMR data, *Q. Rev. Biophys. 19*:115–157 (1987).

163. I. D. Kuntz, J. F. Thomason, and C. M. Oshiro, Distance geometry, *Methods Enzymol. 177*:159–204 (1989).

164. E. A. Torda and W. F. van Gunsteren, Molecular modeling using nuclear magnetic resonance data, *Rev. Comput. Chem. 3*:143–172 (1992).

165. G. M. Crippen, *Distance Geometry and Conformational Calculations. Chemometrics Research Studies Series 1,* Wiley, New York, 1981.

166. G. M. Crippen and T. F. Havel, *Distance Geometry and Molecular Conformation. Chemometrics Research Studies Series 15,* Wiley, New York, 1988.

167. G. M. Crippen, Rapid calculation of coordinates from distance matrices, *J. Comput. Phys. 26*:449–452 (1978).

168. G. M. Crippen and T. F. Havel, Stable calculation of coordinates from distance information, *Acta Crystallogr. A34*:282–284 (1978).

169. A. W. M. Dress and T. F. Havel, Shortest-path problems and molecular conformation, *Discrete Appl. Math. 19*:129–144 (1988).

170. P. L. Easthope and T. F. Havel, Computational experience with algorithm for tetrangle inequality bound smoothing, *Bull. Math. Biol. 51*:173–194 (1989).

171. T. F. Havel and K. Wuthrich, A distance geometry program for determining the structures of small proteins and other macromolecules from nuclear magnetic resonance measurements of intramolecular ^1H–^1H proximities in solution, *Bull. Math. Biol. 46*:673 (1984).

172. W. J. Metzler, D. R. Hare, and A. Pardi, Limited sampling of conformational space by the distance geometry algorithm: Implications for structures generated from NMR data, *Biochemistry 28*:7045–7052 (1989).

173. T. F. Havel, The sampling properties of some distance geometry algorithms applied to unconstrained polypeptide chains: A study of 1830 independently computed conformations; *Biopolymers 29*:1565–1585 (1990).

174. J. Kuszewski, M. Nilges, and A. T. Brunger, Sampling and efficiency of metric matrix distance geometry: A novel partial metrization algorithm, *J. Biomol. NMR 2*:33–56 (1992).

175. W. C. Ripka, W. J. Sipio, and J. M. Blaney, Molecular modeling and drug design: Strategies in the design and synthesis of phospholipase A_2 inhibitors, *Lect. Heterocyclic Chem. 9*:S95 (1987).

176. M. G. M. Thunnissen, E. Ab, K. H. Kalk, J. Drenth, B. W. Dijkstra, O. P. Kuipers, R. Dijkman, G. H. de Haas, and H. M. Verheij, X-ray structure of phospholipase A_2 complexed with a substrate-derived inhibitor, *Nature 347*: 689–691 (1990).

177. F. S. Kuhl, G. M. Crippen, and D. K. Friesen, A combinatorial algorithm for calculating ligand binding, *J. Comput. Chem. 5*:24–34 (1984).

178. A. S. Smellie, G. M. Crippen, and W. G. Richards, Fast drug–receptor mapping by site-directed distances: A novel method of predicting new pharmacological leads, *J. Chem. Inf. Comput. Sci. 31*:386–392 (1991).

179. M. R. Pincus, A. W. Burgess, and H. A. Scheraga, Conformational energy calculations of enzyme–substrate complexes of lysozyme. I. Energy minimization of monosaccharide and oligosaccharide inhibitors and substrates of lysozyme, *Biopolymers 15*:2485–2521 (1976).

180. M. R. Pincus, S. S. Zimmerman, and H. A. Scheraga, Prediction of three-dimensional structures of enzyme–substrate and enzyme–inhibitor complexes of lysozyme, *Proc. Natl. Acad. Sci. USA 73*:4261–4265 (1976).

181. A. R. Leach, Ligand docking to proteins with discrete side-chain flexibility, *J. Mol. Biol. 235*:345–356 (1994).

182. P. Bladon, A rapid method for comparing and matching the spherical parameter surfaces of molecules andd other irregular objects, *J. Mol. Graph. 7*: 130–137 (1989).

183. F. Jiang and S.-H. Kim, Soft docking: Matching of molecular surface cubes, *J. Mol. Biol. 219*:79–102 (1991).

184. R. W. Harrison, I. V. Kourinov, and L. C. Andrews, The Fourier–Green's function and the rapid evaluation of molecular potentials, *Protein Eng. 7*: 359–369 (1994).

185. E. Katchalski-Katzir, I. Shariv, M. Eisenstein, A. A. Friesem, C. Aflalo, and I. A. Vakser, Molecular surface recognition: Determination of geometric fit between proteins and their ligands by correlation techniques, *Proc. Natl. Acad. Sci. USA 89*:2195–2199 (1992).

186. I. A. Vakser and C. Aflalo, Hydrophobic docking: A proposed enhancement to molecular recognition techniques, *Proteins Struct. Funct. Genet. 20*: 320–329 (1994).

187. I. A. Vakser, Protein docking for low-resolution structures, *Protein Eng. 8*: 371–377 (1995).

188. I. V. Kurinov and R. W. Harrison, Prediction of new serine proteinase inhibitors, *Nature Struct. Biol. 1*:735–743 (1994).

189. P. H. Walls and M. J. E. Sternberg, New algorithm to model protein–protein recognition based on surface complementarity, *J. Mol. Biol. 228*:277–297 (1992).

190. I. Motoc, R. A. Dammkoehler, and G. R. Marshall, Three-dimensional structure–activity relationships and biological receptor mapping, *Mathematical and Computational Concepts in Chemistry* (N. Trinajstic, ed.), Ellis Horwood, Chichester, 1986, pp. 222–251.

191. R. A. Dammkoehler, S. F. Karasek, E. F. B. Shands, and G. R. Marshall, Constrained search of conformational hyperspace, *J. Comput. Aided Mol. Design 3*:3–21 (1989).

192. A. R. Leach, K. Prout, and D. P. Dolata, The application of artificial intelligence to the conformational analysis of strained molecules, *J. Comput. Chem. 11*:680–693 (1990).

193. S. S. Zimmerman, M. S. Pottle, G. Nemethy, and H. A. Scheraga, Conformational analysis of the 20 naturally occurring amino acids using ECEPP, *Macromolecules 10*:1–9 (1977).

194. M. Vasquez, G. Nemethy, and H. A. Scheraga, Computed conformational states of the 20 naturally occurring amino acids and of the prototype residue α-aminobutyric acid, *Macromolecules 16*:1043–1049 (1983).

195. S. S. Zimmerman and H. A. Scheraga, Influence of local interactions on protein structure. III. Conformational energy studies of *N*-acetyl-*N'*-methylamides of Gly-X and X-Gly dipeptides. *Biopolymers 17*:1871–1884 (1978).

196. M. Vasquez and H. A. Scheraga, Use of build-up and energy minimization procedures to compute low-energy structures of the backbone of enkephalin, *Biopolymers 24*:1437–1447 (1985).

197. K. D. Gibson and H. A. Scheraga, Revised algorithms for the build-up procedure for predicting protein conformations by energy minimization, *J. Comput. Chem. 8*:826–834 (1987).

198. S. Vajda and C. DeLisi, Determining minimum energy conformations of polypeptides by dynamic programming, *Biopolymers 29*:1755–1772 (1990).

199. K. Gulukota, S. Vajda, and C. DeLisi, Peptide docking using dynamic programming, *J. Comput. Chem. 17*:418–428 (1996).

200. A. R. Leach and K. Prout, Automated conformational analysis: Directed conformational search using the A* algorithm, *J. Comput. Chem. 11*: 1193–1205 (1990).

201. M. H. Lambert and H. A. Scheraga, Pattern recognition in the prediction of protein structure. I. Calculation of tripeptide conformational probabilities from the amino acid sequence, *J. Comput. Chem. 10*:770–797 (1989).

202. B. L. Sibanda and J. M. Thornton, β-Hairpin families in globular proteins, *Nature 316*:170–174 (1985).

203. M. H. Lambert and H. A. Scheraga, Pattern recognition in the prediction of protein structure. II. Chain conformation from a probability-directed search procedure, *J. Comput. Chem. 10*:798–816 (1989).

204. M. H. Lambert and H. A. Scheraga, Pattern recognition in the prediction of protein structure. III. An importance-sampling minimization procedure, *J. Comput. Chem. 10*:817–831 (1989).

205. M. R. Pincus, S. S. Zimmerman, and H. A. Scheraga, Structures of enzyme–substrate complexes of lysozyme, *Proc. Natl. Acad. Sci. USA 74*: 2629–2633 (1977).

206. J. B. Moon and W. J. Howe, Computer design of bioactive molecules: A method for receptor-based de novo ligand design, *Proteins Struct. Funct. Genet. 11*:314–328 (1991).

207. S. Thaisrivongs, A. G. Tomaselli, J. B. Moon, J. Hui, T. J. McQuade, S. R. Turner, J. W. Strohbach, W. J. Howe, W. G. Tarpley, and R. L. Heinrikson, Inhibitors of the protease from human immunodeficiency virus: Design and modeling of a compound containing a dihydroxyethylene isostere insert with high binding affinity and effective antiviral activity, *J. Med. Chem. 34*: 2344–2356 (1991).

208. N. Thanki, J. K. M. Rao, S. I. Foundling, W. J. Howe, J. B. Moon, J. O. Hui, A. G. Tomaselli, R. L. Heinrikson, S. Thaisrivongs, and A. Wlodawer, Crystal structure of a complex of HIV-1 protease with a dihydroxyethylene-containing inhibitor, *Protein Sci. 1*:1061–1072 (1992).

209. J. B. Moon and W. J. Howe, Recent advances in de novo molecular design, *Trends in QSAR and Molecular Modeling 92* (C. G. Wermuth, ed.), *Proceedings of the European Symposium on Structure–Activity Relationships,* ESCOM, 1992, pp. 11–19.

210. F. H. Allen, S. Bellard, M. D. Brice, B. A. Cartwright, A. Doubleday, H. Higgs, T. Hummelink, B. G. Hummelink-Peters, O. Kennard, W. D. S. Motherwell, J. R. Rodgers, and D. G. Watson, The Cambridge Crystallographic Data Centre: Computer-based search, retrieval, analysis and display of information, *Acta Crystallogr. B35*:2331–2339 (1979).

211. Biosym Technologies, *Ligand Design User Guide, Version 2.3,* San Diego CA, 1993.

212. V. J. Gillet, W. Newell, P. Mata, G. Myatt, S. Sike, Z. Zsoldos, and A. P. Johnson, SPROUT: Recent developments in the de novo design of molecules, *J. Chem. Inf. Comput. Sci. 34*:207–217 (1994).

213. R. C. Glen and A. W. R. Payne, A genetic algorithm for the automated generation of molecules within constraints, *J. Comput. Aided Mol. Design* 9:181–202 (1995).

214. Y. Nishibata and A. Itai, Automatic creation of drug candidate structures based on receptor structure: Starting point for artificial lead generation, *Tetrahedron 47*:8985–8990 (1991).

215. R. S. Bohacek and C. McMartin, Multiple highly diverse structures complementary to enzyme binding sites: Results of extensive application of a de novo design method incorporating combinatorial growth, *J. Am. Chem. Soc. 116*:5560–5571 (1994).

216. A. R. Leach, K. Prout, and D. P. Dolata, An investigation into the construction of molecular models by the template joining method, *J. Comput. Aided Mol. Design 2*:107–123 (1988).

217. D. P. Dolata and R. E. Carter, Wizard: Applications of expert system techniques to conformational analysis. 1. The basic algorithms exemplified on simple hydrocarbons, *J. Chem. Inf. Comput. Sci. 27*:36–47 (1987).

218. A. R. Leach and A. S. Smellie, A combined model-building and distance geometry approach to automated conformational analysis and search, *J. Chem. Inf. Comput. Sci. 32*:379–385 (1992).

219. D. P. Dolata, A. R. Leach, and K. Prout, Wizard: AI in conformational analysis, *J. Comput. Aided Mol. Design 1*:73–85 (1987).

220. A. R. Leach, D. P. Dolata, and K. Prout, Automated conformational analysis and structure generation: Algorithms for molecular perception, *J. Chem. Inf. Comput. Sci. 30*:316–324 (1990).

221. A. R. Leach, K. Prout, and D. P. Dolata, Automated conformational analysis: Algorithms for the efficient construction of low-energy conformations, *J. Comput. Aided Mol. Design 4*:271–282 (1990).

222. S. L. Tanimoto, *The Elements of Artificial Intelligence.* Computer Science Press, Rockville MD, 1987.

223. A. R. Leach, Conformational analysis in site-directed molecular design, *New Perspectives in Drug Design* (P. M. Dean, G. Jolles, and C. G. Newton, eds.) Academic Press, New York, 1995, pp. 201–223.

224. J. Desmet, M. De Maeyer, B. Hazes, and I. Lasters, The dead-end elimination theorem and its use in protein side-chain positioning, *Nature 356*:539–542 (1992).

225. I. Lasters and J. Desmet, The fuzzy-end elimination theorem: Correctly implementing the side chain placement algorithm based on the dead-end elimination theorem, *Protein Eng. 6*:717–722 (1993).

226. M. Vasquez, An evaluation of discrete and continuum search techniques for conformational analysis of side chains in proteins, *Biopolymers 36*:53–70 (1995).

227. U. Burkert and N. L. Allinger, *Molecular Mechanics,* American Chemical Society, Washington DC, 1982.

228. P. Dauber-Osguthorpe, V. A. Roberts, D. J. Osguthorpe, J. Wolff, M. Genest, and A. T. Hagler, Structure and energetics of ligand binding to proteins:

Escherichia coli dihydrofolate reductase–trimethoprim, a drug–receptor system, *Proteins Struct. Funct. Genet. 4*:31–47 (1988).

229. J. R. Maple, M. J. Hwang, T. P. Stockfisch, U. Dinur, M. Waldman, C. S. Ewig, and A. T. Hagler, Derivation of class II force fields. Methodology and quantum force field for the alkyl functional group and alkane molecules, *J. Comput. Chem. 15*:162–182 (1994).

230. M. L. Connolly, Analytical molecular surface calculation, *J. Appl. Crystallogr. 16*:548–558 (1983).

231. G. Perrot, B. Cheng, K. D. Gibson, J. Vila, K. A. Palmer, A. Nayeem, B. Maigret, and H. A. Scheraga, Mseed: A program for the rapid analytical determination of accessible surface areas and their derivatives, *J. Comput. Chem. 13*:1–11 (1992).

232. M. H. Lambert, manuscript in preparation.

233. S. J. Wodak and J. Janin, Analytical approximation to the accessible surface are of proteins, *Proc. Natl. Acad. Sci. USA 77*:1736–1740 (1980).

234. I. K. Roterman, M. H. Lambert, K. D. Gibson, and H. A. Scheraga, A comparison of the charmm, amber and ecepp potentials for peptides. II. ϕ, ψ maps for *N*-acetyl alanine *N'*-methyl amide: Comparisons, contrasts and simple experimental tests, *J. Biomol. Struct. Dynam. 7*:421–453 (1989).

235. M. V. Milburn, A. M. Hassell, M. H. Lambert, S. R. Jordan, A. E. I. Proudfoot, P. Graber, and T. N. C. Wells, A novel dimer configuration revealed by the crystal structure at 2.4 Å resolution of human interleukin-5, *Nature 363*: 172–176 (1993).

236. T. N. Wheeler, S. G. Blanchard, R. C. Andrews, F. Fang, Y. Gray-Nunez, C. O. Harris, M. H. Lambert, M. M. Mehrotra, D. J. Parks, J. A. Ray, and T. L. Smalley, Jr., Substrate specificity in short-chain phospholipid analogs at the active site of human synovial phospholipase A_2, *J. Med. Chem. 37*: 4118–4129 (1994).

237. B. A. Lovejoy, A. Cleasby, A. M. Hassell, K. Longley, M. A. Luther, D. Weigl, G. McGeehan, A. B. McElroy, D. Drewry, M. H. Lambert, and S. R. Jordan, Structure of the catalytic domain of fibroblast collagenase complexed with an inhibitor, *Science 263*:375–377 (1994).

238. S. A. Acheson, M. H. Lambert, S. C. Brown, and P. W. Jeffs, Solution structures of α- and β-amanitin via distance geometry calculations and a relaxation matrix analysis of nuclear Overhauser effect spectra, *J. Magn. Reson. B101*:44–51 (1993).

239. D. van Vliet, M. H. Lambert, and F. K. Brown, Design of libraries based on the binding site: The merging of de novo design and combinatorial chemistry, Presented at the ACS National Meeting, Anaheim CA, 1995.

9

An Introduction to De Novo Ligand Design

Mark A. Murcko
Vertex Pharmaceuticals Incorporated, Cambridge, Massachusetts

I. INTRODUCTION AND OVERVIEW

Protein structural information is becoming ever more available. Advances in molecular biology and protein biochemistry have greatly reduced the difficulty of achieving large quantities of highly purified protein. Crystallographic and nuclear magnetic resonance (NMR) techniques (hardware, software, and fundamental methodology) have also advanced rapidly. Thus, there are many more targets of biological interest for which structural information is available.

In the past decade, various drug companies have published research that highlights the usefulness of structural information in drug discovery. Indeed, there are now several drugs, either in development or already marketed, that have benefitted from a structure-based approach (Table 1) [1–11; see also Chap. 1]. One should be careful not to overemphasize the importance of structure-based design—it is one tool among many—but it is clear that having access to structural information and computational methods can facilitate the process of introducing compounds into the clinic.

At the same time, protein homology modeling has made great strides, allowing us to predict the global folds of many targets and to construct reasonably accurate homology models. Moreover, methodology in the area

Table 1 Recent Examples of
Structure-Based Drug Design

Target	Refs.
Carbonic anhydrase II	4,5
Leukocyte elastase	1
HIV-1 protease	4,8,9,11
Influenza sialidase	10
Purine nucleotide phosphorylase	7
Thrombin	1
Thymidylate synthase	4,6

of three-dimensional quantitative structure–activity relationships (3D-QSAR) has advanced, providing both pharmacophore models derived from structure–activity data, as well as low-resolution receptor models [12–14]. Thus, in addition to X-ray and NMR data, homology modeling and 3D-QSAR provide "pseudostructures" for projects without experimental protein structural information. These pseudostructures are obviously lower in accuracy, but they may, nonetheless, provide focus for a research program, especially in the early stages.

Given the tremendous increase in our ability to generate both structures and pseudostructures, novel methods for exploiting this information are increasingly in demand. Specifically, the need grows for a set of computational tools that can analyze receptor sites and suggest compounds that may bind to these sites. These are often called *de novo drug design* methods.

The terms "de novo ligand design," "de novo inhibitor design," and "de novo drug design" are sometimes used interchangeably. Most reported uses of these methods have involved enzymes, because it is much more likely that three-dimensional structural information will be available for those targets. However, because some researchers focus on receptor agonists or antagonists, rather than enzyme inhibitors, we use the term *ligand design* throughout this chapter because it is more general.

De novo drug design is also a little misleading, for two reasons. First, because *drugs* are such complicated chemical entities, it is more accurate to claim that these methods design *ligands*. Second, because these methods are most successful when a portion of a known ligand is used as a starting point, it is inaccurate to refer to them as de novo methods. Despite these formalistic complaints, de novo drug design is still a handy, catch-all phrase that conveys a sense of excitement, and will undoubtedly remain in the lexicon for some time.

A. What Should De Novo Ligand Design Software Do?

Ideally, de novo ligand design methods should meet the following criteria:

1. *Easy to use, preferably with a graphic interface*: The method should be well documented and supported and available to the nonexpert user.
2. *Fast, preferably interactive*: This would encourage users to experiment with the software. For example, they could ask "what if" questions on the fly. Fast programs also allow the computer to evaluate more ideas, increasing the chances of success.
3. *Produce chemically and biologicaly reasonable structures*: Compounds that come out of a de novo program should not include chemically or biologically unstable functional groups. Ideally, the compounds should not be unreasonable to synthesize.
4. *Produce a set of diverse structures*: Rather than generating a single class of compounds, the ideal de novo program would sample "ligand space" more broadly, and generate many chemically diverse structures.
5. *Produce lead molecules with micromolar affinity*: The ideal de novo program would generate not just sound "general" ideas for ligands, but actual ligands with micromolar affinity for the target receptor.
6. *Work well on all classes of receptors*: The method should be able to handle active sites of all shapes, sizes, and chemical properties, including those containing metals, cofactors, experimentally determined waters, and so forth. Ligands that form covalent bonds to the receptor also should be treated properly. In addition, the method should be able to work with "pseudostructures" from homology models and from 3D-QSAR.

B. What Progress Has Been Made?

Many promising approaches toward the goal of automated ligand design have been reported in the literature in the past decade. In particular, there has been an explosion of new methods in the past 3 years, greatly extending the range of approaches to ligand design. As we will see, we have made considerable progress in a short time, but we have some way to go before all the aforementioned criteria are met.

In this chapter, we provide an introduction to the field of de novo drug design. The focus of this review is to highlight critical issues and give representative examples of the kinds of methods that have been devised. Not every reported method is discussed here. However, a pair of highly detailed, back-to-back chapters on this topic have recently appeared [15,16]. They should be viewed as complementary to this chapter. In addition, several earlier, brief reviews of this field also exist [17,18].

It is worth remembering that the field of computational chemistry is quite broad. De novo ligand design is just one out of the many approaches that may be applied to drug discovery. Indeed, successful application of de novo design methods requires a solid understanding of other modeling techniques and topics, such as conformational searching and analysis, hydrogen bonding, the hydrophobic effect, and force-field methods. The interested reader is referred to the many recent reviews on computational methodologies [19–22].

Figure 1 and Table 2 show some of the milestones in the field of de novo ligand design. *The timeline is not intended to show every contribution to the field.* Rather, the intent is to highlight the way this field has progressed. A quick glance at the timeline reveals a few interesting points. First, it is clear that over time, methods have become more complex, in many cases incorporating several approaches into "hybrid" methods. Second, methods today are capable of building a greater diversity of structures and of analyzing structures more quickly than was true only a few years ago. Partially, this is due to improvements in computer hardware, but even more important have been fundamental improvements in the algorithms used. Third, all the early methods in this field came from academic laboratories. The first entry from a pharmaceutical company did not occur until 1991, 9 years after the first DOCK publication. However, more than half the methods published since 1991 have come from pharmaceutical companies. Finally, many of the programs on the list are available, either from the authors directly, or through commercial distributors. This is a welcome trend because of the importance of validating these methods.

C. Classes of Ligand Design Methods

At the simplest level, all de novo design methods fall into one of three categories, as shown in Figure 2:

Methods That Analyze the Active Site

Such methods are used to determine which kinds of atoms and functional groups are best able to interact with the active site. The result of the analysis, for example, may be a set of preferred locations for simple fragments,

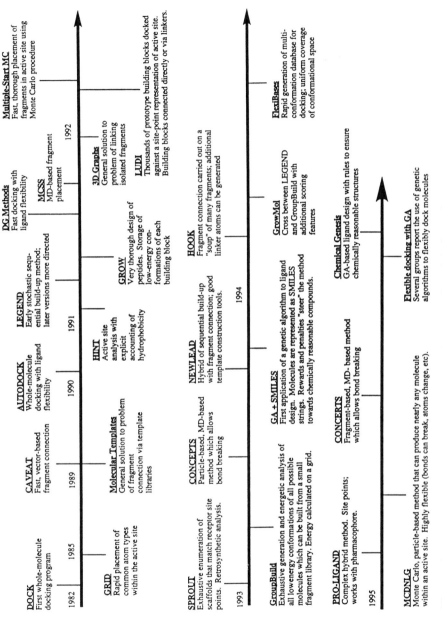

Figure 1 Timeline showing the development of de novo ligand design software.

Table 2   Some Milestones in the Development of
De Novo Drug Design Methods

Year	Method	Category[a]
1982	DOCK	WM
1985	GRID	AA
1989	CAVEAT	FC
1989	Molecular templates	FC
1990	AUTODOCK	WM
1991	LEGEND	SB
1991	MCSS	AA
1991	HINT	AA
1991	GROW	SB
1991	DG methods	WM
1992	LUDI	SP
1992	3D molecular graphs	FC
1992	Multistart MC	AA
1993	SPROUT	SP
1993	GroupBuild	SB
1993	NEWLEAD	SB
1993	GA + SMILES	SB/BB
1993	CONCEPTS	SB/BB
1994	HOOK	FC
1994	GrowMol	SB
1994	FlexiBases	WM
1995	PRO-LIGAND	SB
1995	Chemical Genesis	SB/BB
1995	Flexible docking with GA	WM
1995	CONCERTS	SB/BB
1995	MCDNLG	SB/BB

[a]SB, sequential buildup; WM, whole molecule; FC, fragment connection; SP, site point; AA, active site analysis; "/BB", bonds can be broken.

such as water or benzene. Because fragment location techniques do not directly generate ligands, some researchers would not classify them as true de novo design methods, but rather, a prerequisite for de novo design. However, all researchers would agree that they are essential.

Methods That Dock Whole Molecules

These methods take each proposed ligand, one at a time, and attempt to position it in the active site of the receptor, or match it to a pharmacophore

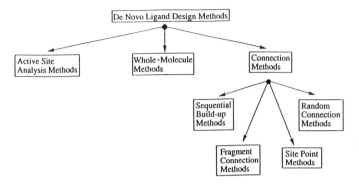

Figure 2 Classifications of ligand design software.

model. Some methods allow the conformation of the ligand to vary while it is being docked; other methods consider multiple conformations for each ligand, and rigidly dock each one. As with methods that analyze the active site, whole-molecule docking software would not be classified by some researchers as true de novo design methods, because they do not design anything—they just attempt to place a ligand in the active site. However, docking of one sort or another is an essential part of most (if not all) de novo methods, and regardless of how they are classified, it makes sense to review them here.

Methods That Connect Molecular Fragments or Atoms Together to Produce a Ligand

These are the methods that everyone agrees are truly de novo design. As shown in Figure 2, these methods fall into a few different categories, depending on the approach used:

1. *Site-point connection methods*: Determine desirable locations of individual atoms ("site points") and then place suitable fragments at those locations.
2. *Fragment connection methods*: Start with previously positioned fragments and find "linkers" or "scaffolds" to connect those fragments without moving them.
3. *Sequential buildup methods*: Construct a ligand atom-by-atom or fragment-by-fragment. The set of building blocks is generally small, and the construction process may be random.
4. *Random connection methods*: A special class of techniques combining some of the features of site-point, fragment connection,

and sequential buildup methods, along with bond-disconnection strategies and other methods to introduce randomness.

It is sometimes hard to classify methods. Some methods are hybrids, combining features from several approaches. Furthermore, most methods may be combined in various ways to produce what are in effect multistep or hybrid approaches. Moreover, some methods can be adapted for alternative uses. For example, a whole-molecule approach may be used with a library of small fragments to determine optimal locations for those fragments, and may thus be viewed as a *fragment placement* method.

D. Factors to Consider When Evaluating a Ligand Design Method

When confronted with a new ligand design method, one first may ask two questions:

1. Into which of the foregoing categories does this method best fit?
2. Is it a hybrid method?

In addition, there are many other questions that can help evaluate the method, including

1. *How is the target represented?* Most methods require the existence of a high-resolution experimental three-dimensional structure or a homology model of the receptor active site into which ligands are fitted. Other methods, however, will work with just a pharmacophore model, or some kind of molecular field or pseudopotential model.

2. *How are the hits scored?* Scoring functions are critical to the results obtained. However, the "scoring function" used by each method is different; no consensus exists in the literature about which function is best. There are two kinds of scoring functions: energy-based and rule-based. Energy-based functions attempt to quantify the contributions from different kinds of interactions between ligand and receptor, such as coulombic, hydrophobic, steric, and others. Rule-based methods analyze databases of structural information (such as the Cambridge Structural Database) and use the frequency of occurrence of various types of contacts to determine the desirability of those contacts. Although a detailed description of scoring functions is beyond the scope of this chapter, the subject has recently been reviewed [23; see also Chap. 10].

3. *Is the method systematic or random?* Some methods produce ligand candidates in a deterministic way wherein all possibilities are considered, and then, a selection is made. Other methods make random changes to the ligand, score the new structure in some fashion, and then decide whether to accept or reject those changes.

4. *Can the method make "anything"?* Some methods produce molecules assembled strictly from preselected blocks. Other methods are more comprehensive in their coverage of compound space and allow a much greater diversity of atom types, bond types, ring systems, and so forth.

5. *Is the method intended to be an "idea generator" or a "ligand generator"?* Some methods are designed to present a broad range of interesting ideas to the user, without claiming to actually generate micromolar quantities of ligands. Other methods suggest specific compounds with the intention that they will actually be potent ligands.

6. *Is the receptor or the ligand flexible?* Some methods construct ligands with greater conformational freedom than others. Likewise, some methods allow the receptor active site to move, althought this is not common. In all known examples for which high-resolution X-ray data is available, there are conformational changes to the receptor on ligand binding. More of a concern is the occasional report of a very large conformational change after ligand binding—sometimes 2 Å or more. Clearly, flexible models are more realistic, and much more desirable, but methods allowing such additional flexibility will be much slower. Occasionally, a compromise is to run a de novo method several times, using different receptor conformations, taken either from molecular dynamics simulations or crystal structures, if more than one structure for the receptor is available.

7. *How fast is the method?* Does it generate a few structures per hour, or a few hundred? The answers to these questions are largely dependent on how the target is represented and how the ligand ideas are scored.

8. *How has the method been validated?* This is a critical issue, and difficult to evaluate. Because of the novelty of ligand design methods, synthetic chemists are understandably hesitant to embark on a complex synthesis simply because a computer program suggests a certain idea. Consequently, only a few substantiated cases exist for which a ligand design program was tested "in the

field" and the results made public. A second, closely related difficulty in evaluating de novo methods is that many of them are
developed in pharmaceutical companies, and these researchers
are frequently unable to reveal the most interesting results, or
even the receptor used in the model simulations. Consequently,
many papers in this field use dihydrofolate reductase (DHFR) as
a model system. Human immunodeficiency virus (HIV) protease
is another enzyme commonly used for control experiments. There
is no doubt that many of the de novo design programs described
in this chapter have been applied to many other targets, and there
is anecdotal evidence of successes which, unfortunately, have not
yet been publicly described.

II. OVERVIEW OF CLASSES OF DE NOVO DESIGN METHODS

A. Category 1. Active Site Analysis Methods

Methods for analysis of the active site do not construct ligands; rather, they
analyze the properties of the active site, and usually determine favorable-
binding locations for individual atoms or small fragments. Although conceptually simple, these approaches are quite useful for successful ligand
design. For example, the fragment connection methods (described later
under Section II.C) require a set of previously docked fragments.

Figure 3 shows an example of how a typical fragment placement
method works. In this example, a collection of benzene rings (for clarity,
the double bonds are not shown) have been placed in a lipophilic pocket
of a receptor-active site, a collection of formaldehyde molecules have been
placed near a hydrogen bond-donor site, and several hydroxyl groups have
been placed near a hydrogen bond-acceptor site.

Methods in this category include GRID [24–31], GREEN [32–34],
HSITE and related programs [35–40]. MCSS [41,42], several Monte Carlo
or simulated annealing-based methods [43–48], HINT [49–53], and
BUCKETS [54].

Several ways exist for scoring and selecting fragments. Some methods are energy-based, using molecular mechanics force fields to evaluate
candidate fragments, whereas others use a rule-based approach, for which
the rules are derived from the analysis of a suitable database of structural
information, such as the Cambridge Structural Database [55]. Energy-based
methods suffer from the disadvantage of being slower, and they depend on
the quality of the energy function(s) used. Furthermore, there are important
issues relating to solvation and other effects that should ideally be consid-

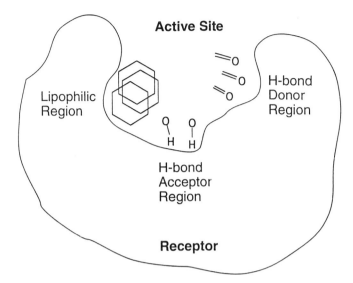

Figure 3 Schematic of fragment-placement methods.

ered, but typically are omitted. On the other hand, rule-based methods are inherently very simplistic, and can be derived only if sufficient raw data are available to invent the rules. The derivation of these rules is also quite time-consuming. Recently, crystallographic soaking experiments have been described that provide evidence for desirable locations of simple organic molecules, such as methanol, within the active site of a receptor [56]. Although interpretation of these results is sometimes difficult, the data may be used to suggest favorable interactions between the receptor and proto-type fragments.

Advantages and Disadvantages

The advantages of fragment placement methods are obvious. First, a small number of well-placed fragments (both lipophilic and hydrogen-bonding) can provide significant binding energy; thus, it is reasonable to first identify such fragments and locations. Second, the more that is known about the range of allowed orientations for those fragments, the more likely it will be that fragment connection methods, described later, will identify ways to connect those fragments. Third, as the diversity of reasonable starting fragments increases, so will the chance of suggesting a synthetically trac-table molecule.

The one limitation of fragment placement methods is that they do not directly propose ligands for testing; rather, they suggest a set of well-placed pieces that can be combined to form a complete ligand. A great deal of additional work must then be done to convert those fragment locations into suggestions for viable ligands.

B. Category 2. Whole-Molecule Methods

The whole-molecule techniques fit entire ligands into a receptor-active site, using either shape complementarity alone, or coupled with electrostatic fitting. The ligands are often taken from well-known databases so that hits may be purchased. Ligand conformational flexibility has been incorporated into several of these methods, generally by allowing selected dihedral angles to adjust. The field of ligand-docking methods has recently been reviewed [57,58].

Whole-molecule methods include DOCK [59–67], perhaps the first computer program in the field of structure-based ligand design. Some variants of DOCK account for ligand flexibility [68,69], whereas others create multiconformation databases and dock those conformers [70–74]. Related techniques use combinations of Monte Carlo and simulated-annealing [43–48] search approaches, such as AUTODOCK [75,76], or distance geometry [77,78] approaches to flexibly fit the ligand. In the past year, several groups have described methods that use genetic algorithms to flexibly dock ligands in a receptor-active site [79–83]. These methods tend to be much slower than those that use rigid structures, but do an excellent job of locating low-energy bound conformations.

The methods in this category are actually quite distinct in their approaches and, therefore, are useful for different purposes. DOCK uses a shape-fitting approach, searching many possible ways to fit ligands into the receptor-active site. Optionally, elecrostatics also may be added to the scoring function. It is designed to search through databases containing thousands of molecules. AUTODOCK, on the other hand, is a conformational search engine, taking a small number of ligands and performing a thorough search of the many conformations that those ligands may adopt. Side chains within the active site also can be allowed to flex. The genetic algorithm-based flexible-docking methods are also useful for carefully docking small numbers of compounds.

Advantages and Disadvantages

A key feature of the whole-molecule methods is that known or synthesizable compounds are generally studied. This is advantageous because any hits produced by the program may readily be tested for activity. A second advantage of some of these methods is that they may also be used to screen large databases of small fragments—in effect, one may use a method such as DOCK for fragment placement analysis. Indeed, one could study larger fragments than are typically used in fragment placement or sequential buildup methods. For example, one could screen a set of low-energy conformations for every possible dipeptide, and then use the best hits as starting points for ligand design. The allowed-binding conformations of such prototype fragments also provide useful ideas for the construction of novel inhibitors. Another advantage shared by some of the whole-molecule methods is their ability to perform an in-depth analysis of all reasonable binding modes for individual compounds. This can be important because it helps the chemist understand the detailed binding orientation of a favored ligand.

A disadvantage is that the fastest of the whole-molecule methods can take up to a week to explore a database of 100,000 compounds. As sample collection and combinatorial libraries reach into the millions of compounds, even docking 100,000 molecules per week is clearly inadequate. A second disadvantage is that rigid-body, whole-molecule fitting is likely to miss many good candidates because the conformation stored in the database represents only one of many reasonable possibilities. When conformational searching is added [79–83], or when multiple conformations are stored for each molecule [70–74], the methods become more reliable, but can be *very* time-consuming. Obviously the development of faster docking algorithms is an important goal.

C. Category 3. Connection Methods

There are four subcategories of connection methods:

Category 3.1. Site-Point Connection Methods

A *site point* is a point in space at which a suitable ligand atom can make favorable interactions with one or more enzyme atoms. For example, in the vicintiy of a phenylalanine side chain, there will be several favorable hydrophobic sites. Site points with appropriate ligand atoms nearby are said to be satisfied. Site-point connection methods attempt to place small fragments in the active site so that one or more site points are satisfied, and fragments are thereby placed in favorable regions. In this sense, fragment placement and site-point methods are similar, and some researchers might argue that site-point connection methods represent a subclass of fragment placement methods. However, the difference is that the methods discussed in this seciton are intended to build up ligands from multiple combinations of fragments, or from fitting entire molecules that match a suitable number of site points. Fragment placement methods have the more limited (but still important!) goal of positioning a simple fragment, such as benzene or water, into a favorable location.

Figure 4 shows how site-point methods work. First, the site points for an active site are generated. Hydrogen bond-acceptor atoms and donor sites are marked with lines, and hydrophobic sites are marked with dots. Then, a small prototype molecule (here, 2-amidinothiophene) is positioned in the active site so that it overlaps with several of the site points. Finally, additional building blocks are attached to the amidinothiophene to make contact with additional site points.

Site-point connection methods include CLIX [84], LUDI [30,31, 85,86], the linked-algorithm approach of Verlinde and co-workers [87], and Klebe's analysis of crystal-field environments [88].

As with fragment placement methods, the site points may be generated with energy-based or rule-based approaches. Site points can also be generated from the output of active site analysis programs. For example, CLIX [84] uses the output from GRID to generate a list of site points and then searches the Cambridge Structural Database for molecules satisfying those site points. Another excellent example is Klebe's analysis of crystal-field environments [88]—that is, his detailed study of the interactions between functional groups in the crystal phase. This research has lead to the generation of rule-based site points that are used in programs such as LUDI.

Advantages and Disadvantages. Site-point connection methods are fast. Only those site points that are near each other are compared, which limits the complexity of the 3D search process, and fragments are selected rapidly. A second advantage of these methods is their versatility. Ligands may be constructed in a fragment-by-fragment fashion; this is essentially a sequential buildup procedure, as described in a later section. Alternatively, site-point connection methods may also be used to find reasonable-bridging groups between two separate pieces. LUDI [85,86] for example, may be used in either mode. A third advantage is that the user may select the number of site points that must be satisfied, allowing a more or less rigorous criterion for compound selection. It is not necessary to match every site point to achieve good binding.

A disadvantage of these methods is their dependence on proper site-point placement. Ligands designed to superimpose on poorly selected site points will most likely be poor ligands. A second problem relates to the "slop factor." If site points need to be matched perfectly, most fragments will miss those site points and be rejected. On the other hand, if large tolerances are allowed for matching the site points, the search may be slowed considerably, and most compounds will not make optimal contacts with the receptor. The key to success is knowing what tolerances to use. Another disadvantage is the lack of flexibility of the individual fragments. As with all kinds of 3D database searching, useful hits are sometimes

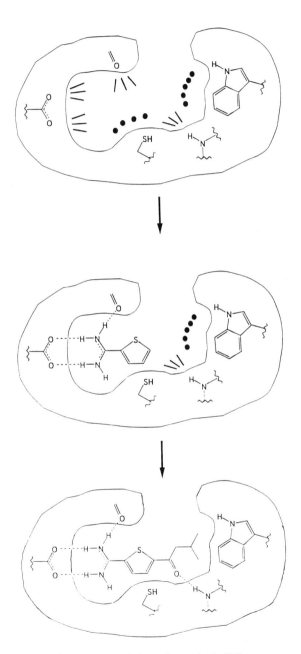

Figure 4 Schematic of site-point methods [17].

missed because the fragments are treated as rigid units. This problem may be overcome by allowing flexible searching, or by storing multiple conformations of each flexible fragment [70–74,89,90].

Category 3.2. Fragment Connection Methods

In fragment connection methods, isolated fragments, which have been selected in a variety of ways, are connected. Often this is done in one step using a single scaffold or linker. This approach relies on the concept that a small number of well-placed fragments, each making favorable interactions with the enzyme, is capable of providing a significant overall binding energy. A key feature of these methods is that, although the linker *may* contribute to binding, favorable contributions from the scaffold are not generally considered a critical part of compound evaluation. Rather an acceptable linker merely needs to avoid bumping into the receptor and possess a suitable geometry to "stitch together" the isolated fragments.

An example of how a fragment connection program works is given in Figure 5. An isolated set of fragments (here, benzene, ammonium, and formaldehyde) are connected together by inserting a tricyclic linker between them.

Methods in this category include the early algorithms of Dean [91,92], Lewis, Leach, and their co-workers [93–97], CAVEAT [98,99], HOOK [100], SPLICE and related programs [101–105], NEWLEAD [106], PRO_LIGAND [107,108], and ELANA [109]. In additon there are various 3D database methods [89,90,110–114].

Fragment connection methods use a variety of database types. Some databases are taken directly from libraries of known compounds, such as the Cambridge Structural Database [55] or the Available Chemicals Directory [115]. Other databases are generated de novo. Examples of this include TRIAD (containing >400,000 reasonable tricyclic systems) and ILIAD (containing >100,000 small, multifunctional fragments), both available for use with CAVEAT. Still other databases are entered by hand and reflect some set of biases of the developers for the optimal set of fragments for use in ligand construction. Finally, some researchers generate many possible linkers "on the fly." For example, Lewis [91–95], Rose [109], and Leach [97], each have developed methods that can generate highly functionalized linkers that connect two fragments. Finally, 3D database searching tools [110–112] allow a specialized kind of fragment-connection method. This field has recently been well reviewed [89,90,113,114] and will not be covered here.

Advantages and Disadvantages. Fragment-connection methods have many advantages. First, information about favorable fragment locations may be obtained from any source. Second, if one already has a set of

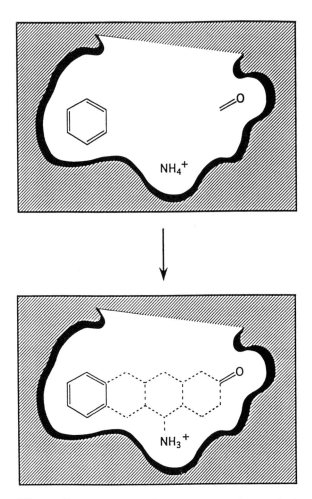

Figure 5 Schematic of fragment connection methods.

candidate fragments placed in the active site, fragment connection methods allow one to quickly stitch together those binding elements. In this way, a pharmacophore hypothesis may be tested. Third, compounds suggested from these methods can be quite rigid when cyclic scaffolds are used (e.g., from the TRIAD database), thereby lowering the overall entropy of the system. Fourth, many choices of scaffolds are available, ranging from rigid polycyclics to completely flexible hydrocarbon chains, and many of these methods take into consideration flexibility of the linkers, or allow multiple conformations to be stored.

Fragment connection methods also have disadvantages. First, they have slow search times for those methods that perform flexible 3D searching or that use very large multiconformational databases. Second, any scaffold, no matter how good it may be in other respects, may be rejected because some portion of it, however small, overlaps the receptor. In Figure 6, one atom of the tricyclic linker (circled) is bumping the receptor; consequently, the scaffold is rejected. This risk can be minimized by the use of "forgiving" scoring functions, but it cannot be completely eliminated. To evaluate the severity of the problem, the geometry of the receptor or ligand may need to be optimized in the hope of relieving steric crowding. A third disadvantage is that the molecules suggested by fragment connection methods are generally rather complicated and, thus, impractical for the medicinal chemist.

Category 3.3. Sequential Buildup Methods

The sequential buildup techniques all share the philosophy that ligands can be constructed piece by piece. The construction need not be linear—in other words, each new piece may be added anywhere on the existing ligand.

Among the atom-by-atom approaches (including those allowing small hydrogen-bonding groups) are LEGEND [116,117], GenStar [118], the artificial intelligence-based method of Cohen and Shatzmiller [119], and GROWMOL [120]. Fragment-by-fragment approaches include GROW

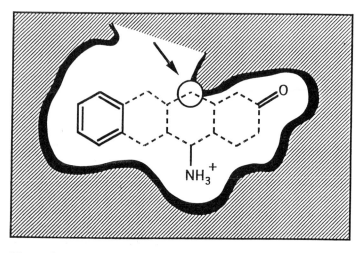

Figure 6 Problems that meay be encountered with fragment connection methods [54].

[121–123], Scheraga's buildup procedure [124], GEMINI [127], Group-Build [54], SPROUT [126–128], and LeapFrog [129].

The general concept of sequential buildup methods is depicted in Figure 7. Here, we begin with just a benzene core fragment on the left-hand side of the active site. In each subsequent panel, an additional functional group is added, until the entire ligand has been assembled.

Significant differences exist among these various approaches. Of prime consideration is the set of building blocks used to construct the ligands. Some techniques use exclusively atoms as their fundamental unit, whereas others use atoms augmented with small hyrogen-bonding frag-

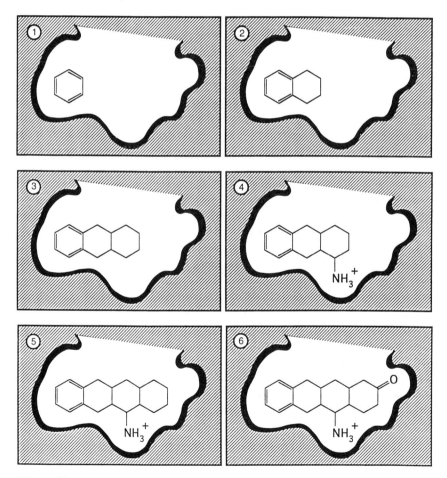

Figure 7 Schematic of sequential buildup methods.

ments; still others allow larger fragments, such as benzene rings or entire amino acids. With conformational searching, again there are significant differences. Some techniques perform conformational searching to optimize the location of new fragments, whereas other techniques arbitrarily select the orientation of candidate fragments. The majority of the sequential buildup procedures use energy-based methods for fragment scoring, although several of the methods use a rule-based approach.

An important issue for sequential buildup methods (as for all de nove approaches) is referred to as "speed versus coverage." If a program builds ligands quickly, it probably does so by sampling poorly—in other words, it fails to consider all possibilities (building blocks, attachment sites, and conformations) as it constructs the new molecule. On the other hand, if a more exhaustive search procedure is used, the method will be fairly slow, because even a few fragments may be attached to a ligand in many locations and orientations and, thus, cover a wide range of possibilities. Each buildup method reflects a choice between speed and coverage.

Advantages and Disadvantages. There are several advantages to sequential buildup procedures. First, because each fragment is selected based on its ability to contribute to enzyme binding, the ligands suggested by these methods should, in principle, be smaller and "more efficient" than molecules derived from fragment connection methods. Second, because each piece is added sequentially, it is possible to perform more detailed conformational analyses, leading to fewer misses.

There are disadvantages as well. The most important of these is the problem of crossing what we call "dead zones"—open spaces of the active site where few enzyme contacts are possible. This problem is depicted in Figure 8. To reach the carbonyl-binding pocket on the right-hand side of the active site, an atom (circled) must be positioned in a region that lacks any favorable interactions, and may never be selected. A second problem with sequential buildup procedures is that they are particularly prone to "combinatorial explosion." In other words, there are a huge number of ways to piece together atoms or small fragments in an active site. Interestingly, despite the problem of combinatorial explosion, many ligands will be impossible to generate because these methods use a finite set of building blocks. Finally, a related issue is synthetic accessibility. The assembly of a ligand from simple building blocks does not guarantee that the ligand will be easy to make. Indeed, unless care is taken in developing suitable rules to guide the ligand construction process, quite often the opposite is true.

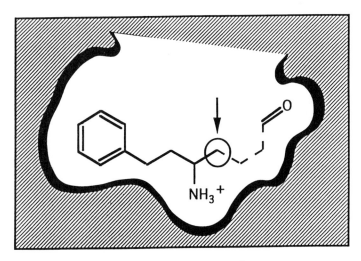

Figure 8 Difficulty in crossing dead zones [54].

D. Category 3.4. Random Connection and Disconnection Methods

This set of methods contains some features of the sequential buildup procedures, but also includes clever methods for altering the bond connectivity of the ligand(s) as they are being constructed. Several of these techniques also employ interesting methods for sampling the allowed conformational space of the fragments from which ligands are constructed.

This category includes genetic algorithm methods [130,131], CONCEPTS [132], CONCERTS [133], the dynamic ligand design (DLD) approach [134,135], MCDNLG [136], and Hahn's RECEPTOR program [137].

Many of these methods begin with a "soup" of building blocks, either individual atoms (particles) or slightly larger fragments. These building blocks may be unconnected at the start of the run, or there may be connections between some or all of the fragments. Regardless of the choice of fundamental building blocks, these methods are all similar in that they slowly construct ligands by making and breaking the connections between building blocks. Although the building blocks can be held fixed, all known methods allow the molecules to move under a molecular dynamics or a Monte Carlo protocol. The particle-based soup methods have the ability to create or annihilate particles, as well as change element type, hybridization type, bonding pattern, and so on. The fragment-based soup methods may or may not permit the modification of the fragments. However, alteration of the connections between fragments is always allowed. In most methods, decisions about whether to accept or reject any changes are not random, but are based on an evaluation procedure. Furthermore, the process of deciding which bonds to alter (make, break, or change) is different in the various methods. For example, some methods simply alter bonds randomly, then decide (using either an energy-based or a rule-based method) whether to keep or reject the change, whereas others simply form a bond whenever two isolated fragments come into appropriate range.

One of the most exciting areas in de novo design is the use of genetic algorithms (GA) to construct ligands. In this approach, a collection of ligands are chosen at random and placed randomly within the active site. Each molecule is described by a string of numbers, analogous to a gene. The genes for pairs of ligands are then crossedover, or recombined, to produce a new generation of ligands. These are scored based on their predicted binding affinity to the receptor, and the highest-scoring ones are retained for further evolution. In addition, individual ligands may be mutated randomly. There are several groups who have published GA-based de novo design work, notably Blaney and associates [78] and Payne and Glen [130]. The topic of genetic algorithms and their use in various other fields of computational chemistry is covered elsewhere [138].

Advantages and Disadvantages

The randomness of these approaches is one of their attractions, in contrast with the more traditional methods that construct a more limited set of molecules. The random connection and disconnection approaches can, in principle, construct any molecule imaginable, and they do so in a manner that is relatively free from bias. Thus, the ability of these methods to explore "drug space" more broadly should be superior to other kinds of methods and, in general, they will generate a more diverse set of suggestions. On the other hand, the sequential buildup methods are already capable of generating a huge variety of compounds, and they do so in a more systematic way. This means that within a given set of building blocks and ways to connect them, the odds of finding productive combinations is probably somewhat higher than with stochastic methods.

III. DETAILS OF A FEW SPECIFIC DE NOVO LIGAND DESIGN METHODS

In this section the details of several ligand design program are described. The intention is to provide a few examples of how a representative sampling of real programs work. The interested reader is referred to other, more detailed reviews of this field to learn more about these and other de novo ligand design methods [15–18].

A. Examples of Active Site Analysis Programs

GRID

Goodford and his colleagues have developed GRID [24–28], which computes the interaction of small organic fragments with an enzyme. The method places probes at regularly spaced grid points within the active site and determines the regions with the most favorable scores. Each probe represents a simple functional group, such as water or methyl, and can be calculated in a few minutes on a typical workstation. Initial tests with hydrofolate reductase (DHFR) were quite favorable; water-binding sites and the placement of hydrogen-bonding groups of inhibitors within the active site were well reproduced. Over the years, a variety of other enzymes have been used to calibrate the functions in GRID and to develop parameters for additional probes [26,27], as well as to carry out de novo design, with good results [28–31]. Recent examples include reproducing the subunit–subunit salt bridge interactions in hemoglobin with an $-NH_3^+$ probe to mimic lysine [28]. Tightly held water molecules in lysozyme also were reproduced [28]. Agouron has successfully applied GRID to the design of thymidilate synthase (TS) inhibitors [6]. The design of PLA_2 inhibitors [29,30] and modified cytochrome $P-450_{CAM}$ substrates [31] were guided by suggestions from GRID and LUDI [85,86]. This marks one of the few examples in the literature during which several ligand design methods were used concurrently.

Multiple-Copy Simultaneous Search (MCSS)

Miranker and Karplus [41] have modified CHARMM so that minimizations and molecular dynamics simulations could be performed without non-bonded interactions between solvent molecules. This allows the solvent molecules to overlap each other in energetically favorable regions and greatly improves the efficiency with which such locations may be identified. Small fragments, such as water and benzene, are used. Typically, 100–1000 copies of each fragment type are used. Following minimization, local searches are carried out in the regions surrounding the low-energy fragment locations. These "fine searches" could be carried out by random sampling or a grid-based approach using a 0.25 Å spacing and rigid rotations at each grid point. A direct comparison of the binding energy of each copy of the fragment type reveals the optimal locations.

Caflisch et al. [42] applied MCSS to the design of HIV-1 protease inhibitors and found that the locations of N-methylacetamide (NMA) fragments corresponded well to the backbone of MVT-101, a submicromolar inhibitor of HIV-1 protease. These NMA fragments were joined together into hexapeptide backbones and clustered, based on conformation, into about 100 families. Additional MCSS runs were then carried out with the side-chain fragments of MVT-101. Low-energy locations for each fragment type were then connected to the backbones and minimized. This process yielded 15 ligands with total energies below an arbitrary cutoff. Monte Carlo minimization (MCM) then was carried out on each of the 15 ligand conformations. One of these conformations was within 2.4 Å of the experimental result for MVT-101, although a considerable amount of variability was seen. The results also allowed the authors to make several suggestions for modifications to MVT-101 to improve its potency.

HINT

Kellogg and co-workers have developed HINT (*h*ydrophoic *int*eractions) to help evaluate and visualize the binding interactions between enzyme and ligand [49–53]. It uses a set of empirical parameters to estimate log*P* or to produce a hydrophobic field that can be added to comparitive molecular field analysis (CoMFA) [13] or other 3D-QSAR treatment [12,14]. It also allows an estimate of all atom–atom pairwise interactions between ligand and receptor (called *microbinding terms*) from which the ligand-binding energy may be estimated. Finally, with the ancillary programs LOCK and KEY it allows the user to map the hydrophobic and polar nature of the active site, as well as the interactions between enzyme and ligand. Regions of greatest lipophilicity calculated with HINT overlap well with the bound conformations of greasy groups in ligands, as determined by X-ray crystallography. The method also does a reasonable job of predicting the K_i for allosteric ligands of hemoglobin [52]. Although HINT is not a de novo drug design program, it is very useful for providing a straightforward, visual map of the properties of the active site, and is thus a valuable tool for fragment placement and analysis. In addition, HINT is one of the few de novo programs that allows the user to visualize both favorable and unfavorable contributions to binding.

B. Examples of Ligand Connection Methods

CLIX

CLIX [84] is a clever demonstration of a hybrid approach that may be viewed as either a site-point or a whole-molecule–docking method. It uses the output from GRID calculations, carried out with a variety of probes, to characterize the receptor site in terms of an ensemble of favorable-binding positions for different groups or fragments. This information is then used to query a chemical database for candidate molecules having good coincidence for individual fragments with members of the ensemble. Mildly repulsive interactions between candidates and the enzyme are relieved by allowing the candidate to relax slightly (without significantly reducing its overlap with the ensemble of binding fragments). The receptor is rigid throughout this process. Binding energy is estimated using the energy information in the GRID interaction energy maps. Also CLIX is able to use the information from the GRID potential maps to suggest possible changes in the structures, derived from the Cambridge Structural Database, to improve their binding. As a test case, sialic acid bound well to a mutant influenza virus hemagglutinin structure, in good agreement with available structural information. Thus, the method may also be viewed as a whole-molecule approach to determine the bound conformation of known ligands, but we generally view CLIX as a site-point method because it relies on fitting ligands to the critical site points obtained from GRID.

LUDI

LUDI [85,86], similar to CLIX, is primarily a method for fitting molecular fragments to site points within an active site. The program was developed by Böhm at BASF and has been widely used as a result of commercial distribution (Molecular Simulations, San Diego CA). Although LUDI accepts the output from GRID in much the same manner as CLIX, LUDI also has the ability to calculate site points suitable for lipophilic interactions or hydrogen bonds. Various approaches may be used to generate the list of site points. The method attempts to distinguish between aliphatic and aromatic lipophilic sites, which is challenging, but can lead to more precise ligand design ideas. Early versions of LUDI used a library of approximately 1000 small functional groups to connect two, three, or four adjacent site points into *fragments*. Then, smaller bridging groups such as $-CH_2-$ and $-CO_2-$ are used to connect these fragments. Both the fragment and the bridging libraries are user-extendable. For the enzyme DHFR, placements of key functional groups in the well-known inhibitor methotrexate were reproduced by LUDI [85]. For trypsin, the rule-based approach to fragment generation failed to reproduce the known conformation of benzamidine; however, the statistical contact pattern method did place this fragment in its proper orientation [85]. LUDI has been well reviewed by Bohm [17].

Analysis of Crystal-Field Environments

Klebe [88] has performed a very careful analysis of the nonbonded contacts observed in the Cambridge Structural Database (CSD). To avoid conformational bias, only intermolecular contacts between neighboring molecules within the unit cell were used. The analysis was carried out for each functional group of interest (carboxylate, amide, sulfate, alcohol, and so on). Because of the large size of the CSD, there are many molecules containing each fragment, thereby providing a large enough data set to infer the statistical distribution of hydrogen bond lengths and angles.

Advances in ligand design methods benefit greatly from fundamental analysis such as this. It was undoubtedly a very complex effort to assemble this database, but the payoff is enormous. For example, the rules thus derived can be used to guide the automatic docking of known ligands as well as to direct a de novo design program. Along the same lines, Bohm [17] and Thornton [125] have found that analysis of the protein database is useful for determining the bound conformations of ligands. Various groups have also found such analysis helpful for deriving empirical scoring functions [17,23; see also Chap. 10].

CAVEAT

CAVEAT, developed by Bartlett and co-workers [98,99], is designed to identify scaffolds that can link together any number of isolated ligand fragments. Bonds are treated as vectors, and the method works by comparing the relation between those vectors in the isolated ligand fragments with those of each molecule in the database. Figure 9 shows the process that CAVEAT follows and, as an example, the way it might be used to design a peptide mimic. Early versions of CAVEAT used the Cambridge Structural Database to identify cyclic spacers to connect fragments already positioned properly in the active site. Later versions added new synthetic databases, such as TRIAD, composed of approximately 400,000 reasonable tricyclic ring systems, and ILIAD, containing nearly 110,000 linkers built from combinations of simple fragments. Both ILIAD and TRIAD are intended to be collections of diverse frameworks—in other words, "idea generators," rather than finished ligand candidates. Much of the translation of these ideas into synthesizable molecules is then up to the medicinal chemist.

Unlike many other fragment connection methods, which work only on pairs of fragments, CAVEAT has been designed to allow any number of isolated ligands to be connected simultaneously with a single scaffold. Postprocessing tools connect the CAVEAT hits to the original ligands, filter out the scaffolds that bump into the receptor (assuming the receptor structure is known), and classify the hits into families (with the ancillary program CLASS). Underlying this entire suite of programs is the philosophy that the method must be very fast (preferably interactive) and easy to use. As a consequence, CAVEAT and CLASS are remarkably fast, handling hundreds of thousands of searches in a matter of seconds. Such tools allow

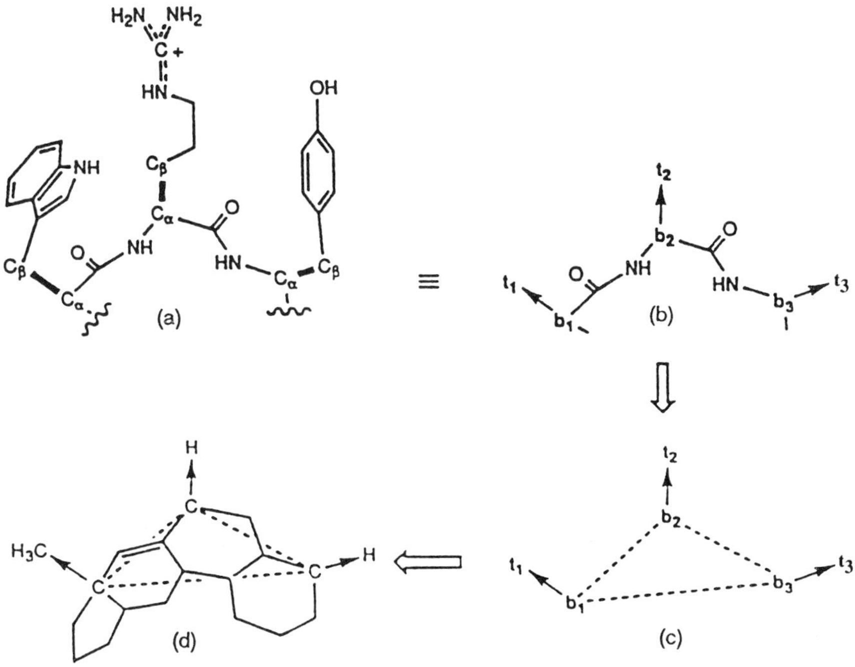

Figure 9 Example of the use of CAVEAT to design a peptide mimic [99].

the modeler to quickly generate many possible ways to connect isolated fragments.

HOOK

Hubbard and co-workers developed HOOK [100], which uses molecular skeletons from a database to connect multiple isolated functional groups. The construction process used by HOOK is shown in Figure 10. Each skeleton has two or more "hooks" which are specific bonds designated as connection points. The skeletons can be selected from various sources, such as the Cambridge Structural Database, or may be generated de novo. Skeletons are treated as rigid, so if a skeleton is actually flexible, it is treated as a set of distinct, rigid conformations. The degree of overlap between the isolated fragments and the skeleton may be controlled by the user. In addition, linkages can occur in several other ways. Functional groups can be linked with unused hooks directly through bond fusion, or an extra methylene group may be used as a spacer to connect the functional group and the hook. After all possible connections have been made between the

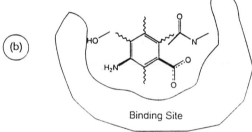

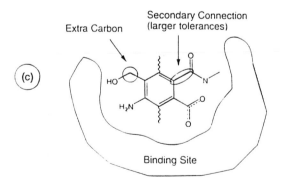

Figure 10 A schematic of the HOOK algorithm [100].

skeleton and the isolated fragments, the resulting molecule is scored using a simple model. The functional groups may have been previously positioned using MCSS [41] or any other fragment placement method.

As a test, the binding of sialic acid to hemagglutinin from the influenza A virus was studied. Sialic acid is a pyranose-based sugar, with a variety of hydrogen-bonding functional groups attached. The functional groups were preserved in the relative orientations they had in the sialic acid–hemagglutinin crystal structure, and the central pyranose ring was removed. A series of molecules similar to sialic acid were regenerated. A second test involved using an MCSS run to generate the functional groups, rather than simply taking them from the sialic acid–hemagglutinin crystal structure. HOOK was then used to link these groups. Approximately 3000 molecules were found that would link together three or more functional groups and fit well into the active site. In a final test, the chloramphenicol-binding site in chloramphenical acetyl transferase (CAT) was filled with fragments from an MCSS run and then connected with HOOK. Again, a large collection of interesting ligand suggestions was assembled.

NEWLEAD

NEWLEAD [106] automatically generates candidate structures by connecting two isolated ligand fragments (the pharmacophoric pieces) with spacers assembled from small chemical entities (atoms, chains, or ring moieties). Details of the method are given in Figure 11. The building blocks for the connecting linker may be single atoms, library spacers, or fused-ring spacers. The library spacers are used to directly connect two pharmacophoric pieces. The single-atom spacers and fused-ring spacers are connected to one of the pieces, and the atoms of the spacer are then used for connection to another pharmacophoric piece with a library spacer. For test cases, known ligands were dissected, key pharmacophoric elements were kept, and the rest of the atoms discarded. Then, NEWLEAD was used to demonstrate that the known ligands could be reproduced. In addition to the expected solutions, the program generated new structures that are chemically unrelated to the reference molecules, providing an unbiased starting point for the design of new generations of lead structures. The treatment is very fast, because only a few bonds are created between building blocks that already have ideal geometries.

PRO-LIGAND

PRO-LIGAND [107,108] employs a *design base* that contains information about the desired structural features of the ligands. This information may be derived from a model or structure of the receptor, or from a pharmacophore model. Next, a *design model* is constructed from the information

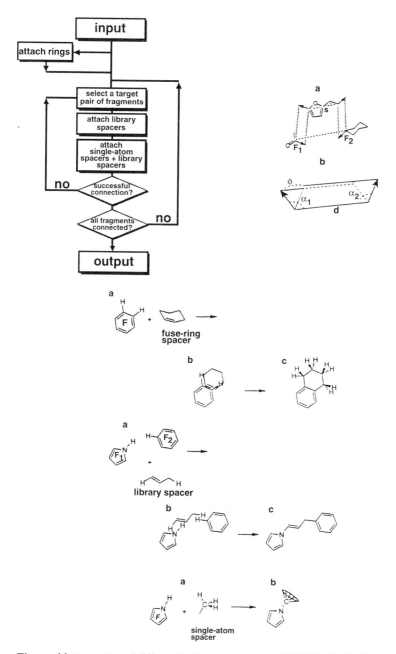

Figure 11 Examples of different linking operations in NEWLEAD [106].

in the design base. This is a 3D template describing the detailed, specific features of the chemical structures to be designed. These features are represented by *interaction sites* in a manner similar to LUDI. Then the *structure generation module* produces ligands consistent with the design model. These structures are created by assembling small molecular fragments that have been preconstructed. Under user control, PRO-LIGAND can grow a ligand in a continuous, linear fashion, or it can be used to bridge between fragments. The assembly process also attempts to eliminate steric conflicts within the ligand being constructed, as well as between the ligand and the receptor. Scoring is based on the number of design features being matched.

PRO-LIGAND was tested by analyzing a set of 35 steroids to produce a pharmacophore for both progestrogen and androgen receptor binding; the method was able to generate a set of novel, nonsteroidal candidate ligands. In a second test, a small set of weakly binding ACE inhibitors was used to generate a pharmacophore, which was then used as the design model. Several compounds were proposed that resembled known ACE inhibitors. To help span the open space between widely separated pharmacophore elements, the open volume was filled with a "wash" of hydrophobic site points to encourage growth across this space. This could help compensate for the dilemma of crossing dead zones (see Fig. 8).

GrowMol

Bohacek and McMartin developed GrowMol [120], which builds ligands one atom or small functional group at a time in linear fashion. At each step in the growth process, the location, atom or functional group, and torsional angle are randomly chosen. Scoring is based on "chemical complementarity" to the receptor, so atoms and groups making good van der Waals contacts or hydrogen bonds are scored highly. Newly grown atoms and groups may also be connected to previously generated portions of the same ligand, leading to polycyclic and fused aromatic systems. Following the generation of ligands, a series of postprocessing steps takes place. First, ligands not making a sufficient number of hydrogen bonds and hydrophobic contacts with the enzyme are eliminated. Next, each molecule is energy-minimized within the active site, and the strain energy of the bound conformation is used to eliminate compounds that are binding in high-energy conformations. Also, near-duplicate structures are eliminated at this point. Next, the potency of each remaining compound is estimated, using a regression equation derived from the experimental data available for that particular receptor. This equation simply counts the number of hydrophobic contacts and hydrogen bonds between the ligand and the enzyme. Finally, the remaining compounds are clustered into families. Tests with thermolysin and HIV protease showed that reasonable suggestions could be made by GrowMol.

GROW

Moon and Howe described GROW, one of the earliest de novo design programs, which uses a buildup procedure to determine the best peptidal ligand or substrate for a given enzyme [121–123]. Unlike the techniques discussed previously, GROW is designed to avoid the difficult problem of connecting isolated fragments by using buildup procedures linearly connecting each fragment to the preceding one. The tradeoff is that a limited set of fragments may be considered. A large predefined library of conformations of each amino acid is used in the construction process. Each conformation of each residue is tested according to a molecular mechanics force field, and the set of N–lowest-energy possibilities is carried along to the next step. Significantly, both conformational (intramolecular) enthalpies and solvation free energies are included in the analysis.

Trial studies with the aspartyl protease rhizopus pepsin were quite successful at reproducing the conformation of a reduced peptide ligand, the structure of which has been determined crystallographically. More recent efforts include the use of a random choice of fragment conformation followed by a metropolis-based decision whether to keep or reject the change. Also, GROW has been extended to include organic ligands by using essentially the same procedure. Methotrexate was divided into three pieces, and its binding to DHFR was well reproduced [123].

GroupBuild

GroupBuild was developed to suggest chemically reasonable structures that efficiently fill the active sites of enzymes [54]. These structures are composed entirely of simple functional groups (also known as *building blocks* or *fragments*) that the program chooses from a small predefined library. The method was designed to propose molecules in which *every* fragment provides the greatest degree of steric and electrostatic contact with the enzyme while existing in a low-energy conformation.

User-selected enzyme seed atom(s) may be used to determine the area(s) where structure-generation begins. Alternatively, GroupBuild may begin with a predocked "ligand core" from which fragments are grown. For each new fragment generated by the program, several thousand *candidates* in a variety of locations and orientations are considered. Each of these candidates is scored with a standard molecular mechanics potential energy function. For efficiency, information about the active site environment is stored in *grids*, which speed program execution by up to two orders of magnitude. The grids contain a list of neighboring enzyme atoms, hydrogen-bonding requirements, and information about the van der Waals and electrostatics interactions. This information may be used, for example, to ensure that hydrogen-bonding fragments are selected only if they make reasonable hydrogen bonds with the enzyme. The selected fragment and its orientation are chosen from among the highest-scoring cases. Optionally, a special-scoring function may be used to ensure that hydrogen-bonding and hydrophobic fragments have equal weighting.

Tests of the method using HIV protease, FK506-binding protein, and human carbonic anhydrase demonstrate that strucures similar to known potent ligands may be generated with GroupBuild. Representative examples are given in Figure 12. For optimal results, the core of a known ligand is generally used as a starting point for running GroupBuild; this is true for both of the examples in Figure 12. Notably, molecules very similar to a class of thiophene-containing HIV protease ligands generated by GroupBuild [54] were later reported [139] to be low-nanomolar inhibitors.

SPROUT

Gillet and co-workers developed SPROUT [126–128], a general-purpose program intended to be useful for a range of applications, including ligand design as well as the design of catalysts and agents for asymmetric synthesis. Figure 13 gives a schematic overview of the program. SPROUT divides the structure-generation process into two phases: primary- and secondary-structure generation. Primary-structure generation produces a 3D molecular graph consistent with the shape of the receptor site and matches *target sites* (i.e., hydrogen-bonding regions). 3D graphs are composed from combinations of *templates*, which represent common building blocks and may be joined in various ways. A unique collection of templates is called a *skeleton*. Skeletons, which are entirely composed of hydrocarbon fragments, are scored based on steric contact with the enzyme, the number of rotatable bonds, the strain energy, and so forth. Secondary-structure generation is the process of converting the graph into a "real" structure with appropriate bonds, atom types, and such. The secondary-structure–generation phase uses information about the active site, such as electrostatics and hydrophobicity.

Early descriptions of SPROUT [126] discussed only primary-structure generation. The method was tested against the APPA binding site of trypsin, and the pepstatin binding site of HIV-1 protease. The trypsin example worked well, but the larger HIV-1 protease active site was more challenging, and SPROUT was unable to reach convergence. A later publication [127] described many further developments of the method, including a graphic user interface; greater user control over the process; the ability to use a pharmacophore hypothesis as input; and a clustering

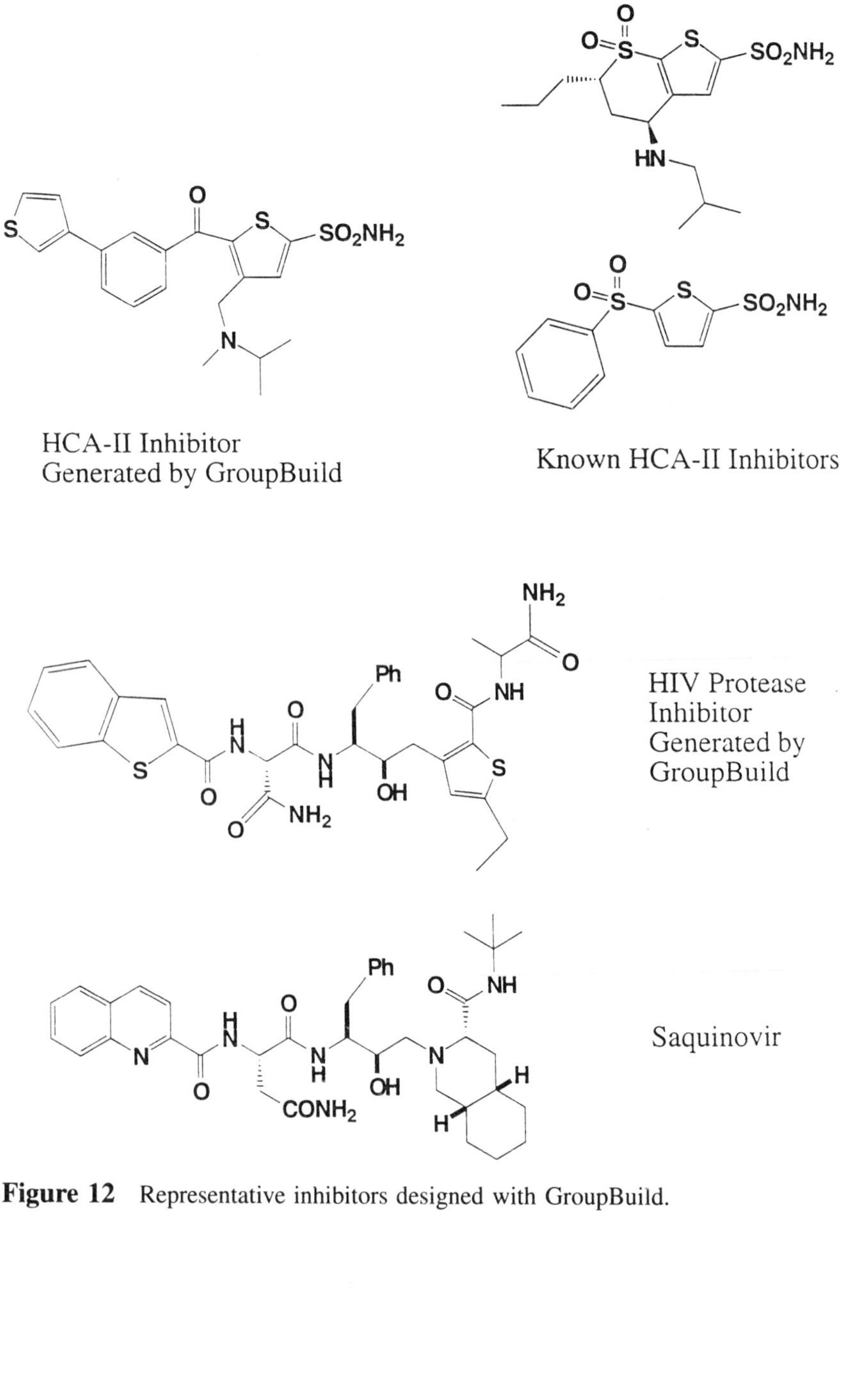

HCA-II Inhibitor
Generated by GroupBuild

Known HCA-II Inhibitors

HIV Protease
Inhibitor
Generated by
GroupBuild

Saquinovir

Figure 12 Representative inhibitors designed with GroupBuild.

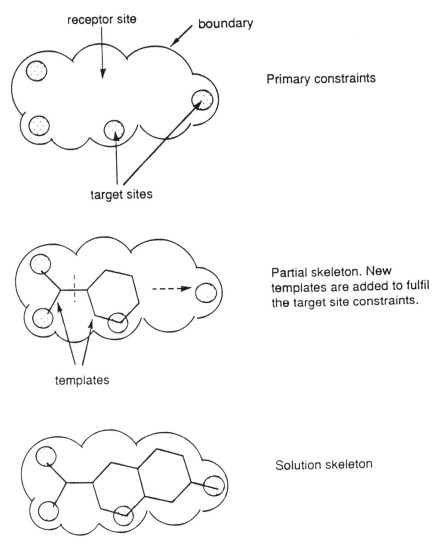

receptor site   boundary

Primary constraints

target sites

Partial skeleton. New
templates are added to fulfil
the target site constraints.

templates

Solution skeleton

Figure 13 The SPROUT program [126].

scheme to simplify browsing through the results. Two other enhancements
merit special mention. Secondary-structure generation in which hydrogen-
bonding atoms are placed at appropriate vertices was added. This allows
SPROUT to actually generate "real-world" ligand suggestions. Finally, an
expert system CAESA is being developed for judging the synthetic acces-

sibility of each proposed ligand. In the second paper two examples are given: the binding of guanidine diphosphate and guanidine triphosphate (GDP and GTP) to p21 *ras* protein, and the binding of morphine to its receptor, based only on a previously proposed morphine agonist model. Finally, a more recent paper [128] has described HIPPO, an active site analysis program to determine the likely orientations of starting fragments.

Genetic Algorithms: Chemical Genesis

Genetic algorithms are probabalistic search techniques based on the principle of evolution and natural selection. In a GA, possible solutions are encoded in a chromosome-like data structure. A group of (typically random) chromosomes are allowed to "evolve," thereby producing a superior set of solutions. The use of GA methods in chemistry has recently been thoroughly reviewed by Judson [138]. Another excellent starting point for learning about these methods is a paper by Payne and Glen [130], who describe GA-based superposition and conformational analysis.

Glen and Payne [140] have also applied genetic algorithms to ligand design. Their method is called Chemical Genesis. Molecular structures are generated that match an enzyme active site or a pharmacophore model. Either random molecules or known ligands may be used as starting points. The algorithm is not limited to structural type; most chemically sensible drug-like structures may be generated. Examples of physicochemical constraints include log$P$, molecular weight, and molecular mechanics strain energy. The method can be initiated from ethane as the seed molecule, or from a series of fragments randomly selected from a library of roughly 30 common building blocks, including benzene, cyclohexane, naphthalene, and the like. Alternatively, a known starting point may be used, which can be frozen in place or allowed to move; it may also be partially frozen by using additional constraints that penalize any changes to the atomic positions or atom types of the fragment. Several mutation operators are available. Mutations that tend to form hydrogen bonds are slightly preferred. After the new molecules have been formed, they are "cleaned up" with molecular mechanics. A number of example problems, including DHFR were used to demonstrate that the method gives satisfactory results.

CONCERTS

Pearlman and Murcko have developed CONCERTS [133], which uses small organic fragments as the basic building blocks. (An earlier program by the same authors, CONCEPTS, had constructed ligands from individual atoms.) These are mixed together in the active site and have only a weak repulsion for each other, so they can come quite close together, but cannot completely overlap. Typically, a dozen fragment types are used, and there are a few hundred copies of each. Alternatively, a smaller number of fragments (methane, benzene, water, ammonia, and formaldehyde) can be used. Molecular dynamics takes place on the fragments with the protein fixed, and whenever two fragments come within reasonable bonding geometry (bond lengths and angles), they are joined. If the energy of the total system goes down, the bond formation is accepted. All energy terms, both inter- and intramolecular, are calculated as in a standard molecular dynamics run. Once joined, two fragments cannot be separated, unless some other compensating bond formation takes place. The method is slow: each run takes about 3 days on a modern Unix workstation and yields dozens of proposed ligands. Tests carried out against HIV-1 protease and FK506-binding protein have been encouraging, with the features of the best-scoring compounds being quite reminiscent of known inhibitors. Because the ligands generated by CONCERTS are not necessarily synthetically accessible, this method definitely falls into the category of idea generators and must be combined with a significant postprocessing effort by both modelers and medicinal chemists.

MCDNLG

When compared with most other methods, the Monte Carlo de novo ligand generator (MDCNLG) [136] is relatively unbiased; for example, it has no fragment library or prestored information about the types of molecules desired. Rather, the method starts with a random collection of atoms packed tightly into the active site of the receptor and slowly anneals it into a chemically stable molecule. Each atom is represented by its element type, hybridization, hydrogen-bonding possibilities, and so on. Changes to the ligand are made randomly from a list and include make–change–break a bond; delete–change–reappear–move a particle; rigidly translate–rotate the ligand; and rotate a bond. Bonds are automatically assumed to exist between two atoms within 2.1 Å. Scoring is based on a combination of intra- and intermolecular force-field terms. The intramolecular strain within the ligand is the sum of the usual terms found in force fields as well as a special term to account for "valence strain" resulting from an incorrect number of valence bonds. This encourages bond formation. Intermolecular interactions between the ligand and the enzyme are handled by a standard Lennard–Jones potential, as well as a hydrogen–bond-counting scheme and a desolvation penalty term for heteroatoms. The latter term is useful to ensure that heteroatoms are placed only in favorable environments.

During the run, a standard metropolis-based Monte Carlo algorithm is used along with a simulated annealing protocol. Typically, several hundred thousand Monte Carlo steps are taken. This procedure takes only a few minutes on a fast workstation. Tests with DHFR, thymidylate synthase

(TS), and HIV-1 protease were carried out [136]. In each test, compounds reminiscent of known inhibitors were generated. Furthermore, MCDNLG was used in a prospective sense with HIV protease. By starting from a known inhibitor, the program made specific suggestions that were later synthesized, occasionally leading to a tenfold increase in potency.

Notably, one compound that resulted from using MCDNLG was later selected for preclinical development. This marks one of the few unambiguous success stories reported in the literature for a de novo design program.

B. Examples of Whole-Molecule Methods

DOCK

One of the best-known and oldest methods for de novo ligand design is DOCK, which uses a fast sphere-matching algorithm to dock compounds from a user-supplied database in an enzyme active site [59–61]. DOCK is covered in detail in Chapter 3 of this volume, so we will not go into the specifics about the method here. It is worth pointing out, however, that DOCK has continued to evolve over the years, and has become much faster and more efficient. For many problems, it now takes less than a week to go through a database of 100,000 compounds on a typical workstation.

DOCK has been used in a wide variety of design projects. Bodian et al. [66] studied the binding of benzoquinones and hydroquinones to influenza hemagglutinin. Ring et al. [67] designed antiparasitic agents using homology models of both the serine protease cercarial elastase and the trophozoite cysteine protease. A screening of the best-scoring compounds yielded low micromolar hits against each enzyme. Other examples are discussed in recent reviews of docking [57,58; see also Chap. 3].

Unfortunately, DOCK still does not provide for ligand flexibility. To overcome this, one can dock a set of conformations for each molecule. Researchers at Merck [70,71] and Vertex [72,73] demonstrated that this approach leads to a much greater hit rate. Klebe also has demonstrated that rapid conformational searching can be carried out efficiently for drug-sized molecules [74]. Therefore, as the technology of conformational searching advances, the use of multiconformational databases in docking should become more commonplace.

Distance Geometry Approaches

Blaney has described an impressive application of distance geometry (DG) to ligand docking [77,78]. The active site is first defined by overlapping spheres of variable radii, in a manner similar to DOCK. With use of DG, the ligand is then generated directly in the binding site in a random orientation and conformation. The fit between the ligand and spheres is then optimized, also using a DG method. The ligand is completely flexible during this process; when the minimization is complete, the entire volume of the ligand is inside the collection of active site spheres. The spheres are then removed and the ligand is further refined with a standard force field.

As a test, the fit of methotrexate (MTX) into DHFR was attempted [78]. Of 100 random trials, 15% are within 2.5 Å of the X-ray structure and the lowest-energy fits were closest to the X-ray structure. Each conformation takes less than a second on a typical workstation.

Genetic Algorithm Approaches

In the past 2 years, several groups have described GA-based methods for docking ligands [79–83]. All these GA methods represent the conformation of the ligand by a set of torsion angles. These methods do an excellent job of reproducing experimentally determined conformations of a variety of ligands while bound to their receptors. For example, Oshiro and associates [81] studied DHFR–MTX, thymidilate–phenolphthalein, and HIV protease–thioketal halopiridol, and in each pair they found low-energy conformations with less than 1 Å rmsd from the crystal structures. Similarly impressive successes have also been reported [79,82,83]. Typically, a GA run will take several minutes, and most of the publications in this field suggest that several runs are required to have a reasonable confidence that conformational space has been adequately sampled. In addition, several researchers have included a desolvation term into their calculations, which further decreases their speed [80]. Flexible GA-based docking procedure can take 100–1000 times longer than a "traditional" rigid DOCK run. This limits the usefulness of the GA-based flexible-docking methods for the analysis of large databases.

IV. GENERAL DISCUSSION OF LIGAND DESIGN APPROACHES

As we have shown, there now exists a wide variety of methods for ligand design, and new methods appear on a regular basis. These methods each have different goals, and they involve a range of underlying assumptions about the best way(s) to design drugs. All show promise.

There are a number of obvious limitations to current de novo ligand design methods. First, they are still rather slow and inefficient; they generate small numbers of (we hope) good ideas. Second, most methods are simplistic: they use simplified models for the ligand–receptor system, and simple-scoring functions. Third, most methods are hard or impossible for the nonexpert to use.

On the bright side, many methods have demonstrated that even with these limitations, they can be useful in the drug discovery process. Even simple methods can "capture" a great deal of the essential character of the active site, and point out good, solid ideas that can be used as starting points. Furthermore, it is clear that combinations of methods may be used profitably to overcome limitations in any one particular method. It makes sense to be creative and flexible in one's use of these techniques.

It is obvious that because of the limitations of current de novo methods, successful applications will require the medicinal chemists to play an essential role—providing creative input, filtering out synthetically intractable ideas, and so forth. It is our experience that without a committed synthetic chemist who is willing to play this role, de novo methods are essentially useless. At the same time, the more practical the suggestions that come out of the computer, the more likely the synthetic chemist will be interested. For example, compound suggestions that are not entirely "de novo," but that retain significant features from earlier compound classes, and allow the chemist to apply the existing structure–activity data to the problem, are more likely to be well received.

In the coming years, it will be important for de novo methods to improve in several areas. They must become much faster and efficient; they must use more realistic models for the receptor and better scoring functions; and they must take synthetic accessibility into consideration. Just as importantly, a more standardized set of test cases should be devised to ensure that new methods (as well as old ones) are actually meeting their objectives.

Finally, it is also useful to keep the topic of de novo design in perspective. To quote one the most successful medicinal chemists of our time, Ralph Hirschmann [144]:

> Activity in relevant in vitro and in vivo assays does not mean that a compound is a drug. Rather, a drug is a substance approved by a regulatory agency in a medically sophisticated country. Many a promising compound has failed in safety studies, or in the clinic, because of poor bioavailability, rapid metabolism, species difference, and so forth. Discovering an active compound is relatively easy, but discovering an important new drug remains unbelievably difficult.

In other words, even when all the difficulties of *ligand* design software have been overcome, there will be many other issues facing the *drug* design team. A good ligand is not necesarily a good drug. This highlights what is perhaps the most critical issue in computational chemistry that faces us in the pharmaceutical community: How does one more fully integrate computational methods into the entire drug discovery process? As our understanding of pharmacology, toxicology, metabolism, basic biology, and other disciplines becomes more sophisticated, it will, perhaps, be possible to create de novo ligand design tools that anticipate some of the "downstream" developmental issues and suggest actual drugs. This day will not arrive soon, but it is a worthy goal for the coming decades.

ACKNOWLEDGMENTS

I thank many of the researchers whose work is cited in this review for sending me materials in advance of publication, and for many helpful discussions. I also thank my colleagues at Vertex, Sergio Rotstein, David Pearlman, Guy Bemis, Govinda Rao, Pat Walters, Scott Thomas, and Matt Stahl for their many helpful discussions and for their comments on the manuscript. Thanks also to Paul Charifson for his careful reading of the manuscript.

REFERENCES

1. M. A. Navia and M. A. Murcko, The use of structural information in drug design, *Curr. Opin. Struct. Biol.* 2:202–210 (1992).
2. M. D. Walkinshaw, Protein targets for structure-based drug design, *Med. Res. Rev.* 12:317–372 (1992).
3. P. M. Colman, Structure-based drug design, *Curr. Opin. Struct. Biol.* 4: 868–874 (1994).
4. J. Greer, J. W. Erickson, J. J. Baldwin, and M. D. Varney, Application of the three-dimensional structures of protein target molecules in structure-based drug design, *J. Med. Chem.* 37:1035–1054 (1994).
5. J. J. Baldwin, G. S. Ponticello, P. S. Anderson, M. E. Christy, M. A. Murcko, W. C. Randall, H. Schwam, M. F. Sugrue, J. P. Springer, P. Gautheron, J. Grove, P. Mallorga, M.-P. Viader, B. M. McKeever, and M. A. Navia, Thienothiopyran-2-sulfonamides: Novel topically active carbonic anhydrase inhibitors for the treatment of glaucoma, *J. Med. Chem.* 32:2510–2513 (1989).
6. K. Appelt, R. J. Bacquet, C. A. Bartlett, et al., Design of enzyme inhibitors using iterative protein crystallographic analysis, *J. Med. Chem.* 34: 1925–1934 (1991).
7. J. A. Montgomery, S. Niwas, J. D. Rose, J. A. Secrist 3d, Y. S. Babu, C. E. Bugg, M. D. Erion, W. C. Guida, and S. E. Ealick, Structure-based design of inhibitors of purine nucleoside phosphorylase. 1. 9-(Arylmethyl) derivatives of 9-deazaguanine, *J. Med. Chem.* 36:55–69 (1993).
8. J. W. Erickson, D. J. Neidhart, J. VanDrie, et al., Design, activity, and 2.8 Å crystal structure of a C_2-symmetric inhibitor complexed to HIV-1 protease, *Science* 249:527–533 (1990).

9. P. Y. Lam, P. K. Jadhav, C. J. Eyermann, et al. Rational design of potent, bioavailable, nonpeptide cyclic ureas as HIV protease inhibitors, *Science* *263*:380–384 (1994).

10. M. von Itzstein, W. Y. Wu, G. B. Kok, et al. Rational design of potent sialidase-based inhibitors of influenza virus replication, *Nature 363*:418–423 (1993).

11. E. E. Kim, C. T. Baker, M. D. Dwyer, M. A. Murcko, B. G. Rao, R. D. Tung, and M. A. Navia, Crystal-structure of HIV-1 protease in complex with VX-478, a potent and orally bioavailable inhibitor of the enzyme, *J. Am. Chem. Soc. 117*:1181–1182 (1995).

12. H. Kubinyi, ed., *3D QSAR in Drug Design*, ESCOM, Leiden, 1993.

13. R. D. Cramer, D. E. Patterson, and J. D. Bunce, Comparative molecular field analysis (CoFMA). 1. Effect of shape on binding of steroids to carrier proteins, *J. Am. Chem. Soc. 110*:5959–5967 (1988).

14. R. S. Pearlman, 3D molecular structures: Generation and use in 3D searching, *3D QSAR in Drug Design* (H. Kubinyi, ed.), ESCOM, Leiden, 1993, pp. 41–79.

15. D. E. Clark, C. W. Murray, and J. Li, Current issues in de novo molecular design, *Reviews in Computational Chemistry*, Vol. 11 (K. B. Lipkowitz and D. B. Boyd, eds.), VCH, New York, 1997.

16. M. A. Murcko, Recent advances in ligand design methods, *Reviews in Computational Chemistry*, Vol. 11 (K. B. Lipkowitz and D. B. Boyd, eds.) VCH, New York, 1997.

17. H.-J. Bohm, Ligand design. *3D-QSAR in Drug Design* (H. Kubinyi, ed.), ESCOM, Leiden, 1993.

18. R. A. Lewis and A. R. Leach, Current methods for site-directed structure generation, *J. Comput. Aided Mol. Design 8*:467–475 (1994).

19. L. M. Balbes, S. W. Mascarella, and D. B. Boyd, A perspective of modern methods in computer-aided drug design, *Reviews in Computational Chemistry*, Vol. 5 (K. B. Lipkowitz and D. B. Boyd, eds.), VCH, New York, 1994, pp. 337–380.

20. W. C. Guida, Software for structure-based drug design, *Curr. Opin. Struct. Biol. 4*:777–781 (1994).

21. N. C. Cohen, J. M. Blaney, C. Humblet, P. Gund, and D. C. Barry, Molecular modeling software and methods for medicinal chemistry, *J. Med. Chem. 33*: 883–894 (1990).

22. R. S. Bohacek, C. McMartin, and W. C. Guida, The art and practice of structure-based drug design: A molecular modeling perspective, *Med. Chem. Rev. 16*:3–50 (1996).

23. Ajay and M. A. Murcko, Computational methods to predict binding free energy in ligand-receptor complexes, *J. Med. Chem. 38*:4953–4967 (1995).

24. P. J. Goodford, A computational procedure for determining energetically favorable binding sites on biologically important macromolecules, *J. Med. Chem. 28*:849–857 (1985).

25. D. N. A. Boobbyer, P. J. Goodford, P. M. McWhinnie, and R. C. Wade, New hydrogen-bond potentials for use in determining energetically favorable binding sites in molecules of known structure, *J. Med. Chem.* 32:1083–1094 (1989).

26. R. C. Wade, K. J. Clark, and P. J. Goodford, Further development of hydrogen bond functions for use in determining energetically favorable binding sites on molecules of known structure. 1. Ligand probe groups with the ability to form two hydrogen bonds, *J. Med. Chem* 36:140–147 (1993).

27. R. C. Wade and P. J. Goodford, Further development of hydrogen bond functions for use in determining energetically favorable binding sites on molecules of known structure. 2. Ligand probe groups with the ability to form more than two hydrogen bonds, *J. Med. Chem.* 36:148–156 (1993).

28. R. Wade, Molecular interaction fields, *3D-QSAR in Drug Design* (H. Kubinyi, ed.), ESCOM, Leiden, 1993.

29. M. T. Pisabarro, A. R. Ortiz, A. Palomer, F. Cabre, L. Garcia, R. C. Wade, F. Gago, D. Mauleon, and G. Carganico, Rational modification of human synovial fluid phospholipase A_2 inhibitors, *J. Med. Chem.* 37:337–341 (1994).

30. M. T. Pisabarro, A. Palomer, A. R. Ortiz, R. C. Wade, F. Gago, D. Mauleon, and G. Carganico, Rational drug design: GRID- and LUDI-based structural modifications of a human synovial fluid phospholipase A_2 inhibitor leading to enhanced activity, *J. Mol. Graph.* 12:72–80 (1994).

31. V. Helms, E. Deprez, E. Gill, C. Barret, B. Hui Bon Hoa, and R. C. Wade, Improved binding of cytochrome $P450_{cam}$ substrate analogs designed to fill extra space in the substrate binding pocket, *Biochemistry* 35:1485–1499 (1996).

32. N. Tomioka, A. Itai, and Y. Iitaka, A method for fast energy estimation and visualization of protein–ligand interactions, *J. Comput. Aided Mol. Design* 1:197–210 (1987).

33. N. Tomioka, A. Itai, and Y. Iitaka, Real-time estimation and visualization of protein-ligand interaction on 3D graphics display, *Three-Dimensional Structures and Drug Action* (Y. Iitaka and A. Itai, eds.), University of Tokyo Press, Tokyo, 1987, pp. 186–194.

34. N. Tomioka, and Itai, A. GREEN: A program package for docking studies in rational drug design, *J. Comput. Aided Mol. Design* 8:347–366 (1994).

35. D. J. Danziger and P. M. Dean, Automated site-directed drug design: A general algorithm for knowledge acquisition about hydrogen-bonding regions at protein surfaces, *Proc. R. Soc. Lond. B* 236:101–113 (1989).

36. D. J. Danziger and P. M. Dean, Automatic site-directed drug design: The prediction and observation of ligand point positions at hydrogen-bonding regions on protein surfaces, *Proc. R. Soc. Lond. B* 236:115–124 (1989).

37. E. N. Baker and R. E. Hubbard, Hydrogen bonding in globular proteins, *Prog. Biophys. Mol. Biol.* 44:97–179 (1984).

38. C. S. Poornima and P. M. Dean, Hydration in drug design. 1. Multiple hydrogen-bonding features of water molecules in mediating protein–ligand interactions, *J. Comput. Aided Mol. Design 9*:500–512 (1995).

39. C. S. Poonima and P. M. Dean, Hydration in drug design. 2. Influence of local site surface shape on water binding, *J. Comput. Aided Mol. Design 9*: 513–520 (1995).

40. C. S. Poornima and P. M. Dean, Hydration in drug design. 3. Conserved water molecules at the ligand-binding sites of homologous proteins, *J. Comput. Aided Mol. Design 9*:521–531 (1995).

41. A. Miranker and M. Karplus, Functionality maps of binding sites: A multiple copy simultaneous search method. *Proteins Struct. Funct. Genet. 11*:29–34 (1991).

42. A. Caflisch, A. Miranker, and M. Karplus, Multiple copy simultaneous search and construction of ligands in binding sites: Applications to inhibitors of HIV-1 aspartic proteinase, *J. Med. Chem. 36*:2142–2167 (1993).

43. T. N. Hart and R. J. Read, A multiple-start Monte-Carlo docking method, *Proteins Struct. Funct. Genet. 13*:206–222 (1992).

44. S.-Y. Yue, Distance-constrained molecular docking by simulated annealing, *Protein Eng. 4*:177–184 (1990).

45. S. R. Wilson and F. Guarneri, Calculation of rotational states of flexible molecules using simulated annealing, *Tetrahedron Lett. 32*:3601–3604 (1991).

46. F. Guarnieri and W. C. Still, A rapidly convergent simulation method: Mixed Monte Carlo/stochastic dynamics, *J. Comput. Chem. 15*:1302–1310 (1994).

47. A. Caflisch, P. Niederer, and M. Anliker, Monte Carlo docking of oligopeptides to proteins, *Proteins Struct. Funct. Genet. 13*:223–230 (1992).

48. Z. Li and H. A. Scheraga, Monte-Carlo minimization approach to the multiple-minima problem in protein folding, *Proc. Natl. Acad. Sci. USA 84*: 6611–6615 (1987).

49. D. J. Abraham and G. E. Kellogg, Hydrophobic fields, *3D-QSAR in Drug Design* (H. Kubinyi, ed.), ESCOM, Leiden, 1993, pp. 506–522.

50. G. E. Kellogg, S. F. Semus, and D. J. Abraham, HINT: A new method of empirical hydrophobic field calculation for CoMFA, *J. Comput. Aided Mol. Design 5*:545–552 (1991).

51. G. E. Kellogg, G. S. Jjoshi, and D. J. Abraham, New tools for modeling and understanding hydrophobicity and hydrophobic interactions, *Med. Chem. Res. 1*:444–453 (1992).

52. F. C. Wireko, G. E. Kellogg, and D. J. Abraham, Allosteric modifiers of hemoglobin. 2. Crystallographically determined binding sites and hydrophobic binding/interaction analysis of novel hemoglobin oxygen effectors, *J. Med. Chem. 34*:758–767 (1991).

53. D. J. Abraham and G. E. Kellogg, The effect of physical organic properties on hydrophobic fields, *J. Comput. Aided Mol. Design 8*:41–49 (1994), and references therein.

54. S. H. Rotstein and M. A. Murcko, GroupBuild: A fragment-based method for de novo drug design, *J. Med. Chem. 36*:1700–1710 (1993).

55. F. H. Allen, O. Kennard, and R. Taylor, Systematic analysis of structural data as a research technique in organic chemistry, *Acc. Chem. Res. 16*: 146–153 (1983).

56. D. Ringe, What makes a binding site a binding site? *Curr. Opin. Struct. Biol. 5*:825–829 (1995).

57. T. P. Lybrand, Ligand–protein docking and rational drug design, *Curr. Opin. Struct. Biol. 5*:224–228 (1995).

58. G. Jones and P. Willett, Docking small-molecule ligands into active sites, *Curr. Opin. Biotechnol. 6*:652–656 (1995).

59. I. D. Kuntz, J. M. Blaney, S. J. Oatley, R. Langridge, and T. E. Ferrin, A geometric approach to macromolecule–ligand interactions, *J. Mol. Biol. 161*: 269–288 (1982).

60. R. L. DesJarlais, G. L. Seibel, I. D. Kuntz, P. S. Furth, J. C. Alvarez, P. R. O. De Montellano, D. L. DeCamp, L. M. Babé, and C. S. Craik, Structure-based design of nonpeptide inhibitors specific for the human immunodeficiency virus 1 protease, *Proc. Natl. Acad. Sci. USA 87*:6644–6648 (1990).

61. R. L. DesJarlais, R. P. Sheridan, G. L. Seibel, J. S. Dixon, I. D. Kuntz, and R. Venkataraghavan, Using shape complementarity as an initial screen in designing ligands for a receptor binding site of known three-dimensional structure, *J. Med. Chem. 31*:722–729 (1989).

62. E. C. Meng, D. A. Gschwend, J. M. Blaney, and I. D. Kuntz, Orientational sampling and rigid-body minimization in molecular docking, *Proteins 7*: 266–278 (1993).

63. E. C. Meng, B. K. Shoichet, and I. D. Kuntz, Automated docking with grid-based energy evaluation, *J. Comput. Chem. 13*:505–524 (1992).

64. R. L. DesJarlais and J. S. Dixon, A shape- and chemistry-based docking method and its use in the design of HIV-1 protease inhibitors, *J. Comput. Aided Mol. Design 8*:231–242 (1994).

65. B. K. Shoichet and I. D. Kuntz, Matching chemistry and shape in molecular docking, *Protein Eng. 6*:723–732 (1993).

66. D. L. Bodian, R. B. Yamasaki, R. L. Buswell, J. F. Stearns, J. M. White, and I. D. Kuntz, Inhibition of the fusion-inducing conformational change of influenza hemagglutinin by benzoquinones and hydroquinones, *Biochemistry 32*:2967–2978 (1993).

67. C. S. Ring, E. Sun, J. H. Mckerrow, G. K. Lee, P. J. Rosenthal, I. D. Kuntz, and F. E. Cohen, Structure-based inhibitor design by using protein models for the development of antiparasitic agents, *Proc. Natl. Acad. Sci. USA 90*: 3583–3587 (1993).

68. R. L. DesJarlais, R. P. Sheridan, J. S. Dixon, I. D. Kuntz, and R. Venkataraghavan, Docking flexible ligands to macromolecular receptors by molecular shape, *J. Med. Chem. 29*:2149–2153 (1986).

69. A. R. Leach and I. D. Kuntz, Conformational analysis of flexible ligands in macromolecular receptor sites, *J. Comput. Chem. 13*:730–748 (1992).
70. S. K. Kearsley, D. J. Underwood, R. P. Sheridan, and M. D. Miller, FlexiBases: A way to enhance the use of molecular docking methods, *J. Comput. Aided Mol. Design 8*:565–582 (1994).
71. M. D. Miller, S. K. Kearsley, D. J. Underwood, and R. P. Sheridan, FLOG: A system to select quasi-flexible ligands complementary to a receptor of known three-dimensional structure, *J. Comput. Aided Mol. Design 8*: 8153–8174 (1994).
72. W. P. Walters, M. R. Stahl, and D. Dolata, WIZARD III: A new model building conformational search program, *J. Chem. Inf. Comput. Sci.*, (in press).
73. W. P. Walters, Developing an integrated set of tools for identifying potential drug candidates, 211th ACS National Meeting, New Orleans LA, 1996.
74. G. Klebe and T. Mietzner, A fast and efficient method to generate biologically relevant conformations, *J. Comput. Aided Mol. Design 8*:583–606 (1994).
75. D. S. Goodsell and A. J. Olsen, Automated docking of substrates to proteins by simulated annealing, *Proteins Struct. Funct. Genet. 8*:195–202 (1990).
76. D. S. Goodsell, H. Lauble, C. D. Stout, and A. J. Olsen, Automated docking in crystallography: Analysis of the substrates of aconitase, *Proteins Struct. Funct. Genet. 17*:1–10 (1993).
77. J. M. Blaney, A distance geometry-based approach for docking conformationally flexible molecules from 2D or 3D-chemical databases, American Chemical Society National Meeting, Symposium on 3D Chemical Structure Handling, New York, NY, Aug. 28, 1991.
78. J. M. Blaney and J. S. Dixon, Distance geometry in molecular modeling, *Reviews in Computational Chemistry*, Vol. 5 (K. B. Lipkowitz and D. B. Boyd, eds.), VCS Publishers, New York, 1994, pp. 299–335.
79. K. P. Clark, Ajay, Flexible ligand docking without parameter adjustment across 4 ligand-receptor complexes, *J. Comput. Chem. 16*:1210–1226 (1995).
80. R. S. Judson, Y. T. Tan, E. Mori, C. Melius, E. P. Jaeger, A. M. Treasurywala, and A. Mathiowetz, Docking flexible molecules—a case-study of 3 proteins, *J. Comput. Chem. 16*:1405–1419 (1995).
81. C. M. Oshiro, I. D. Kuntz, and J. S. Dixon, Flexible ligand docking using a genetic algorithm, *J. Comput. Aided Mol. Design 9*:113–130 (1995).
82. G. Jones, P. Willett, and R. C. Glen, Molecular recognition of receptor-sites using a genetic algorithm with a description of desolvation, *J. Mol. Biol. 245*:43–53 (1995).
83. D. K. Gehlhaar, G. M. Verkhivker, P. A. Rejto, C. J. Sherman, D. B. Fogel, L. J. Fogel, and S. T. Freer, Molecular recognition of the inhibitor AG-1343 by HIV-1 protease—conformationally flexible docking by evolutionary programming, *Chem. Biol. 2*:317–324 (1995).

84. M. C. Lawrence and P. C. Davis, CLIX: A search algorithm for finding novel ligands capable of binding proteins of known three-dimensional structure, *Proteins Struct. Funct. Genet. 12*:31–41 (1992).

85. H.-J. Bohm, The computer program LUDI: A new method for the de novo design of enzyme inhibitors, *J. Comput. Aided Mol. Design 6*:61–78 (1992).

86. H.-J. Bohm, Rule-based automatic design of new substituents for enzyme inhibitor leads, *J. Comput. Aided Mol. Design 6*:593–606 (1992).

87. C. L. M. J. Verlinde, G. Rudenko, and W. G. J. Hol, In search of new lead compounds for trypanosomiasis drug design: A protein structure-based linked-fragment approach, *J. Comput. Aided Mol. Design 6*:131–147 (1992).

88. G. Klebe, The use of composite crystal-field environments in molecular recognition and the de novo design of protein ligands, *J. Mol. Biol. 237*: 212–235 (1994).

89. G. M. Downs and P. Willett, Similarity searching in databases of chemical structures, *Reviews in Computational Chemistry.* Vol. 7 (K. B. Lipkowitz and D. B. Boyd, eds.), VCH Publishers, New York, 1995, pp. 1–66.

90. A. C. Good and J. S. Mason, Three-dimensional structure searches, *Reviews in Computational Chemistry,* Vol. 7 (K. B. Lipkowitz and D. B. Boyd, eds.), VCH Publishers, New York, 1995, pp. 67–118.

91. R. A. Lewis and P. M. Dean, Automated site-directed drug design: The concept of spacer skeletons for primary structure generation, *Proc. R. Soc. Lond. B 236*:125–140 (1989).

92. R. A. Lewis and P. M. Dean, Automated site-directed drug design: The formation of molecular templates in primary structure generation, *Proc. R. Soc. Lond. B 236*:141–162 (1989).

93. R. A. Lewis, Automated site-directed drug design: Approaches to the formation of 3D molecular graphs, *J. Comput. Aided Mol. Design 4*:205–210 (1990).

94. R. A. Lewis, D. C. Roe, C. Huang, T. E. Ferrin, R. Langridge, and I. D. Kuntz, Automated site-directed drug design using molecular lattices, *J. Mol. Graph. 10*:66–78 (1992).

95. R. A. Lewis, Automated site-directed drug design: A method for the generation of general 3D molecular graphs, *J. Mol. Graph. 10*:131–143 (1992).

96. S. R. Kilvingon and A. R. Leach, An algorithm for connecting docked fragments, Molecular Graphics Society Meeting, University of York, UK, Mar. 28, 1993.

97. A. R. Leach and R. A. Lewis, A ring-bracing approach to computer-assisted ligand design, *J. Comput. Chem. 15*:233–240 (1994).

98. P. A. Bartlett, G. T. Shea, S. J. Telfer, and S. Waterman, CAVEAT: A program to facilitate the structure-derived design of biologically active molecules, *Molecular Recognition in Chemical and Biological Problems, Spec. Pub. R. Chem. Soc. 78*:182–196 (1989).

99. G. Lauri and P. A. Bartlett, CAVEAT: A program to facilitate the design of organic molecules, *J. Comput. Aided Mol. Design 8*:51–66 (1994).

100. M. B. Eisen, D. C. Wiley, M. Karplus, and R. E. Hubbard, HOOK: A program for finding novel molecular architectures that satisfy the chemical and steric requirements of a macromolecule binding site, *Proteins Struct. Funct. Genet. 19*:199–221 (1994).

101. C. M. Ho and G. R. Marshall, SPLICE: A program to assemble partial query solutions from three-dimensional database searches into novel ligands, *J. Comput. Aided Mol. Design 7*:623–647 (1993).

102. C. M. Ho and G. R. Marshall, FOUNDATION: A program to retrieve all possible structures containing a user-defined minimum number of matching query elements from three-dimensional databases, *J. Comput. Aided Mol. Design 7*:3–22 (1993).

103. C. M. W. Ho and G. R. Marshall, De novo design of ligands, Proceedings 27th Hawaiian International Conference on Systems Sciences, Biotechnology Computing, Vol. 5, IEEE Computer Society Press, Los Alamitos CA, 1994, pp. 213–222.

104. C. M. W. Ho and G. R. Marshall, DBMAKER: A set of programs designed to generate three-dimensional databases based upon user-specified criteria, *J. Comput. Aided Mol. Design 9*:65–86 (1995).

105. C. M. W. Ho and G. R. Marshall, Cavity search: an algorithm for the isolation and display of cavity-like binding regions, *J. Comput. Aided Mol. Design 4*:337–354 (1990).

106. V. Tschinke and N. C. Cohen, The NEWLEAD program: A new method for the design of candidate structures from pharmacophoric hypotheses, *J. Med. Chem. 36*:3863–3870 (1993).

107. D. E. Clark, A. D. Frenkel, S. A. Levy, J. Li, C. W. Murray, R. Robson, B. Waszkowycz, and D. R. Westhead, PRO-LIGAND: An approach to de novo drug design. 1. Application to the design of organic molecules, *J. Comput. Aided Mol. Design 9*:13–32 (1995).

108. B. Waszkowcycz, D. E. Clark, D. Frenkel, J. Li, C. W. Murray, B. Robson, and D. R. Westhead, PRO-LIGAND: An approach to de novo molecular design. 2. Design of novel molecules from molecular field analysis (MFA) models and pharmacophores, *J. Med. Chem. 37*:3994–4002 (1994).

109. P. W. Rose, Exhaustive search for molecular linkers in structure-based drug design. ACS National Meeting, Mar. 1994, San Diego CA, COMP 50.

110. R. P. Sheridan, A. Rusinko III, R. Nilakantan, and R. Venkataraghavan, Searching for pharmacophores in large coordinate databases and its use in drug design, *Proc. Natl. Acad. Sci. USA 86*:8165–8169 (1989).

111. J. H. Van Drie, D. Weininger, and Y. C. Martin, ALADDIN: An integrated tool for computer-assisted molecular design and pharmacophore recognition from geometric, steric, and substructure searching of three-dimensional molecular structures, *J. Comput. Aided Mol. Design 3*:225–251 (1989).

112. S. E. Jakes and P. Willett, Pharmacophoric pattern matching in files of 3-D chemical structures: Selection of interatomic distance screens, *J. Mol. Graph. 4*:12–20 (1986).

113. Y. C. Martin, 3D database searching in drug design, *J. Med. Chem. 35*: 2145–2154 (1992).

114. Y. C. Martin, M. G. Bures, and P. Willet, Searching databases of three-dimensional structure, *Reviews in Computational Chemistry*, Vol. 1 (K. B. Lipkowitz and D. B. Boyd, eds.), VCH, New York, 1990, pp. 213–264.

115. The *Available Chemicals Directory* (ACD) and a variety of other 3D chemical databases are available from MDL Information Systems, San Leandro CA.

116. Y. Nishibata and A. Itai, Automatic creation of drug candidate structures based on receptor structure—starting point for artificial lead generation, *Tetrahedron 47*:8985–8995 (1991).

117. Y. Nishibata and A. Itai, Confirmation of usefulness of a structure construction program based on three-dimensional receptor structure for rational lead generation, *J. Med. Chem. 36*:2921–2928 (1993).

118. S. H. Rotstein and M. A. Murcko, GenStar 1.0: A method for de novo drug design. *J. Comput. Aided Mol. Design 7*:23–43 (1993).

119. A. A. Cohen and S. E. Shatzmiller, Structure design: An artificial intelligence-based method for the design of molecules under geometrical constraints, *J. Mol. Graph. 11*:166–173 (1993).

120. R. S. Bohacek and C. McMartin, Multiple highly diverse structures complementary to enzyme binding sites: Results of extensive application of de novo design method incorporating combinatorial growth, *J. Am. Chem. Soc. 116*: 5560–5571 (1994).

121. J. B. Moon and W. J. Howe, Computer design of bioactive molecules: A method for receptor-based de novo ligand design, *Proteins Struct. Funct. Genet. 11*:314–328 (1991).

122. J. B. Moon and W. J. Howe, Recent advances in de novo molecular design, *Trends QSAR Molecular-Modelling 92* (C.-G. Wermuth, ed.), ESCOM, Leiden, 1993, pp. 11–19.

123. J. B. Moon and W. J. Howe, Automated receptor-based ligand design: development of the GROW program, American Crystallographic Society/Molecular Graphics Society Meeting, Albuquerque NM, May 1993.

124. K. D. Gibson and H. A. Scheraga, Revised algoriths for the build-up procedure for predicting protein conformations by energy minimization, *J. Comput. Chem. 8*:826–834 (1987).

125. J. Singh, J. Saldanha, and J. M. Thornton, A novel method for the modeling of peptide ligands to their receptors, *Protein Eng. 4*:251–261 (1991).

126. V. Gillet, A. P. Johnson, P. Mata, S. Sike, and P. Williams, SPROUT: A program for structure generation, *J. Comput. Aided Mol. Design 7*:127–153 (1993).

127. V. J. Gillet, W. Newell, P. Mata, G. Myatt, S. Sike, Z. Zsoldos, and A. P. Johnson, SPROUT: Recent developments in the de novo design of molecules, *J. Chem. Inf. Comput. Sci. 34*:207–217 (1994).

128. V. J. Gillett, G. Myatt, Z. Zsoldos, and A. P. Johnson, SPROUT, HIPPO, and CAESA: Tools for de novo structure generation and estimation of syn-

thetic accessibility, *Perspectives in Drug Discovery and Design*, Vol. 3 (K. Müller, ed.), ESCOM, Leiden, 1995.

129. Leapfrog manual, SYBYL version 6.1, Tripos Associates, St. Louis MO.

130. A. W. Payne and R. C. Glen, Molecular recognition using a binary genetic search algorithm, *J. Mol. Graph. 11*:74–91 (1993).

131. J. M. Blaney, D. Weininger, and J. S. Dixon, Conformationally flexible docking and evolution of molecules to fit a binding site of known structure, Molecular Graphics Society Meeting, University of York, UK, Mar. 28, 1993.

132. D. A. Pearlman and M. A. Murcko, CONCEPTS: New dynamic algorithm for de novo drug suggestion, *J. Comput. Chem. 14*:1184–1193 (1993).

133. D. A. Pearlman and M. A. Murcko, Concerts—dynamic connection of fragments as an approach to de-novo ligand design, *J. Med. Chem. 39*: 1651–1663 (1996).

134. A. Miranker and M. Karplus, Ligand perturbation space: An algorithm for de novo ligand design, Molecular Graphics Society Meeting, University of York, UK, Mar. 28, 1993.

135. A. Miranker and M. Karplus, An automated-method for dynamic ligand design, *Protein Struct. Funct. Genet. 23*:472–490 (1995).

136. D. K. Gehlhaar, K. E. Moerder, D. Zichi, C. J. Sherman, R. C. Ogden, and S. T. Freer, De Novo design of enzyme inhibitors by Monte Carlo ligand generation, *J. Med. Chem. 38*:466 (1995).

137. M. A. Hahn, Receptor surface models as a guide to drug discovery, ACS National Meeting, Apr. 2–6, 1995, Anaheim CA, COMP 107.

138. R. Judson, The use of genetic algorithms in chemistry, *Reviews in Computational Chemistry*, Vol. 10 (K. B. Lipkowitz and D. B. Boyd, eds.), VCH Publishers, New York, 1997.

139. S. Y. S. Cho, L. N. Jungheim, and A. J. Baxter, Novel HIV-1 protease inhibitors containing a β-hydroxy sulfide isostere, *Bioorg. Med. Chem. Lett. 5*:715–720 (1994).

140. R. C. Glen and A. W. Payne, A genetic algorithm for the automated generation of molecules within constraints, *J. Comput. Aided Mol. Design 9*: 181–202 (1995).

141. R. Hirschmann, Medicinal chemistry in the golden age of biology: Lessons from steroid and peptide research, *Angew. Chem. Int. Ed. Engl. 30*: 1278–1301 (1991).

10

Recent Advances in the Prediction of Binding Free Energy

Ajay and Mark A. Murcko
Vertex Pharmaceuticals Incorporated, Cambridge, Massachusetts

Pieter F. W. Stouten
The DuPont Merck Pharmaceutical Company, Wilmington, Delaware

I. INTRODUCTION

Most biological processes depend on the ability of molecules to bind and discriminate between one another. Molecular association is essential for many functions [1]. Enzyme catalysis, transport and storage of small molecules, immune protection, and cell growth and differentiation, all are examples that highlight the importance of binding.

Thermodynamics governs the basic physical principles of molecular recognition. The fundamental processes involved in the binding of two or more molecules are similar to those for the folding of proteins. Binding, however, should be a simpler problem compared with folding because a smaller number (10–30) of amino acids, mostly in the active site, are involved. The affinity of two molecules that form a noncovalent complex is described by the change in enthalpy and entropy of the *system*; in other words, by the change in the *free energy* of the system. The system consists of the molecules and solvent (before complex formation) and the complex and solvent (Fig. 1). In general, molecular association depends on the ionic strength and pH of the solution [e.g., see Ref. 2].

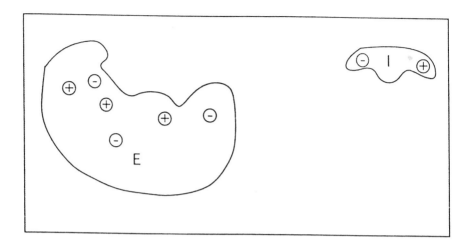

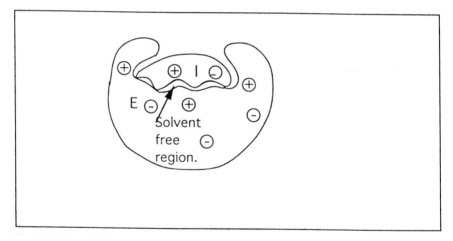

Figure 1 The process of general complex formation in solution: E is the enzyme and I the ligand. Note that both the ligand and the protein change conformation after binding. There is also an associated charge redistribution. Some of the ligand–water and protein–water interactions are replaced by ligand–protein interactions.

Kauzmann's 1959 review [3] can still be profitably read to understand the physical and thermodynamic basis for the contributing factors that govern binding. In early work, Page and Jencks [4,5] attempt a quantitative understanding of the entropic contributions to binding; namely, rotational and translational entropy losses and the loss in entropy on freezing bond rotations. Janin and Chotia [6], in 1978, also contributed to the understanding of binding and protein folding using both entropic contributions and surface area burial (in an attempt to account for the "hydrophobic forces" involved in the reactions).

Structural information gathered over the past three decades has helped us understand many complexes at the molecular level, providing a detailed description of protein–protein, protein–DNA, and enzyme–ligand interactions. Binding can be remarkably sensitive to even small differences in structure. A quantitative knowledge of the binding process is, therefore, essential to understanding molecular recognition. A prediction of binding affinities would be of immense benefit to rational drug design and for protein redesign. To obtain such a prediction we need a detailed understanding of the physical forces involved in the interaction and to be able to predict the importance of each of the forces (electrostatics, van der Waals, hydrophobic, entropic, and so forth) that contribute to the reaction. The major difficulty with all prediction methods is that no general statements can be made about the importance of any single force that is valid for all the complexes that can be formed.

In this chapter we will review some of the recent attempts at predicting binding affinities. Our primary focus is on noncovalent interactions between molecules; hence, the binding of aspirin, for example, will not be considered. Molecular mechanics—one of the fundamental tools for theoretical calculations—cannot treat the formation and breaking of covalent bonds (i.e., the electronic structure) correctly; therefore, the absolute-binding energy of covalent inhibitors will be poorly represented. We do not cover attempts to predict binding energies based on semiempirical quantum calculations in this chapter [7]. Another aspect of ligand binding that we do not address is metal ion binding. Ion binding can often be important for the stability and function of a variety of proteins. For zinc-binding proteins, it appears that sequence homology is sufficient to determine the binding domain [8]. However, different calcium-binding proteins reveal strikingly different folds [9]. Theoretical calculations on ion binding are plagued by very drastic approximations of hydration effects.

Almost all of the methods reviewed here use structural information on the complex. The structure is known either through X-ray or nuclear magnetic resonance (NMR) methods, or it can been modeled using computational methods (experimentally determined structures are preferable).

As such, the binding prediction methods form an integral part of structure-based drug design protocols. Examples of such structure-based design include human immunodeficiency virus (HIV) protease [10] for anti-AIDS agents, thymidylate synthase [11] for anticancer agents, trypanosomal GAPDH [12] for antiparasitic agents, elastase [13] for the treatment of emphysema, glycogen phosphorylase [14] for the treatment of diabetes, and others.

This chapter is organized as follows: We begin with a brief overview of the concepts involved in binding; namely, the binding constant and free energy. Next we discuss the thermodynamics of binding. This is followed by a detailed description of the different contributions to the free energy of binding, including the role of water, conformational strain, specific protein–ligand interactions and so forth. This is followed by a detailed description of the salient features of some of the newer empirical approaches to obtaining the free energy of binding. Throughout our description we concentrate on the assumptions, and, hence, some of the limitations, of the methods. We conclude this chapter with a look at the immediate future of the prediction methods.

II. DEFINING BINDING AFFINITY

Interactions between proteins and ligands involve physical contact between the two species for a certain time period. These contacts are specific and result in an attractive force. The receptor–ligand interactions, in general, are, dependent on the concentration of the ligand, protein, and salts in the solution.

$$RL \underset{k_{-1}}{\overset{k_{+1}}{\rightleftharpoons}} R + L \tag{1}$$

represents a chemical interaction. Here, R is the receptor, L the ligand, RL the receptor–ligand complex, k_{-1} is the association rate constant for the reaction R + L going to RL, and k_{+1} is the dissociation rate constant for the reaction RL going to R + L.

An equilibrium constant (the dissociation constant, k_{+1}/k_{-1}) can now be defined as

$$K_d = \frac{[R][L]}{[RL]} \tag{2}$$

Note that when the magnitude of K_d is small the tendency of RL to dissociate is small (i.e., RL tends to remain as a complex).

A fundamental thermodynamic relation relates free-energy change to changes in enthalpy and entropy,

$$\Delta G = \Delta H - T\Delta S \tag{3}$$

where ΔG is the change in free energy of a reaction, ΔH and ΔS are the corresponding changes in enthalpy and entropy, and T is the temperature of the system. The experimentally measured equilibrium dissociation constant can be related to the free-energy change of the formation of the RL [15] complex by,

$$\Delta G = \Delta G^0 - RT \ln K_d \tag{4}$$

Here R the gas constant and T the absolute temperature. ΔG^0 is the free-energy change associated with the reaction under standard conditions (all reactants and products are present at 1-M concentration, $T = 298$ K, and pressure is 1 atm). At equilibrium we have $\Delta G = 0$, therefore,

$$\Delta G^0 = RT \ln K_d \tag{5}$$

For model (ideal) systems K_d is only a function of temperature; hence, the name equilibrium constant.

The following points must be kept in mind relative to the foregoing discussion.

- Equation (2) shows that K_d has units of moles per liter, but Eq. (5) implies that K_d is unitless. The apparent contradiction is resolved by noting that Eq. (5) should really read as

$$\Delta G^0 = RT \ln \frac{K_d}{c^0} \tag{6}$$

  where, c^0 is the ratio of the activities of each chemical species in the standard state [16]. Therefore, ΔG^0 depends on c^0, the standard state; therefore, when comparing ΔG^0 values, we should be aware of the standard states used in the calculations.
- To be accurate, the quantities [X] (X = R, L, RL) in Eq. (2), are only equal to concentration for ideal solutions. In real systems, concentrations have to be replaced by activities. However, because of the very dilute solutions in which these measurements are made, the conditions of ideality are closely approximated; hence, the differences are often ignored.
- The error in K_d measurements is usually about 10–20%, implying an error in ΔG^0 of 0.1–0.25 kcal mol^{-1} at room temperature (Table 1). Experimental data on enthalpies and heat capacities usually have larger errors.
- An important point is that ΔH is independent, whereas both ΔG and ΔS are dependent on the definition of standard state [15].

Table 1 Importance of Small Differences in Binding Energy for Binding Constant Values at Room Temperature

Change in binding energy (kcal/mol^{-1})	Change in binding constant
0.5	2×
1.0	5×
1.5	13×
2.0	29×
2.5	68×
3.0	158×

In the rest of the chapter, we drop the superscript "0" from all thermodynamic quantities, with the implicit understanding that they always refer to standard states.

It is instructive to note the quantitative relation between a particular change in ΔG_{bind} and the corresponding change in K_i (see Table 1). Notice that a prediction of ΔG with an error of 2 kcal mol^{-1} (not considered unreasonable for most methods) implies an error of about 30-fold in K_i at room temperature!

A. The Measurement of Binding Affinity

Kinetic experiments are used to measure K_i. An important issue to keep in mind concerning K_i measurements is that experiments that involve both the substrate and the inhibitor are not equilibrium measurements unless steady-state kinetics is assumed. More direct K_i measurements (usually called K_d measurements) that do not involve competition with the substrate, however, are equilibrium measurements. All theoretical calculations strive to calculate the ensemble averaged free-energy change. Therefore, all comparisons with experimental numbers should ideally take place when the experiments are done under equilibrium conditions. This condition is often ignored, but this may not be inappropriate, given the current limitations in the theoretical calculations and general difficulties with the experiments.

An IC_{50} value may also be used to measure the interaction of the ligand with a protein [17]. IC_{50} measures the concentration of the inhibitor required to reduce the binding of a ligand (or rate of reaction) by half. However, it is not very suitable for theoretical studies, for it depends on the amount of ligand available to the receptor, and this makes comparisons between data obtained under different conditions impossible. The binding constants (K_i and K_d), on the other hand, can be compared more easily. In principle, $K_i = K_d$. Determination of binding constants requires more data than is needed for the calculation of IC_{50}. The binding constant is usually expressed in terms of a dissociation constant. K_d is defined as the ligand concentration at which 50% of the receptor sites are occupied in a one-to-one complex. IC_{50} values are not true inhibition constants. Therefore, the ratio of two IC_{50} values for two enzymes are equivalent to K_i ratios *only* when the assays are performed under the same conditions and the enzymes have the same K_s (Michaelis constant) values. In general quantification of inhibition is complicated by small values of K_s, substrate inhibition, low values of K_i, multiple conformations of the protein, and rate transients during assays.

Inhibitors bind to enzymes in several ways. Binding may be reversible or irreversible; furthermore, the ligand may bind competitively, noncompetitively, or uncompetitively relative to the substrate. If the ligand competes with the substrate for active site binding, it is *competitive inhibition*. If the ligand binds at a site other than the substrate-binding site (resulting in conformational change in the enzyme and, hence, inhibition of substrate turnover) then it is *noncompetitive inhibition*. If the ligand binds to the enzyme–substrate complex and not to the enzyme it is called *uncompetitive inhibition*. In principle, the binding constants in all these processes are independent of ligand or substrate concentration [18]. Accordingly, comparisons across laboratories can be reliably made.

III. THE THERMODYNAMICS OF BINDING

The free-energy difference between the bound and the free states is the quantity of interest in determining binding constants. We will use superscripts to designate the relevant part of the system, and subscripts to designate the nature of contribution.

$$\Delta G = G^c - G^u \tag{7}$$

where, the superscripts c and u are complexed and uncomplexed, respectively.

The calculation of free energy of binding is not yet an exact science. One of the basic steps that is often used is the factorization of the binding free energy into components:

1. The interaction energy between ligand and protein: Crystallographically identified water molecules are often integral to this. A major portion of the interaction energy is electrostatic. One important factor in a quantitative evaluation of the electrostatic interaction strength is the microscopic dielectric constant, which

is almost never known. The greater the dielectric constant, the smaller the strength of the electrostatic interactions. Many different approximations are made for the dielectric constant for the interior of the protein.

2. *Hydrophobic effect* (i.e., the entropy gain of water owing to the binding of the ligand): The optimization of molecular interactions after a hydrocarbon has been removed from water has less entropic cost than the optimization of molecular interactions with the hydrocarbon in water.

3. Changes in steric interaction energy on binding.

4. Change in conformational energy of the receptor and ligand on binding.

5. The entropy loss in both the enzyme and the ligand owing to rotational constraints about single bonds on complex formation.

6. Overall loss in entropy caused by association: that is, the loss in translational and rotational entropy (ligand and receptor are thought of as rigid entities). The changes in vibrational degrees of freedom also contribute.

The role of crystallographically identified water molecules, or water molecules with a large mean residence time in NMR experiments [19], is often very difficult to interpret, but these water molecules can play an important role in determining binding affinity. For example, noncovalent extensions of DNA bases by water molecules serve as selective recognition sites for specific protein–DNA interactions [20].

The basic assumption in most of the work that is reviewed in this chapter is that different contributions to free energy of binding can be calculated separately and that they are additive. For example, we could separate out the electrostatic and nonpolar contributions, calculate each, and combine the results to obtain the net change in free energy (an approach adopted by the Honig group; later discussion). There are other ways to dissect the interaction energies. Various researchers have adopted different approaches based on the importance of specific contributions to binding in the particular system under study and because of differences in the nature of these interactions.

A common practice (following the model adopted in force fields) is to write the free energy of binding as an additive interaction of different parts. We call this the "master equation." We do this in the following series of equations by first writing it out conceptually.

$$\Delta G_{bind} = \Delta G_{solvent} + \Delta G_{conf} + \Delta G_{int} + \Delta G_{motion} \tag{8a}$$

This accounts for the contributions from (a) the solvent, (b) conformational changes in the protein and the ligand, (c) the specific protein–ligand interactions that comes from their proximity, and (d) the "motion" in the protein and ligand once they are proximal.

$$\Delta G_{solvent} = \Delta G_{hyd} \tag{8b}$$

ΔG_{hyd} is the hydration free energy.

$$\Delta G_{conf} = \Delta G^r + \Delta G^l \tag{8c}$$

ΔG^r is the change in free energy of the receptor on complex formation, ΔG^l is the same quantity for the ligand.

$$\Delta G_{int} = \Delta G^{rl}. \tag{8d}$$

ΔG^{rl} is the change in free energy caused by specific (electrostatics and van der Waals) interactions between the ligand and the receptor.

$$\Delta G_{motion} = \Delta G_{rot} + \Delta G_{t/r} + \Delta G_{vib} \tag{8e}$$

ΔG_{rot} is the free energy contribution from the freezing of the internal rotations of the receptor and ligand, $\Delta G_{t/r}$ is the change in translational–rotational free energy, and ΔG_{vib} is the change in vibrational free energy owing to complexation.

We reiterate that this is just *one* of many ways in which the free energy of binding can be partitioned. Care should be taken, however, to avoid double counting the contribution of certain interactions; these complications can arise when accounting for hydration interactions (discussed later).

Many assumptions are usually made to simplify the analysis. We will detail them in the following. Parenthetically, the assumptions used in free-energy perturbation methods are different from those now listed (see Section IV).

- All the quantities in Eq. (8) should be ensemble averages, for the complex, the free protein, and the ligand are dynamic entities. Flexibility of the molecules is often required for biological activity. However, the most common assumption is that ensemble averages can be replaced by values corresponding to a single stable structure in evaluating the terms in Eq. (8).
- The ligand–protein complex itself is almost always assumed to be a unique structure; that is, it is assumed that the dynamic nature of the complex will not significantly affect binding constants.

- The receptor before complexation is also assumed to be a unique structure; that is, ΔG^r and ΔG^{rl} are the change in free energy on going from a single uncomplexed receptor conformation to a single complexed receptor conformation.
- The ligand is sometimes assumed to be rigid. If the ligand is considered flexible then both ΔG^l and ΔG_{hyd} should involve conformational averages.
- ΔG_{rot} is usually approximated solely by entropy changes. In principle, enthalpy does make some contribution, but it appears that most of the rotational free energy contribution derives from the changes in entropy; hence, enthalpic contributions are ignored.
- $\Delta G_{t/r}$ is often assumed to be a constant, because it varies slowly with mass or moment of inertia. The entropic contribution to this comes from the loss of six degrees of freedom (three translations and three rotations each for the receptor and ligand reduces to six degrees of freedom for the complex). The enthalpy loss comes mainly from the loss in the three degrees of rotational freedom.
- New vibrational modes created on complex formation are either ignored or approximated in a somewhat ad hoc manner.
- The errors and approximations in the force fields (CHARMM [21], AMBER [22], ECEPP [23]) used for estimating the enthalpic and entropic (through Monte Carlo or molecular dynamics simulations) contributions are ignored.
- Strictly, there is a difference between enthalpy and energy. The additional $P\Delta V$ term, however, is negligible in solution.

The term *energy* is used loosely, and often imprecisely, by different authors at different times. *Free energy* is the total energy of the system, and includes both an enthalpic and entropic component (see Eq. [3]). Some experiments yield the free energy of a system or a chemical process, whereas other experiments give energy or enthalpy (spectroscopic and calorimetric experiments are notable examples of the latter case). Often, this distinction is overlooked by theoreticians. For example, molecular mechanics ("force field") calculations do not generally include the effects of zero-point energy, vibrational effects, or entropy; they should best be thought of as energies, rather than enthalpies or free energies. However, the parameters that are developed for these force fields are derived from fitting experimental enthalpies or free energies. Thus, the force field parameters must implicitly be accounting for these effects in some manner.

Both enthalpic and entropic terms contribute to the master equation. The ΔG^r and ΔG^l terms are unfavorable for binding because, in general, the conformational enthalpy of the uncomplexed receptor and ligand will often be lower than that of the complex. The term, ΔG^{rl} favors binding and is entirely enthalpic. The solvation energy (ΔG_{hyd}) is usually favorable for binding at room temperature. The rotational constraints in the term ΔG_{rot}, arising on binding are unfavorable primarily because of the entropic cost of "freezing" the molecule into its bound conformation. However, there is both an entropic and enthalpic part to this, and some of the enthalpic release of heat to the surroundings can be taken up by new vibrational modes (ΔG_{vib}) in the complex. $\Delta G_{t/r}$, which gives the change in translational and rotational free energy, is also unfavorable to binding. The vibrational contribution ΔG_{vib} is favorable to binding (see Sec. V.D).

IV. NONPARTITIONING METHODS: FREE ENERGY PERTURBATION

Free-energy difference methods, such as free-energy perturbation (FEP) and thermodynamic integration (TI), are the only approaches that, in their basic formulation, do not start by partitioning the free energy of binding into different parts (as was done in the foregoing master equation). The basic idea derives from statistical mechanics, and it relates the free energy of a system and the ensemble average of an energy function that describes the system. There have been many excellent reviews of this method in the past few years [see e.g., Refs. 24–26, and references therein], and so we will not go into many details. The method has been reasonably successful in rationalizing many experimental observations and in predictions for ligands binding to proteins [27] and less often for DNA-binding ligands [28]. This is the only method that even attempts to deal seriously with calculating ensemble averages. In addition, it treats solvent molecules and ions explicitly.

Free-energy difference methods suffer from three main drawbacks: sampling difficulties, errors in the force-field, and many "adjustable" parameters. On a microscopic level, equilibrium is ill-defined: one needs to sample a representative section of conformational space at every step of the way. However, in practice, sampling difficulty is effectively a technical problem in the sense that, with better algorithms and faster computers, the major problem of keeping the system in equilibrium during the simulation can be achieved. Also, it is conceivable that better-sampling methods will be devised that, strictly speaking, do not represent a true equilibrium. The force-field errors are more fundamental and reflect, among other things, our inadequate understanding of electrostatics in water. However, progress is being made on this front. One promising direction is the technique of using Ewald sums [29,30], or better still cell-multiple methods [31], to calculate electrostatic contributions without truncation. Another is the attempt to incorporate polarizability through nonadditive potential functions [32,33]. Another phenomenon that requires study is the coupling between the force fields of the explicit solvent and the solute [34]. Torsion parameters and point charges account for most of the "adjustable" parameters in FEP calculations [35]. Of the three, the sampling problem is probably the most important.

Sampling problems and difficulties with parameterization (of atom and bond types and atomic charges) make the routine use of free-energy perturbation methods difficult. However, this is a very promising method with immense potential.

V. INDIVIDUAL TERMS IN THE MASTER EQUATION

In this section we will consider each term in the master equation [see Eq. (8)], and explain the methods adopted to evaluate them. Table 2 summarizes the approach of the different groups.

Our discussion of the master equation approach follows Eq. (8). First we look at the methods adopted to account for the interactions of water molecules. Next we explore methods to account for the conformational contribution to binding. This has two parts: (a) conformational changes in the protein and (b) conformational changes in the ligand. The following section accounts for the interactions between the protein and the ligand once they are in close proximity to one another. Finally, we concentrate on accounting for molecular motion once the ligand and protein are in close proximity to one another.

A. Calculating the Influence of Water

Both the protein and the ligand are solvated before complexation, and they lose their respective solvation shell on complex formation (Fig. 2). Consequently, all protein–ligand interactions compete with interactions with water. But the role of water molecules is still very difficult to characterize accurately. The properties of water do not make it amenable to simple pairwise additive interactions [36]. This has been one of the sources of theoretical difficulty. Both the bulk (long-range hydrophobic effect and dielectric shielding) and specific (hydrogen-bonding) interactions of water are important in elucidating binding. This section is devoted to an overview of some of the attempts to relate the bulk properties of water with a description at the molecular level.

The total free energy of interaction between two molecules can be written as

Table 2 Overview of Recent Work on Prediction of Binding Free Energy[a]

Study/refs.	Methods used and results
Master equation-based methods	
Honig et al. [60,96]	Total free energy change is sum of electrostatic change and hydrophobic interactions.
	Electrostatics obtained from solving Poisson–Boltzmann equation.
	Hydrophobic interactions calculated based on surface area.
Novotny and others [47,69]	Fixed receptor.
	Fixed ligand.
	Surface area-based hydrophobic cost.
	Molecular mechanics-based electrostatic interaction energy (no van der Waals contribution).
	Constant entropic conformational penalty.
	Constant translation–rotation penalty.
	Cratic entropy correction
Shen and Wendoloski [104]	P–B method for electrostatics.
	Surface area-based desolvation entropy.
	No adjustable parameters.
	Only a set of very similar ligands examined.
	No accounting of conformational penalty.
Vajda et al. [71]	Fixed receptor.
	Ensemble average of ligand conformations.
	Molecular mechanics interaction energy (no van der Waals contribution).
	Conformational entropy cost based on X-ray data.
	ASP-based hydration free energies.
	Constant T/R contribution.
	No explicit vibrational contribution.
Williams [70,80] and others [79]	Fixed receptor.
	Fixed ligand.
	van der Waals interactions for hydrocarbons and intrinsic binding constants for polar groups.
	Entropic loss for freezing rotors—a constant.
	Constant for translation–rotation.
	Surface area-based hydration free energy.
	The Andrews work accounts for the terms differently from that of Williams' group.

Table 2   Continued

Study/refs.	Methods used and results
	Regression methods
Böhm [82]	Uses multiple linear regression to estimate the contributions of hydrogen bonding, ionic bonding, surface area buried, number of rotatable bonds in the ligand and a constant. Parameters estimated from crystal structure and experimental K_i values.
Marshall's group [111]	A approach similar to Böhm's. Uses a different set of terms for the regression, a larger database, and two different regression techniques.
Horton [58]	Interaction energy calculated by an extension of the Eisenberg and McLachlan method to separate out atoms involved in hydrogen bonding from those not involved. Constant rotational–translational penalty.
Grootenhuis [93], Holloway [94], Ortiz [95]	Use multiple linear regression based on a molecular mechanics potential function. The details of the terms included and regression methods differ substantially among the three groups.

[a]See text for details.

$$\Delta G(r) = U(r) + \Delta G_s(r) \tag{9}$$

Here $U(r)$ is the direct interaction in the absence of solvent and $\Delta G_s(r)$ is the contribution induced by the solvent. High-level quantum mechanical (gas-phase) calculations for dispersion and electrostatic forces are reasonably accurate, with errors probably in the range of 5–25%. However, water will modify both the electrostatic and dispersion interactions that are observed in the gas phase. As a consequence, for theoretical calculations on the influence of water, there are disagreements, even in the sign of the effect. The effects of approximations are most egregious in estimating solvation contributions.

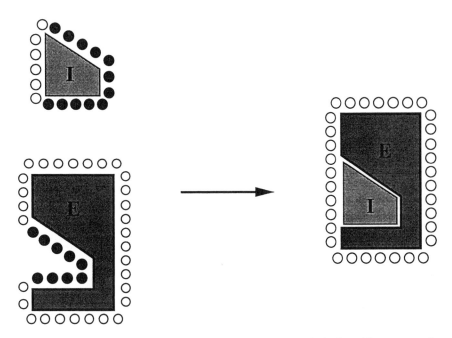

Figure 2 Representation of the desolvation process of binding: The enzyme is labeled E, and the inhibitor is labeled I. The small circles are water molecules. The filled circles are water molecules that are displaced during the binding process. This desolvation process has important energetic consequences.

Experimental Data and Its Interpretation

Changes in free energy, enthalpy, entropy, and heat capacity are measured on transferring compounds from organic liquids to water (experiments have also been done with vacuum-to-water transfer and solid phase-to-water). Almost all of the experimental knowledge of solvation is obtained by these so-called transfer experiments. There is a large literature in this area [e.g., see Ref. 37]. Interestingly, over 30 different scales (based on different model systems) are well correlated [38], suggesting that all of them capture similar information. Another method to evaluate the hydrophobic contributions to the stability of proteins is by introducing conservative point mutations that replace large hydrophobic side chains by smaller ones. The difference in stability can be related to free-energy change. Interestingly, extraction of atomic solvation parameters (see following section) from these methods yield numbers twice as large as those from octanol–water transfer experiments. Attempts to resolve the discrepancy have not been very successful [39, and references therein]. One reason for the discrepancy may be that octanol is not a good model for protein interiors.

Difficulties abound in interpreting these experiments. For example, the amino acid analogue or small organic molecule is assumed to have the same conformation in the two phases, and there is dispute over whether or not (and if so, how?) to account for the entropy of mixing (also known as the Gibbs paradox). This controversy involves the extraction of solvation energies from transfer experiments [see Refs. 40–42 for details].

There are many different methods that have been adopted to account for solvation free energies. For a recent review of some of the ways solvation is modeled see Smith and Pettitt [43] and references therein. We will outline what we consider to be the most promising of these.

Estimating Solvation Effects Based on Surface Area

Many researchers have made the intriguing empirical observation that the enthalpy, entropy, and heat capacity of solvation are strongly correlated with solvent-exposed surface area [44–46]. Attempts at a microscopic explanation of this connection are not entirely convincing [40,42].

Both, ΔC_p, and ΔS_{solv} (the change in entropy of hydration) can be described within experimental error by changes in water-accessible surface area. The relations usually take two forms. The first [46],

$$\Delta S_{solv} = 0.32 \Delta A_{np} \ln\left(\frac{T}{386}\right) \tag{10}$$

relates the entropy from the hydrophobic effect to the nonpolar surface area buried. In Eq. (10) ΔA_{np} is the nonpolar surface area buried in square angstroms, T is in degrees Kelvin, and entropy is in calories per degrees Kelvin per mole (cal K^{-1} mol^{-1}). It says that the complex is stabilized by a constant amount of 0.03 kcal mol^{-1} for every square angstrom of nonpolar area that is buried. A second variant,

$$\Delta G_{hyd} = 25 \, A_{contact}(\text{in calories}) \tag{11}$$

simply relates the hydration free energy to contact surface area on binding [47].

When using surface area-based methods, it is not always clear in the published papers which buried surface area is being measured: (a) just the protein, (b) just the ligand, or (c) both the ligand and the protein. From our master equation point of view, we are interested in the surface area buried in both.

Atomic Solvation Parameters: An Elaborate Surface Area Method

The atomic solvation parameters (ASP) method is a refinement of surface area-based method, described in the previous section. Here, $\Delta G_{hyd} = \sum_i \sigma_i A_i$, where σ_i are the atomic solvation parameters for different types of atoms (five for the Eisenberg and McLachlan model [48]; seven for the Ooi et al. [49] model), and A_i is the averaged solvent exposed surface area for each type of atom. The same formulation is also used by Stouten et al. [50] and Kang et al. [51], in which instead of accessible surface areas, atomic occupancies (volume) are used. It is unclear which of these methods is better. The volume methods seem to have an edge in terms of the speed of calculations, as no complicated derivatives of the surface area relative to atomic coordinates have to be calculated. Also, it is possible to store the appropriate values on a grid [52]. The σ_i is calculated from experimental transfer energies, either from octanol-to-water or gas phase-to-water. This method of calculating ΔG_{hyd} includes both enthalpic and entropic contributions for the least-squares fit; adopted to obtain averaged values of σ_i, is obtained from experimental free energy data. Complications arise when this data is incorporated into binding prediction schemes, because most of the σ_i approaches do not allow for straightforward disentangling of conformational entropy and the entropy water. And even if it were straightforward, partitioning entropy in solvation and conformational contributions cannot be justified from a statistical mechanics perspective.

The original paper by Eisenberg and McLachlan [48] was parameterized such that it could not be used in conjunction with a molecular mechanics potential function. However, Ooi et al. [49] generated parameters that could be used in conjunction with a molecular mechanics (MM) potential function (data from water–gas-phase transfer experiments were used). In addition, fewer assumptions were made by Ooi et al., especially for conformational changes owing to the transfer. Wesson and Eisenberg [53], in later work, also generated parameters that could be used with an MM potential function.

One can make two major objections to ASP-based methods. The first is that, in general, polar (or charged) groups in the interior of the protein would have different hydration energies than groups on or close to the surface [54]. The second, is that hydration free energy of a group depends both on the hydration shell and the *entire* interface between protein and water [55]. The physical meaning of the numeric values obtained from the regression for each atom type is ambiguous. Another problem with the ASP parameters is that they may not complement the molecular mechanics force-field parameters. For details on both these points, see Schiffer et al.

[56]. More fundamentally, the validity of partitioning of solvation free energy into atomic contributions cannot be rigorously justified from a statistical mechanics perspective [57].

It is important to point out an attempt by Horton and Lewis [58] to predict binding. They used two criteria: (a) surface area term from Eisenberg and McLachlan and (b) loss of entropy on complex formation to fit experimental free energy of association of 15 protein complexes. By recognizing that the surface area terms for polar atoms should have different contributions, depending on whether or not they take part in hydrogen bonding or ionic interactions, they assign two additional parameters to the fitting procedure to account for this difference. The contribution by surface area for atoms that take part in hydrogen bonds is assessed separately from the contribution by the surface area of nonpolar atoms. The parameters for each of these and the entropy loss were accounted for by using a linear regression procedure. Excellent agreement (within a couple of kilocalories per mole) was obtained. Note, however, that a double-fitting procedure (one by Eisenberg and McLachlan and the other by Horton and Lewis) is not as reliable as a single one.

An Approximate Nonempirical Treatment of Electrostatics in Water

Still et al. [59] adopt the so-called generalized Born model (the GB/SA model). Here the electrostatic contribution to hydration free energy is modeled by the standard coulombic interaction in addition to a polarization term of the two-charge system,

$$\Delta G_{el} = \Delta G_{coul} + \Delta G_{pol} \tag{12}$$

The coulombic part is given by,

$$\Delta G_{coul} = 166 \sum_{i \neq j} \frac{q_i q_j}{r_{ij}} \tag{13}$$

where q_i is the charge on atom i and r_{ij} is the distance between atoms i and j and the units are kilocalorie per mole (kcal mol^{-1}). The polarization function is,

$$\Delta G_{pol} = -166 \left(1 - \frac{1}{D_0} \right) \sum \sum \frac{q_i q_j}{f_{ij}} \tag{14}$$

where, $f_{ij} = r_{ij}$ for $i \neq j$ and $f_{ij} = a_i$ for $i = j$, q_i is the charge on atom i and r_{ij} is the distance between atoms i and j, a_i is the Born radius of atom i and the units are kilocalorie per mole.

This is an approximate continuum model (see the next item) formulation and avoids repeated solution of the Poisson equation. Next, a fitting procedure is adopted to determine the adjustable parameter in Eq. (14) to approximate the total hydration energy of two atoms in any molecule. It appears that this fitting procedure yields more accurate results for polar molecules than for ionic molecules. To reproduce hydration energies of simple hydrocarbons, Still et al. introduced another term proportional to the surface area, $\Delta G_{cav} = \sigma \sum A_i$, (with a constant of proportionality σ independent of the atom type). The ΔG_{cav} term is added to the ΔG_{el} term to obtain the total contribution of the hydration effect. They refer to ΔG_{cav} as the free energy of cavity formation which, strictly speaking, should be positive and increases with solute size and does not include the dispersion interactions between the solute and water. However, Still et al. use it to represent the total hydration free energy of transfer of nonpolar solutes from gas phase to water.

A Detailed Theoretical Treatment of Electrostatics in Water: The Continuum Model

A very substantial effort has been mounted to understand electrostatics in water over the past decade. The Honig group [60] has been one of the pioneers in this area (the program DELPHI is a contribution from this group). This is an important field, because proteins are polar and an adequate understanding of inter- and intramolecular interactions require models that correctly reflect electrostatics. Most of the recent work focuses on continuum descriptions of solvent or protein–solvent systems and uses the boundary element method (BEM) or finite difference method (FDM). In a continuum description, water molecules are not treated explicitly; instead, the emphasis is on a realistic treatment of the protein– or ligand–solvent boundary.

Most BEM applications solve the Poisson equation and FDM approaches solve the linearized Poisson–Boltzmann (PB) equation. Absolute values of electrostatic energies are very hard to determine with these methods owing to the approximations required to make the numeric methods tractable. One of the major problems with both these methods for calculating solvation energies is the errors induced because of the finite size of the grid; the grid points at which polarization charges are calculated may be at incorrect distances from the respective charged atom. It also appears that the PB approach, as is often used, may not be able to predict the electrostatic contribution to the difference in solvation free energy to better than 2 kcal mol^{-1} [61]. A nice feature of this approach is that it is capable of dealing approximately with both polarization of functional groups and the ions present in the solvent. More details about the FDM approach can be found (see Sec. VII.A).

Bound Water Molecules in Hydration Free-Energy Calculations

The role of bound water molecules can be quite important in elucidating binding free energies. Continuum models may adequately describe bulk water, but they fail where individual isolated water molecules are concerned. Therefore, an alternative approach must be found that properly accounts for the enthalpic and entropic effects of burying water. This is a very difficult and important issue to resolve. Recently, from experimental data on anhydrous and hydrated inorganic salts, Dunitz [62] estimated the entropic cost of a single strongly bound water molecule to be roughly 2 kcal mol^{-1} at 300 K. This number has been disputed by Bryan [63], who showed that much larger increases (up to 6 kcal mol^{-1} at 300 K) are possible. He also suggests that both the entropy of the protein and water can decrease. In our opinion, this contribution will be the hardest to calculate theoretically, compared with all the other contributions to binding free energy. The reason is that distinctions between strongly bound and not-so-strongly bound water molecules are extremely difficult even in experiments.

B. Evaluating the Effects of Conformational Changes

In this section we review the methods adopted to account for contributions stemming from changes in conformation of the protein and ligand owing to their interactions. Figure 3 shows an example of the kinds of changes that can take place.

Protein Conformational Changes (ΔG^r)

In many complexes, the conformation of the receptor does not change much from the uncomplexed structure. In others (e.g., HIV protease), the situation is different, and the protein goes through a large change in its conformation on inhibitor binding.

The process of conformational change of the protein on binding involves the burial of hydrophobic surfaces (desolvation); which enhances binding, and a change in entropy owing to conformational changes (both backbone and side chain); which discourages binding. Its enthalpic component can be obtained by changes in energy from the molecular mechanics potential function. The basic form of a molecular mechanics potential function is,

$$E = E_{bond} + E_{angle} + E_{torsion} + E_{vdW} + E_{coulombic} \qquad (15)$$

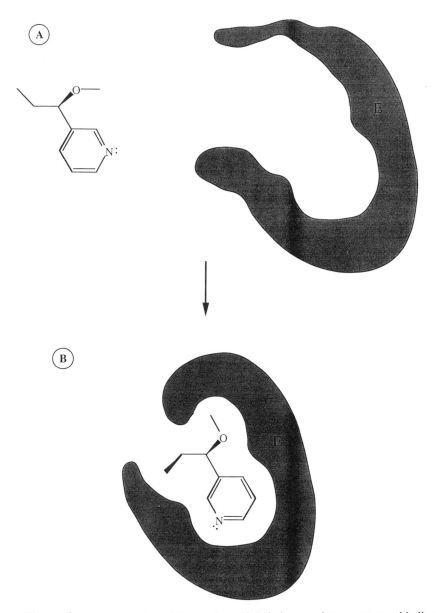

Figure 3 Representation of the conformational changes that accompany binding: The enzyme is labeled E. Both the enzyme and the inhibitor change their conformation on binding. These changes in conformation have important energetic consequences.

The desolvation effects are modeled in two different ways, either using the atomic solvation parameters (ASPs; see Sec. V.A) or by treating this contribution as purely entropic (ΔS_{solv}, the hydrophobic entropy) and estimating it from the change in heat capacity (see Sec. V.A).

Many empirical observations about protein structure can be used in evaluating conformational changes of the protein. For example, certain residues have preferences for different conformational states (α-helix, β-sheet, and such). However, there is controversy over the underlying reasons. Four factors have been identified for bringing about the observed preferences: (a) conformational entropy [64,65], (b) steric factors [66], (c) hydrophobic effects [67], and (d) electrostatics [68]. Knowing which of these factors is most important in a given system would simplify modeling the conformational changes on binding.

Ligand Conformational Changes (ΔG^l)

If it is assumed that a single conformation dominates the free ligand (note that we have already assumed that the bound conformation of the ligand is unique, and structural fluctuations of the bound ligand contribute negligible amounts to the free energy of binding) then the change in the self-energy of the ligand can be calculated in a fashion parallel that of the receptor, as described in the previous section [69,70].

However, in general, it is incorrect to assume that the free ligand has a single dominant conformation in solution. Therefore, ensemble averages (which are relatively easier to calculate here than for the receptor) become important for calculating the internal energy change, the backbone entropy change, and the hydrophobic transfer free-energy change [71].

Statistical mechanics provides a recipe for calculating ensemble averages through the partition function,

$$\langle \Delta E^l \rangle = \frac{\sum_i \Delta E_i^l \exp[-\Delta E_i^l / RT]}{Z} \tag{16}$$

where Z is the partition function [72] and the subscript i is for an individual conformation. A rigorous evaluation of the partition function is almost impossible in a system of reasonable size. However, the average in Eq. (16) can be approximated by sampling a large enough number of conformations of the ligand. If a molecular mechanics potential function is used with explicit waters then the enthalpic contribution, ΔE^l, to ΔG^l can be evaluated. The solvation contribution can also be accounted for using these conformations; that is, the ΔG_{hyd}^l (hydration free energy of the ligand) part of ΔG_{hyd} [see Eq. (8)]. If ASPs are used to account for the solvation contribution, then we have to remember that they are based on the assumption that the conformation of the amino acid residues does not change in the transfer experiments used to derive them. Therefore, an additional entropic term for the torsional freezing, $T\Delta S$, is also present. These entropies are evaluated using the microscopic definition of entropy,

$$S = -R \sum_j p_j \ln p_j \tag{17}$$

where, R is the gas constant, and p_j is the probability for conformation j, and hence $\sum_j p_j = 1$. The estimation of entropies can, again, be based on extensive simulation data, or may be based on experimentally observed distributions, with the probabilities being calculated for each fragment of the ligand [69,71,73]. Such entropy calculations are approximate owing to difficulties in determining p_j.

C. Intermolecular Interaction Energy

The ΔG^{rl} term in Eq. (8) represents the interaction energy. This is purely an enthalpic contribution, so ΔG is being replaced by ΔE. Therefore, $\Delta E^{c,rl}$, the interaction energy in the complex is $E^{c,rl} - E^{f,r} - E^{f,l}$, where $E^{c,rl}$ is the total energy of the complex, $E^{f,r}$ is the energy of the free protein and $E^{f,l}$ the energy of the free ligand. Figure 4 shows one possible set of interactions.

There are two major contributions to the interaction energy, electrostatics and van der Waals interactions. The simplest way to calculate electrostatic interactions is to use Coulomb's law with atom-centered point charges. This is the standard molecular mechanics approach. There are also charge–dipole and dipole–dipole interactions, which are weaker individually, but are larger in number. In general, complex formation can also be accompanied by charge redistribution. Such charge redistribution results in a net attractive force. It is called polarization if it takes place within the ligand or the receptor, and it is called charge transfer, if it takes place between the ligand and the receptor. Almost all calculations based on molecular mechanics potential functions, however, are restricted to charge–charge interactions. The interaction between nonpolar molecules are parameterized as van der Waals interactions. This is a balance between attractive dispersion forces and short-range repulsion.

What Dielectric Constant?

An important issue in treating electrostatic interactions is the answer to the question, "what is the dielectric constant ϵ in the active site?" Many answers to this question have been proposed, ranging from a constant value ($\epsilon = 1$ for vacuum, and $\epsilon = 78$ for bulk water), to being proportional to

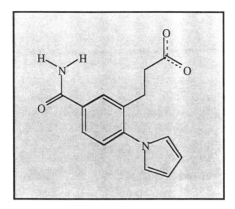

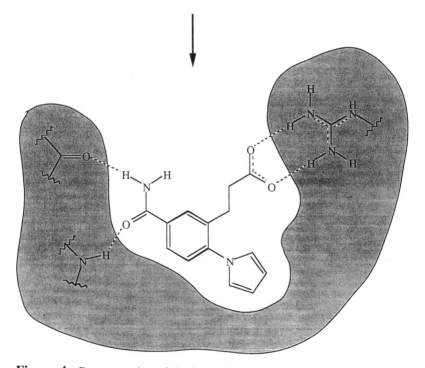

Figure 4 Representation of the interaction energies that drive the binding process: Initially, the ligand and enzyme are each surrounded by water. When the enzyme–inhibitor complex forms, specific hydrogen bonds and van der Waals interactions are made. Some of these interactions are move favorable than those the enzyme and inhibitor were able to make in water. This, in turn, drives the binding process.

the distance between the atoms (a "distance-dependent" dielectric, $\epsilon = r$) and more complicated functional forms [74–76]. The interaction energies can change quite drastically as a result of changes in the dielectric constant. Different researchers use different values for mostly arbitrary reasons. There is neither a theoretically sound nor an experimentally compelling reason to prefer one value of dielectric constant over another. The same is true for the different distance-dependent functional forms that attempt to model the notion of an "effective dielectric constant" [77]. It appears that none of the functional forms in use today can model all the different pair interactions in DNA [78]. On the experimental front, gas-phase, solution-phase, and solid-phase data may be used to justify different dielectrics. Most of the theoretical work has been done in improving the calculation of the electrostatic contribution, including the desolvation effect (see Sec. V.A). Interestingly, the question of the form of the dielectric function has turned out to be important in our docking studies. For example, it is almost impossible to regenerate the docked conformation of methotrexate bound to dihydrofolate reductase (DHFR) if we use $\epsilon = 4r$. However, on using $\epsilon = r$, it is relatively easy to find low-energy conformations close to the crystal structure.* Another complication arises from the differences in the details of the different molecular mechanics potential energy functions. For example, the potential function may describe hydrogen bonds as purely electrostatic, or there may be an additional geometric term.

The Contribution of a Functional Group

Some of the published work replaces the electrostatic contribution to ΔG^{rl} by $\sum_i \Delta G_i$, where ΔG_i is the so-called intrinsic (or apparent) binding energy [4] of the ith functional group in the ligand. Andrews et al. [79] have calculated the average-binding energies of ten functional groups (CO_2^-, OH, CO, sp^2 C, halogens, and such) from 200 drugs and enzyme inhibitors. They assumed that all of the translational and rotational degrees of freedom of the ligand were lost completely on binding. This led to the assignment of unusually large values of intrinsic-binding affinity to the functional groups, unlike in the work of Williams' groups (see later). Usually, ΔG_i contains all the interactions between polar groups, with the assumption that these values are transferable to any ligand interacting with any receptor (perhaps with the restriction of similar environment and solvent). The major motivation for this approach is to be able to answer the

---

*The AMBER molecular mechanics force field has been used for these studies. Note, however, that docking studies are not necessarily a good guide for developing algorithms to predict K_i. For example, it is possible to obtain the correct binding orientations without including the crystallographically observed water molecules.

following question: What is the change in binding energy if a particular functional group has been added to the ligand?

Experimentally, the intrinsic-binding energy for a functional group is obtained by comparing the binding energies for pairs of compounds that differ only in the functional group, with the added assumption (or knowledge) that the two compounds bind similarly (for details, see Williams et al. [70]). The van der Waals contribution is calculated separately, following the molecular mechanics framework. Another feature of this approach is the implicit accounting of the enthalpic contribution when estimating the contribution from desolvation effects. Therefore, care should be maintained to calculate only the entropic contributions to desolvation effects. Williams' group has been very active in the field of binding energy prediction methods using the notion of intrinsic-binding energy of functional groups (see Searle et al. [80] and references therein). They have also contributed to the elucidation of the entropic costs of the translational, rotational, and conformational constraints. One of the peculiarities of attributing free energies to specific functional groups is that the specific values depend strongly on whether vibrational contributions on complex formation (see Sec. V.D) are assigned to functional groups or are treated along with the loss of translational, rotational entropies. It is unclear why an explicit accounting of ΔG_{vib} has not been performed to address this redundancy. One very nice feature of their work (that is not found often in other work) is that they attempt to asses the influence of error in one contribution on the calculation of other contributions. Another important conclusion of the work by Williams' group is that the loss of entropy on binding is significantly smaller than that estimated by Page (i.e., significant vibrational entropy remains in the complex; see the following discussion of ΔG_{vib}).

Some workers [69,71] assume that protein–ligand, protein–solvent, and ligand–solvent interfaces are well packed and, hence, neglect any changes in the van der Waals interaction energy. Others assume that van der Waals interactions can be different in a complex and, therefore, explicitly include them. Incorporation of van der Waals interactions depends on exactly how the other quantities are accounted for (e.g., Williams et al. [70] take into consideration only the nonpolar–nonpolar interactions as the well-packed polar–polar interactions are assumed to be accounted for in the ΔG_i calculations).

Crystallographic Water Molecules

Explicit accounting of crystallographically well-defined water molecules as part of the protein can turn out to be very important for certain systems (e.g., the "flap-water" in HIV protease). Another example is the recent work by Weber et al. [81], who attempt to explain the streptavidin–biotin binding by the number of crystallographic water molecules displaced. Therefore, hydrogen bonding and van der Waals interactions should incorporate the location of the water molecules. The presence of the water molecules should also be accounted for in the calculation of desolvation penalties, although the difference here may not be too significant. Individual water molecules play a role in drug design when functional groups are modified, which could lead to either the creation or removal of cavities large enough to accommodate water.

D. Accounting for Molecular Motion: The Nonstatic Picture of Molecular Interaction

This section considers the methods adopted to incorporate the effects of molecular motion. The approximations involved are underscored by the fact that in various methods the contributions are constant for a given ligand. Loss of torsional freedom (owing to binding) is covered first and then translational, rotational, and vibrational contributions are considered.

The Loss of Torsional Freedom On Binding (ΔG_{rot})

The formation of a complex is associated with the freezing of the internal rotations of both the protein and the ligand. Hence, there is a cost to free energy. This effect is mainly due to the adverse entropic change, although there is some contribution due to enthalpy (changes in kinetic energy). This effect is usually incorporated using a constant [69–71,82] value per dihedral angle that is frozen. Different constant values have been used. One approach to evaluate the loss of conformational entropy of immobilized side chains is to consider that there are three equal states (i.e., three equienergetic states (*trans* and $\pm$ *gauche*) per rotatable bond, therefore,

$$T\Delta S_{rot} = -RT \ln 3 \qquad (18)$$

from Eq. (17) or (19). This leads to a value of approximately 0.7 kcal mol^{-1}. Usually, the rotations of terminal CH_3 and NH_2 groups are not considered.

A third method, developed for treating peptides, but generally applicable, is to approximate the entropy of the free state using,

$$S_i = -R \sum_j p_{ij} \ln(p_{ij}) \qquad (19)$$

where p_{ij} is probability of side chain i to be in state j. Note that this is similar to Eq. (17). These have been estimated using observed frequencies of side-chain conformations by Pickett and Sternberg [83], Sternberg and Chickos [73] who also attempt to estimate the errors involved in their calculations. Creamer and Rose [64] have also built a consistently calibrated conformational entropy scale using Monte Carlo simulations. This conformational entropy scale is consistent with that of the hydrophobicity scale used in ASP formulations, in that the desolvation effects of binding are incorporated separately from the conformational effects. These calculations, as is true for all accounts of solvation contribution, have their own controversies (see e.g., the conclusions in Sternberg and Chickos [73]). There is a difference of approximately five times between using experimental values for the entropy of fusion of small organic compounds [73] and entropy of hydration [45] on the calculated conformational entropy estimates for proteins.

Krystek et al. [69] argue that use of Eq. (18) would be an *underestimate* of the real loss in entropy, based on the argument that restricting one torsional angle would also restrict some others. However, from the analysis of Pickett and Sternberg [83], one finds a range of values for the *effective* number of equienergetic states for amino acid side chains. Interestingly, it turns out that the Krystek et al. [69] value is, in fact, an *overestimate*. This points out the difficulties with qualitative arguments. One important and useful lesson that points out the difficulties in K_i prediction schemes can be found in the Pickett and Sternberg [83] data. Errors generated in estimating ΔG_{rot} by using the Krystek et al. [69] approach can be as large as 1.5 kcal mol^{-1}. Overall the Krystek et al. results are quite good. One possible reason for this is the enthalpy–entropy compensation phenomenon (see Sec. IX for details).

Calculations of backbone entropy that uses an approach similar to the calculation of side-chain entropy are hard to justify. In general, the backbone entropy is a function of the length and the particular sequence of amino acid residues involved, the presence of disulfide bonds, or steric hindrance from side chains.

Translation, Rotation, and Vibrational Changes

The fundamental reason for treating all three contributions together is that often the translational and rotational degrees of freedom of the ligand and enzyme in the unbound state became mixed into the many vibrational states of the complex. However, we continue with the additive assumption. An extreme example of ligand mobility in the complex is exemplified by some very interesting experimental results on the binding of thiocamphor and other ligands to cytochrome P-450$_{CAM}$. Raag and Poulos [84] show that the lack of hydrogen bonds and complementary van der Waals interactions leads to higher mobility of the ligand in the complex; the evidence being provided by the higher temperature factors in the crystal structures than in the camphor complex, and the numerous hydroxylation sites.

When two molecules bind, there is a loss of three rotational and three translational degrees of freedom. There is an enthalpic and entropic contribution to this free-energy loss. The enthalpic contribution can be reasonably expected to be about $3RT$ ($RT/2$ for each degree of freedom). This is usually assumed to be a constant value, independent of the size of the ligand. The entropic contribution, however, is not simple to evaluate accurately. It appears that an overall contribution between 7 and 11 kcal mol^{-1} is agreed on, irrespective of the ligand [4,70,80]. The exact value of this contribution, however, is important only for absolute values of the binding free energy. This contribution would cancel out when comparing different ligands binding to the same receptor.

It is relatively simple to calculate rotational and translational free energies for small molecules, and immensely difficult for larger ones (see, e.g., Hill [72], who has given expressions for translational, rotational, and vibrational entropies in the gas phase). It is believed to be a reasonable approximation to use gas-phase equations to study solution behavior [4,85,86].

1. On complex formation, parts of the translational and rotational freedom appear as new normal modes, namely six new internal vibrational modes. In addition to these six new modes, there can also be a change in the vibrational density of states (the frequency of the vibrational normal modes are altered). It has also been suggested that the complex has lower-frequency modes than those of the uncomplexed protein [4]. A general principle that could be kept in mind is that looser complexes have a larger vibrational entropy than tighter ones.

2. Finkelstein and Janin [85] evaluate that about half of the loss in translational and rotational entropy is compensated by new vibrational modes on binding of bovine pancreatic trypsin inhibitor (BPTI). This results in a net loss of approximately 15 kcal/mol. However, this number appears to be quite large when protein-cleaving experiments are considered [87]. Proteins can be cleaved at one or two sites without loss of stability. If the Finkelstein and Janin estimate of the loss of translational and rotational entropy is correct, what compensates for the loss of 15–30 kcal mol^{-1} in entropy?

3. Conformational entropy: Karplus and Kushick [88] found that both dihedral angle and bond angle variations contribute significantly to the entropy of proteins. However, see detailed criticism of their methods by Edholm and Berendsen [89].

4. The vibrational entropy should be treated quantum mechanically, whereas the translational and rotational contributions can be treated semiclassically. The vibrational contribution can be obtained by calculating the normal modes of the protein before and after complexation (assuming that the anharmonic components cancel). However, this approach completely neglects protein motion. Vibrational contribution to binding is, to a very good approximation, independent of the size of the ligand. This is not true for the solvation effects considered earlier. Therefore, for small ligands that have small solvation contribution, accurate evaluation of the vibrational entropy would be important in accessing binding free energies.

In an early attempt, Page and Jencks [4] derived unfavorable $T\Delta S$ contribution at room temperature in solution of 12–17 kcal mol^{-1} (if one of the components is about 100 to less than 1000 mass units). This value comes from reducing the 12 degrees of freedom (rotations and translations before association) to 6. This number, has held up even in recent work with minor modifications [70]. The loss of the 3 rotational degrees of freedom also results in an enthalpy loss of about 1 kcal mol^{-1}. The translational degrees of freedom do not contribute to enthalpy, for the average translational kinetic energy of a molecule is $3RT/2$ irrespective of whether it is in a gas, liquid, or solid phase. The reason is that on going from the gas to the liquid phase the molecule's motion becomes restricted to a narrower region of space.

VI. QSAR-TYPE APPROACHES

In the previous section we discussed approaches based on the master equation. Here, we discuss a very different phenomenological (rather than physical) method: methods that average-out the contributions from many complexes. The simplest of these procedures have some value from an applications perspective owing to their computational efficiency.

One of the oldest methods that attempts to rationalize the binding of different molecules to a receptor is quantitative structure–activity relations (QSAR). The basic idea is to build a regression model for the biological activity of a number of related compounds, given the physical and chemical properties of the ligands. Many different properties have been used to build regression models [90]. To incorporate the three-dimensional (3D) nature of the binding process the notion of building regression models based on the spatial properties of the ligands (e.g., electrostatics) has been introduced. There is now a large body of research on 3D-QSAR methods [91].

3D-QSAR can be quite powerful and useful. However, there are two major reasons why a regression model in 3D-QSAR can be misleading:

1. The binding mode of a given ligand is not known, a priori. This effectively has to be guessed either by aligning similar ligands based on their properties, or by aligning them based on the receptor interactions that are present (if known). Obviously, the regression will be more predictive if the alignment is done based on the properties of the receptor-binding site.
2. The problem is underdetermined (i.e., there are a much larger number of possible regressors compared with the ligands). This implies that standard regression methodology will yield incorrect results and some kind of biased regression method has to be used [the term *biased* is used here in a strict statistical sense and is not meant in the literal sense of the word], the most common one being partial least-squares (PLS). Usually, many equivalent models can be built using the regression approach. A method that has been recently developed that combines these different models [92] to build a higher-level model could be useful to enhance predictive power.

A. Predictions Based on Molecular Mechanics Energy

Recently, there have been attempts to generate QSAR-type regression equations based on a molecular mechanics energy function [93–95] yielding reasonable results. These methods ignore (a) the influence of the solvent almost completely and (b) the influence of difference between bound and unbound conformations of the ligands to different degrees. These procedures assume that the bound conformation of the ligand and protein are known or can at least be well approximated. There are fundamental limits to this approach that arise from the neglect of entropic penalities and solvation contributions. Therefore, the success of these methods depends on the ability to carefully define the set of ligands on which predictions will be applied which, in turn, is difficult to accomplish a priori. An interesting conclusion (stated without any details) in the Holloway et al. [94] work is that "attempts to incorporate these [flexibility of ligand and receptor, solvation] effects into a prediction model have been thus far unsuccessful in improving the observed correlation." In any event, it appears that the purely molecular mechanics-based approaches may be useful in a congeneric series.

VII. THE NEW EMPIRICAL FUNCTIONS APPROACH

All approaches to prediction of binding affinity are empirical. The degree and nature of empiricism differs. For example, free-energy perturbation uses the parameters developed for a particular force field. In a similar vein, the Poisson–Boltzmann approach requires adjustment of van der Waals radii and atomic charges so that solvation free energies are reproduced. Such indirectly generated parameters are then used within a particular scheme to predict binding free energies. Other methods, directly parameterize an equation by regressing on the binding affinity for a series of complexes. In this section we provide a brief and critical overview of some of the recent literature in the field.

A. Master Equation-Based Methods

Contributions from Honig's Group

The very compute-intensive free-energy perturbation and integration methods aside, the approach to calculating binding affinities that is most solidly rooted in physics and statistical mechanics is probably the one taken by the Honig and Sharp groups [60,96]. They separate the binding free energy into electrostatic and nonpolar contributions. The electrostatic interactions and solvation contributions are evaluated by numerically solving the Poisson–Boltzmann (PB) equation, whereas the nonpolar contributions are calculated using a surface area term. Fast multigrid methods [97] and other approaches are available to solve the PB equation. One of the big advantages is that a physical model (including ionic strength) lies at the basis of this approach, and its functional form is not arbitrarily chosen (as in several of the approaches detailed later), but within the limitations of the approximations derives directly from the physical description. The problem with arbitrary functions is that they may fit well the training data, but may break down as soon as the function is applied to situations outside the training set. Indeed, several of the more empirical regression approaches work well for only one receptor with a set of very similar ligands. The choice for a "physically realistic" or phenomenological approach depends on whether one aims for a general method to predict binding affinities a priori, even for systems for which no experimental data are available, or for an ad hoc method that quickly and specifically derives a prediction model from available experimental data. A disadvantage of Honig and Sharp's PB approach is that they assume only two dielectrics, one for the explicitly described solute ($\epsilon = 1$ or 2) and one for the continuum solvent, with a sharp boundary between them. They also disregard atomic polarizability of the solute, which may be very important at the surface. Furthermore, they scale the point charges (derived from ab initio data or taken from existing force fields) and atomic radii of the solute to reproduce experimental solvation free energies, leading to average errors of 0.4 kcal mol^{-1} for the test set of 67 small molecules and 0.1 kcal mol^{-1} for amino acid side chain and peptide backbone analogues. Fitting charges and radii may be justified as long as one does not allow any internal degrees of freedom within the solutes, but when adding their solvation–electrostatics description to a molecular mechanics force field, the balance of the different terms may be upset. It seems that if one takes atomic polarizability into account in some form this will eliminate several of the drawbacks of their approach, and it may well be essential for a proper description of solute–solvent boundaries. Note that this criticism applies much more severely to several other approaches described here, which are generally much more simplistic and approximate than Honig and Sharp's.

The description of nonpolar contributions by Honig and Sharp is somewhat empirical. They attempt to let their microscopic hydrophobic treatment resemble a physically realistic macroscopic model. Their model is based on the observation that the transfer free energy of unbranched alkanes from vacuum to water varies linearly with their solvent-accessible surface areas, as calculated with a very accurate, modified Shrake and Rupley algorithm [98]. The proportionality constant, γ would be comparable with the marcroscopic surface tension. However, Flory [99] and Huggins [100] have shown that solute volume as well as surface may contribute to solubility of alkanes. Interestingly, at different temperatures the entropy–enthalpy balance of hydrocarbon solubility differs, but the free energy of transfer varies little. The most serious shortcoming of Honig and Sharp's method is that it applies only to static structures. It cannot be combined with a molecular mechanics force field in a straightforward manner. Therefore, enthalpic and entropic consequences of any conformational changes occurring on binding of a ligand to a receptor cannot be accounted for. Efforts are underway [Gilson, personal communication] to calculate PB derivatives so that combination with a molecular mechanics force field becomes possible.

Contributions from Novotny and Co-workers

Novotny and others [47,69] partitioned their binding or complexation (free) energy in electrostatic interactions with molecular mechanics charges, an entropic conformational penalty, a surface area-based hydrophobic term, and constant translational–rotational and cratic entropic contributions. They use a distance-dependent dielectric, that although widely used has no sound physical basis. They did not consider intramolecular (strain) or van der Waals dispersive and repulsive energies. Therefore, their approach suffers from drawbacks similar to Honig and Sharp's approaches, detailed in the foregoing, in that they will be able to calculate binding free energies only when the binding mode of the ligand to the receptor is known. That binding mode can have been determined either by X-ray crystallography or NMR, or modeled using, for example, a regular molecular mechanics approach. In principle, strain and van der Waals terms could easily be added to Novotny's method. That this was not done may be due to any combination of the following: (a) a priori, van der Waals and internal strain contributions are expected to be relatively small, especially when one uses energy-minimized, properly resolved crystal structures; (b) many force fields, even fairly sophisticated ones, still have problems reproducing energy minima of a simple tetrapeptide [101]; (c) taking these contributions into account did not improve the correspondence with experimental data. With their rigid ligand as well as receptors, they also had to make assumptions about the differences in mobility of their solutes before and after complexation to be able to assess the conformational entropy penalty. Indeed, they assume that single bonds became locked in one of three equi-energetic states (*gauche-*, *gauche+*, or *trans*) as a result of surface side-chain immobilization on binding. For each bond that is frozen, an entropic penalty of $RT \ln 3$ is paid. Better, but more expensive, methods would involve conformational sampling of the free solutes and of the complex using techniques, such as molecular dynamics, Monte Carlo, or exhaustive sampling of a limited set of rotatable bonds.

The hydrophobic term is proportional to the amount of buried hydrophobic surface. The gain in free energy on burial is 25 cal mol^{-1} A^{-2} [102]. The translational–rotational and cratic entropic contributions are assumed to be constant for the association of two molecules. The free-energy increase of the complex owing to the loss of translational and rotational degrees of freedom has been estimated by Page and Jencks [4] as 7–11 kcal mol^{-1}. Novotny et al. use the median value of 9 kcal mol^{-1}. The absolute entropy of a compound in solution depends on its concentration (recently very clearly explained by Janin [103]). The cratic entropy term of 2 kcal mol^{-1} accounts for the fact that all calculations are carried out for molecules that are assumed to be in their standard states (1 mol L^{-1}), whereas the experimental values refer to (ideally) infinite dilution. Note that this cratic entropy calculation assumes a 1:1 binding stoichiometry [3].

When comparing the association of different ligands and receptors (i.e., when calculating $\Delta\Delta G$ values), those entropic contributions cancel out each other. However, calculating absolute binding or association free energies aids in assessing whether the calculated components of the binding free energy add up to a value that is comparable with experimental data. With X-ray coordinates, Novotny et al. applied their method to the calculation of binding free energies of antigen–antibody and inhibitor–enzyme complexes. Ignoring two clear outliers, the deviations from experimental values were on the order of 2 kcal mol^{-1}, consistent with the estimated error of 4 kcal mol^{-1} in the calculated binding free energies. It should be noted, however, that these results imply errors in calculated K_i of a factor of 100–300. The structure of one of the two outliers (kallikrein–BPTI) was determined at very low pH, and the discrepancy between measured and calculated binding free energy was attributed to the protonation of an unknown number of carboxylates that were considered to be deprotonated in the calculations. The electrostatic free energy of the complex is markedly more negative in this instance than for the other complexes. One would expect that if the experimental structure was indeed affected by the low pH, the electrostatic interactions in the complex would be optimal of that pH and, if anything, the calculated electrostatic energy would be less favorable when incorrect protonation states are assumed. The second outlier concerns trypsinogen–BPTI. Here, too, the favorable-binding free energy calculated is an overestimation. The authors speculate that trypsinogen must undergo a conformational change before binding to BPTI. Because no intramolecular contributions are taken into account, this could not have been predicted on the basis of their calculations. Most (if not all) other methods would also fail in situations during which considerable conformational changes occur. The authors conclude that their method gives semiquantitative results. Some interesting biologically relevant observations were made as well: (a) decomposition of ΔG into component terms suggested that only a small number of amino acids contribute actively to binding energetics; (b) the most productive enzyme-contacting residues in all inhibitors were found in analogous positions on their respective binding loops; thus, the calculations revealed a functional, energetic motif that parallels the structural similarity of the binding loops; and (c) amino acids with side chains that incur no conformational entropic penalty on complex formation (Pro, Ala, Gly) are abundant in the interfaces of several inhibitor–enzyme complexes, whereas aromatic and polar side chains predominate on binding surfaces of antibodies. This suggests that different classes of molecules harness the free energy of binding in different ways.

Contribution by Shen and Wendoloski

An interesting, very basic approach has been presented by Shen and Wendoloski [104]. Their premise is that the two major contributions to binding affinity are electrostatics and desolvation entropy. This implies that a good steric fit is assumed a priori. The finite difference Poisson–Boltzmann Program UHBD [105] is used to describe the electrostatics, whereas the solvation entropy is taken to vary linearly with solvent-accessible surface, independently of the (polar or nonpolar) nature of that surface. Their method, which contains no fittable parameters, was applied to binding affinity prediction of a series of 13 phosphorus-containing partially peptidic thermolysin inhibitors. The rms deviation between observed and predicted relative-binding affinities was 1.12 kcal mol^{-1}. This good correspondence is because the inhibitors are very similar and probably bind in similar fashions, with comparable conformational strain and entropy. In fact, in the only example for which conformational flexibility may play a substantial role (an inhibitor leucine-to-phenylalanine mutation), the deviations are considerably larger (1.9–2.3 kcal mol^{-1}). Also, on repositioning of the phenylalanine side chain and subsequent energy minimization, the deviation became larger, which exemplifies the problem of using different techniques and tools for docking and for evaluation of binding affinities. The authors attribute the deviation for the leucine-to-phenylalanine mutant partly to errors in the solvation entropy estimate: the experimental value for the solvation of propane is greater in absolute magnitude than that of benzene, but the surface area-based solvation entropy term gives the reverse. Free-energy perturbation calculations had been carried out previously for two inhibitor mutations also studied by Shen and Wendoloski. The affinity differences calculated by the present method for these mutations are of an accuracy comparable with the FEP calculations. Interestingly, by analyzing the binding contributions of individual residues, the authors show that the energy of a hydrogen bond is not confined to the donor and acceptor. Shen and Wendoloski have demonstrated that, in a well-behaved system, the electrostatic energy and empirically derived solvation entropy can account for most of the binding energy differences between fairly similar inhibitors, but we suspect that in its present form their method will not be able to predict binding affinity differences for arbitrary systems.

Contributions from Vajda and Co-workers

Vajda et al. [71] follow a scheme that is very reminiscent of Novotny's [69], but that remedies some of its drawbacks. The contributions to the binding free energy in their scheme are electrostatic energy with $\epsilon = 4r$, an entropic backbone and side chain conformational penalty, a surface area-based solvation term, and constant translational–rotational and cratic entropic contributions. They assume a rigid receptor, but to properly account for flexibility of the ligand, they calculate ensemble averages of the differences in ligand solvation free energy and internal energy over numerous conformations. They assume (as Novotny does) that the system of solvent and solutes is well packed; therefore, the van der Waals interaction energies can be neglected, even though this might not necessarily be justified [106]. Moreover, this assumption need not be made unless incorporating van der Waals terms leads to undesired side effects, but we are not aware of such effects. Vajda et al. use a more sophisticated scheme than Novotny to estimate side-chain and backbone entropic differences on binding. Pickett and Sternberg [83] had estimated the entropy of amino acid side chains in the free state based on an analysis of crystal structures. The entropy S_j of side chain type j is defined in Eq. (19). Vajda et al. assumed that the entropy loss is proportional to the side-chain surface area that becomes buried. For the loss of backbone entropy on binding, they used a similar formalism. Similar to Novotny et al., they use constant translational–rotational and cratic entropic penalties (of 7 and 2 kcal mol^{-1}, respectively).

They employ a solvation term (similar to Eisenberg's [48,53]) that relates the total free energy of solvation (hydrophobic and hydrophilic, enthalpic and entropic contributions) to exposed surface areas. The experimental solvation free energies used to derive the solvation parameters represent an average overall water configurations and over all conformations of the ligand. Although done by many authors, it is unclear what the consequences are if one adds such a solvation term to a method that generates conformations explicitly and subsequently reaverages solvation free energies over many conformations. They used octanol–water partition coefficients to derive solvation parameters (i.e., proportionality constants that relate the surface area to the free energy of solvation). To be able to use octanol–water, rather than vacuum–water, transfer free energies, they again have to make the assumption that van der Waals contributions can be ignored. It is unclear why they do not use vacuum–water transfer free energies. The Vajda approach is different from Novotny et al., who used a solvation term that accounted for only the hydrophobic effect. Novotny's implicit assumption was probably that a dielectric of $4r$ attenuates the coulombic interactions, especially the longer-range ones, and thus, in an average fashion, accounts for desolvation of polar groups. It is doubtful, however, that any simple dielectric scheme will properly describe solvation effects. Vajda's results indicate that his approach is not likely to circumvent the electrostatics–solvation problem either (e.g., exhibiting itself in the tendency of exposed side chains of opposite polarity to move toward each other, rather than to stick into solvent). In fact, improper treatment of electrostatics and solvation are probably responsible for most of the problems in generating atomically realistic-binding modes of ligands to receptors and accurately evaluating the associated binding free energy.

To evaluate their method, the authors elegantly applied it to three data sets for which increasingly general methods are required. The first set is Novotny's endopeptidase–protein inhibitor complexes [69]. This set consists of proteins that do not change conformation on binding and for which the major contribution to the solvation free energy is entropic. Disregarding the two outliers (kallikrein–BPTI and trypsinogen–BPTI), the rmsd between the experimental and calculated binding free energy is 1.3 kcal mol^{-1} with Vajda's method and 2.4 kcal mol^{-1} with Novotny's. Vajda et al. observe a similar discrepancy between experimental and calculated values for trypsinogen–BPTI; however, their calculated value for kallikrein–BPTI is much closer to experimental data. It appears that small errors in force-field parameters had led to an unrealistic, highly favorable electrostatic interaction in Novotny's structure. This is a strong indication that defects in force fields may constitute a serious problem in predicting binding modes and affinities. The second data set compares the binding free energies of biotin and two analogues to streptavidin. Here, the structures are also rigid, but the solvation free energy needs to include both enthalpic (polar) and entropic components. Encouragingly, the predicted free-energy differences are approximately the same as those obtained by free-energy perturbation techniques, and differ from the experimental values by only 0.2 and 0.5 kcal, respectively. The final application is a comparison with the measured stabilities of 13 different major histocompatibility complex (MHC) receptor–peptide complexes. Here both enthalpic and entropic effects play a role as well as flexibility of the small peptidic ligands. The authors show that flexibility contributes 30–50% of the free-energy change and find a correlation of 0.88 between predicted free energies and peptide dissociation times. It is gratifying to see that their method does so well on increasingly more complicated problems. One might hope that the method is general enough that, with some additional modifications, even more difficult problems can be tackled.

Contributions from Williams' Group

In contrast with some of the previously described approaches that mainly focused on protein–protein interactions, Williams et al. [70,80] studied dimerization of small molecules and binding of very short peptides to antibiotics. In principle, this should allow more precise pinpointing of problems in predicting affinities of small molecular nonpeptidic ligands to macromolecular receptors than the other approaches. They partition binding free energy in translational–rotational terms (including cratic entropy), an entropic conformational penalty (0.8–1.2 kcal mol^{-1} per frozen rotor), a surface area-based hydrophobic term (-48 cal mol^{-1} A^{-2} of ligand buried), and a term that accounts for polar interactions. They note that differences in conformational strain and van der Waals interactions between the free and bound ligands play a role, but in their calculations they do not allow flexibility in the receptor or ligand, and they assume unstrained binding and van der Waals interactions that are always optimal and do not depend on the state (i.e., free or bound) of the ligand. Their partitioning is very much like Novotny's [69], but rather than an explicit coulombic term, Williams et al. use intrinsic binding energies (ΔG_p) that represent polar interactions between functional groups at a geometry that is supposed to be optimal for binding. The intrinsic-binding energy for each pair of interacting polar groups can be derived from experimental values after the other (translational, rotational, conformational, and hydrophobic) contributions have been subtracted. The advantage of this formalism over a coulombic description is that the ΔG_p values implicitly account for the desolvation of polar groups (a term that is largely absent in Novotny's approach). The disadvantages are that for each pair of polar interaction types ΔG_p values must be fitted to experimental data, that there is no a priori reason to assume that these ΔG_p values are transferable between environments (e.g., as noted by Böhm [personal communication], in practice, very different coulombic energies are associated with exposed and buried polar interactions), and that it is very difficult to account for suboptimal binding modes.

Williams et al. found that considerable residual relative motions remain in the complex after association. For crystallization of diketopiperazine from aqueous solution (as a model for biomolecular association) they concluded that the molecule loses only about 38% of its translational and rotational free energy (G_{t+r}). ΔG_p values are intended to be transferable and to apply equally well to monomolecular (e.g., protein folding) and bimolecular association. Therefore, the entropic contributions of the residual motions should not be incorporated in the ΔG_p parameters. These contributions were estimated on the basis of literature data on the fusion, sublimation, and dissolution of model compounds. Williams et al. argued that the translational and rotational free energies (G_{t+r}) of the free ligand and the free energy associated with its residual motions in the complex are both proportional to the logarithm of the ligand's mass. Therefore, to a first approximation, the net increase in G_{t+r} is independent of the ligand's mass. However, this leads to an apparent paradox: dimerization of γ-butyrolactam, δ-valerolactam, and ϵ-caprolactam in CCl_4 has $T\Delta S$ values ranging from -2.4 to -6.7 kcal mol^{-1}, whereas on the basis of the foregoing reasoning, one would have expected very similar values. In this instance, however, there are also compensating large differences in dimerization enthalpies leading to overall dimerization free energies with a much smaller range (-3.1 to -3.6 kcal mol^{-1}). The enthalpy–entropy compensation observed here for the lactam dimerizations (i.e., the greatest exotherm interaction paying the largest entropic penalty) is a well-known phenomenon that is of general relevance to binding interactions of biological importance. If we recall that ΔG_p is defined as the polar interaction at optimum-binding geometry, it is evident that to calculate ΔG_p values not only the residual motions in the complex should be taken into account, but also an enthalpic term that accounts for deviation from ideality. It is noteworthy, however, that within this formalism, one cannot replace ΔG_p terms with actual coulombic interaction terms. Using ΔG_{t+r} values that were properly corrected, idealized free energies (i.e., ΔG_p values) for amide–amide hydrogen bond formation in a lactam dimer and in peptide–antibiotic complexes were obtained that are in good agreement with the range of -0.5 to -2 kcal mol^{-1} derived from protein-engineering experiments [107,108]. However, the values they obtained ranged from -0.2 to -3 kcal mol^{-1}. No explanation was given for this deviation, but it may well be that the description in terms of ΔG_p referring to ideal hydrogen bonds without any possibility to account for deviations from ideality (as that is made an implicit part of ΔG_{t+r}) is one of the causes. Williams et al. also varied two of the less precisely determined parameters (hydrophobic solvation parameter and entropic loss per frozen rotor) between reasonable values and obtained average values for ΔG_p ranging from -0.2 to -1.7 kcal mol^{-1}. The numeric results do not seem precise enough to have any predictive value, but a very useful comparison between the calculated values and data stemming from many different sources was made and qualitative agreement was obtained. The careful analysis of all possibly relevant contributions to binding free energies provide great insight in the issues involved. Williams et al. have written a set of truly pioneering papers, with interesting, novel approaches.

B. Regression-Based Methods

Contribution by Böhm

Böhm [82] has made an interesting and ambitious attempt to adopt a linear regression approach to describe binding with five well-chosen variables. He partitioned the binding free energy $\Delta G_{binding}$ as following:

$$\Delta G_{binding} = \Delta G_0 + \Delta G_{hb} + \Delta G_{ion} + \Delta G_{hyd} + \Delta G_{rot}$$

$$\Delta G_{hb} = k_{hb} \sum_{hbonds} w(r,\alpha)$$

$$\Delta G_{ion} = k_{ion} \sum_{ionic} w(r,\alpha) \tag{20}$$

$$\Delta G_{hyd} = k_{hyd} A_{hyd}$$

$$\Delta G_{rot} = k_{rot} N_{rot}$$

All ΔG values on the right-hand side are parameters to be fitted by linear regression. ΔG_0 represents loss of overall rotational and translational degrees of freedom. ΔG_{hb} and ΔG_{ion} are the free energies of ideal hydrogen-bonded and ionic interactions, respectively, whereas the weighting function $w(r,\alpha)$ depends on the deviation from the ideal interaction geometry. ΔG_{hyd} is the free energy owing to burying hydrophobic surface area (A_{hyd} is the size of this surface area). ΔG_{rot} is the free energy loss for freezing the rotatable bonds in the ligand (N_{rot} is the number of bonds that become frozen). The k values and ΔG_0 are determined by linear regression and the function $w(r,\alpha)$ is predefined. Böhm and Williams [70] use similar terms in their binding free-energy equations, but where Williams predetermines all but one parameter (with substantial uncertainties) and attempts to fit the final parameter (that accounts for polar interactions) to binding energy data, Böhm optimizes all parameters simultaneously by fitting to binding data. Also, Williams did not differentiate between ionic and neutral hydrogen-bonded interactions, which turn out to be associated with substantially different free energies in Böhm's free-energy (or scoring) function.

Böhm used binding affinities, and models or crystal structures of 45 protein–ligand complexes to derive his parameters. His function reproduces the binding free energies (ranging from -2.2 to -18.2 kcal mol^{-1}) of the data set, with a standard deviation of 1.9 kcal mol^{-1}, corresponding to 1.4 orders of magnitude in binding affinity. The parameters take on the following values: $\Delta G_0 = +1.3$ kcal mol^{-1} (± 2 kcal mol^{-1}; the least precise parameter); $k_{hb} = -1.1$ kcal mol^{-1}; $k_{ion} = -2.0$ kcal mol^{-1}; $k_{hyd} = -41$ cal mol^{-1} A^{-2}; $k_{rot} = +0.33$ kcal mol^{-1}. Although in principle, physically unrealistic values can result from an unbiased-fitting procedure, that does not seem true here: an ideal hydrogen bond was earlier found to give about -1.3 kcal mol^{-1}; [81,107,108]. Williams [80] had estimated ΔG_{hyd} as -48 cal mol^{-1} and the present ΔG_{rot} value is not unreasonable, if one assumes that typically only 30–40% of the free energy of rotors is lost on freezing. The equation obtained also seems to have reasonable predictive ability in the examples considered. Böhm's function is very simple, and it has obvious limitations. For example, regression methods, such as Böhm's, cannot predict complexes that fall well outside its training set. One reason for this derives from unpaired buried polar groups in the protein–ligand interface that are strongly adverse to binding, will generally not be observed, and consequently, will not be part of the training set of those regression methods. The same reasoning applies to (potentially severe) steric clashes and internal strain energy. Regression methods will not put a penalty on such binding modes, and their binding affinities will be overestimated. Böhm's function has a tolerance for certain types of poor interactions, and if one intends to use his scoring function in a predictive capacity, one has to prescreen binding modes and either accept or reject them (as Böhm does with his program LUDI [109]), or use a hybrid method with standard molecular mechanics bonded and van der Waals terms (as Marshall et al. next section). On the other hand, the advantage of having some tolerance is that predictions on the basis of model complexes (rather than crystal structures) do not suffer from the assumption of a rigid receptor. A good example is given in Böhm's paper: 3PTB is the crystal structure of trypsin plus benzamidine. Benzamidine does not fit well in trypsin from 2PTC (trypsin plus BPTI), for which (through induced fit) narrower S1 pocket accommodates the slimmer lysine side chain. A standard molecular mechanics energy evaluation found benzamidine in 3PTB trypsin much more favorable than in 2PTC trypsin. Böhm's scoring function ranks them equally well: the calculated 3PTB and 2PTC K_i are 3.3 and 3.0 M, respectively. Also, in our experience [and Böhm's, personal communication], the strength of contributions of different terms in the equation is highly dependent on the complexes included in building the regression. The method seems to well predict changes in free energy caused by changes in surface area burial, but predicts the effects of changes in hydrogen bonds less well. The contribution toward a hydrogen bond in the Böhm scheme depends on the details of the radial and angular interactions and, therefore, will be very dependent on how the hydrogens are added to donor atoms. In addition, the contribution to binding (or stability) of hydrogen bond formation depends highly on the environment in which the hydrogen bond is formed (e.g., due to different local dielectrics) and values ranging from -2 to -10 kcal mol^{-1} have been obtained (see Dill [110] for details on the difficulty of estimating this number). To remedy some of the defects described here, Böhm has more recently developed an improved scoring function that is based on 82 protein–ligand complexes of known 3D-structure and associated binding constants. This new function differentiates between buried and solvent-exposed hydrogen bonds on a continuous scale and takes into account the replacement of water molecules from the binding site. It reproduces the binding constants of the data set with a standard deviation of 1.7 kcal mol^{-1} [Böhm, personal communication].

Contribution by Marshall's Group

Head et al. [111] have taken an approach that bears some resemblance to Böhm's [82], but is different in several aspects. Their aim, just as Böhm's, is to derive a universally applicable function for the prediction of the affinity of ligands for receptors of known three-dimensional structure. This function should be especially useful in the early stages of the ligand design process, when one often lacks a set of diverse ligands with measured affinities to calibrate traditional QSAR methods. Böhm identified a small set of independent parameters that should cover all aspects of binding and obtained physically realistic values for those parameters. Heat et al. use a set of 12 (potentially dependent) properties, that all seem to capture various portions of the binding free energy to various extents. These properties were analyzed with partial least-squares and neural network techniques. No results using standard multiple linear regression procedures were reported. Three of the properties are directly based on a molecular mechanics force field. Two of these are pairwise nonbonded terms: a coulombic function E_{coul} that uses Amber charges and a relative dielectric of 1; and an r^6/r^{12} van der Waals term E_{vdW}. The third term ΔE_{strain} is the difference in internal conformational energy between the bound ligand and the free ligand. It is assumed that the free ligand is adequately represented by a single conformation obtained from an energy minimization of the bound ligand using the Amber force field [22] with the generalized Born solvation area solvation model [59]. Four terms account for various types of contact surface areas (CSA): (1) nonpolar, (2) favorable polar (opposite charges), (3) unfavorable polar (like charges), and (4) polar–nonpolar (unfavorable). These areas are calculated by taking into consideration all receptor atoms that are in contact with each ligand surface point. Surprisingly, the predictive power of the model improves when one adds two more surface area terms that are equivalent to $CSA1$ (nonpolar) and $CSA3$ (unfavorable polar), but that consider, at the most, one receptor atom as being in contact with any ligand surface point. This may well be related to the observation by Flory [99] and Huggins [100] that both the solute surface and the volume play a role in solubility. The remaining three terms are the number of frozen rotatable bonds, the steric fit, and an adjusted partition coefficient. The steric fit parameter provides a means to penalize van der Waals overlap and empty spaces between the ligand and receptor, but to a large extent, the van der Waals term E_{vdW} and the surface terms $CSA1$ and $CSA2$ should be able to account for steric fit aspects. Indeed, the steric fit contributes only 1% to the predicted-binding free energy. The adjusted partition coefficient is the calculated water–octanol $\log P$ of the ligand, multiplied by $+1$ if, overall, the receptor site is lipophilic and by -1 if it is hydrophilic. Head et al. mention that $\log P$ is a measure of the energetic and entropic effects of removing the ligand from bulk water. As the interactions between the receptor and ligand are described explicitly, but the interactions with bulk solvent are not, the partition coefficient would be considered the equivalent of a regular solvation term. In that event, there is no obvious reason to adjust it for the character of the binding site unless the fitting procedure indicates otherwise. In fact, when both binding site and ligand are hydrophilic, instead of paying a substantial desolvation penalty, an energy bonus is given.

Even if one wants to differentiate between different types of receptor-binding sites, rather than using two discrete values, it seems logical to use a continuous scale proportional to the percentage of the receptor site that is lipophilic. An interesting conclusion of this work is that the correlation between the electrostatic energy and binding was very weak in the regression equation. This may be due to a combination of reasons: (a) the single-atom $CSA3$ and multi-atom $CSA2$ and $CSA3$ terms can account for a large part of the coulomb interactions, and (b) a coulombic term with nonpolarizable point charges and a uniform relative dielectric of 1 and without explicit desolvation, may be inadequate. The authors suggest that ab initio-derived multipoles may improve the electrostatics description, but it is our view that more is to be gained at substantially lower computational cost by simply taking into account the degree of exposure of interacting polar atoms (using, e.g., a local dielectric that depends on the environment or a dielectric gradient). Interestingly, the second and third largest contributions (after the multi-atom lipophilic contact surface area $CSA1$) came from intramolecular properties: entropy loss owing to freezing rotatable bonds and strain energy. Most methods described before ignore one or the other, but Head et al.'s results strongly suggest that both properties should be taken into account.

Overall, both the neural network and the PLS method yield similar results. It would appear that different statistical procedures for eliminating unimportant variables would lead to different equations with similar predictive behavior, but this analysis was not performed. The ability of the model to predict the affinity of novel complexes not included in the training set was demonstrated with three independent test sets. The first set of 14 complexes of known three-dimensional structure, including three DNA complexes, was predicted with an rms error of 1.3 kcal mol^{-1}. Although neither the ligands nor the receptors of this test were part of the training set, thrombin and trypsinogen (in the test set) are similar to trypsin (in the training set). The second set consisted of 13 HIV protease inhibitors, energy-minimized in the HIV protease active site. The rms error in the prediction was 1.2 kcal mol^{-1}, whereas the actual binding affinities spanned a range of only 5.9 kcal. Although 15 of the 51 structures in the training set were HIV protease complexes, in contrast with the "generic" test set 1, the slope between actual and predicted affinities deviated considerably from 1. The third set consisted of 11 thermolysin inhibitors fit to thermolysin. The rms error was 2.6 kcal mol^{-1} with a maximum error of 4.2 kcal mol^{-1}. This is most likely due to the well-known problem that molecular mechanics force fields have to do with treating transition metals, and to using energy minimization only in docking the inhibitors to the enzyme. Head et al. have presented an interesting method with reasonable predictive power. In the examples for which it does not perform well, the generation of complex structures, rather than the prediction method, itself may be the main culprit.

VIII. SOME PRACTICAL CONSIDERATIONS

Apart from enhancing our fundamental understanding of molecular interactions, reliable calculations of the free energy of binding also contribute to the drug design process. To be of real value to drug design, the free-energy predictions have to be accurate (and reliably so) as well as fast in terms of computational resources. The FEP method is reliable, but requires huge computational resources. Therefore, in practice there is a compromise that needs to be reached between accuracy of prediction and the speed of calculation. As examples, the Böhm method can calculate about a 100 compounds per minute on a fast workstation, with an estimated accuracy of about 70%. The method VALIDATE, on the other hand, takes a few minutes per molecule with an estimated accuracy of about 78%. A word of caution about the concept of estimated accuracy is in order here: these estimates are from cross-validation studies on a limited number of complexes. There are many known problems with cross-validation on small data sets. To our knowledge, there are, unfortunately, no systematic studies that estimate accuracy in a more reliable fashion. Clearly, in the initial stages of drug design process Böhm's method is quite useful. Regrettably, all methods that significantly improve the cross-validated accuracy demand much higher computational resources. There is still lack of a proved method that will come in useful at later stages of the drug design process when we can afford to spend higher computational resources, but would result in a significantly higher estimated accuracy, say over 85–90% in carefully constructed studies. It would also be interesting to know how much of the improvement from Böhm's work with VALIDATE came about because of the larger set of complexes and the addition of extra parameters.

IX. DISCUSSION AND OUTLOOK

Both theorists and experimentalists use rules and theories for rationalizing and interpreting data. Rules for estimating binding affinity (however approximate) play an important role in designing new and potent inhibitors because, as often occurs, the binding affinity of every possible modification cannot be measured experimentally, or the measurement is difficult.

Most contributions to protein–ligand interactions are electrostatic [36]. Major nonelectrostatic contributions arise from chemical bonds, short-range repulsion from the Pauli principle, and partially entropic forces owing to differences in the number of substates. The least well-understood, theoretically or experimentally, are solvation effects. A nice illustration of some of the contradictory conclusions that can be reached using different experimental setups is given in Table 1 of Connelly [112], in which different model systems used to mimic protein folding or protein–ligand binding predict opposite signs for contributions from the same interaction (ΔC_p, ΔH, ΔS, and ΔG).

We mentioned in the introduction that ligand binding should be a simpler problem to understand than protein folding. There is usually a large exchange of ideas between the two communities; therefore it is useful to study some of the newer approaches in protein folding. One of these is the method of Sippl [113] that starts by constructing a potential function based on crystal structures. The basic aim is to guarantee that the minimum of that potential function is the crystal structure; this is not true for molecular mechanics potential energy functions. Because this approach involves extensive averaging to determine the probability distribution of different configurations (and depends critically on such averaging for its success), it will become more attractive as the number of X-ray or NMR determined structures of complexes increases.

One of the first attempts to understand the thermodynamics of protein–ligand and protein–protein interaction was by Janin and Chotia [6]. They used two criteria: (a) surface area buried on complexation and (b) loss of rotational–translational entropy. They obtained reasonable results. However, Finkelstein and Janin [85] noted that the earlier calculations neglected the effect of vibrational entropy (as large as 15 kcal mol^{-1}), hence, this would significantly change the original results. This example, to our mind, exemplifies the difficulties that have plagued attempts at predicting free energy of binding.

In all of the analyses presented in the foregoing, it has been implicitly assumed that free energy can be broken up into components *meaningfully*. Recently, Mark and van Gunsteren [114] criticized this assumption by showing that free energy is a state function, but the components of the free energy are not. However, with careful interpretation, the individual components of the free energy can be used in enhancing our understanding of the chemical process under study [115]. In particular, the choice of the path projects the free energy change on different terms in the potential function and each decomposition provides an alternative but valid interpretation [115]. Janin [116] provided an overview of some of the questions that are (a) usually assumed to be significant, but are not, and (b) important to keep in mind while predicting free energies of binding.

Although the issues raised by Mark and van Gunsteren and Janin are relevant, we do believe that there is usefulness in the attempts to understand free energies as described in this chapter based on the following two reasons:

1. Despite severe approximations, some of the empirical schemes that we have described work remarkably well.
2. As stated earlier, even approximate rules can be useful for gaining a measure of understanding of the relevant issues.

The qualitative and quantitative information thus obtained provides a rational handle for selecting and prioritizing compounds to be synthesized in the context of a drug design program and, in doing so, speeds up the discovery process substantially.

We would like to point out that "back-of-the-envelope" calculations of binding affinity are not necessarily very predictive when hydrogen bonds and salt bridges are involved in the binding process. For example, it is often believed that binding affinity increases about one order of magnitude per hydrogen bond. The glycogen phosphorylase–glucose complex [14] shows that despite many hydrogen bonds to the protein, the ligand exhibits only a very weak binding. The primary reason for this is that desolvation costs can entirely compensate for hydrogen bonds. These desolvation penalties, as we have seen, depend on the microscopic environment of the hydrogen-bonding groups.

Typically, there is some correlation (empirically observed) between the number of hydrogen bonds formed and the K_i; similarly there is some correlation between K_i and the lipophilic surface area buried. Neither correlation is perfect, as evidenced by the results of Horton and Lewis [58] and Böhm [82]. It is possible, for example, that certain lipophilic groups on ligands stabilize the bound conformation of the ligand in solution, even though the lipophilic area buried does not change.

An approach that is often used to improve binding is specific rigidification of the ligand. Ku et al. [117] provide an example of the successful design of a potent nonpeptide fibrinogen receptor antagonist by analogy with a low-activity constrained peptide. On the other hand, the work by Weber et al. [118] provides a counterexample. They found that for synthetic azobenzene ligands of streptavidin, ligand flexibility in the bound state contributes to the overall binding.

We have described the controversies involved in both the theoretical calculations and experimental interpretations of data. This is especially true relative to the role of water. The question that becomes immediately obvious is, what are the reasons for the published successes? These are not immediately apparent. It is clear that the methods work under certain conditions (e.g., when there is a large amount of fortuitous cancellations among the contributions that are neglected). This could be related to the enthalpy–entropy compensation in aqueous solutions that lets us predict the total free energy even though the components cannot be predicted reliably [119]. In other words, increasing the enthalpic contribution to binding would require very specific positioning of functional groups which, in turn, would increase the entropic cost for binding. Under these conditions, incorrect predictions of components of the free energy of binding may not lead to large inaccuracies in the prediction of binding free energies.

In our opinion there are three steps that will be important in the immediate future to enhance our understanding of the quality of our prediction algorithms:

1. A more careful estimation of prediction error.
2. Setting up a database of ligand–receptor complexes chosen to emphasize differences in (a) magnitude of K_i and (b) major contributions to binding that can be used to analyze and compare the performance of all the available prediction algorithms. This database should contain both flexible and rigid ligands, ligands that differ in one or more hydrogen- or ionic-bonding possibilities, and ligands that have different amounts of polar and nonpolar surface area buried. A series of complexes that span a range of functionally and structurally different proteins will also be needed.
3. Finally, only a limited number of microcalorimetric measurements that measure both the enthalpy and entropy changes exist. More data along these lines will surely enhance theoretical studies because, given a protein, different ligands can bind either through enthalpically or entropically driven processes; an example is biotin binding to streptavidin is enthalpy driven, whereas azobenzene ligands binding to streptavidin is entropy driven [81,118].

The basic conclusions from our analysis are as follows:

- Rule-of-thumb methods do not always work well for hydrogen bonding. They are better for lipophilic interactions.
- Straightforward forcefield methods are too simplistic except for congeneric series.
- The free-energy perturbation method holds great promise if the convergence problems can be solved.
- Solvation effects are still not well understood.

    1. It constitutes the largest source of error in predictions.
    2. It has bulk effects on the environment of the active site.

3. Conformational preferences for ligands are often different in solution and vacuum.
4. Specific water-mediated hydrogen bonds are hard to predict and their effects hard to quantify.
5. Addition of explicit water molecules really slows down calculations.

• Ligand flexibility is essential. It allows estimating,

1. Entropy of binding (how many conformations are likely)
2. Strain energy on binding

• Protein flexibility is important, although it is often neglected. It is computationally intensive, but allows estimating the consequences of

1. Major conformational changes
2. Many side-chain motions

• The vibrational states of the complex and unbound protein and ligand are different in general. Accounting for these differences is difficult.

Finally, it is clear that considerable progress has already been made toward improving our understanding of ligand–receptor-binding affinities. During the past 3 years, there has been an explosion of interest in this area, which continues to grow rapidly.

We expect that as this field matures, more careful and robust statistical analysis will be carried out on K_i prediction methods, increasing our confidence in their usefulness. In addition, a great deal more structural information will become available during the next decade, and computers should continue to rapidly increase in speed. Taken together, all these factors lead us to be optimistic about the prospects of significant improvements in the coming decade.

REFERENCES

1. T. E. Creighton, *Proteins: Structures and Molecular Properties*, 2 ed. W. H. Freeman, New York, 1993.
2. J. Gómez and E. Freire, Thermodynamics of inhibitor binding to endothiapepsin, *J. Mol. Biol. 252*:337–350 (1995).
3. W. Kauzmann, Some factors in the interpretation of protein denaturation, *Adv. Protein Chem. 14*:1–63 (1959).

4. M. I. Page and W. P. Jencks, Entropic contributions to rate accelerations in enzymic and intramolecular reactions and the chelate effect, *Proc. Natl. Acad. Sci. USA 68*:1678–1683 (1971).

5. W. P. Jencks, Binding energy, specificity, and enzymic catalysis: The circe effect, *Adv. Enzyme Related Areas Mol. Biol. 43*:219–410 (1975).

6. J. Janin and C. Chotia, Role of hydrophobicity in the binding of coenzymes. Appendix. Translational and rotational contribution to the free energy of dissociation, *Biochemistry 17*:2943–2948 (1978).

7. C. J. Cramer and D. G. Truhlar, AM1-SM2 and PM3-SM3 parameterized SCF solvation models for free energies in aqueous solution, *J. Comput. Aided Mol. Design 6*:629–666 (1992).

8. J. M. Berg, Zinc finger domains: Hypotheses and current knowledge. *Annu. Rev. Biophys. Biophys. Chem. 19*:405–421 (1990).

9. N. C. J. Strynadka and M. N. G. James, Crystal structures of the helix–loop–helix calcium-binding proteins, *Annu. Rev. Biol. 58*:951–998 (1989).

10. E. E. Kim, C. T. Baker, M. D. Dwyer, M. A. Murcko, B. G. Rao, R. D. Tung, and M. A. Navia, Crystal structure of HIV-1 protease in complex with VX-478, a potent and orally bioavailable inhibitor of the enzyme, *J. Am. Chem. Soc. 117*:1181–1182 (1995).

11. S. H. Reich, M. A. Fuhry, D. Nguyen, el al., Design and synthesis of novel 6,7-imidazotetrahydroquinoline inhibitors of thymidylate synthase using iterative protein crystal, *J. Med. Chem. 35*:847–858 (1992).

12. C. L. Verlinde, E. A. Merritt, F. V. den Akker, H. Kim, I. Feil, L. F. Delboni, S. C. Mande, S. Sarfaty, P. H. Petra, and W. G. Hol, Protein crystallography and infectious diseases, *Protein Sci. 3*:1670–86 (1994).

13. C. A. Veale, P. R. Bernstein, C. Bryant, et al., Nonpeptidic inhibitors of human leukocyte elastase. 5. Design, synthesis, and X-ray crystallography of a series of orally active 5-aminopyrimidin-6-one-containing trifluoromethyl ketones, *J. Med. Chem. 38*:98–108 (1995).

14. K. A. Watson, E. P. Mitchell, L. N. Johnson, et al., Design of inhibitors of glycogen phosphorylase: A study of alpha- and beta-*d*-glucosides and 1-thio-beta-*d*-glucose compounds, *Biochemistry 33*:5748–58 (1994).

15. J. de Heer, *Phenomenological Thermodynamics with Applications to Chemistry*, Prentice Hall, Englewood Cliffs NJ, 1986.

16. P. W. Atkins, *Physical Chemistry*, 4 ed., W. H. Freeman, New York, 1990.

17. Y. C. Martin, *Quantitative Drug Design: A Critical Introduction*, Marcel Dekker, New York, 1978.

18. A. Fersht, *Enzyme Structure and Mechanism*, 2 ed., W. H. Freeman, New York, 1985.

19. M. Levitt and B. H. Park, Water: Now you see it, now you don't. *Structure 1*:223–226 (1993).

20. Z. Shakked, G. Guzikevich-Guerstein, F. Frolow, D. Rabinovich, A. Joachimiak, and P. B. Sigler, Determinants of repressor/operator recognition from the structure of the *trp* operator binding site, *Nature 368*:469–473 (1994).

21. B. R. Brooks, R. E. Bruccoleri, B. D. Olafson, D. J. S. S. Swaminathan, and M. Karplus, Charmm: A program for macromolecular energy minimization, and dynamics calculations, *J. Comput. Chem.* 4:187–217 (1983).
22. S. J. Weiner, P. A. Kollman, D. T. Nguyen, and D. A. Case, An all atom force field for simulations of proteins and nucleic acids, *J. Comput. Chem.* 7:230–252 (1986).
23. G. Nemethy, M. S. Pottle, and H. A. Scheraga, Energy parameters in polypeptides. 9. Updating the geometrical parameters, nonbonded interactions, and hydrogen bond interactions for the naturally occurring amino-acids. *J. Phys. Chem.* 87:1883–1887 (1983).
24. T. P. Straatsma, Free energy by molecular simulation, *Reviews in Computational Chemistry*, Vol. 9 (D. B. Boyd, and K. B. Lipkowitz, eds.), VCH Publishers, New York, 1996, pp. 81–127.
25. P. Kollman, Free energy calculations—applications to chemical and biochemical phenomena, *Chem. Rev.* 93:2395–2417 (1993).
26. A. E. Mark and W. F. van Gunsteren, Free energy calculations in drug design: A practical guide, *New Perspectives in Drug Design* (G. Jolles, P. M. Dean, and C. G. Newton, eds.), Academic Press, London, 1995, pp. 185–200.
27. B. G. Rao, R. F. Tilton, and U. C. Singh, Free energy perturbation studies on inhibitor binding to HIV-1 proteinase, *J. Am. Chem. Soc.* 114:4447–4452 (1992).
28. S. B. Singh, Ajay, D. E. Wemmer, and P. A. Kollman, Relative binding affinities of distamycin and its analog to d(CGCAAGTTGGC) d(GCCAACTTGCG): Comparison of simulation results with experiment, *Proc. Natl. Acad. Sci. USA* 91:7673–7677 (1994).
29. H. Schreiber and O. Steinhauser, Cutoff size does strongly influence molecular dynamics results on solvated polypeptides, *Biochemistry* 31:5856–60 (1992).
30. D. M. York, T. A. Darden, and L. G. Pedersen, The effect of long range electrostatic interactions in simulations of macromolecular crystals: A comparison of Ewald and truncated list methods, *J. Phys. Chem.* 99:8345–8348 (1993).
31. L. F. Greengard, Fast algorithms for classical physics, *Science* 265:909–914 (1994).
32. J. W. Caldwell and P. A. Kollman, Cation–pi interactions—nonadditive effects are critical in their accurate representation, *J. Am. Chem. Soc.* 117:4177–4178 (1995).
33. Y-P. Liu, K. Kim, B. J. Berne, and R. A. Friesner, Polarizable force field for water from ab initio quantum mechanics, (submitted; 1996).
34. P. E. Smith and W. F. van Gunsteren, Translational and rotational diffusion of proteins, *J. Mol. Biol.* 236:629–636 (1994).
35. Y. Y. Shi, A. E. Mark, C. X. Wang, F. Huang, H. J. Berendsen, and W. F. van Gunsteren, Can the stability of protein mutants be predicted by free energy calculations? *Protein Eng.* 6:289–95 (1993).

36. J. N. Israelachvili, *Intermolecular and Surface Forces*, Academic Press, London, 1985.

37. J. L. Fauchere and V. Pliska, Hydrophobic parameters π of amino acid side-chains from the partitioning of N-acetyl-amino acid amides, *Eur. J. Med. Chem. 18*:369–375 (1983).

38. J. L. Cornette, K. B. Cease, H. Margalit, J. L. Spouge, J. A. Berzofsky, and C. DeLisi, Hydrophobicity scales and computational techniques for detecting amphipathic structures in proteins, *J. Mol. Biol. 195*:659–685 (1987).

39. B. Lee, Estimation of the maximum change in stability of globular proteins upon mutation of a hydrophobic residue to another of smaller size, *Protein Sci. 2*:733–738 (1993).

40. K. A. Sharp, A. Nicholls, R. Friedman, and B. Honig, Extracting hydrophobic free energies from experimental data: Relationship to protein folding and theoretical models, *Biochemistry 30*:9686–9697 (1991).

41. H. S. Chan and K. A. Dill, Solvation—effects of molecular size and shape, *J. Chem. Phys. 101*:7007–7026 (1994).

42. A. Ben-Naim and R. M. Mazo, Size dependence of the solvation free-energies of large solutes, *J. Phys. Chem. 97*:10829–10834 (1993).

43. P. E. Smith and B. M. Pettitt, Modeling solvent in biomolecular systems, *J. Phys. Chem. 98*:9700–9711 (1994).

44. P. L. Privalov and G. I. Makhatadze, Contribution of hydration and noncovalent interactions to the heat capacity effect on protein unfolding, *J. Mol. Biol. 224*:715–723 (1992).

45. P. L. Privalov and G. I. Makhatadze, Contribution of hydration to protein folding thermodynamics. II. the entropy and Gibbs energy of hydration, *J. Mol. Biol. 232*:660–669 (1993).

46. R. S. Spolar and M. T. Record, Jr., Coupling of local folding to site-specific binding of proteins to DNA, *Science 263*:777–784 (1994).

47. J. Novotny, R. E. Bruccoleri, and F. A. Saul, On the attribution of binding energy in antigen–antibody complexes MCPC 603, d1.3 and hyhel-5; *Biochemistry 28*:4735–4749 (1989).

48. D. Eisenberg and A. D. McLachlan, Solvation energy in protein folding and binding, *Nature 319*:199–203 (1986).

49. T. Ooi, M. Oobatake, G. Nemethy, and H. A. Scheraga, Accessible surface area as a measure of the thermodynamic parameters of hydration of peptides, *Proc. Natl. Acad. Sci. USA 84*:3086–3090 (1987).

50. P. F. W. Stouten, C. Frommel, H. Nakamura, and C. Sander, An effective solvation term based on atomic occupancies for use in protein simulations, *Mol. Simul. 10*:97–120 (1993).

51. Y. K. Kang, K. D. Gibson, G. Nemethy, and H. A. Scheraga, Free energies of hydration of solute molecules. 4. Revised treatment of the hydration shell model, *J. Phys. Chem. 92*:4739–4742 (1988).

52. B. A. Luty, Z. R. Wasserman, P. F. W. Stouten, C. N. Hodge, M. Zacharias, and J. A. McCammon, A molecular mechanics/grid method for evaluation of ligand–receptor interactions, *J. Comput. Chem. 16*:454–464 (1995).

53. L. Wesson and D. Eisenberg, Atomic solvation parameters applied to molecular dynamics of proteins in solution, *Protein Sci. 1*:227–235 (1992).

54. A. A. Rashin, Continuum electrostatics and hydration phenomena, *Int. J. Quant. Chem. Quant. Biol. Symp. 15*:103–118 (1988).

55. I. Klapper, R. Hagstrom, R. Fine, K. Sharp, and B. Honig, Focusing of electric fields in the active site of Cu–Zn superoxide dismutase: Effects of ionic strength and amino-acid modification, *Proteins 1*:47–59 (1986).

56. C. A. Schiffer, J. W. Caldwell, P. A. Kollman, and R. M. Stroud, Protein structure prediction with a combined solvation free energy–molecular mechanics force field, *Mol. Simul. 10*:121–149 (1993).

57. A. Ben-Naim, *Solvation Thermodynamics*, Plenum Press, New York, 1987.

58. N. Horton and M. Lewis, Calculation of the free energy of association for protein complexes, *Protein Sci. 1*:169–181 (1992).

59. W. C. Still, A. Tempczyk, R. C. Hawley, and T. F. Hendrickson, Semianalytical treatment of solvation for molecular mechanics and dynamics, *J. Am. Chem. Soc. 112*:6127–6129 (1990).

60. B. Honig, K. Sharp, and A.-S. Yang, Macroscopic models of aqueous solutions: Biological and chemical applications, *J. Phys. Chem. 97*:1101–1109 (1993).

61. S. W. Rick and B. J. Berne, The aqueous solvation of water: A comparison of continuum methods with molecular dynamics, *J. Am. Chem. Soc. 116*: 3949–3954 (1994).

62. J. D. Dunitz, The entropic cost of bound water in crystals and biomolecules, *Science 264*:670–670 (1994).

63. W. P. Bryan, The entropic cost of binding water to proteins, *Science 266*: 1726 (1994).

64. T. P. Creamer and G. D. Rose, Side-chain entropy opposes alpha-helix formation but rationalizes experimentally determined helix-forming propensities, *Proc. Natl. Acad. Sci. USA 89*:5937–5941 (1992).

65. S. Padmanabhan and R. L. Baldwin, Straight-chain nonpolar amino acids are good helix-formers in water, *J. Mol. Biol. 219*:135–137 (1991).

66. J. Hermans, A. G. Anderson, and R. H. Yun, Differential helix propensity of small apolar side chain studied by molecular dynamics simulation, *Biochemistry 31*:5646–5653 (1992).

67. A. Horowitz, J. M. Matthews, and A. Fersht, alpha-Helix stability in proteins II. Factors that influence stability at an internal position, *J. Mol. Biol. 227*: 560–568 (1992).

68. F. Avbelj and J. Moult, Role of electrostatic screening in determining protein main chain conformational preferences, *Biochemistry 34*:755–764 (1995).

69. S. Krystek, T. Stouch, and J. Novotny, Affinity and specificity of serine endopeptidase–protein inhibitor interactions, *J. Mol. Biol. 234*:661–679 (1993).

70. D. H. Williams, J. P. L. Cox, A. J. Doig, M. Garner, U. Gerhard, P. T. Kaye, A. R. Lal, I. A. Nicholls, C. J. Salter, and R. C. Mitchell, Toward the se-

miquantitative estimation of binding constants. Guides for peptide–peptide binding in aqueous solution, *J. Am. Chem. Soc. 113*:7020–7030 (1991).

71. S. Vajda, Z. Weng, R. Rosenfeld, and C. DeLisi, Effect of conformational flexibility and solvation on receptor–ligand binding free energies, *Biochemistry 33*:13977–13988 (1994).

72. T. L. Hill, *Statistical Mechanics: Principles and Selected Applications*, Dover Publisher, New York, 1987.

73. M. J. E. Sternberg and J. S. Chickos, Protein side-chain conformational entropy derived from fusion data—comparison with other empirical scales, *Protein Eng. 7*:149–155 (1994).

74. B. E. Hingerty, R. H. Ritchie, T. L. Ferrel, and J. E. Turner, Dielectric effects in biopolymers: The theory of ionic saturation revisited, *Biopolymers 24*: 427–439 (1985).

75. R. Lavery, H. Sklenar, K. Zakrzewski, and B. Pullman, The flexibility of the nucleic acids (II) The calculation of internal energy and applications to mononucleotide repeat DNA, *J. Biomol. Struct. Dyn. 3*:989–1014 (1986).

76. E. von Kitzing, Modeling DNA structures, *Proc. Nucl. Acid Res. Mol. Biol. 43*:87–108 (1992).

77. M. E. Davis and J. A. McCammon, Electrostatics in biomolecular structure and dynamics, *Chem. Rev. 90*:509–521 (1990).

78. R. A. Friedman and B. Honig, The electrostatic contribution to DNA base-stacking interactions, *Biopolymers 32*:145–152 (1988).

79. P. R. Andrews, D. J. Craik, and J. L. Martin, Functional group contributions to drug–receptor interactions, *J. Med. Chem. 27*:1648–57 (1984).

80. M. S. Searle, D. H. Williams, and U. Gerhard, Partitioning of free energy contributions in the estimation of binding constants: Residual motions and consequences for amide–amide hydrogen bond strengths, *J. Am. Chem. Soc. 114*:10697–10704 (1992).

81. P. C. Weber, J. J. Wendoloski, M. W. Pantoliano, and F. R. Salemme, Crystallographic and thermodynamic comparison of natural and synthetic ligands bound to streptavidin, *J. Am. Chem. Soc. 114*:3197–3200 (1992).

82. H-J. Böhm, The development of a simple empirical scoring function to estimate the binding constant for a protein–ligand complex of known three-dimensional structure, *J. Comput. Aided Mol. Design 8*:243–356 (1994).

83. S. D. Pickett and M. E. Sternberg, Empirical scale of side-chain conformational entropy in protein folding, *J. Mol. Biol. 231*:825–839 (1993).

84. R. Raag and T. L. Poulos, Crystal structure of cytochrome P-450$_{CAM}$ complexed with camphane, tiocamphor, and adamantane: Factors controlling P-450 substrate hydroxylation, *Biochemistry 30*:2674–2684 (1991).

85. A. V. Finkelstein and J. Janin, The price of lost freedom—entropy of bimolecular complex formation *Protein Eng. 3*:1–3 (1989).

86. C. Chotia and J. Janin, Principles of protein–protein recognition, *Nature 256*: 705–708 (1975).

87. J. Sancho and A. R. Fersht, Dissection of an enzyme by protein engineering—the N-terminal and C-terminal fragments of barnase form a

native-like complex with restored enzymic activity, *J. Mol. Biol.* *224*: 741–747 (1992).

88. M. Karplus and J. N. Kushick, Method for estimating the configurational entropy of macromolecules, *Macromolecules 14*:325–332 (1981).

89. O. Edholm and H. J. C. Berendsen, Entropy estimation from simulations of non-diffusive systems, *Mol. Phys. 51*:1011–1028 (1984).

90. C. Hansch, P. G. Sammes, and J. B. Taylor, eds., *Comprehensive Medicinal Chemistry: The Rational Design, Mechanistic Study and Therapeutic Application of Chemical Compounds*, Pergamon Press, New York, 1990.

91. H. Kubinyi, et., *3D QSAR in Drug Design*, ESCOM, Leiden 1993.

92. Ajay, On better generalization by combining 2 or more models—a quantitative structure activity relationship example using neural networks, *Chem. Int. Lab. Syst. 24*:19–30 (1994).

93. P. D. J. Grootenhuis and S. P. van Helden, Rational approaches towards protease inhibition: Predicting the binding of thrombin inhibitors, *Computational Approaches in Supramolecular Chemistry* (G. Wipff, ed.), Kluwer Academic, Boston, 1994, pp. 137–149.

94. M. K. Holloway, J. M. Wai, T. A. Halgren, et al. A priori prediction of activity for HIV-1 protease inhibitors employing energy minimization in the active site, *J. Med. Chem. 38*:305–317 (1995).

95. A. R. Ortiz, M. T. Pisabarro, F. Gago, and R. C. Wade, Prediction of drug binding affinities by comparative binding energy analysis, *J. Med. Chem. 38*: 2681–2691 (1995).

96. D. Sitkoff, K. A. Sharp, and B. Honig, Accurate calculation of hydration free energies using macroscopic solvent models, *J. Phys. Chem. 98*: 1978–1988 (1994).

97. H. Oberoi and N. M. Allewell, Multigrid solution of the non-linear Poisson–Boltzmann equation and calculation of titration curves, *Biophys. J. 65*:48–55 (1993).

98. A. Shrake and A. J. A. Rupley, Environment and exposure to solvent of protein atoms. Lysozyme and insulin, *J. Mol. Biol. 79*:351–371 (1973).

99. P. J. Flory, *Phys. Chem. 9*:660–671 (1941).

100. M. L. Huggins, *J. Phys. Chem. 9*:440–449 (1941).

101. M. D. Beach, D. Chasman, R. B. Murphy, T. A. Halgren, and R. A. Friesner, Accurate ab initio quantum chemical determination of the relative energetics of peptide conformations and assessment of empirical force fields, (*preprint* 1996).

102. C. Chotia, Hydrophobic bonding and accessible surface area in proteins, *Nature 248*:338–339 (1974).

103. J. Janin, For Guldberg and Waage, with love and ceatic entropy, *Proteins 24*:i–ii (1996).

104. J. Shen and J. Wendoloski, Binding of phosphorus-containing inhibitors to thermolysin studied by the Poison–Boltzmann method, *Protein Sci. 4*: 373–381 (1995).

105. M. E. Davis, J. D. Madura, B. A. Luty, and J. A. McCammon, Electrostatic diffusion of molecules in solution: Simulation with the University of Houston Brownian Dynamics Program, *Comput. Phys. Commun.* 62:187–190 (1991).
106. C. M. Roth, B. L. Neal, and A. M. Lenhoff, van der Waals interactions involving proteins, *Biophys. J.* 70:977–987 (1996).
107. A. R. Fresht, The hydrogen bond in molecular recognition, *Trends Biochem. Sci.* 12:301–304 (1987).
108. B. A. Shirley, P. Stanssens, U. Hahn, and C. N. Pace, Contribution of hydrogen bonding to conformational stability of ribonuclease t1, *Biochemistry* 31:725–732 (1992).
109. H-J. Böhm, The computer program LUDI: A new method for the de novo design of enzyme inhibitors. *J. Comput. Aided Mol. Design* 6:61–78 (1992).
110. K. A. Dill, Dominant forces in protein folding, *Biochemistry* 29:7133–7155 (1990).
111. R. D. Head, M. L. Smythe, T. I. Oprea, C. L. Waller, S. M. Green, and G. R. Marshall, Validate: A new method for the receptor-based prediction of binding affinities of novel ligands, *J. Am. Chem. Soc.* 118:3959–3969 (1995).
112. P. R. Connelly, Acquisition and use of calorimetric data for prediction of the thermodynamics of ligand-binding and folding reactions of proteins, *Curr. Opin. Biotechnol.* 5:381–388 (1994).
113. M. J. Sippl, Boltzmann's principle, knowledge-based mean fields and protein folding. An approach to the computational determination of protein structures, *J. Comput. Aided Mol. Design* 7:473–501 (1993).
114. A. E. Mark and W. F. van Gunsteren, Decomposition of the free energy of a system in terms of specific interactions, *J. Mol. Biol.* 240:167–176 (1994).
115. S. Boresch and M. Karplus, The meaning of component analysis: Decomposition of the free energy in terms of specific interactions, *J. Mol. Biol.* 254:801–807 (1995).
116. J. Janin, Elusive affinities, *Proteins Struct. Funct. Genet.* 21:30–39 (1995).
117. T. W. Ku, F. E. Ali, et al., Direct design of a potent non-peptide fibrinogen receptor antagonist based on the structure and conformation of a highly constrained cyclic RGD peptide, *J. Am. Chem. Soc.* 115:8861–8862 (1993).
118. P. C. Weber, M. W. Pantoliano, D. M. Simons, and F. R. Salemme, Structure-based design of synthetic azobenzene ligands for streptavidin, *J. Am. Chem. Soc.* 116:2717–2724 (1994).
119. B. Lee, Enthalpy–entropy compensation in the thermodynamics of hydrophobicity, *Biophys. Chem.* 51:271–277 (1994).

11

Long-Range Electrostatic Effects

Ulrich Essmann*
University of North Carolina, Chapel Hill, North Carolina

Thomas A. Darden
National Institute of Environmental Health Sciences,
Research Triangle Park, North Carolina

I. INTRODUCTION

The importance of a careful treatment of long-range coulombic forces in molecular simulations has long been appreciated by the liquid simulation community [1]. In contrast, with few exceptions (e.g., [2,3]), the biomolecular simulation community has until recently chosen to ignore the problem. Undoubtedly, the major reason for this decision was because the methods that accounted for long-range forces were computationally too expensive for macromolecular systems; hence, it was not possible to rigorously test if they made a difference. However, the decision to ignore long-range forces by using nonbonded cutoffs has also been justified a priori in the literature. These justifications were typically one or more of the following:

*Current affiliation: German National Research Center for Information Technology, Schloss Birlinghoven, Sankt Augustin, Germany.

1. Errors owing to truncation of coulombic interactions at a modest cutoff radius (8–10 A) are probably small compared with errors in the empirical force fields currently in use.
2. Because biological macromolecules are typically dissolved in water, which has a high dielectric constant, the coulombic interactions between charged groups are strongly shielded. This shielding effect is especially pronounced when counterions are present, such as at psychological salt concentrations, in which case coulombic interactions can be treated as if they were short-ranged.
3. It is currently impossible to correctly account for long-range coulombic interactions, so it is better not to include them.

On the relatively short time scale (less than 100 ps) of the simulations that were possible until recently, little or no evidence emerged to indicate problems with the cutoff scheme. Lately, however, evidence has mounted indicating severe artifacts associated with truncation of coulombic forces. In retrospect, we can criticize the foregoing statements (1) and (2), and examine the validity of statement (3). In particular, statement (1) may be correct for the errors in the instantaneous interactions, but recent results show that it is certainly quite wrong for time-averaged interactions, such as potentials of mean force. For example, from the calculation of the potential of mean force Dang and Pettitt [4] predicted that CL^- ions form pairs with a separation of 3.4 A. Later, Hummer and associates [5] were able to attribute this result to the use of cutoff methods. Simulations with Ewald summation [6] showed no sign of Cl^-–Cl^- pairing in agreement with experimental expectations [7]. A more striking observation was made by Bader and Chandler [8]. They observed a strong attractive well for the potential of mean force for Fe^{2+}–Fe^{3+} pairs when a cutoff was used, and a purely repulsive mean force, with the correct dielectric shielding, when Ewald summation was used. Certainly this latter cutoff artifact far exceeds any deficiencies in the empirical potentials used in the study. Moreover, even when artifacts caused by the use of cutoffs are not this dramatic, it seems prudent to first address them before modifying the force field to improve agreement with experimental data.

For statement (2), note that it is the time-averaged interactions, such as potentials of mean force, that are thus shielded, whereas molecular dynamics uses instantaneous interactions, which are not shielded. Furthermore, the foregoing argument would lead one to believe that cutoff schemes should work better when counterions are present, whereas our experience and that of others shows the opposite. Consider, for instance, the solution simulations of bovine pancreatic trypsin inhibitor (BPTI) by Levitt et al., which are discussed in Daggett and Levitt [9]. Their simulation of "neutral" BPTI without counterions had a time-averaged backbone root-mean-square (rms) deviation from the crystal structure of approximately 0.8 A, whereas an otherwise similar simulation of "standard" (i.e., net charge + 6) BPTI, including six chloride counterions led to an rms deviation nearly twice as large. Recently, Auffinger and Beveridge [10] simulated a system of 1531 H_2O molecules plus 29 NaCl pairs. Even though the cutoff was 16 A, the radial distribution functions of the ion pairs revealed a strong tendency for ions of the same charge to be separated by distances close to the cutoff distance, whereas ion pairs of opposite charge showed a corresponding depletion at the cutoff. This clearly shows that counterions do not correctly screen interactions in molecular dynamics simulations that use cutoffs. Moreover Kitson et al. [11] demonstrated similar problems for pairs of charged residues within proteins. In their calculations, use of a larger cutoff seemed to ameliorate the problem. We had similar experiences simulating the highly charged *p21* H-*ras* and prothrombin fragment 1 proteins [12–14]. However, when trying to simulate DNA, we and others were unable to produce stable trajectories using any cutoff distance. In contrast, several groups have reported successful simulations of DNA using Ewald sums [15–18].

Schreiber and Steinhauser [19] demonstrated a strong influence of the choice of cutoff on the stability of a 17-residue α-helical model peptide in solution, including four chloride counterions. Using a 6- or 14-A charge group-based cutoff the α-helix unwound within 90 ps. Surprisingly, the stability of the helix was not a monotonic function of the cutoff radius, because the application of a 10-A cutoff improved the stability. Thus, it is not always clear how to decide when a cutoff is "big enough." Use of Ewald summation in this study led to a stable helix.

These results as well as others [20–34] clearly demonstrate the importance of a proper treatment of coulombic forces in computer simulations. Artifacts caused by an improper treatment should actually be more dramatic in systems containing counterions, contrary to the foregoing screening argument, for the instantaneous interaction energy decays asymptotically as $1/r$. In systems containing only neutral charge groups, the interactions decay more rapidly and so the effects are probably not as pronounced [2]. However, calculations of the dielectric constant of water have shown [35] that, even here, cutoff effects change the results.

For statement (3), because it is not possible to simulate macroscopic systems, some artifactual behavior owing to the choice of boundary conditions is inevitable. However, from the foregoing discussion, we believe that truncation of coulombic interactions is no longer a tenable option in many situations, so it is necessary to explore methods that can account for long-range interactions.

The liquid simulation community has developed techniques for approximating long-range interactions, such as Ewald summation [1,6,36] and the reaction field method [37]. So far, to our knowledge, no artifacts caused by their use in liquid simulations have been identified, despite early concerns [38,39]. It remains to be seen if they will prove as successful in biomolecular simulations, although our early results using Ewald summation have led us to be hopeful. Meanwhile, other techniques appropriate for various boundary conditions have been developed. In parallel, during the last several years various fast algorithms have been developed that allow these techniques to be applied to macromolecular systems, with only a small to moderate increase in computer time, compared with cutoff schemes. Because of the importance of long-range forces, many of the modern simulation packages now incorporate one or more of these long-range force techniques, together with fast algorithms for their computation. The present chapter attempts to review the long-range force techniques and relevant fast algorithms that are currently available. Only the basic ideas will be given, together with references to the original literature for a detailed discussion.

The choice of the boundary conditions for coulombic interactions in a simulation is heavily influenced by the treatment of the solvent. Vacuum simulations, in which solvent is ignored completely, and continuum methods, which treat the solvent implicitly, naturally lead to the use of nonperiodic boundary conditions. In contrast, simulations involving explicit solvent molecules are typically performed using periodic boundary conditions, although several methods for simulating such systems under nonperiodic conditions have been proposed. Accordingly, although the focus of the current chapter is to describe the various methods for treating long-range electrostatics, along with a discussion of their advantages and disadvantages, it is convenient to organize the chapter along the lines of the treatment of solvent. The various methods for treating long-range electrostatics can then be discussed in this context.

The outline of the rest of the chapter is as follows: In the next section we first consider simulations in which solvent is completely ignored (i.e., vacuum simulations) and then models that ignore the molecular nature of solvent (i.e., continuum methods). At the next level of approximation to full atomic detail are the models with minimal explicit solvation, in which the solute is surrounded by a thin layer of explicit water molecules. This approach attempts to avoid the computational cost and possible artifacts of full atomic simulations using periodic boundary conditions, while providing atomic details close to the solute, where the limitations of continuum methods should be most pronounced. While reviewing these methods, we also discuss the recent fast multipole method and related tree-based algorithms, which are most natural for large systems under nonperiodic boundary conditions.

To eliminate the severe artifacts caused by surface effects in small systems Monte Carlo simulations as well as molecular dynamics simulations, which involve explicit solvent molecules, are often performed using periodic boundary conditions. In the final section we discuss explicit solvent simulations under periodic boundary conditions. A variety of methods for treating long-range forces are used in this context, including cutoff methods (with a wealth of variations), reaction field methods, and the Ewald sum and grid-based fast-algorithm methods for computing it.

In preparing this chapter we were helped immensely by our reading of several recent comprehensive reviews of various aspects of this subject [40–47], although our viewpoint may not always coincide with that expressed therein.

II. IMPLICIT TREATMENT OF SOLVENTS

A. Distance-Dependent Dielectric Functions

The earliest molecular dynamics simulations of biomolecular systems [48] were performed in a vacuum, primarily to reduce the system size. To treat coulombic interactions a simple distance-dependent dielectric function $\epsilon = r$ was used, for two reasons. First, it reduced computational cost, because nonbond energies and forces could be computed using only even powers of the Cartesian distances, thus avoiding the square root. Secondly, it mimicked the expected dielectric behavior of water over short distances.

To discuss distance-dependent dielectric functions in general, it is useful to introduce the idea of an effective dielectric constant [43]. For a given pair of charges q_1 and q_2, separated by a distance r_{12}, in a system of interest, the *effective dielectric constant* is defined as the ratio of the vacuum electrostatic energy, $q_1 q_2 / 4 \pi \epsilon_0 r_{12}$, to the measured energy of interaction in a dielectric medium. From this perspective, the distance-dependent dielectric function is an attempt to model the dielectric response of the surrounding medium, which in general depends on the positions of each of the pair of charges (i.e., is a function of six Cartesian variables), by a smooth function of a single variable, the distance between the pair.

The foregoing definition of the effective dielectric constant involves a conceptual problem [43]. The electrostatic force between a charge pair is obtained from the derivative of the energy, which involves the derivative of the effective dielectric constant, as well as that of the $1/r$ term. Therefore, the ratio of the vacuum electrostatic force to the measured force of interaction in a dielectric medium will, in general, not be equal to the foregoing ratio of energies, which makes the definition of the effective dielectric constant somewhat arbitrary.

Although the simple function $\epsilon = r$ for approximating solvent screening is still widely used, several alternative functional forms have been proposed [49–53]. Hingerty [49] and Lavery [50] have used sigmoidal forms for the effective dielectric, which approach 1 as r_{12} approaches zero and 78 (the dielectric of bulk water) for r_{12} greater than 20 A. The Debye–Hückel theory (discussed later) leads to an effective dielectric constant that increases exponentially with distance. To model the screening in ionic solutions, dielectric functions based on this functional form have been proposed [51,52].

The distance-dependent dielectric function attempts to model the effective dielectric constant, a function of all six coordinates of two particles, by a function of the interparticle distance. In an inhomogeneous system, the association of a dielectric constant with a certain particle distance is problematic because the strength of the interaction between two charges is dependent on their environment. The interior of a protein has a dielectric constant between 2 and 5, whereas that of the surrounding water is approximately 78. Even if both charges are buried within the protein, it is misleading to assume that the interactions are reduced by a factor of only 2–5. By modeling the protein as a sphere, with a dielectric constant of 2 imbedded in an ionic continuum solvent with electrostatics approximated by a modified Tanford–Kirkwood approach, Gilson et al. [54] were able to obtain the electrostatic pair interactions explicitly. The resulting effective dielectric constant between two charges occasionally exceeded a value of 100, whereas other pairs separated by the same distance produced values closer to 10.

A more realistic test of the use of distance-dependent dielectric functions was provided by Friedman and Honig [55]. They applied the more complete (although more computationally intensive) Poisson–Boltzmann theory of solvent screening (see later) to calculate the interactions in B-DNA. These calculations showed that interaction energies between phosphates could be modeled by effective dielectrics of the Debye–Hückel type, whereas the sigmoidal form of Hingerty is more appropriate for interactions between base atoms. None of the existing distance-dependent dielectric functions were able to model all of the relevant pair interactions in DNA. Thus, it seems that effective screening functions should be applied with caution in modeling studies. Nevertheless, their simplicity and computational efficiency are appealing, and they will probably continue to be used when rapid approximate energies are needed, such as in docking studies.

Simulations done under vacuum conditions, using effective dielectric constants modeled as in the foregoing, have exhibited two major deficiencies. First, the effects of the solvent on the dynamics of the macromolecule have not been accounted for. The solvent provides random thermal excitations, as well as viscous damping forces. The net result seems complex and difficult to model [47,56–58]. The second major deficiency in early vacuum simulations was the excessive intramolecular hydrogen-bonding between polar groups on the surface of the molecule, owing to the lack of a "self-energy" term accounting for interactions of polar or charged groups with the high-dielectric solvent. Consequently, significant qualitative differences were found between the potential energy surface of alanine dipeptide in vacuum, using a distance-dependent dielectric term, and the potential of mean force energy surface in explicit solvent [59–61]. Furthermore, vacuum potential energies are unable to distinguish between correctly folded and misfolded proteins [62].

B. Atomic Solvation Energy Correction

To address this latter deficiency in vacuum potential energies, Eisenberg and McLachlan [63] developed an approximation to the protein–solvent interaction component of the free energy of protein folding, which is not treated in the foregoing described vacuum simulations. Their method expresses this protein–solvent interaction component as the sum of individual atomic contributions. An atom's contribution, which represents the free energy of transfer of that atom from the interior of the protein to its surface, is assumed to be proportional to the extent of its interaction with solvent; in particular, by the size of its first solvation shell, which for simplicity is estimated by its solvent-accessible surface area. The constants of proportionality, called the atomic solvation parameters, are specific to each atom type. Eisenberg and McLachlan obtained these parameters by fitting their model to experimental octanol-to-water transfer free energies for amino acid analogues [64]. Given the atomic coordinates, they were able to approximate the contribution of the protein–solvent interaction to the free energy of protein folding. With this approach, they were able to distinguish between correctly folded and misfolded protein structures in their example set. This result was verified by Chiche et al. [65], and Novotny et al. [66]; however Chiche et al. found some example proteins for which the solvation energy criterion barely distinguished folded from misfolded structures.

The entropic contribution of the hydrophobic effect provides the dominant term in the free energy of biological complex formation [67]. This free-energy contribution is proportional to the amount of nonpolar solvent-accessible surface area removed on complex conformation, with a proportionality constant of approximately 25 cal mol^{-1} A^{-2} at room temperature. Other contributions, such as specific hydrogen bonds or other coulombic interactions, are insignificant in comparison. With this, together with estimates of conformational entropy in peptide folding, the free-energy gain on forming a more extensive complementary interface surface is sufficient to explain the "induced fit" of most of the site-specific DNA recognition by proteins [67]. Misra and Honig [68] examined DNA–ligand interactions, using the nonlinear Poisson–Boltzmann equation (see Sec. II.D) to model the electrostatic contribution to the free energy of complex formation. They also concluded that the electrostatic contribution was small in comparison with that provided by burial of hydrophobic surface area.

Ooi et al. [69] developed a similar approach to that of Eisenberg and McLachlan, using data from vapor-to-solution free energies of transfer. Thus, their atomic solvation energy term represents the free energy of transfer of an atom from vapor phase to solution. These atomic solvation energies were then added to the internal energies from the ECEPP force field [70] to allow calculation of solvation free energies of flexible solutes, using Boltzmann-weighted energies of accessible conformations. Wesson and Eisenberg [71], using CHARMM [72], and Schiffer et al. [73], using AMBER [74], later adopted this version of atomic solvation energies to provide solvation corrections to vacuum molecular mechanics calculations. They also explored its use in molecular dynamics simulations. For this purpose, it is necessary to calculate derivatives of the solvent-accessible surface area relative to atomic positions. Fortunately, several fast algorithms for approximate [75] or exact [71,76,77] analytic solvent-accessible surface areas, together with the appropriate gradients, have recently become available.

A potential problem with adding atomic solvation energy terms of this type to vacuum empirical force fields is that the scale of the solvation terms may not be appropriate to a specific force field, that is, the expanded force field may not be "balanced," so some parameter adjustment may be necessary. For example, from the studies of Spolar and Record [67] as well as Misra and Honig [68], one would expect that the surface energy terms should be much larger than other potential energy contributions, whereas this is not always true in the foregoing solvation-corrected force fields. In addition this approach still uses distance-dependent dielectric functions when calculating interactions between charge pairs in the solute, which, as we noted earlier, should be applied with caution. On the other hand, given the recent progress in fast algorithms for calculating the solvent-accessible surface, together with its derivatives relative to atomic position, this simple continuum approach should be very efficient for large biomolecular systems, when compared with the more sophisticated models of solvation.

C. Born Solvation Model

A particularly simple model for the explicit treatment of ionic solvation is the Born model [78]. In this model a spherical charge q within a spherical cavity of radius R is immersed into a dielectric medium with a dielectric constant ϵ_s. For this simple model it is possible to solve the Poisson equation [Eq. (5)] and, thereby, calculate the work of charging the ion in a vacuum as well as in the dielectric medium, and in this manner calculate the free energy of solvation:

$$\Delta G = \frac{q^2}{8\pi R} \left(\frac{1}{\epsilon_0} - \frac{1}{\epsilon_s} \right) \qquad (1)$$

This model has been successfully applied to the calculation of the solvation free energy of ions. However, the application of this formula involves choosing the size of the cavity radius R. The original treatment by Born used crystallographic radii, which resulted in substantial errors. Clearly, the free energy depends sensitively on the choice of this radius, and so it is not surprising that accurate values are easily obtained by minor adjustments to the Born values. For example Latimer [79] added 0.85 A to the cation radii and 0.1 A to the anion radii to reproduce experimental results for alkali cations and univalent anions. Rashin and Honig [80], instead, multiplied the covalent ionic radii by an adjustable parameter to obtain similar results.

The question of the physical meaning of these atomic radii has engendered a lively debate [81–86]. In particular, Rick and Berne [83] demonstrate that the linear response assumption of continuum solvation models is incorrect, and then show how adjustments to the atomic radii can improve the fit to solvation energies at the cost of worse fits to other properties. Because the same sensitivity for atomic radii is seen in all of the continuum electrostatics models, the accuracy achieved in a fit to solvation free energies for a set of compounds is not necessarily a predictor of its success with other compounds or in other modeling contexts. That is, the cautions appropriate to any statistical fitting procedure should be invoked.

In the vicinity of strongly charged solutes, the dielectric response of water is no longer a linear function of the applied field, but rather, becomes saturated. Bontha and Pintauro [86] explored the effect of dielectric saturation on the Born solvation energies. They found that a combined use of the Laplace equation with the Booth equation, which models the dielectric saturation close to the ion, together with a consideration of solvent reorganization energy, allowed them to accurately fit ionic solvation data without the statistical parameter adjustments needed by other groups.

In the context of explicit solvent simulations, the Born model has been used to correct free energies for finite cutoffs [87]. The use of a finite cutoff implies neglect of all ion–solvent interactions beyond the cutoff radius r_c. Therefore, using Eq. (1) and setting $R = r_c$ corrects for the free-energy contribution of the charge interacting with the (bulk) medium beyond r_c. The question of continuum corrections for cutoff effects has been discussed more thoroughly by Wood [88]. Besides the Born solute–solvent cutoff correction, he provides additional continuum corrections owing to the cutoff of solvent–solvent interactions, as well as the (small) corrections by the use of periodic boundary conditions.

Unfortunately, the Born model cannot be used for calculating solvation free energies of molecules or for calculating intermolecular interactions, because in these cases, the problem loses its spherical symmetry. Therefore, the foregoing simple formula [Eq. (1)] cannot be applied.

A more general approach to solvation free energies was described by Still et al. [89]. They express the solvation free energy G_{sol} as a sum of a solute–solvent cavity term G_{cav}, a solute–solvent van der Waals term G_{vdW}, and a solute–solvent polarization term G_{pol}:

$$G_{sol} = G_{cav} + G_{vdW} + G_{pol} \qquad (2)$$

The solvation free energies for saturated hydrocarbons are approximately linearly related to their solvent-accessible surface areas. Because here, G_{sol} is approximately equal to $G_{cav} + G_{vdW}$, Still et al. assume that the cavity plus van der Waals energy $G_{cav} + G_{vdW}$ is, in general, directly proportional to solvent accessible surface area, with a single proportionality constant for all atom types. The polarization energy, which is the electrostatic free energy in a dielectric medium minus that in a vacuum can be evaluated explicitly for a system of n widely separated particles. The result is

$$G_{pol} = -\frac{1}{8\pi}\left(\frac{1}{\epsilon_0} - \frac{1}{\epsilon_s}\right)\sum_{i=1}^{n}\sum_{j=1}^{n}\frac{q_i q_j}{f_{ij}} \qquad (3)$$

where $f_{ij} = r_{ij}$ for $i \neq j$ and $f_{ii} = R_i$, the Born radius for particle i. By generalizing the form of f_{ij} to give appropriate values for three limiting cases of interatomic distance, Still et al. extended this result to charged molecules. The atomic radii R_i in the model are obtained by fitting Born solvation energies to results of a calculation by Poisson's equation of the free energy of charging an individual atom within the molecule. More efficient empirical procedures for obtaining these radii have since been developed [42,90]. During conformational searches these radii are updated periodically. Solvation energies obtained using this method appear to be comparable with those from the more computationally intensive Poisson–Boltzmann approach, and equal to or better than those obtained with explicit solvent free-energy perturbation calculations, which are far more computationally intensive.

Still et al. [89] note that their method is quite sensitive to the partial charges employed, a weakness that is shared by other empirical continuum methods [91,42]. Furthermore, the assumption of a linear relation between $G_{cav} + G_{vdW}$ and solvent-accessible surface area, which is employed in many recent continuum approaches, has been criticized by Simonson and Brünger [92] (see later discussion). Finally, although the generalized Born approach has worked well for small convex-shaped molecules, it remains to be seen if it can be applied to more complex-shaped solutes.

D. Poisson–Boltzmann Approach

A very different technique for ionic solutions was developed on the basis of ideas of Gouy and Chapman [93] and later Debye and Hückel [94], the so-called Poisson–Boltzmann approach [95]. To discuss this approach we first introduce more carefully the Poisson equation in dielectric media. Given a continuous charge distribution with charge density $\rho(r)$ as a function of position r within a vacuum or other material with dielectric constant ϵ_0, applying Gauss' law together with the divergence theorem of calculus we have [96]

$$\nabla \cdot E(r) = \frac{\rho(r)}{\epsilon_0} \tag{4}$$

The electric field $E(r)$ and the electrostatic potential satisfy $E(r) = -\nabla\phi(r)$, by definition. Combining this with Eq. (4) we have Poisson's equation

$$\Delta^2\phi(r) = \frac{-\rho(r)}{\epsilon_0} \tag{5}$$

When the charge density exists within a dielectric medium having a relative dielectric constant different from 1, and possibly depending on position, the situation becomes more complex [96]. In addition to the given charge density, now denoted the free-charge density, surface charge distributions are induced at dielectric boundaries and volume charge densities are induced within the dielectric medium if the dielectric constant $\epsilon(r)$ is not uniform. Under these circumstances, Poisson's equation becomes [96]

$$\nabla \cdot [\epsilon(r)\nabla\phi(r)] = -\rho_{free}(r) \tag{6}$$

Next, we introduce the concept of the potential of mean force, which is related to the ionic pair distribution function. The probability per unit volume of finding an ion of species i at the origin and an ion of species j at position r_j is given by:

$$P(r_i = 0, r_j) = \frac{N_i}{V} \frac{N_j}{V} \exp\left(-\frac{w_{ij}}{k_B T}\right) \tag{7}$$

where N_i, N_j are the numbers of ions of species i and j in the system, V is the system volume, T is the temperature in degrees Kelvin, k_B is Boltzmann's constant, and where w_{ij} is the potential of mean force between ion species i and j, defined as the work required to bring ions i and j into the given configuration in the presence of solvent and all other ions.

The basic assumption of the Poisson–Boltzmann approach is that the potential of mean force w_{ij} is equal to the electrostatic potential energy: $w_{ij} = eZ_j\phi_i(r_j)$, where e is the electronic charge in the appropriate units, Z_j is the formal charge of the ions of species j, and $\phi_i(r_j)$ is the electrostatic potential at r_j caused by ion i at the origin and all the other ions in the system. Under this assumption the charge density can be written as:

$$\rho(r) = \sum_\alpha eZ_\alpha \frac{N_\alpha}{V} \exp\left[-\frac{eZ_\alpha\phi_i(r)}{k_B T}\right] \tag{8}$$

where the summation runs over all ion species α. This equation implies that the concentration of counterions close to the ion of interest is high, but that it decreases with increasing distance.

By using this Boltzmann distribution of the counterions to express the charge density in the Poisson equation, we arrive at the Poisson–Boltzmann equation:

$$\nabla \cdot (\epsilon\nabla\phi_i) = -\sum_\alpha eZ_\alpha \frac{N_\alpha}{V} \exp\left[-\frac{eZ_\alpha\phi_i}{k_B T}\right] \tag{9}$$

Note that this equation is a nonlinear differential equation. To account for short-range repulsive interactions, we assume that counterions cannot penetrate into the ion i. That is, we exclude a sphere of radius a for such ions. The charge of the ion is distributed over the surface of the sphere, whereas the charge inside is zero and the dielectric is a constant. Therefore, for $r \leq a$ we obtain:

$$\Delta^2\phi_i = 0 \tag{10}$$

Under conditions of low ionic strength and constant dielectric outside the central ion we can expand the right-hand side of the Poisson–

Boltzmann equation in a Taylor series to arrive at a more tractable equation. By using the fact that the system is electrically neutral, we have that $\Sigma_\alpha e z_\alpha N_\alpha / V = 0$ (i.e., the zeroeth-order term vanishes). By truncating the series after the first-order terms, we then derive the so-called linearized Poisson–Boltzmann equation:

$$\Delta^2 \phi_i = \kappa^2 \phi_i \tag{11}$$

The constant κ, which is called the Debye screening distance, has the dimension of an inverse length and is defined as:

$$\kappa^2 = \frac{e^2}{\epsilon k_B T} \sum_\alpha Z_\alpha^2 \frac{N_\alpha}{V} \tag{12}$$

For physiological ionic strengths $1/\kappa$ has values of the order of 10 A.

The linearized Poisson–Boltzmann equation can now be solved using spherical symmetry, yielding the well known Debye–Hückel result:

$$\phi_i(r) = \frac{Z_i e}{4\pi\epsilon} \frac{\exp(\kappa a)}{1 + \kappa a} \frac{\exp(-\kappa r)}{r} \tag{13}$$

From this solution of the linearized Poisson–Boltzmann equation it is possible to calculate the chemical potential of an ion in solution by charging up a sphere of radius $R = a$ from zero to $q = Z_i e$. The free energies obtained in this way correctly predict the behavior of dilute solutions such as the limiting-law value [95].

In the Debye–Hückel approximation, the potential decays exponentially with distance and with a decay length for physiological ion concentrations of approximately 10 A. This expression for the counterion charge density leads naturally to the aforementioned distance-dependent dielectric of von Kitzing and Dieckmann [52]. Because of its origin, it should be most appropriate for ionic solutions.

The basic assumption of the Poisson–Boltzmann approach is that the potential of mean force can be written as $w_{ij} = e Z_j \phi_i(r_j)$. This assumption is rather strong, because it implies neglect of nonelectrostatic interactions between ions, such as short-ranged repulsion. Correlations between the central ion and surrounding ions are partially accounted for by defining the radius a of the ion from which all other ions are excluded. However, repulsive interactions between these other ions are ignored altogether. Inclusion of these interactions between the counterions would give rise to an oscillatory behavior of the counterion density, well known from the theory of simple liquids. Actually, this line of thought leads to a deeper understanding of the limitations of the Poisson–Boltzmann approach. Because of the linear superposition principle of classic electrostatics, the representation: $w_{ij} = eZ_j\phi_i(r_j)$ implies automatically that the potential of mean force for triplets is the sum of pair potentials of mean forces: $w_{ijk} = w_{ij} + w_{jk} + w_{ki}$. However, from liquid theory, it is well known that this relation is valid only in the limit of infinite dilution. This consideration affects the nonlinear as well as the linear Poisson–Boltzmann equation; for concentrations in excess of 10^{-3} M, the Poisson–Boltzmann approach to ionic solution theory becomes inaccurate [95].

Various attempts have been made to extend the simple Poisson–Boltzmann theory by including correlation effects between ions. Perhaps the simplest is the Bjerrum pair theory [97], in which some ion pairs form at higher concentrations to reduce the number of free ions participating in the electrostatic potential. Modern approaches to this problem have involved mainly the integral equation methods of liquid state theory. These techniques have been applied only sparingly by the biomolecular simulation community [98–100] and, unfortunately, are beyond the scope of this chapter.

The Poisson–Boltzmann approach has been extended to organic solutes, including macromolecules. Following the earlier work of Tanford and Kirkwood [101], the solute is treated as a region of low dielectric constant, containing fixed atomic partial charges, and surrounded by a solvent of high dielectric constant, containing a continuous distribution of counterions, the charge density of which satisfies the foregoing approximation involving the electrostatic potential energy. The linearized Poisson–Boltzmann equation is solvable in closed form in some simple situations, such as in the Debye–Hückel theory for ions, or cylindrical polyion models for DNA [102]. Several approximate analytic approaches are available in other situations, stemming mainly from the early work of Tanford and Kirkwood [101], and these have been well described [43]. Recently, some new, highly efficient variants of these have been developed, based on inducible multipoles [103], a modified image charge method [104], and a generalized Born approach [105]. The latter uses a continuous gaussian density to represent the volume occupied by atoms within the solute. A similar approach was used previously [106] as an efficient alternative to the use of atomic solvent-accessible surface areas, in calculating solvation free energies.

Although the foregoing analytic approximations are very promising, particularly in the context of energy minimization and molecular dynamics simulations requiring atomic forces, accurate solutions of the Poisson–Boltzmann equation for organic solutes require numeric approaches, such as have been developed for other partial differential equations. Warwicker and Watson [107] pioneered the use of finite-difference numeric solutions of the Poisson equation in the context of proteins, demonstrating the importance of dielectric boundary effects. Honig and co-workers extended this approach to the linear [108] and nonlinear [109] Poisson–Boltzmann equation, and are largely responsible for demonstrating and promoting the usefulness of these methods in biomolecular investigations. These finite-difference Poisson–Boltzmann techniques (FDPB), which have recently grown in popularity, are available to the chemistry community through the widely used DelPhi [110,111] and GRASP [112] programs from the Honig group.

Several alternative numeric techniques are available (e.g., the variational approach [113–115]), but owing to its simplicity and widespread use, we discuss (briefly) only the FDPB technique, which converts the foregoing partial differential equation into a set of coupled linear equations that are typically solved by an iterative technique. This requires first a spatial discretization of the problem, where the molecule is placed inside a larger cubic cell representing the solvent. The cell is gridded, with typical grid spacings at or below 1 A. To represent the interior of the molecule as a medium with a low dielectric constant, one has furthermore to calculate the surface of the molecule. The region inside this surface is assigned a low value of the dielectric constant (2–4). For the outside medium a dielectric constant of 78–80 is assigned, and an ionic strength has to be chosen. Atomic partial charges are interpolated onto the neighboring grid points, and the dielectric constant at midpoints of grid edges is assigned by whether it is inside or outside the molecular surface. Finally, boundary conditions at the edge of the system must be chosen. This is usually done in stages. At first the electrostatic potential at the boundary is assigned according to some reasonable a priori assumption (e.g., that given by a superposition of Debye–Hückel potentials due to the atomic charges). After solving the linear equations for these boundary conditions, using a coarse grid, the resulting potential at the boundary of a subcube that still contains the molecule is used as the boundary conditions for a subsequent finite difference calculation at finer grid density over this subcube. This "focusing" procedure may be repeated one or more times to arrive at a final solution. A good description is given in Gilson et al. [110].

Substantial numeric errors can be associated with the finite difference algorithms. Tests for the error are done by carrying out a series of FDPB calculations in which the molecule is slightly shifted relative to the grid. In addition to the brute force approach to error reduction by using final grid spacings of 0.25 A or smaller, the use of "dielectric smoothing" [116] "charge smearing" [117], and removal of the self-energy term [118] have led to more stable calculations. Multigrid techniques [119,120] appear promising as a method of efficiently adjusting grid density, based on the required local accuracy. Sometimes, as in binding free-energy calculations of receptor–ligand complexes, the errors owing to discretization can be made to largely cancel by carrying out the various calculations with the ligand and receptor frozen relative to the grid [121].

To assess the accuracy of the Poisson–Boltzmann approach Simonson and Brünger calculated the free energy of transfer, from vapor or cyclo-hexane to water, of a variety of small organic molecules, using a three-step thermodynamic cycle [92]. First, a molecule in vacuum or cyclohexane is discharged. The free energy associated with this process is called (for the vacuum) $\Delta G_{\text{vac}}(q \to 0)$, and is estimated by solving the Poisson equation numerically. Next, the free energy of inserting the neutral molecule into water is estimated using an empirical relation between the free energy $\Delta G_{h\Phi}$, the atomic solvent accessible-surface area A_j, and the atomic surface tension γ_j:

$$\Delta G_{h\Phi} = c + \sum_j \gamma_j A_j \tag{14}$$

Finally, the molecule is charged again within the aqueous medium. The free energy $\Delta G_{\text{wat}}(0 \to q)$ of this charging step is estimated with the finite difference Poisson–Boltzmann equation.

Simonson and Brünger assume a single surface tension term γ for all atoms, although they did explore more complex models. For vacuum-to-water transfer they take c to be zero, and γ to be 6 cal mol^{-1} A^{-2} for all atoms. For cyclohexane-to-water transfer they take c to be -0.56 kcals and γ to be 19 cal mol^{-1} A^{-2}. Note, in comparison, that Still et al. [89] used 7.2 cal mol^{-1} A^{-2} for transfer from vapor to water, whereas Spolar and Record [67] used a value of approximately 25 cal mol^{-1} A^{-2}, with no constant term c, to model the free-energy contribution of burial of hydro-phobic surface area, arguing for the applicability of a "liquid hydrocarbon" model based on free energy of transfer from water to pure liquid phase.

In a detailed analysis of the errors involved in the three-stage process, Simonson and Brünger focus attention on the empirical surface tension approximation for solvation of uncharged molecules. They point out that, although in general, it is safe to assume that the free energy of solvation of a neutral solute, such as a saturated hydrocarbon, is linearly related to its solvent-accessible surface area, there are remarkable exceptions, such as cyclooctane and cycloheptane. These have a free energy of approxi-mately 1.5 kcal mol^{-1} lower than expected. Thus, it is possible that this empirical surface tension expression could lead to substantial errors for larger and more complex surfaces, such as interfacial surfaces in protein–protein complexes. There have been some attempts to apply more complex approximations [112], but the correct treatment of this hydrophobic surface energy term seems to us to be an important future area for research. Simonson and Brünger also assign an error of approximately 1–2 kcal to their electrostatic calculations, leading to an overall error of the order of 1–2 kcal mol^{-1}. This was comparable with the error in a simple three-parameter empirical model [122].

Simonson and Brünger also studied the application of continuum models to the potential of mean force of molecular pair interactions in water, and concluded that, for these applications, the method has serious shortcomings, in particular, relative to local water-mediated interactions that may be critical in biomolecular complex formation.

The Poisson–Boltzmann approach has long been used to model the electrostatic contribution to the thermodynamics of colloidal suspensions in electrolyte solutions. A consensus has emerged [114,115] that although the Poisson–Boltzmann equation accurately represents the electrostatic potential in the bulk solvent many angstroms away from charged macromolecular surfaces, it is unable to represent the ion distribution close to these surfaces. That is, the Poisson–Boltzmann approach accurately represents long-range electrostatics, but fails to account for the short-range effects that depend on atomic details of solvation. Warwicker [123] has suggested that the use of more complex descriptions of the solvent dielectric response can improve the accuracy of estimated charge–charge interactions in proteins. He recommends including a saturating dielectric function, similar to that used by Bontha and Pintauro [86] (discussed earlier), as well as the use of two solvent probe radii, the larger to represent bulk water clusters that are excluded from the immediate vicinity of the solute. In contrast, Hecht et al. [124] found that their estimates of electrostatic potentials near the surface of DNA were most accurate when bulk dielectric behavior was assumed immediately outside the DNA; that is, accounting for local dielectric saturation was not helpful.

The Poisson–Boltzmann equation has been applied to many questions of biochemical interest, such as the salt-dependence of DNA–ligand-binding equilibria, the contribution of salt bridges to protein stability, calculations of pKa in proteins, and calculation of electrostatic potentials near proteins and DNA. These applications have been recently reviewed [44,46]. Graphic display of solutions of the Poisson–Boltzmann equation, using, for example, the widely used program GRASP [112], provides a powerful qualitative tool for understanding electrostatic phenomena in macromolecules. For example, it is now possible to consider "electrostatic homology modeling." This application as well as other biological applications have also been recently reviewed [125].

In summary, despite the foregoing theoretical shortcomings, the Poisson–Boltzmann equation and related approaches are rapidly becoming very important in the biomolecular simulation field. Given the inherent inaccuracies in the empirical force fields currently in use, it has not yet been demonstrated that the additional approximations introduced by these simplistic continuum theories contribute substantially to the errors in modeling. Meanwhile, they are far more efficient than the more computationally demanding explicit solvent simulations, which argues for their use when quick estimates are required. Of the methods discussed so far, the Poisson–Boltzmann treatment of electrostatics certainly seems better founded than the simple surface energy-corrected vacuum simulations discussed earlier, or the generalized Born approach, owing to its better treatment of the solvent screening of pair interactions. We have not, however, seen unambiguous evidence of better accuracy in practice.

E. Langevin Dipole Model

Warshel et al. [126–128] argued that the most important problem for the reliable calculation of thermodynamically relevant quantities is the proper sampling of the phase space. The ability of water molecules to form four tetrahedrally arranged hydrogen bonds and, therefore, three-dimensional hydrogen bond networks, clearly has important consequences for structural properties and details of the solvation of individual groups. However, the properties of the hydrogen bond network are not directly related to any thermodynamic properties. The use of detailed water models is accompanied by a large increase in computational cost. To improve the sampling of the phase space, these authors proposed a simplified representation of the solvent, consisting of dipoles located at crystallographic water positions which, however, has more microscopic detail than the continuum representations. They argue that the simplification of representing water molecules by dipoles introduces only a second-order error into thermodynamic calculations.

Warshel and Levitt elaborated these ideas into the protein dipoles Langevin dipoles (PDLD) methodology [126]. For example, to simulate a protein in solution, they divide the whole system into three regions: Region I contains the charge group under study; here the electrostatic interactions are represented by fractional charges q_i. Region II includes the permanent dipoles—represented by charges—and induced dipoles of the remainder of the protein. Region III is formed by the surrounding solvent molecules. Up to, for example, 12 A from the center of the protein the solvent molecules are represented by Langevin dipoles and beyond that distance by a continuum model. The model can be further elaborated in region I by the inclusion of a quantum mechanical treatment of part of the molecule. A further elaboration of the model in region III is to represent the solvent molecules close to region I by explicit water molecules.

The charges in regions I and II are either taken from some parameter set or are fitted by a quantum mechanical calculation. The dipoles in region II are calculated in a self-consistent way by an iterative procedure. In region III a Langevin dipole is assigned to grid points farther than 2.6 A away from any protein atom and inside the 12-A sphere around the reaction center. The spacing between the grid points is usually 3 A. The orientation of the Langevin dipoles is calculated in a mean field approximation using the local electrostatic field. Because the Langevin dipole influences the local field, these equations also have to be solved iteratively until self-consistency. Interactions with nearest neighbors (i.e., for separations smaller than 3.2 A) are excluded.

Russell and Warshel [129] tested this procedure by calculating the solvation free energies of four acidic groups of BPTI. Despite the differences in the structure of the groups, the solvation free energies for all four groups are on the order of -70 kcal mol^{-1}. With this procedure, Russell and Warshel were able to reproduce the experimental values to within 7 kcal mol^{-1}. Recently Xu et al. [130] were able to improve the procedure and reduce this error to approximately 3 kcal mol^{-1}.

F. Continuum Corrections to Quantum Mechanics

Cramer and Truhlar [42] summarize the free energy of solvation as being due to electronic, nuclear, and polarization (ENP) terms, as well as to cavitation, dispersion, and solvent dispersion (CDS) terms. The first set of terms accounts for electronic and nuclear polarization of the solute by the solvent, and polarization of the bulk dielectric solvent by the solute. The second set accounts for the specific effects associated with the first solvation layer, and are only crudely accounted for in current continuum models, through the use of atomic "surface tensions." For the first set of terms, whereas all of the foregoing continuum approaches account for the polarization of the bulk solvent by the solute, they differ in their treatment of the electronic and nuclear polarization of the solute.

The importance of nuclear polarization effects—that is, conformational rearrangement induced by solute–solvent interactions—is underscored by the study of Antosiewicz et al. [131]. In attempting to predict protonation equilibria in proteins by a Poisson–Boltzmann approach, they were forced to assume a dielectric constant of approximately 20 within the solvent-excluded volume. Presumably, this provides a crude estimate of the effect of dipolar reorientation within the protein. A more accurate treatment would require weighted averages over the conformations visited by the protein during the process in question, which is not yet computationally feasible in macromolecules. However, conformational averaging to estimate nuclear polarization effects is possible in smaller organic solutes [132].

Electronic polarization of the solute is usually accounted for only very crudely in the foregoing continuum models, by assigning a dielectric constant of 2–4 to the solvent-excluded volume. At present, most biomolecular simulation packages for explicit solvent simulations do not attempt to account for solute or solvent electronic polarizability either, although it is possible to extend them by reparameterization. The protein dipole Langevin dipole approach allows for a somewhat improved treatment of this ENP term. As Cramer and Truhlar point out, however, only a quantum mechanical approach, involving the addition of solvation terms to the electronic Hamiltonian operator, allows a complete and rigorous treatment of the mutual polarization of solute and solvent, within the continuum approximation. These methods also allow one to attack the very interesting question of the effect of solvation on transition-state energies.

Several methods for incorporating continuum solvation effects into the self-consistent iterative procedures of quantum chemistry are under development. By using either ab initio or semiempirical Hamiltonian functions, these include reaction field approaches using the standard molecular monopole and dipole terms, as well as high-order multipolar expansions, and the polarized continuum model, in which the reaction field is represented by induced charges on the surface of the solvent-excluded cavity. These methods are discussed thoroughly (with many references) by Cramer and Truhlar [42]. Although the BKO (Born, Kirkwood, Onsager) approach, which incorporates the reaction field caused by the molecular monopole and dipole in an approximating spherical solute cavity, is very appealing because of its simplicity, it has only limited accuracy. Modifications involving higher-order multipoles unfortunately converge very slowly relative to multipole order. The use of distributed monopoles seems more efficient. More complex cavity shapes have also been used. The polarized continuum approach appears to be quite promising. Cramer and Truhlar also discuss their simulation model (SMx, x standing for version number) approach, which augments a semiempirical Hamiltonian function with a generalized Born term for the effect of solvent. As with the other quantum models incorporating continuum solvation, the free-energy contribution of the solvent must be determined self-consistently in parallel with the Fock matrix and the density matrix. At each iteration of the self-consistent procedure, the generalized Born solvation free-energy contributes to the energy functional being minimized. The atomic partial charges needed in this generalized Born contribution are determined from the valence charges (the nuclear charges minus the number of core electrons) together with the density matrix. The atomic radii are determined by a procedure similar to that of Still et al. [89]. Finally, the CDS terms appear to couple into the procedure through their dependence on bond orders.

After reviewing the extant methods, Cramer and Truhlar compare several continuum approaches relative to experimental free energies of solvation. In addition to pointing out the need for a treatment of the CDS contributions, they demonstrate the sensitivity of the FDPB approach to the partial charge parameters used. In the SMx approach, the partial charges are not arbitrary parameters, but rather emerge, along with the atomic radii, as part of the self-consistent solution (although there are other parametric aspects of the method). The SMx methods compare very favorably with the other approaches tested. Finally Cramer and Truhlar illustrate the use of the SMx approach in the modeling of solvent effects on conformational and tautomeric equilibria, as well as on organic reaction rates.

III. FINITE MODELS WITH EXPLICIT SOLVENT

Water plays an important role in the interactions between biological macromolecules. Although the foregoing continuum approaches are able to capture much of the long-range electrostatic effects as well as some of the hydrophobic effects of water, there is increasing evidence of the importance of water's molecular nature. Israelachvilli and Wennerström have recently reviewed the role of water structure in the interactions between surfaces in aqueous solution [133], giving various examples of the subtleties involved. For example, the measured forces of interaction between mica surfaces in aqueous KCl solution, when plotted as a function of the distance of separation, show oscillations, with a period of 2.5 A, indicating the presence of water layers that must be displaced as the surfaces approach. Israelachvilli and Wennerström ascribe the strong repulsions between lipid membranes at close distances to excluded volume effects involving the tightly held first layer of solvent as well as the finite size of hydrated counterions. Furthermore, they point out that the strongly oriented dipolar array of the first layer of solvent, when strongly bound to a surface, can give rise to either repulsive or attractive interactions with another such surface, depending on the atomic details of solute and solvent.

Recently, Grubmüller et al. [134] have carried out molecular dynamics simulations of an atomic force microscopy experiment measuring the streptavidin–biotin rupture force. The protein and ligand were immersed in a sphere of water molecules, and equilibrated for 500 ps. Water molecules at the surface were subjected to a boundary potential (see Sec. III.C), and long-ranged interactions were accounted for using a fast multipole algorithm (see Sec. III.D). After equilibration, the biotin ligand was subjected to a harmonic force, pulling it out of its binding pocket. The simulations suggest that water bridges that form during the rupture substantially enhance the stability of the complexes.

Crystallographic as well as thermodynamic studies have pointed to the importance of water bridges in the complex between *trp* repressor and its DNA target [135,136]. Interestingly, this complex does not appear to fit Spolar and Record's buried hydrophobic surface area model of protein–DNA energetics. That is, although there are no conformational rearrangements on binding, the change in heat capacity on complexation, as calculated by Spolar and Record's method, is only half the measured value. Ladbury [137] suggests that restriction of vibrational modes in the complex-specific bound water molecules may account for the discrepancy. Dunitz [138] has estimated that bound water molecules can contribute approximately 2 kcal mol^{-1} each to a binding free energy.

Thus, there seems to be increased interest among structural biologists in the structure of water around proteins and other biological macromolecules [139]; accordingly, the inclusion of at least some explicit solvent in biomolecular simulations will doubtless become increasingly important in the future. In addition, studies such as Chan and Lim's [85] have shown that inclusion of a layer of water can greatly reduce the problems associated with boundaries in continuum studies. However, the traditional approach in molecular simulations of immersing a solute into the solvent and then replicating the system by periodic boundary conditions has the unfortunate consequence that the number of solvent atoms often far exceeds the number of solute atoms. Therefore, the simulation program spends most of the time calculating the solvent–solvent interactions, which are of secondary interest. In addition, some theoreticians, on principle, have objected to the use of periodic boundary conditions [38,39]. To avoid such artifacts and to speed up calculations, while still accounting for the effects of explicit solvent, numerous schemes have been developed.

A. Free Boundary Conditions

The most straightforward approach to including explicit solvent without using periodic boundary conditions is to simply surround the solute with a limited number of water molecules, and to run the combined system as a vacuum simulation. This choice is deemed *free boundary conditions* and seems to have first been tried by Bossis [140], who simulated a two-dimensional disk of water to calculate the dielectric constant. He restricted the simulation to two dimensions to minimize artifacts caused by the vacuum interface. A priori, there appear to be two major artifacts associated with this approach. First, there is severe surface tension at the vacuum–water interface, causing the water molecules near this boundary to have properties very different from those in the bulk. Second, the dielectric properties of the bulk solvent are not accounted for. Nonetheless, the simplicity of this approach is attractive and, in practice, the artifacts may be less severe than anticipated. A recent example of this approach is a study of Steinbach and Brooks [56]. They solvated BPTI with varying numbers of water molecules, ranging from zero to 3830. By measuring the radius of gyration, the rms deviation from the crystal structure, and the length anisotropy of the BPTI molecule, they found that, with 350 added water molecules, the protein is fully hydrated. This number corresponds closely to the number derived from experiments [141]. At this hydration level, the water forms a patchwork of water clusters, rather than a uniform monolayer. The water molecules concentrate around the charged groups, leaving 37% of the surface uncovered. On further hydration the protein–water system becomes more spherical. Up to the hydration level of 350 water molecules, the interaction between protein and water dominates over the tendency of the surface tension to reduce the surface.

Guenot and Kollman [34] have advocated the use of a simple distance-dependent dielectric variable in simulations under free-boundary conditions, because the artifactual effects of cutoffs are less than with the use of a constant dielectric value, and the effects of the "dielectric boundary" at the vacuum–water interface are reduced. Although trajectories appear to be more stable with this protocol, it has been criticized by Steinbach and Brooks [21] because it causes suppression of fluctuations.

B. Stochastic Boundary Conditions

Many simulations of finite systems are performed using stochastic boundary conditions. Stochastic boundary conditions were invented by Berkowitz and McCammon [142] and were initially applied to the simulation of a Lennard-Jones system. In this approach the whole system is divided into three regions: The central region, within 10-A distance of the atom closest to the center of the system, is called the reaction region. The trajectories for the particles in the reaction region are calculated from the forces created by all the particles in the system in the standard molecular dynamics fashion. The surrounding shell of 1-A thickness around the reaction region is called the bath or buffer region. Particles in this region move according to a Langevin equation that includes, besides the forces from other particles, a friction force and a random force. The shell of 4-A thickness around the bath region is called the reservoir or boundary region. In this region the positions of the particles are fixed. As the system evolves, particles can move between the different regions. For Lennard-Jones systems, this method led to accurate values for the radial distribution function as well as the velocity autocorrelation function [142].

The same basic ideas have been adapted to more complex systems, such as BPTI [143] and lipid membranes [144–146]. For BPTI, the division of the system into reaction region, buffer region, and reservoir region was performed on a residue basis and was dependent on its distance to an "active site" [143]. Whenever any atom of a residue is closer than 7 A to any atom of the active site, the whole residue belongs to the reaction region. Residues belong to the reservoir region if all atoms are separated by more than 9 A from any atom of the active site. The residues between reaction and reservoir region belong to the buffer region. To increase the stability of the protein, the atoms in the buffer region are restrained, by harmonic forces, to their initial positions. The disadvantage of this procedure is that only high-frequency motions are included owing to the harmonic constraints [143]. This limitation might be solvable by considering more complex Langevin-type forces.

Juffer and Berendsen revisited this approach and modified it in several ways [147]. The boundary atoms were placed on the sites of a regular polygon. The boundary atoms are fixed by harmonic forces to their initial positions. Furthermore, the Lennard-Jones parameters between two boundary atoms and a boundary atom and a "normal" Lennard-Jones atom can be chosen differently. By adjusting these parameters, the distance between the boundary atoms and the strength of the harmonic forces, Juffer and Berendsen were able to reproduce thermodynamic properties of periodic boundary simulations of Lennard-Jones, such as pressure, chemical potential number density, pair correlation function, and velocity autocorrelation function.

C. Boundary Potential Methods

In their simulations of water clusters, Belch and Berkowitz [148] used a method similar to the foregoing stochastic boundary conditions. However, they replaced the boundary region by a half-harmonic restraining force to prevent molecules from evaporating, and the random force by a simple temperature rescaling technique. By a detailed analysis, they found that the structure of the water close to the surface is similar to the structure of water next to a hydrophobic wall [149]. These perturbations can penetrate deep into the interior of the cluster [148]. Apparently, the vacuum outside the cluster acts as a hydrophobic medium and induces density oscillations and artificial orientational correlations. Many attempts have been made to design special potentials to compensate for the structure-inducing effect of the interface, allowing calculation of "bulk-like" quantities with as few solvent molecules as possible. The foregoing discussed stochastic boundary condition simulations are examples of such attempts.

The most obvious arrangement for a system in which a solute molecule is surrounded by a few solvent molecules is to make the total system a sphere. For this, a spherical half-harmonic potential, such as that of Belch and Berkowitz [148], can preserve the integrity of the system. However, if the solute molecule is nonspherical, this procedure requires innumerable solvent molecules to complete the sphere. To avoid this excess of solvent molecules Beglov and Roux [150] designed a potential that maintains a thin "skin" of solvent molecules around the solute. Specifically, they proposed a harmonic potential between solvent molecule i and the closest solute atom j:

$$U_{shell}(r_{ij}, R_{shell}) = \begin{cases} \frac{1}{2}K_{shell}x^2 \\ 0 \end{cases} \tag{15}$$

where $x = (r_{ij} - R_{vdw}^{(j)} - R_{shell})$ and $R_{vdw}^{(j)}$ denotes the van der Waals radius of solute atom j and r_{ij} the distance to that solute atom j for which $r_{ij} - R_{vdw}^{(j)}$ is the smallest. The shell parameter R_{shell} can fluctuate in response to the forces within the confined space. Typically this radius is rather small, with a value of approximately 5 A. Because of the small shell Beglov and Roux needed only 43 water molecules to solvate an alanine dipeptide, and only 50 water molecules to solvate an alanine tripeptide [150].

To assess the validity of this approach Beglov and Roux [150] calculated the free-energy difference between the C_{7ax} and α_L conformations of alanine dipeptide in vacuum and with the shell model, and compared these results with previous bulk simulations [151,152]. The free-energy differences using the shell model agreed much better with bulk simulations than did the vacuum simulations [150]. Furthermore, the free-energy difference between the closed and open reverse β-turn conformations of the alanine tripeptide, calculated using bulk simulations, was also reproduced using the shell model. These examples suggest that the shell model is able to capture the solvent's dominant contribution to the free energy. Thus free-energy calculations may be possible using only a few solvent molecules. Beglov and Roux also suggest the interesting possibility of combining the shell model with the Poisson–Boltzmann approach to account for "dielectric boundary" effects at the vacuum interface.

In an attempt to decrease the surface tension effects at the droplet–vacuum interface [148], Essex and Jorgensen proposed more complicated restraining functions than the foregoing harmonic potentials [153]. Specifically, these authors addressed the problem that water molecules are excessively ordered at the system interface. They propose a surface potential that is not only a (complicated) function of the position of the water molecule within the cluster, but also is a function of the orientation of the water's dipole vector and a function of the orientation of the vector perpendicular to the plane of the water molecule [153].

By monitoring local density and the relative orientations of the water molecules as a function of their relative position within the cluster during a droplet simulation, Essex and Jorgensen demonstrate that this approach greatly reduces the ordering effect of the interface, when compared with a simple harmonic potential. Furthermore, the calculated free energy of converting a water molecule into a methane molecule agrees much better with bulk simulations than do results of a simulation with a harmonic potential.

A disadvantage of the approach of Essex and Jorgensen is that the restraining potential is rather complicated and requires parameterization for the particular situation. To avoid these ambiguities Wang and Hermans [154], following the earlier work of Rullmann and van Duijnen [155], proposed a completely different approach, based on Friedman's [38] image charge approximation to the reaction field model. The basic idea of this approach is that the electrostatic variable of a spherical water droplet in vacuum can be treated as that of a spherical region of high-dielectric constant ϵ_1 within a medium having a low-dielectric constant ϵ_2. For this instance, Friedman had shown that the full solution to the electrostatic boundary problem can be efficiently approximated by placing virtual "image charges" outside the sphere. If a charge q_i is at the position r_i within the spherical cavity of radius R, then the strength of the image charge, q'_i, can be calculated according to

$$q'_i = -\frac{\epsilon_2 - \epsilon_1}{\epsilon_2 + \epsilon_1} \left(\frac{R}{r_i}\right) q_i \qquad \qquad (16)$$

This image charge is at the location r'_i:

$$\mathbf{r}'_i = \left(\frac{R}{r_i}\right)^2 \mathbf{r}_i \qquad \qquad (17)$$

In addition to the image charges, Wang and Hermans employed a soft-restraining harmonic potential that confines the water molecules to the spherical cavity.

By analyzing the local density and the orientation properties of water molecules, the authors found a surprisingly small effect of the reaction field on the physical properties of the cluster, when compared with that of a simple harmonic potential. Furthermore, free-energy calculations of charging up a cation showed that the free energy agrees with that calculated by bulk simulations, if the cation is in the center of the system. However, the calculated free energies are sensitive to the relative position of the cation within the cluster, indicating that the reaction field does not help remedy the positional dependence of the hydration free energy. This result may reflect the singularity inherent in Eqs. (16) and (17) as the charge approaches the cavity boundary. By neglecting certain interactions Wang and Hermans were able to significantly improve the results. However, because a physical basis for the neglect of these interactions has not been found, it is still unclear whether this interesting approach can be significantly improved.

D. The Fast Multipole Method

If cutoff methods are not employed, the computation of the electrostatic energy of system of N charges requires consideration of all charge pairs, an order N^2 calculation. For large systems this calculation becomes prohibitive. Similar problems are encountered in a host of other problems of physical interest, such as cosmologic simulations involving the formally similar forces of gravitation. Consequently, several approximate algorithms aimed at reducing the computational cost to order N or $N \log(N)$ have been developed. In this section we review methods based on the recursive grouping of distant particles into multipoles, culminating in the fast multipole method (FMM) of Greengard and Rokhlin [156]. Later, in the context of periodic boundary conditions, we discuss methods based on Fourier expansion of the singularity free portion of the pair potential. Recently, Greengard [157] has given a general overview of these as well as other fast summation algorithms, such as multigrid methods, and illustrated their use in a variety of physical problems.

Appel [158] described an early "divide-and-conquer" or hierarchical tree approach to calculating the energies and forces in a system of N particles. Barnes and Hut [159] introduced a more refined version of Appel's algorithm that was amenable to error analysis. Saito [31] implemented it in the context of solvated macromolecular simulations, using a spherical boundary potential. A simple tree algorithm, based on these ideas, is described by Esselink [160]. This simple algorithm, developed for astronomic simulations, is not appropriate for electrostatic interactions, for it represents distant groups of particles by a simple monopole approximation. Nevertheless, because of its simplicity, it provides a good introduction to tree algorithms. Before detailing the algorithm, we first describe the octal tree construction. Assume the particles are contained in a cube. The cube itself is the level zero or root cell. This cell is divided evenly in half in each of the x, y, and z directions to produce the eight, level 1 cells that are the children of the level zero cell. Similarly, each level 1 cell is divided evenly to produce eight, level 2 cells, for a total of 64 level 2 cells. This process is continued to produce a succession of levels. The cells at level l are the parents of cells at level $l + 1$, and the children of cells at level $l - 1$. The cells at the finest subdivision level are called the leaves. For simplicity, assume these leaf cells contain either zero or one particle.

Next we describe the pair interaction algorithm for two cells at the same level. If the two cells are sufficiently well separated (i.e., if the cell diameters divided by the distance between their centers are both less than some tolerance), the energy of interaction is simply that of a pair of particles, each representing one of the cells. The particle masses are given by the total mass within their cells, and their positions given by the center of mass of the cells. [Note that the total mass and center of mass of a cell are easily computed recursively by the mass and center of mass of its children (i.e., without considering all particles within it). This gives a hint of the more complex recursive calculation of multipole moments in the upward pass of the Greengard–Rokhlin fast multipole algorithm, discussed in the following.] If the two cells are not well separated, their pair interaction is arrived at by summing the 64 pair interactions involving the eight children of one cell with the eight children of the other. The pair interaction for leaf cells is the standard pair potential energy for the actual particle positions.

Finally we describe the cell energy algorithm. If a cell is a leaf cell, its energy is zero, because it contains either zero or one particle. Otherwise its energy is given by the sum of the energies of its children, plus the sum of the 28 pair interactions between its children. The total energy of the system is then given by the energy of the root cell.

This simple algorithm illustrates the basic features of the tree algorithms. Minor modifications permit treatment of systems of charges, as well as calculation of forces. Barnes and Hut [159] mentioned the possibility of higher-order expansions, up to quadrupole, to more accurately represent the particles in a cell. Note that, in these algorithms, the forces on particles within a cell are computed particle by particle; that is, the individual particles interact with other cells, either through a multipole approximation, as in the foregoing center of mass approximation, or through recursive interactions with the child cells. Therefore, these algorithms are sometimes referred to as body–cell algorithms, as opposed to cell–cell algorithms, such as the fast multipole algorithm, which we describe next. In cell–cell algorithms, a local or Taylor expansion, valid for an entire cell is derived. Far field forces for the particles in the cell are obtained by evaluating the local expansion at the particle position. In body–cell algorithms, each particle force requires $O[\log(N)]$ evaluations (owing to the number of cells examined), whereas in cell–cell algorithms, each particle requires only $O(1)$ evaluations. In addition, these body–cell algorithms usually use low-order Cartesian multipole expansions, whereas cell–cell algorithms often involve high-order multipole expansions. These are usually expressed in terms of spherical harmonics, rather than Cartesian multipoles, because expansions in spherical harmonics are far more efficient at higher orders. Thus, these tree algorithms are usually faster, but less accurate. Salmon and Warren [161] give an example of the serious consequences of too loose a criterion for "well separatedness," and argue for a more rigorous error analysis.

The FMM algorithm begins with the foregoing octal tree construction. The leaf cells now contain typically 10–20 particles, instead of 1. Given a cell at level l, other cells at the same level are said to be well separated if they are not one of the (at most) 124 nearest or next nearest neighbor cells. The potentials and forces for particles in the leaf cells are obtained by first directly calculating the interactions involving particles in leaf cells that are not well separated. These results are added to the potentials and forces resulting from the local Taylor expansion about the center of the cell, which accounts for the particles in well-separated leaf cells. Efficient computation of these local expansions is the main thrust of the Greengard FMM, and involves a two-pass procedure.

In the first, or upward pass, multipole moments are formed for every cell in the tree. The multipole moments for the leaf cells are obtained by straightforward calculation, using the center of the cell as the origin of the expansion. Rather than repeat the procedure to calculate the multipole moments of the parent cell, which involves expansion about a different origin, Greengard employs translation operators to shift the center of expansion of a multipole moment from a cell's center to that of its parent. Thus, the contribution of a cell to its parent's multipole moments involves a linear combination over its own multipole moments, with coefficients given by these translation operators. The contributions of the eight children are summed together to give the multipole moments of the parent. In this way the multipole moments of the root cell are eventually formed.

In the second, or downward pass, local Taylor expansions are formed out of the previously computed multipole moments. Given a cell A at level l the local expansion about A's center accounts for the contribution of all well-separated cells at level l. This local expansion can be shifted to the centers of A's children using translation operators similar to those employed in the upward pass. Similarly A inherits some of its local expansion from that of its parent. This part accounts for the contributions of level

$l - 1$ cells that are well separated from A's parent and, hence, the contributions of their level l children. The remaining cells that must be considered are the (at most) 875 level l cells that are well separated from A, but that are children of level $l - 1$ cells that are not well separated from A's parent. These latter level l cells make up the interaction list. To obtain the local expansion accounting for their contribution, Greengard introduced operators that convert a multipole expansion about the center of a cell B in the interaction list into a local expansion about the center of A. The separate local expansions from these interaction list cells are added together and combined with the contribution of A's parent to arrive at the complete local expansion for A. This, as noted earlier, is translated to the centers of each of A's children to continue the downward pass. In this way the local expansions for the leaf cells are eventually formed.

The mathematical details of the foregoing algorithm are easier to understand in two dimensions, because complex multiplication and division can be employed to conveniently reexpress the relevant expansions. This case is discussed fully in Greengard's thesis [162]. In three dimensions the mathematics is much more complex. Although this example is also discussed in Greengard's thesis, a more concise description is given by White and Head-Gordon [163].

The Greengard algorithm has been extended to periodic systems, as described in Section IV; thus, it is more general than the Fourier-based methods discussed later. Because it has been proved to be of order N, rather than $N \log (N)$, as in the tree codes and Fourier-based methods, it also must be faster above some system size. The question of its actual performance has been somewhat controversial. When compared with direct pairwise evaluation, the breakeven point, or the point at which the FMM becomes faster, depends on the accuracy required. For a reasonable relative rms force error of approximately 5×10^{-4}, which is standard for simulations using Ewald sums (discussed later), the early results of Schmidt and Lee [164] obtain a breakeven point of approximately 20,000. This level of accuracy requires multipole expansions up to order 8. Ding et al. [165] derived a much faster algorithm, called Cartesian multipole method (CMM), by using Cartesian multipole expansions, rather than spherical harmonics, and by including only low-order expansions that, however, lead to much greater force errors. Board and co-workers [166] parallelized the FMM while deriving a faster serial version than Schmidt and Lee. They obtain a breakeven point of approximately 3500 particles at similar accuracy. White and Head-Gordon report a slightly lower breakeven point. They also illustrate a couple of interesting and possibly disturbing aspects of the performance. First, the number of levels in the tree is not a continuous function of the number of particles. For a range of system sizes encompassing a fixed tree depth, the number of particles in the leaf nodes grows linearly, leading to local quadratic growth in computational cost, owing to the direct interactions. Second, the relative rms force errors produced by a fixed order of multipole expansion tend to grow with system size. This growth in error can be seen clearly in Table 2 of Zhou and Berne [167].

Other factors also need to be considered when examining reports of FMM performance. First, the accuracy is affected by the choice of "well-separatedness." Some workers have considered cells to be well separated if they are not immediate neighbors, whereas others, such as Greengard, rule out second neighbors, as in our foregoing description. This results in greater accuracy at the cost of more time in the direct sum routine, and a more pronounced local quadratic growth in computational effort as a function of system size (as noted by White and Head-Gordon). Second, the FMM scales linearly in system size, but its cost scales as p^4 where p is the order of the multipole expansion. This becomes very costly for large p. Greengard and Rokhlin [168] suggested the use of the fast Fourier transform (FFT) in the foregoing translation operators, which reduces this cost to $p^2 \log(p)$, but which increases memory needs. Shimada et al. [169] implemented a very efficient variant of this idea in the CMM context, called particle–particle mesh multipole expansion (PPM/MPE), which reduces the computational cost of evaluating distant interactions by a factor of 10 or more. A different approach was used by Lustig et al. [170]. The CMM, which uses Cartesian multipole expansions, is faster at low accuracy as well as easier to program than the FMM. However, as noted by Lustig et al. (see also Shimada et al. [169]) the computational cost grows as p^6 which proves prohibitive for high-accuracy simulations. They advocate the use of "Chebyshev economization" to retransform the multipole expansion into a series with fewer terms, leading to a substantial reduction in computing time.

That the Legendre polynomials are bounded by unity leads to simple bounds for the error owing to truncating multipole expansions at order p, which are sufficient to establish the basic asymptotic costs of the FMM. Much more precise bounds for the worse-case error are derived by Petersen et al. [171]. When using these, they propose another type of optimization, in which the multipole expansion for distant cells is truncated at lower values of p. They report that this variant, called the very fast multipole method (VFMM) [172] is two to three times as fast as the standard FMM.

When considering questions of accuracy, we should point out that it is presently unclear what level of error is actually acceptable in the evaluation of long-range interactions. As we pointed out in the introduction, cutoff methods can lead to far more dramatic errors in the time-averaged forces than in the instantaneous forces, so perhaps comparisons of potentials of mean force would be more enlightening.

Finally, the computational cost of these methods can be ameliorated by a multiple time step approach. For example, Windemuth [173] has implemented a distance class multiple time step [174] variant of Board's algorithm wherein the full pairwise interactions are calculated by the FMM only every 20 steps, whereas the short-range coulombic terms out to 7 A are updated along with the van der Waals terms every step. Grubmüller et al. [134] also employ the distance class multiple time step algorithm; however, they use an adaptive variant of the FMM [175]. A much more satisfying approach is given by Zhou and Berne [167], who combine the FMM with the reversible reference system propagator (r-RESPA) approach [176] to obtain an efficient algorithm that conserves energy. Energy conservation should be a required property for any viable algorithm. This requirement puts an upper limit on the cost savings that can be achieved by infrequent calculation of the full pairwise interactions.

IV. SIMULATIONS UNDER PERIODIC
BOUNDARY CONDITIONS

The presence of a vacuum interface can lead to severe artifacts. Despite the progress just reported in developing boundary potentials for these situations, the use of periodic boundary conditions still seems the most straightforward way to eliminate these artifacts. The system to be simulated comprises a simulation cell, for example a cube. This cube is then replicated infinitely in all directions. Thus, each particle i at position r within the cube has an infinite number of "image" particles at positions $r + (n_1L, n_2L, n_3L)$ where n_1, n_2, n_3 are integers and L is the length of the cube. The interaction of particle i with j in periodic boundary conditions is evaluated by summing that of i with j and all its images. For interactions, such as Lennard-Jones, that die off faster than the inverse third power of distance, this infinite series converges absolutely, and there are no ambiguities associated with this choice of boundary condition. In that event, as noted in the following, it is usually acceptable to truncate the series at the "minimum image" term, that is for i to only feel that image of j that is closest to it. However, for coulombic interactions, it is not obvious a priori how to properly evaluate this pair interaction. In the following, we review the use of truncation methods, including switch functions, reaction field approaches, and finally the Ewald method, which emerges from a careful treatment [36,177] of the full lattice sum of image interactions.

A. The Use of Switch Functions in Periodic Boundary Simulations

The first molecular dynamics simulations used very simple systems, such as the hard sphere fluid and the Lennard-Jones fluid. For these potential functions, the range of interactions is rather short. Therefore, it seemed appropriate to calculate the interactions as minimum image interactions, and then only up to a given cutoff distance r_c, and either to neglect all interactions beyond the cutoff, or to estimate them by a homogeneous continuum. In combination with the Verlet neighbor list, this method saved a significant amount of computer time [1]. For short-range potentials, such as the Lennard-Jones, this procedure is a good approximation, even if the cutoff distance is as small as $r_c = 2.5\sigma$. To understand this we should recall that the time evolution of the system is determined by the forces. In a condensed liquid or solution, the Lennard-Jones density is fairly homogeneous and, therefore, the force on a particle i from a particle j at position $r_i + r_{ij}$ is on average compensated by forces from particles near $r_i - r_{ij}$. However, for quantities such as potential energy and pressure the contributions from r and $-r$ are additive; therefore, for these one has to correct for the neglect of long-ranged interactions. This can be achieved by representing the particles outside the cutoff by a homogeneous Lennard-Jones fluid and obtaining the correction analytically.

With the attempt to study more complex fluids, such as water [178–181], cutoff methods were also adapted to these cases. (Interestingly, Rahman and Stillinger [179] recognized clearly that it would be desirable to use Ewald sums, but they dismissed this possibility on the grounds of computational expenses.) Complex fluids, such as water and aqueous biomolecular solutions, are commonly represented by a combination of intra- and intermolecular interactions. The intramolecular interactions reflect the chemical bonding within the molecules, and once the potential form and potential parameters are chosen, that are straightforward to compute. The intermolecular potential is usually a combination of Lennard-Jones and coulomb interactions. To represent the electrostatic field caused by the molecules, partial charges are assigned to each atom. Application of the cutoff procedure on an atom–atom basis causes severe problems. Although the long-range behavior of a Lennard-Jones potential is dominated by the $1/r^6$ term the charge–charge interaction vanishes only as $1/r$. For liquid water, a simple improvement is possible by applying the cutoff condition to the molecule–molecule interaction (i.e., whenever the oxygen–oxygen distance is smaller than r_c the interaction is calculated; otherwise, it is neglected). Because water molecules are neutral, the lowest nonzero multipole is the dipole term; hence, for large r the interactions decay like

$1/r^3$ instead of $1/r$ (thus, they are almost short-ranged, the sums almost converge absolutely). Consequently, artifacts caused by the cutoff procedure are substantially reduced. Recently, however, Steinbach and Brooks [21] have criticized this choice, because energy is not a state function when it is employed.

For biomolecular systems, the use of the cutoff procedure has been widely adopted to save computer time [40]. To minimize artifacts, the foregoing idea of applying cutoffs on a molecule–molecule basis has been modified for this case, by introducing the concept of charge groups. The idea behind this procedure is that the exchange of charge within molecules is rather localized; therefore, it is possible to identify neutral groups (except, e.g., for ions or charged residues in proteins or DNA). To apply the cutoff condition, it is necessary to define the "distance" between charge groups. One possible choice has been implemented into the program GROMOS [182]. The interactions between two charge groups are neglected if the distance between reference points belonging to the groups is larger than r_c. For a "solute" charge group the reference point is the center of geometry, whereas for a "solvent" charge group it is the position of the first atom of the solvent molecule.

An entirely different definition of the distance between charge groups is implemented into the program package AMBER [74]; namely, the minimum distance between any two atoms, one from each group. The definition used in AMBER clearly increases the amount of computer time because the distance between reference points is in general larger, but on the other hand, this definition should be more accurate. For large charge groups, a cutoff criterion based on reference points can lead to a situation in which individual atoms of the groups are close to each other, but do not interact owing to the distance between their reference points. Subsequently, if the relative motion of the groups brings the reference points within cutoff distance, these proximate interactions can lead to significant jumps in energy and atomic forces.

Conversely, the cutoff criterion used in AMBER can lead to ambiguities in the application of the minimum image convention. If a charge group is large, or if one of the box lengths is rather small, two charge groups might be within the cutoff distance of each other in two ways: by translating one of the charge groups by plus or by minus one box length.

At the cutoff distance the potential energy jumps from a nonzero value to value of zero. The force associated with the potential jump should be described by a δ-function. Because this δ-function is usually omitted, the energy conservation in a molecular dynamics simulation is destroyed, leading to a slow heating of the system. (Because of the neglect of the

δ-function the equivalence of the Monte Carlo method and molecular dynamics method is also lost.)

To avoid the discontinuity in the potential energy, a switch function $S(r)$ has frequently been applied [40]. A popular choice is a simple polynomial that switches the potential from full strength at $r = r_1$ to zero at $r = r_c$, with vanishing derivatives at r_1 and r_c. Oftentimes r_1 is chosen close to r_c, leading to a rather steep potential function. Because the forces are the gradient of the potential, they become artificially large in the switch region, causing strong artifacts [40,30]. Recently, Steinbach and Brooks [21] analyzed the artifacts associated with switching of the potential energy, and recommend the use of larger cutoffs and switch regions (e.g., 12-A cutoffs and 4-A switch regions. These authors also recommend switching or shifting forces, rather than the potential energy, or alternatively, if a group-based method is used, shifting the potential function before a switch function is applied. They devise numerous functions for these purposes. The force-shifting function for example has the functional form:

$$ F(r) = \frac{q_i q_j}{r^2} \left[1 - \left(\frac{r}{r_c} \right)^{\beta + 1} \right] \frac{r}{r} \, \theta(r_c - r) \qquad (18) $$

Where θ is the Heaviside step function and β is some integer. This shift function is identical [30] with the reaction field expression (see the following) of Hummer et al. [183,184] if $\beta = 2$. This observation provides a physical basis for the otherwise rather arbitrary selection of a shift function.

In the Ewald method, the direct interactions are switched off by the *erfc* or complementary error function. However, it is misleading to view the *erfc*-function as a switch function in the same sense as the functions discussed earlier. The contributions neglected in the direct sum are accounted for in the reciprocal sum. As a result the total potential energy is independent of how fast the *erfc*-function switches off the direct sum. It seems more appropriate to view the *erfc*-function as a tuning function that divides the computational effort between direct and reciprocal sum.

Because the interactions neglected in the direct sum are accounted for in the reciprocal sum the *erfc*-function should be applied on an atom–atom basis, which makes the programming easier and removes ambiguities associated with group-based switching.

B. Reaction Field Method

To calculate the dielectric constant of liquids, Onsager [185,186] developed the idea of using a reaction field to represent the long-ranged interactions.

Originally, this theory was developed for liquids that are composed of molecules with a permanent and an induced dipole. A given dipole in the liquid is surrounded by other dipoles that produce an electric field at the position of the dipole under consideration. This dipole, in turn, generates an electric field that acts on the surrounding dipoles. The rearrangement of the surrounding dipoles further alters the electric field at the location of the dipole under consideration. To describe this feedback mechanism of the dipole on the electric field at its own position, Onsager introduced the concept of the reaction field.

To arrive at an analytical result, Onsager considered a spherical cavity of radius a around the dipole $\vec{\mu}$. The system outside the cavity is described as a uniform dielectric medium with a dielectric constant ϵ. To calculate the electrostatic potential inside and outside the cavity, the field equations as well as the boundary conditions have to be specified. Because the dielectric medium outside the cavity contains no free charges, the potential can be described by the Laplace equation: $\nabla^2 \phi = 0$. Inside the cavity the potential is a superposition of a dipole potential: $\phi = $ wm; $/r^2 \cos \theta$, plus a potential that satisfies the Laplace equation. The potential ϕ in these two regions must satisfy the following three conditions: (a) The potential outside the cavity vanishes at infinity: $\lim_{r \to \infty} \phi = 0$. (b) At the boundary the potential is continuous: $\lim_{r \to a^-} \phi = \lim_{r \to a^+} \phi$; and (c) the radial component of the electric displacement changes continuously: $\lim_{r \to a^-} (\partial \phi / \partial r) = \epsilon \cdot \lim_{r \to a^+} (\partial \phi / \partial r)$.

The field of the dipole in the cavity is axially symmetric; therefore the solutions to the Laplace equation can be expanded in Legendre polynomials. Because the Legendre polynomials form an orthogonal set of functions, the coefficients have to fulfill the field equations term by term. This procedure leads to zero coefficients except for the $n = 1$ term, which contains the dipole contribution (note the Legendre polynomial of degree 1 is just $\cos \theta$), and as a result the field produced by the polarization of the dielectric medium induces a dipole field in the cavity. This reaction field is opposed to the original field and has a magnitude of $\vec{R} = (1/a^3) [2(\epsilon - 1)/(2\epsilon + 1)]\vec{\mu}$.

The original derivation of Onsager is valid only for dipolar systems. It has been generalized to many different physical situations. The reaction field of an ion in a dielectric medium at infinite dilution was calculated by Hummer et al. [187]. Mathematically this result can be obtained in a manner similar to the foregoing, except, here, a charge, rather than a dipole is placed at the center of the cavity. The functional form of the pair interaction is given in Eq. (18), with $\beta = 2$.

Alper and Levy [188] proposed a generalized reaction field based on calculations of Tanford and Kirkwood [101] for a set of charges in a low-dielectric cavity embedded in a high-dielectric medium. The electric field outside the cavity is described by the Poisson equation. Alper and Levy [188] calculated the dielectric constant of water from the Kirkwood G_k factor. The authors find an improved convergence compared with the traditional reaction field and obtain results in good agreement with bulk simulations. Furthermore, they showed that the charging free energy of ions is well reproduced if the ion is in the center of the system. A problem arises in this method, however, because fixed boundary conditions are employed, and the results of the free-energy calculations are sensitive to where the particles are located relative to these boundaries.

To apply the reaction field method to ionic solutions, Tironi et al. [189] modified the basic assumptions in two ways: (a) Within the cavity the dipole field is replaced by a coulombic law. (b) Because it is assumed that the concentration of ions in the system is nonzero, the electric field outside the cavity is described by a Poisson–Boltzmann equation, instead of a Laplace equation. As in the original reaction field method, the solution is expanded with the aid of Legendre polynomials. The final result of this treatment provides a simple expression for the reaction field that is a function not only of the dielectric constant, but also of the ionic strength. The calculation of the reaction field contribution requires only a minor overhead over conventional truncation methods [189]. To test the validity of this procedure Tironi et al. [189] calculated the ion–ion pair distribution of a 1 M NaCl solution and compared the results to simulations with a simple cutoff scheme and Ewald summation. Although the simple cutoff scheme reproduced the remarkable buildup, at the cutoff, in the ion–ion pair correlation functions for like ions observed by Auffinger and Beveridge [10] (discussed in Sec. I), the results of the reaction field simulation produce significantly better results, comparable with those using Ewald summation. However, the results are sensitive to the reaction sphere radius used, indicating that it should be greater than the 9-A radius used in this study [190].

Reaction field methods are, in a sense, the strict opposite of Ewald summation methods, because the long-range isotropy is build into the theory, whereas Ewald summation methods are strictly lattice sums, and thus, anisotropic. Therefore, reaction field methods seem particularly appropriate to liquid simulations. However, it should be emphasized that the approach is valid only if the cavity for which the direct interactions are calculated is much larger than the largest correlation length within the system. Only then, could one expect that the medium outside the cavity behaves as a uniform dielectric continuum. Especially for proteins or supermolecular aggregates, this correlation length might be quite large, forcing a large diameter for the cavity.

C. Ewald Summation and Other Lattice Summation Techniques

Evaluation of pair interactions under periodic boundary conditions leads to consideration of infinite lattice sums, unless one uses one of the foregoing approximate treatments. Because the coulombic interactions do not decay fast enough to provide absolutely converging series (see later discussion) and, hence, unambiguous evaluation methods, we are forced to consider more carefully what we are modeling. Although the traditional Ewald sum can be arrived at fairly easily by the artifice of applying gaussian counter- and coion clouds to each charged particle [1,191], this approach does not come to grips with the inherent difficulties. Instead, as discussed by Cichocki et al. [192], the correct approach to this problem is to consider a large, but finite, periodic array of unit cells, immersed in a dielectric continuum. Without going too deeply into the mathematics, we will try to discuss the source of the difficulties, and how, using the foregoing model of a large but finite crystal, the asymptotic result emerges.

Suppose there are N point charges $q_1, q_2, \ldots, q_N$ at positions $r_1, r_2, \ldots, r_N$ within the unit cell U satisfying $q_1 + q_2 + \cdots + q_N = 0$. For simplicity, assume the unit cell is a cube of length L (the method generalizes to arbitrary unit cells, however). The charges interact according to Coulomb's law with periodic boundary conditions. Thus, a point charge q_i at position r_i interacts with other charges $q_j, j \neq i$ at positions r_j as well as with all of their periodic images at positions $r_j + (n_1 L, n_2 L, n_3 L)$ for all integers n_1, n_2, n_3. It also interacts with its own periodic images at $r_i + (n_1 L, n_2 L, n_3 L)$ for all such integers n_α with n_1, n_2, n_3 not all zero. The electrostatic energy of the unit cell U can then be written:

$$E(r_1, \ldots, r_N) = \frac{1}{2} {\sum_n}' \sum_i \sum_j \frac{q_i q_j}{|r_i - r_j + n|} \qquad (19)$$

where the outer sum is over the vectors $n = (n_1 L, n_2 L, n_3 L)$, the prime indicating that terms with $i = j$ and $n = 0$ are omitted.

To appreciate the problems involved, consider the simple lattice sum

$$\sum_{n \neq 0} \frac{1}{|n|^p} \qquad (20)$$

where the lattice vectors n are as just defined. If $p > 3$ this sum converges, whereas if $p \leq 3$ it diverges to infinity. This result is the origin of the distinction between short-range and long-range interactions. Thus, if there were only a single positive charge in the unit cell, replicated by periodic boundary conditions, the unit cell electrostatic energy would be infinite, even though, by symmetry, the particle would experience no force. Similarly, if the unit cell were not neutral, the sum in Eq. (19) would diverge. Oddly enough, the forces actually converge (conditionally) here, as we will see later, even though they are long-ranged as well.

If the unit cell is neutral, the sum in Eq. (19) converges, albeit only conditionally. This latter statement means that the result obtained depends on how the limit to infinity is taken. A simple example of a conditionally convergent series is the one-dimensional series $1 - 1/2 + 1/3 - 1/4 + 1/5 + \ldots$. The series converges, meaning the sequence of its partial sums converges to some number. However if we rearrange the series as follows: $1 + 1/3 - 1/2 + 1/5 + 1/7 - 1/4 + \ldots$, that is, two positive terms followed by a negative term, then it now converges to a different limit [193]. This peculiar result cannot happen if a series is absolutely convergent; that is, if the series with all terms replaced by their absolute values were to converge. The same kind of problem can be expected for the sum in Eq. (19), because it is not, in general, absolutely convergent, by the foregoing criterion [see Eq. (20)] (i.e., coulombic interactions are long-ranged). If, for example, you perform the summation by slabs, making n_3 the outer sum, and first taking the infinite sum over n_1 and n_2 for each fixed n_3, you will not generally obtain the same answer as if you compute the sum by gathering the lattice points n into spherical shells and summing this way; nor will the forces agree.

One approach to obtaining limits to conditionally convergent series is to use "convergence factors." That is, one multiplies the terms of the original series c_n by factors $f(n, s)$, $s > 0$, so that the new series converges absolutely to some limit $L(s)$, and then takes the limit of $L(s)$ as s approaches zero. DeLeeuw et al. [36] showed how different orders of summation in Eq. (19) could be expressed in terms of different choices of convergence factors. They then derived an explicit form for the limit, in terms of the standard Ewald sum (see later) plus a correction term, depending on the dipole moment of the unit cell. If the array of unit cells is immersed in a dielectric fluid, the dipole moment term is modified to look like a reaction field term. In particular, if the fluid has infinite dielectric ("tinfoil") boundary conditions, it vanishes, leaving the original Ewald sum.

Later Smith [177] developed a more direct approach. For a large, but finite crystal, the shape can be specified in terms of a specified region. For example, for a spherical order of summation, consider the crystal consisting of the original unit cell, centered about the origin, plus all translations by vectors $n = (n_1 L, n_2 L, n_3 L)$ satisfying $|n| \leq R$. Consider the electrostatic energy of the central unit cell within this crystal, given by

$$E_R(r_1, \ldots, r_N) = \frac{1}{2} \sum_{|n| \leq R}' \sum_i \sum_j \frac{q_i q_j}{|r_i - r_j + n|} \qquad (21)$$

and then consider the limit as R tends to infinity.

To evaluate this energy, Smith uses a theta transform technique, similar to that previously used by Ewald [6] and DeLeeuw et al. [36], to express $1/|r|$ as a "direct space" contribution $erfc(\beta|r|)/|r|$ plus an integral over "reciprocal space." The breakup looks similar to that employed in Kittel [191]. However, when using this expression, the behavior of the reciprocal space integrand near the origin becomes important. Neutrality of the unit cell is critical, and in the limiting process a dipolar contribution, not present in the original Ewald sum, emerges. The result for a spherical order of summation is:

$$E(r_1, \ldots, r_N) = \frac{1}{2} \sum_n' \sum_i \sum_j \frac{q_i q_j \, erfc(\beta|r_i - r_j + n|)}{|r_i - r_j + n|}$$
$$+ \frac{1}{2\pi L^3} \sum_{m \neq 0} \frac{\exp(-\pi^2 m^2/\beta^2)}{m^2} S(m)S(-m) \qquad (22)$$
$$- \frac{\beta}{\sqrt{\pi}} \sum_i q_i^2 + \frac{2\pi}{3L^3} M^2$$

where M is the dipole moment of the unit cell, given by

$$M = \sum_{j=1}^N q_j r_j \qquad (23)$$

and $S(m)$, for $m = (m_1/L, m_2/L, m_3/L)$ are the structure factors, given by

$$S(m) = \sum_{j=1}^N q_j \exp(2\pi i m \cdot r_j) \qquad (24)$$

A more detailed version of this derivation, including the generalization to other reciprocal powers of distance, is given in Appendix A of Essmann et al. [194]. Deem et al. [195] derive dipole contributions for more complex summation orders.

Smith [196], has considered the case of a large spherical crystal immersed in a dielectric medium and subject to short-ranged external surface pressure. By rigorously defining a Hamiltonian function for this system, imposing periodic boundary conditions by a constrained Lagrangian function [197], he arrives at limiting expressions for the forces caused by particle–particle short-range and coulombic interactions, as well as polarization effects by the medium. The dipolar contribution reduces to the familiar Onsager reaction field term. To correctly compute this dipole, one must not employ wrapping of particles. Finally, Smith obtains a limiting expression for the pressure tensor in this situation.

Caillol [198] arrived at similar conclusions about the correct limiting Hamiltonian function by providing a physical interpretation to the convergence factor approach of DeLeeuw et al. [36]. Specifically, he considers central particles at positions $r_{j\,0}$ and having charge q_j and mass m_j, together with an infinite array of image particles at positions $r_{j\,0} + n$ having charge $q_j \exp(-s\,|n|^2)$ and mass $m_j \exp(-s\,|n|^2)$. A similar scaling can be applied (e.g., to the Lennard-Jones well-depth parameter). Imposing the same velocity constraints as Smith [196], he arrives at a Hamiltonian function that factorizes as a scalar $K(s)$ that diverges as s approaches infinity times a Hamiltonian of the central system, which itself converges to the same limit as Smith's for spherical summation order. Caillol also concludes that the correct way to calculate the dipole in the Ewald formula is to use unwrapped coordinates.

One frequent source of confusion is how to treat periodic boundary conditions if the unit cell is not neutral. Examining Eqs. (2.7a) in Caillol [198], one sees that the singularity in the pair potential, as s approaches zero, is independent of particle positions; that is, the forces converge even if the unit cell is not neutral. However, the total dipole moment depends on the choice of reference in this instance, so it would seem that tinfoil boundary conditions should be used. Because the forces can be identified here, there is no conceptual difficulty with molecular dynamics. However, the energy diverges. The accepted solution for this is to imagine a uniform neutralizing plasma. Note that this addition will not affect the forces, but will lead to an extra constant term in the Ewald unit cell energy, namely $Q^2\pi/2\beta^2 L^3$, where $Q = q_1 + q_2 + \ldots + q_N$. Hummer et al. [199] show how, when this extra term is used, reasonable values for solvation free energies of ions can be obtained. Figuerido et al. [200] also discuss the case of nonneutral systems, and isolate a finite system effect when charging free energies of ion pairs.

The Ewald sum is relatively simple to program. A Fortran routine to perform it is described in Allen and Tildesley [1]. It has been extended to other potentials, such as Lennard-Jones [201]. Because it is so heavily used, various techniques for speeding the evaluation have been developed [202]. The computational cost grows as the $3/2$ power of the number of particles [203,204]. Errors caused by truncation of the direct and reciprocal sum have been analyzed [205–207], and the computational cost at fixed accuracy as a function of system size has been compared with alternative techniques, such as FMM- and the FFT-based methods (see later discussion). Toukmaji and Board [208] have provided a very nice review of many of these developments. Cichocki et al. [192] proposed a very accurate method, based on expansion of the Wigner potential in spherical harmonics, but at lower accuracy it does not appear to be competitive with Ewald summation. Although the Ewald sum breaks the coulombic interaction into direct and reciprocal sums using the *erfc*-switching function, this choice is not mandatory. Natoli and Ceperley [209] investigated a class of switching functions that is expressed in terms of spline basis functions and derived a least-squares criterion to arrive at an optimal switching function. They report a factor of 2 performance gain over conventional Ewald summation. Finally, as in the foregoing FMM methods, the computational cost of the Ewald sum can be ameliorated by a multiple time step method. Procacci and Marchi [210] have designed an r-RESPA algorithm that provides a fourfold or more speedup for large systems while conserving energy and reproducing the density of states.

Schmidt and Lee [164] extended the FMM to periodic boundary conditions by considering lattice sums in the multipole moments of the unit cell, which emerge at the end of the "upward" pass. Ding et al. [211] replace the computationally complex multipole Ewald sums by representing the unit cell by a "reduced cell" of a small number of particles for which the multipoles, up to a fixed order, agree with that of the cell. Because their CMM is a low-accuracy method anyway, this may not introduce any additional error. Recently Lambert et al. [212] introduced a technique wherein the unit cell itself becomes part of a large finite array of copies, as in the setup of Smith [177]. The unit cell becomes a child cell within the array, and recursion techniques similar to those in the conventional FMM are used to evaluate interactions. The method is thus a numeric technique to investigate convergence to the limit, for a large selection of summation orders.

Because these techniques are all order (N) with system size, they are certain to outperform Ewald summation at some point. The question of the breakeven point has been somewhat controversial. Depending on accuracy considerations, various groups have estimated breakeven points of 300 [211], a few thousand [164], more than 23,000 (for regular Greengard–Rokhlin; i.e., without the use of FFTs in translations [169]), and close to 100,000 [160,171].

Hockney and Eastwood [213] developed a method called particle mesh (PM), wherein the coulombic potential at particles was obtained by solving Poisson's equation in periodic boundary conditions. The charges were interpolated onto a regular grid, and the discretized Poisson's equation was solved by expanding in a discrete Fourier transform. For a regular grid, this transform is evaluated using the fast Fourier transform (FFT), resulting in a very efficient algorithm. However, the estimated interactions for nearby particles were poorly represented. Subsequently they developed the particle–particle particle–mesh (P3M) approach, wherein the interaction is split into short- and long-range contributions using switching functions, and the long-range potential is obtained by gridding the charges and employing the FFT as before. To obtain higher accuracy, they modify the form of the solution, using an optimal "influence function," obtained by a least-squares approach. More recently, Shimada et al. [214] and Luty et al. [215,216] have taken up this approach to apply it to molecular systems. The method appears to be very efficient; however, because it involves low-order interpolation and numerical differentiation to obtain the forces, it is unclear if it can efficiently achieve high accuracy [214]. Furthermore, the computationally expensive least-squares approach may be inconvenient when changing unit cell shapes.

Rather than use arbitrary-switching functions to split interactions into short- and long-range components, the particle mesh Ewald (PME) algorithm [194,217] began with the conventional split of the Ewald sum into direct and reciprocal sums. By choosing the convergence coefficient β large enough, the direct sum can be made to converge within a conventional cutoff of, for example, 8–10 A. Unfortunately, the reciprocal sum now requires a large number of terms for convergence. The reciprocal sum is expressed in terms of structure factors, which are obtained as Fourier series involving the particle positions. By using Lagrangian [217] or B-spline [194] interpolation of the trigonometric functions involved, the structure factors can be efficiently approximated using FFTs. The approximation becomes progressively worse for high-frequency structure factors, but these are damped exponentially in the reciprocal sum. As a result, the method can easily be adjusted to obtain any accuracy desired [194]. The original PME method [217] was implemented independently by Petersen [206], who provides a rigorous error analysis and a comparison with Ewald summation. He obtains a breakeven point of approximately 10,000, whereas we later [194] found a breakeven of close to 1,000 particles. This discrepancy probably is mainly due to differences in the efficiencies of the Ewald and FFT codes used. Petersen also pointed out that the PME method behaved similarly to Ewald summation relative to the ratio between the maximal atomic force error and the rms force error, unlike methods based on the FMM, which gave much higher ratios.

The foregoing P3M methods typically employ quadratic interpolation, in which the charge for each particle is distributed over 27 grid points, whereas the PME method may require cubic interpolation (64 grid points) to achieve comparable accuracy at the same grid density. In other respects, the computational costs should be very close, for the algorithms are formally very similar. The importance of the relative cost (order 64 N versus order 27 N, where N is the number of particles) of the charge gridding and potential and force interpolation steps depends on the size of the cutoff used. Typically, in these FFT-based methods, the cost of the long-range reciprocal part of the calculation is less than the short-range part, unlike the FMM algorithms. The PME method thus trades a small loss of efficiency for generality, because it avoids the least-squares optimization procedure and also extends easily to high accuracy, arbitrary cell shape, and other interaction potentials, such as Lennard-Jones, that can be written in terms of a rapidly converging sum over structure factors. Recently, Procacci et al. [218] have implemented an r-RESPA multiple time step variant of the PME algorithm, leading to a two- to threefold improvement in computational cost. These multiple time step methods should eventually blur the differences in efficiency between algorithms.

Finally, the reciprocal Ewald sum is the solution to Poisson's equation in periodic boundary conditions, with gaussian charge densities as sources. York and Yang [219] developed a method to solve Poisson's equation directly using the FFT, by sampling these charge densities onto the grid, rather than using interpolation. This results in accurate electrostatic potentials and fields at the grid points. Rather than use interpolation to obtain atomic potentials and forces, leading to lower accuracy, they were able to obtain the desired quantities in terms of interactions of a continuous gaussian centered at the particle, plus a correction. They were able to achieve very high accuracy using this approach, but it is currently more costly in computer time than the other FFT-based methods, because it involves a large number of grid points per particle. However, it should generalize more easily to consideration of continuous charge distributions.

V. SUMMARY AND CONCLUSIONS

In this chapter we have tried to review recent developments in the treatment of long-range coulombic interactions, as well as providing some background material to the various methods, where needed. As we have seen, the methods often reflect a balance between computational efficiency and physical rigor. We organized the presentation according to the treatment of solvent, presenting the various approaches in the context of the solvent model employed.

For optimal computational efficiency, it seems clear that rapid approximate continuum methods, such as the generalized Born method, or perhaps the methods based on atomic solvation coefficients, will be the methods of choice, barring any major breakthrough in solving the Poisson–Boltzmann equation. Vacuum simulations, in which solvent is ignored completely seem too severe an approximation because desolvation plays such a major role in biomolecular complex formation [67]. Optimal algorithms to compute atomic solvent accessible surface areas (or equivalent measures of solvation) and their gradients relative to atomic coordinates still seem like a worthwhile research pursuit. To be useful in modeling complex formation, these rapid continuum methods need to be supplemented by methods to estimate conformational entropy [220]. These rapid methods are still saddled with possibly impossible conformational search problems for some applications, such as estimation of pK_a [131].

Methodologically, for long-range electrostatic effects, the Poisson–Boltzmann approach seems most satisfying, because it can account for both dielectric and ionic effects in a mean field manner, which should be adequate for distant pair interactions. However, we are skeptical that the continuum approach can be used to accurately model these effects at distances close to a group of interest, for it omits entirely the finite size effects of solvent molecules and counterions.

The methods based on finite shells of solvent are of great interest because they explicitly account for solvent close to the biomolecule of interest, without invoking periodic boundary conditions that may involve artifacts as well as much larger total system sizes. With the advent of fast hierarchical methods, such as the fast multipole method, together with multiple time step methods, such as r-RESPA [167], these nonperiodical systems no longer require the use of cutoffs for efficient simulations. Particularly interesting would be methods that can account for the bulk medium surrounding the finite water layer in a manner similar to the Poisson–Boltzmann approach. However, the explicit water molecules do increase the computational cost of free-energy estimates because their conformational substates must be fully sampled. At present, these methods all suffer from artifactual behavior of explicit water molecules near the vacuum interface. These problems seem difficult to overcome [153]. One approach is to simply include more layers of water, but this involves larger system sizes and, hence, more computational work in averaging.

Finally, there are the methods based on the use of periodic boundary conditions. One great advantage of these methods is the ease with which they can emulate bulk behavior. For example, in pure water simulations under periodic boundary conditions, there is no special position within the system, unlike in cluster simulations. For long-range interactions, we feel that the reaction field methods are probably best used for simulations involving small solutes, owing to the assumption of bulk-like behavior outside the cutoff. The intrinsic periodicity is best expressed through the use of Ewald summation, in which bulk-like behavior is only assumed at large distances. With the advent of the FFT-based methods discussed earlier, the Ewald sum is competitive with cutoff-based methods for computational expense. There have been occasional complaints against Ewald sums owing to a priori concerns about "enhanced correlations" [39], but little if any evidence of artifacts has yet emerged. This situation could change, but it is clear that the dominant effects in electrostatics under periodic conditions are due to the minimum image interactions. In some ways this concern about explicit periodic boundary conditions (i.e., Ewald summation) is reminiscent of the concerns some scientists have had about the validity of crystallographic structures. To obtain a reliable diffraction pattern, long-range positional correlations, similar to those involved in periodic boundary conditions, must be in place. Nonetheless, proteins in the crystal have frequently retained their normal biochemical properties. For example some enzymes are fully active in the crystal. Moreover, the structures deduced by crystallographers are usually very close to solution structures found by NMR techniques. The differences, caused by crystal-packing effects, are ascribed to immediate contacts with neighboring macromolecules, not some mysterious long-range effects. Consequently, the use of periodic boundary conditions in solution simulations, which do not involve direct contact with other macromolecules, should not lead to serious artifacts in structural studies. Questions remain about finite size effects for some other quantities, such as free energies of solvation and pair interaction energies [190;199,200].

In conclusion, the importance of a careful treatment of long-range coulombic interactions now seems well established. There are a variety of approaches available to choose from, with efficient algorithms for their implementation, so that computational cost should no longer be a reason for excluding a method. One hopes that, over time, a consistent picture of the consequences of using a particular method will emerge, so that, for example, its effects on structural and energetic quantities can be estimated. This will be important, especially during force field development and other situations for which experimentally measured quantities are compared with the results of simulations. Finally, although we have not discussed methods for improving on the static atomic partial charge description of molecular charge distributions, it is clear that a consistent treatment of this problem will require consideration of the long-range coulombic aspects. We believe that a successful attack on this problem will lead to a major improvement in the ability of molecular modelers to describe and predict important biomolecular interactions.

ACKNOWLEDGMENTS

The authors would like to acknowledge Anthony Nicholls and Christophe Lambert for their careful reading of the manuscript. Uli Essmman would like to acknowledge the support by the Office of Naval Research during the course of this work.

REFERENCES

1. M. P. Allen and D. J. Tildesley, *Computer Simulation of Liquids*, Clarendon Press, Oxford, 1987.

2. C. L. Brooks, B. M. Pettitt, and M. Karplus, Structural and energetic effects of truncating long ranged interactions in ionic and polar fluids, *J. Chem. Phys. 83*:5897–5908 (1985).

3. H. J. C. Berendsen, Treatment of long-range forces in molecular dynamics, *Molecular Dynamics and Protein Structure* (J. Hermans, ed.), Polycrystal Book Service, (Western Springs IL), 1985.

4. L. X. Dang and B. M. Pettitt, Chloride ion pairs in water, *J. Am. Chem. Soc. 109*:5531–5532 (1987).

5. G. Hummer, D. M. Soumpasis, and M. Neumann, Computer simulations do not support Cl–Cl pairing in aqueous NaCl solution, *Mol. Phys. 81*: 1155–1163 (1993).

6. P. Ewald, Die Berechnung optischer and elektrostatischer Gitterpotentiale, *Ann. Phys. 64*:253–287 (1921).

7. E. C. Zhong and H. L. Friedman, Self-diffusion and distinct diffusion of ions in solutions, *J. Phys. Chem. 92*:1685–1692 (1988).

8. J. S. Bader and D. Chandler, Computer simulation study of the mean forces between ferrous and ferric ions in water, *J. Phys. Chem. 96*:6423–6427 (1992).

9. V. Daggett and M. Levitt, Realistic simulations of native-protein dynamics in solution and beyond, *Annu. Rev. Biophys. Biomol. Struct. 22*:353–380 (1993).

10. P. Auffinger and D. L. Beveridge, A simple test for evaluating the truncation effects in simulations of systems involving charged groups, *Chem. Phys. Lett. 234*:413–415 (1995).

11. D. H. Kitson, F. Avbelj, J. Moult, D. T. Nguyen, J. E. Mertz, D. Hatzi, and A. T. Hagler, On achieving better than 1 angstrom accuracy in a simulation of a large protein: *Streptomyces griseus* protease A, *Proc. Natl. Acad. Sci. USA 90*:8920–8924 (1993).

12. M. Frech, T. A. Darden, L. G. Pedersen, C. K. Foley, P. S. Charifson, M. W. Anderson, and A. Wittinghofer, Role of glutamine-61 in the hydrolysis of GPT by $p21^{H-ras}$: An experimental and theoretical study, *Biochemistry 33*:3237–3244 (1994).

13. N. Hamaguchi, P. Charifson, T. Darden, L. Xiao, L. Padmanabhan, A. Tulinsky, R. Hiskey, and L. Pedersen, Molecular dynamics simulation of bovine prothrombin fragment 1 in the presence of calcium ions, *Biochemistry 31*: 8840–8848 (1992).

14. L. Li, T. Darden, C. Foley, R. Hiskey, and L. Pedersen, Homology modeling and molecular dynamics simulation of human prothrombin fragment 1, *Protein Sci.* 4:2341–2348 (1995).

15. S. Weerasinghe, P. E. Smith, V. Mohan, Y. K. Cheng, and B. M. Pettitt, Nanosecond dynamics and structure of a model DNA triple helix in saltwater solution, *J. Am. Chem. Soc.* 117:2147–2158 (1995).

16. T. E. Cheatham III, J. L. Miller, T. Fox, T. A. Darden, and P. A. Kollman, Molecular dynamics simulations on solvated biomolecular systems: The particle mesh Ewald method leads to stable trajectories of DNA, RNA, and proteins, *J. Am. Chem. Soc.* 117:4193–4194 (1995).

17. H. Lee, T. A. Darden, and L. G. Pedersen, Molecular dynamics simulation studies of a high resolution Z-DNA crystal, *J. Chem. Phys.* 102:3830–3834 (1995).

18. D. M. York, W. Yang, T. Darden, and L. G. Pedersen, Towards the accurate modeling of DNA: The importance of long-range electrostatics, *J. Am. Chem. Soc.* 117:5001–5002 (1995).

19. H. Schreiber and O. Steinhauser, Cutoff size does strongly influence molecular dynamics results on solvated polypeptides, *Biochemistry* 31:5856–5860 (1992).

20. R. J. Loncharich and B. R. Brooks, The effects of truncating long-range forces on protein dynamics, *Proteins Struct. Funct. Genet.* 6:32–45 (1989).

21. P. J. Steinbach and B. R. Brooks, New spherical cutoff methods for long-range forces in macromolecular simulation, *J. Comput. Chem.* 15:667–683 (1994).

22. J. D. Madura and B. M. Pettitt, Effects of truncating long-range interactions in aqueous ionic solution simulations, *Chem. Phys. Lett.* 150:105–108 (1988).

23. P. E. Smith and B. M. Pettitt, Peptides in ionic solutions: A comparison of the Ewald and switching function techniques, *J. Chem. Phys.* 95:8430–8441 (1991).

24. H. E. Alper, D. Bassolino, and T. R. Stouch, Computer simulation of a phospholipid monolayer-water system: The influence of long range forces on water structure and dynamics, *J. Chem. Phys.* 98:9798–9807 (1993).

25. K. F. Lau, H. E. Alper, T. S. Thacher, and T. R. Stouch, Effects of switching functions on the behavior of liquid water in molecular dynamics simulations, *J. Phys. Chem.* 98:8785–8792 (1994).

26. M. Belhadji, H. E. Alper, and R. M. Levy, Molecular dynamics simulations of water with Ewald summation for the long range electrostatic interactions, *Chem. Phys. Lett.* 179:13 (1991).

27. J. E. Roberts and J. Schnitker, How the unit cell surface charge distribution affects the energetics of ion–solvent interaction in simulations, *J. Chem. Phys.* 101:5024–5031 (1994).

28. J. E. Roberts and J. Schnitker, Boundary conditions in simulations of aqueous ionic solutions: A systematic study, *J. Phys. Chem.* 99:1322–1331 (1995).

29. G. S. D. Buono, T. S. Cohen, and P. J. Rossky, Effects of long-range interactions on the dynamics of ions in aqueous solution, *J. Mol. Liquids 60*: 221–236 (1994).

30. L. Perera, U. Essmann, and M. L. Berkowitz, Effect of the treatment of long-range forces on the dynamics of ions in aqueous solutions, *J. Chem. Phys. 102*:450–456 (1995).

31. M. Saito, Molecular dynamics simulations of proteins in water without the truncation of long-range coulomb interactions, *Mol. Simul. 8*:321 (1992).

32. M. Saito, Molecular dynamics simulations of proteins in solution: Artifacts caused by the cutoff approximation, *J. Chem. Phys. 101*:4055–4061 (1994).

33. K. Tasaki, S. McDonald, and J. W. Brady, Observations concerning the treatment of long-range interactions in molecular dynamics simulations, *J. Comput. Chem. 14*:278–284 (1993).

34. J. Guenot and P. Kollman, Conformational and energetic effects of truncating nonbonded interactions in an aqueous protein dynamics simulation, *J. Comput. Chem. 14*:295–311 (1993).

35. O. Steinhauser, On the dielectric theory and computer simulation of water, *Chem. Phys. 79*:465–482 (1983).

36. S. W. DeLeeuw, J. W. Perram, and E. R. Smith, Simulation of electrostatic systems in periodic boundary conditions I: Lattice sums and dielectric constants, *Proc. R. Soc. Lond. A 373*:27–56 (1980).

37. J. A. Barker and R. O. Watts, Monte Carlo studies of the dielectric properties of water-like models, *Mol. Phys. 26*:789–792 (1973).

38. H. Friedman, Image approximation to the reaction field, *Mol. Phys. 29*: 1533–1543 (1975).

39. J. P. Valleau and S. G. Whittington, A guide to Monte Carlo for statistical mechanics: 1. Highways, *Statistical Mechanics*, Part A: *Equilibrium Techniques* Vol. 5 (B. J. Berne, ed.), Plenum, New York, 1977.

40. H. J. C. Berendsen, Electrostatic interactions, *Computer Simulation of Biomolecular Systems*, Vol. 2 (W. F. van Gunsteren, P. K. Weiner, and A. J. Wilkinson, eds.), ESCOM, Leiden, 1993, pp. 161–181.

41. C. L. Brooks, Methodological advances in molecular dynamics simulations of biological systems, *Curr. Opin. Struct. Biol. 5*:211–215 (1995).

42. C. J. Cramer and D. G. Truhlar, Continuum solvation models: Classical and quantum mechanical implementations, *Reviews in Computational Chemistry* Vol. 6 (K. Lipkowitz and D. B. Boyd, eds.), VCH Publishers, New York, 1995.

43. M. E. Davis and J. A. McCammon, Electrostatics in biomolecular structure and dynamics, *Chem. Rev. 90*:509–521 (1990).

44. M. K. Gilson, Theory of electrostatic interactions in macromolecules, *Curr. Opin. Struct. Biol. 5*:216–223 (1995).

45. S. C. Harvey, Treatment of electrostatic effects in macromolecular modeling, *Proteins 5*:78–92 (1989).

46. K. A. Sharp, Electrostatic interactions in macromolecules, *Curr. Opin. Struct. Biol. 4*:234–239 (1994).

47. P. E. Smith and B. M. Pettitt, Modeling solvent in biomolecular systems, *J. Phys. Chem. 98*:9700–9711 (1994).
48. J. A. McCammon, P. G. Wolynes, and M. Karplus, Picosecond dynamic of tyrosine side chains in proteins, *Biochemistry 18*:927–942 (1979).
49. B. E. Hingerty, R. H. Ritchie, T. L. Ferrel, and J. E. Turner, Dielectric effects in biopolymers: The theory of ionic saturation revisited, *Biopolymers 24*: 427–439 (1985).
50. R. Lavery, H. Sklenar, K. Zakrzewski, and B. Pullman, The flexibility of the nucleic acids. (II) The calculation of internal energy and applications to mononucleotide repeat DNA, *J. Biolmol. Struct. Dyn. 3*:989–1014 (1986).
51. A. Sarai, J. Mazur, R. Nussinov, and R. L. Jernigan, Origin of DNA helical structure and its sequence dependence, *Biochemistry 27*:8498–8502 (1988).
52. E. von Kitzing and S. Diekmann, Molecular mechanics calculations of $dA_{12} \cdot dT_{12}$ and the curved molecule $d(GCTCGAAAAA)_4 \cdot d(TTTTTCGAGC)_4$, *Eur. Biophys. J. 15*:13–26 (1987).
53. E. von Kitzing, Modelling DNA structures, *Prog. Nucleic Acid Res. Mol. Biol. 43*:87–108 (1992).
54. M. K. Gilson, A. Rashin, R. Fine, and B. Honig, On the calculation of electrostatic interactions in proteins, *J. Mol. Biol. 184*:503–516 (1985).
55. R. A. Friedman and B. Honig, The electrostatic contribution to DNA base-stacking interactions, *Biopolymers 32*:145 (1988).
56. P. J. Steinbach and B. R. Brooks, Protein hydration elucidated by molecular dynamics simulation, *Proc Natl Acad Sci. USA 90*:9135–9139 (1993).
57. P. J. Steinbach and B. R. Brooks, Hydrated myoglobin's anharmonic fluctuations are not primarily due to dihedral transitions, *Proc. Natl. Acad. Sci. USA 93*:55–59 (1996).
58. M. K. Gilson, J. A. McCammon, and J. D. Madura, Molecular dynamics simulation with a continuum electrostatic model of the solvent, *J. Comput. Chem. 16*:1081–1095 (1995).
59. B. M. Pettitt and M. Karplus, The potential of mean force surface for the alanine dipeptide in aqueous solution: A theoretical approach, *Chem. Phys. Lett. 121*:194–201 (1985).
60. W. F. Lau and B. M. Pettitt, Conformations of the glycine dipeptide, *Biopolymers 26*:1817–1831 (1987).
61. A. G. Anderson and J. Hermans, Microfolding: Conformational probability map for the alanine dipeptide in water from molecular dynamics simulations, *Proteins Struct. Funct. Genet. 3*:262–265 (1988).
62. J. Novotny, R. Bruccoleri, and M. Karplus, An analysis of incorrectly folded protein models. Implications for structure prediction, *J. Mol. Biol. 177*: 787–818 (1984).
63. D. Eisenberg and A. D. McLachlan, Solvation energy in protein folding and binding, *Nature 319*:199–203 (1986).
64. R. Wolfenden, L. Anderson, P. M. Cullis, and C. C. Southgate, Affinities of amino acid side chains for solvent water, *Biochemistry 20*:849–855 (1981).

65. L. Chiche, L. M. Gregoret, F. E. Cohen, and P. A. Kollman, Protein model structure evaluation using the solvation free energy of folding, *Proc. Natl. Acad. Sci. USA 87*:3240–3243 (1990).

66. J. Novotny, A. A. Rashin, and R. Bruccoleri, Criteria that discriminate between native proteins and incorrectly folded models, *Proteins Struct. Funct. Genet. 4*:19–30 (1988).

67. R. S. Spolar and M. T. Record, Coupling of local folding to site-specific binding of proteins to DNA, *Science 263*:777–784 (1994).

68. V. K. Misra and B. Honig, On the magnitude of the electrostatic contribution to ligand–DNA interactions, *Proc. Natl. Acad. Sci. USA 92*:4691–4695 (1995).

69. T. Ooi, M. Oobatake, G. Nemethy, and H. A. Scheraga, Accessible surface areas as a measure of the thermodynamic parameters of hydration of peptides, *Proc. Natl. Acad. Sci. USA 84*:3086–3090 (1987).

70. F. A. Momany, R. F. McGuire, A. W. Burgess, and H. A. Scheraga, Energy parameters in polypeptides. VII Geometric parameters, partial atomic charges, nonbonded interactions, hydrogen bond interactions, and intrinsic torsional potentials for the naturally occurring amino acids, ⟨J. Phys. Chem. 79⟩:2361–2381 (1975).

71. L. Wesson and D. Eisenberg, Atomic solvation parameters applied to molecular dynamics of proteins in solutions, *Protein Sci. 1*:227–235 (1992).

72. B. R. Brooks, R. E. Bruccoleri, B. D. Olafson, D. J. States, S. Swaminathan, and M. Karplus, CHARMM: A program for macromolecular energy, minimization and dynamics calculations, *J. Comput. Chem. 4*:187–217 (1983).

73. C. A. Schiffer, J. W. Caldwell, R. M. Stroud, and P. A. Kollman, Inclusion of solvation free energy with molecular mechanics energy: Alanyl dipeptide as a test case, *Protein Sci. 1*:396–400 (1992).

74. U. C. Singh, P. K. Weiner, J. W. Caldwell, and P. A. Kollman, *AMBER (Version 3.1)*, Dept. Pharmaceutical Chemistry, University of California, San Francisco, 1988.

75. T. F. H. W. Hasel and W. C. Still, A rapid approximation to the solvent accessible surface area of atoms, *Tetrahedron Comput. Methodol. 1*:103 (1988).

76. F. Eisenhaber and P. Argos, Improved strategy in analytic surface calculation for molecular systems: Handling of singularities and computational efficiency, *J. Comput. Chem. 14*:1272–1280 (1993).

77. S. Sridharan, A. Nicholls, and K. A. Sharp, A rapid method for calculating derivatives of solvent accessible surface areas of molecules, *J. Comput. Chem. 16*:1039–1044 (1995).

78. M. Born, Volumen der Hydratationswärme der Ionen, *Z. Phys. Chem. 1*: 45–48 (1920).

79. W. M. Latimer, K. S. Pitzer, and C. M. Slansky, The free energy of hydration of gaseous ions, and the absolute potential of the normal calomel electrode, *J. Chem. Phys. 7*:108–111 (1939).

80. A. A. Rashin and B. Honig, Reevaluation of the Born model of ion hydration, *J. Phys. Chem.* *89*:5588–5593 (1985).

81. F. Hirata, P. Refern, and R. M. Levy, Viewing the Born model for ion hydration through a microscope, *Int. Quant. Chem. Quant. Biol. Symp.* *15*: 179–190 (1988).

82. L. R. Pratt, G. Hummer, and A. E. Garcia, Ion pair potentials-of-mean-force in water, *Biophys. Chem.* *51*:147–165 (1994).

83. S. W. Rick and B. J. Berne, The aqueous solvation of water: A comparison of continuum methods with molecular dynamics, *J. Am. Chem. Soc.* *116*: 3949–3954 (1994).

84. G. Hummer, L. R. Pratt, and A. E. Garcia, Hydration free energy of water, *J. Phys. Chem.* *99*:14188–14194 (1995).

85. S. L. Chan and C. Lim, Reducing the uncertainty in the Born radius in continuum dielectric calculations, *J. Phys. Chem.* *98*:692–695 (1994).

86. J. R. Bontha and P. N. Pintauro, Prediction of ion solvation free energies in a polarizable dielectric continuum, *J. Phys. Chem.* *96*:7778–7782 (1992).

87. T. P. Straatsma and H. J. C. Berendsen, Free energy of ionic hydration: Analysis of a thermodynamic integration technique to evaluate free energy differences by molecular dynamics simulations, *J. Chem. Phys.* *89*: 5876–5886 (1988).

88. R. H. Wood, Continuum electrostatics in a computational universe with finite cutoff radii and periodic boundary conditions: Correction to computed free energies of ionic solvation, *J. Chem. Phys.* *103*:6177–6187 (1995).

89. W. C. Still, A. Tempczyk, R. C. Hawley, and T. Hendrickson, Semianalytical treatment of solvation for molecular mechanics and dynamics, *J. Am. Chem. Soc.* *112*:6127–6129 (1990).

90. D. D. Humphreys, R. A. Friesner, and B. J. Berne, Simulated annealing in a continuum solvent by multiple-time-step molecular dynamics, *J. Phys. Chem.* *99*:10674–10685 (1995).

91. V. Mohan, M. E. Davis, J. A. McCammon, and B. M. Pettitt, Continuum model calculations of solvation free energies: Accurate evaluation of electrostatic contributions, *J. Phys. Chem.* *96*:6428–6431 (1992).

92. T. Simonson and A. Brünger, Solvation free energies estimated from macroscopic continuum theory: An accuracy assessment, *J. Phys. Chem.* *98*: 4683–4694 (1994).

93. T. J. Sluckin, Applications of the density functional theory of charged fluids, *J. Chem. Soc. Faraday Trans.* *77*:575–586 (1981).

94. P. Debye and E. Hückel, Zur Theorie der Elektrolyte, *Phys. Z.* *24*:185–206 (1923).

95. R. S. Berry, S. A. Rice, and J. Ross, *Physical Chemistry*, John Wiley & Sons, New York, 1980.

96. D. J. Griffiths, *Introduction to Electrodynamics*, Prentice-Hall, Englewood Cliffs NJ, 1989.

97. L. Onsager, Theories of concentrated electrolytes, *Chem. Rev.* *3*:73–89 (1933).

98. P. E. Smith, B. M. Pettitt, and M. Karplus, Stochastic dynamics simulations of the alanine dipeptide using a solvent-modified potential energy surface, *J. Phys. Chem.* *97*:6907–6913 (1993).

99. G. Hummer, A. E. Garcia, and D. M. Soumpasis, Hydration of nucleic acid fragments: Comparison of theory and experiment for high-resolution crystal structures of RNA, DNA and DNA-drug complexes, *Biophys. J.* *68*: 1639–1652 (1995).

100. P. J. Rossky, The structure of polar molecular liquids, *Annu. Rev. Phys. Chem.* *36*:321–346 (1985).

101. C. Tanford and J. G. Kirkwood, Theory of protein titration. I. General equations for impenetrable spheres, *J. Am. Chem. Soc.* *79*:5333–5339 (1957).

102. T. L. Hill, Approximate calculation of the electrostatic free energy of nucleic acids and other cylindrical macromolecules, *Arch. Biochem. Biophys.* *57*: 229–239 (1955).

103. M. E. Davis, The inducible multipole solvation model: A new model for solvation effects on solute electrostatics, *J. Chem. Phys.* *100*:5149–5159 (1994).

104. R. Abagyan and M. Totrov, Biased probability Monte Carlo conformational searches and electrostatic calculations for peptides and proteins, *J. Mol. Biol.* *235*:983–1002 (1994).

105. M. Schaefer and M. Karplus, A comprehensive analytical theory of continuum electrostatics, *J. Phys. Chem.* *100*:1578–1599 (1996).

106. P. F. W. Stouten, C. Frömmel, H. Nakamura, and C. Sander, An effective solvation term based on atomic occupancies for use in protein simulations, *Mol. Simul.* *10*:97–120 (1993).

107. J. Warwicker and H. C. Watson, Calculation of electric potential in the active site cleft due to α-helix dipoles, *J. Mol. Biol.* *157*:671–679 (1982).

108. I. Klapper, R. Hagstrom, R. Fine, K. Sharp, and B. Honig, Focusing of electric fields in the active site of Cu–Zn superoxide dismutase: Effects of ionic strength and amino-acid modification, *Proteins Struct. Funct. Genet.* *1*:47–59 (1986).

109. B. Jayaram, K. A. Sharp, and B. Honig, The electrostatic potential of B-DNA, *Biopolymers* *28*:975–993 (1989).

110. M. K. Gilson, K. A. Sharp, and B. H. Honig, Calculating the electrostatic potential of molecules in solution: Method and error assessment, *J. Comput. Chem.* *9*:327–335 (1988).

111. A. Nicholls and B. Honig, A rapid finite difference algorithm, utilizing successive overrelaxation to solve the Poisson–Boltzmann equation, *J. Comput. Chem.* *12*:435–445 (1991).

112. A. Nicholls, K. A. Sharp, and B. Honig, Protein folding and association: Insights from the interfacial and thermodynamic properties of hydrocarbons, *Proteins Struct. Funct. Genet.* *11*:281–296 (1991).

113. T. J. You and S. G. Harvey, Finite element approach to the electrostatics of macromolecules with arbitrary geometrics, *J. Comput. Chem.* *14*:484–501 (1993).

114. E. S. Reiner and C. L. Radke, Variation approach to the electrostatic free energy in charged colloidal suspensions: General theory for open systems, *J. Chem. Soc. Faraday Trans.* *86*:3901–3912 (1990).

115. T. J. Sluckin, Applications of the density-functional theory of changed fluids, *J. Chem. Soc. Faraday. Trans.* 2:77, 575–586 (1981).

116. M. E. Davis and J. A. McCammon, Dielectric boundary smoothing in finite difference solutions of the Poisson equation: An approach to improve accuracy and convergence, *J. Comput. Chem.* *12*:909–912 (1991).

117. R. E. Bruccoleri, Grid positioning independence and the reduction of self-energy in the solution of the Poisson–Boltzmann equation, *J. Comput. Chem.* *14*:1417–1422 (1993).

118. Z. Zhou, N. Kuhn, P. Payne, M. Vazquez, and M. Levitt, Finite difference solution of the Poisson–Boltzmann equation: Complete elimination of the self-energy, *J. Comput. Chem.* *17*:1344–1359 (1996).

119. M. Holst and F. Saied, Multigrid solution of the Poisson–Boltzmann equation, *J. Comput. Chem.* *14*:105–113 (1993).

120. M. Holst, R. E. Kozack, F. Saied, and S. Subramaniam, Treatment of electrostatic effects in proteins: Multigrid-based Newton iterative method for solution of the full Poisson–Boltzmann equation, *Proteins Struct. Funct. Genet.* *18*:231–241 (1994).

121. J. Shen and J. Wendoloski, Electrostatic binding energy calculation using the finite difference solution to the linearized Poisson–Boltzmann equation: Assessment of its accuracy, *J. Comput. Chem.* *17*:350–357 (1996).

122. Y. Marcus, Linear solvation energy relationships. Correlation and prediction of the distribution of organic solutes between water and immiscible organic solvents, *J. Phys. Chem.* *95*:8886–8891 (1991).

123. J. Warwicker, Improved continuum modelling in proteins, with comparison to experiment, *J. Mol. Biol.* *236*:887–903 (1994).

124. J. L. Hecht, B. Honig, Y. K. Shin, and W. L. Hubbell, Electrostatic potentials near the surface of DNA: Comparing theory and experiment, *J. Phys. Chem.* *99*:7782–7786 (1995).

125. B. Honig and A. Nicholls, Classical electrostatics in biology and chemistry, *Science* *268*:1144–1149 (1995).

126. A. Warshel and M. Levitt, Theoretical studies of enzymatic reaction: Dielectric, electrostatic and steric stabilization of the carbonium ion in the reaction of lysozyme, *J. Mol. Biol.* *103*:227–249 (1976).

127. A. Warshel and S. T. Russell, Calculation of electrostatic interactions in biological systems and in solutions, *Q. Rev. Biophys.* *17*:283–422 (1984).

128. A. Warshel, S. T. Russell, and A. K. Churg, Macroscopic models for studies of electrostatic interactions in proteins: Limitations and applicability, *Proc. Natl. Acad. Sci. USA* *81*:4785–4789 (1984).

129. S. T. Russell and A. Warshel, Calculation of electrostatic energies in proteins, the energetics of ionized groups in bovine pancreatic trypsin inhibitor, *J. Mol. Biol.* *185*:389–404 (1985).

130. Y. W. Xu, C. X. Wang, and Y. Y. Shi, Improvements on the protein–dipole Langevin–dipole model, *J. Comput. Chem.* *13*:1109–1113 (1992).

131. J. Antosiewicz, J. A. McCammon, and M. K. Gilson, Prediction of pH-dependent properties of proteins, *J. Mol. Biol. 238*:415–436 (1994).

132. T. A. Ewing and T. P. Lybrand, A comparison of perturbation methods and Poisson–Boltzmann electrostatics calculations for estimation of relative solvation free energies, *J. Phys. Chem. 98*:1748–1752 (1994).

133. J. Israelachvili and H. Wennerström, Role of hydration and water structure in biological and colloidal interactions, *Nature 379*:219–225 (1996).

134. H. Grubmüller, Predicting slow structural transitions in macromolecular systems: Conformational flooding, *Phys. Rev. E 52*:2893–2906 (1995).

135. T. Haran, A. Joachimiak, and P. Sigler, The DNA target of the *trp* repressor, *EMBO J. 11*:3021–3030 (1992).

136. J. E. Ladbury, J. G. Wright, J. M. Sturtevant, and P. Sigler, A thermodynamic study of the *trp* repressor–operator interaction, *J. Mol. Biol. 238*:669–681 (1994).

137. J. E. Ladbury, Counting the calories to stay in the groove, *Structure 3*: 635–639 (1995).

138. J. Dunitz, The entropic cost of bound water in crystals and biomolecules, *Science 264*:670–670 (1994).

139. M. Levitt and B. H. Park, Water: Now you see it, now you don't, *Structure 1*:223–226 (1993).

140. G. Bossis, Molecular dynamics calculation of the dielectric constant without periodic boundary conditions, *Mol Phys. 38*:2023 (1979).

141. X. Cheng and B. P. Schoenborn, Hydration in protein crystals. A neutron diffraction analysis of carbonmonoxymyoglobin, *Acta Crystallogr. B 46*: 195–208 (1990).

142. M. L. Berkowitz and J. A. McCammon, Molecular dynamics with stochastic boundary conditions, *Chem. Phys. Lett. 90*:215–217 (1982).

143. C. L. Brooks III, A. Brünger, and M. Karplus, Active site dynamics in protein molecules: A stochastic molecular–dynamics approach, *Biopolymers 24*: 843–865 (1985).

144. H. D. Loof, S. C. Harvey, J. P. Segrest, and R. W. Pastor, Mean field stochastic boundary molecular dynamics of a phospholipid in a membrane, *Biochemistry 30*:2099–2113 (1991).

145. H. Heller, M. Schaefer, and K. Schulten, Molecular dynamics simulation of a bilayer of 200 lipids in the gel and in the liquid–crystal phases, *J. Chem. Phys. 97*:8343–8360 (1993).

146. F. Zhou and K. Schulten, Molecular dynamics study of a membrane–water interface, *J. Phys. Chem. 99*:2194–2207 (1995).

147. A. H. Juffer and H. J. C. Berendsen, Dynamic surface boundary conditions. A simple boundary model for molecular dynamics simulations, *Mol. Phys. 79*:623–644 (1993).

148. A. C. Belch and M. L. Berkowitz, Molecular dynamics simulations of TIPS2 water restricted by a spherical hydrophobic boundary, *Chem. Phys. Lett. 113*: 278–282 (1985).

149. C. Y. Lee, J. A. McCammon, and P. J. Rossky, The structure of liquid water at an extended hydrophobic surface, *J. Chem. Phys. 80*:4448–4455 (1984).

150. D. Beglov and B. Roux, Dominant solvation effects from the primary shell of hydration: Approximation for molecular dynamics simulations, *Biopolymers 35*:171–178 (1995).

151. D. J. Tobias and C. L. Brooks III, Conformational equilibrium in the alanine dipeptide in the gas phase and aqueous solution: A comparison of theoretical results, *J. Phys. Chem. 96*:3864–3870 (1992).

152. D. Beglov and B. Roux, Finite representation of an infinite bulk system: Solvent boundary potential for computer simulations, *J. Chem. Phys. 100*: 9050–9063 (1994).

153. J. W. Essex and W. L. Jorgensen, An empirical boundary potential for water droplet simulations, *J. Comput. Chem. 16*:951–972 (1995).

154. L. Wang and J. Hermans, Reaction field molecular dynamics simulation with Friedman's image charge method, *J. Phys. Chem. 99*:12001–12007 (1995).

155. J. A. C. Rullmann and P. T. van Duijnen, Analysis of discrete and continuum dielectric models; application to the calculation of protonation energies in solution, *Mol. Phys. 61*:293–311 (1987).

156. L. Greengard and V. Rokhlin, A fast algorithm for particle simulations, *J. Comput. Phys. 73*:325–348 (1987).

157. L. F. Greengard, Fast algorithms for classical physics, *Science 265*:909–914 (1994).

158. A. W. Appel, An efficient program for many-body simulations, *SIAM J. Sci. Stat. Comput. 6*:85–103 (1985).

159. J. Barnes and P. Hut, A hierarchical $O(N\log N)$ force-calculation algorithm, *Nature 324*:446–449 (1986).

160. K. Esselink, A comparison of algorithms for long-range interactions, *Comput. Phys. Commun. 87*:375 (1995).

161. J. K. Salmon and M. S. Warren, Skeletons from the treecode closet, *J. Comput. Phys. 111*:1 (1994).

162. L. F. Greengard, *The Rapid Evaluation of Potential Fields in Particle Systems*, MIT Press, Cambridge, MA, 1988.

163. C. A. White and M. Head-Gordon, Derivation and efficient implementation of the fast multipole method, *J. Chem. Phys. 101*:6593–6605 (1994).

164. K. E. Schmidt and M. A. Lee, Implementing the fast multipole method in three dimensions, *J. Stat. Phys. 63*:1223–1235 (1991).

165. H. Q. Ding, N. Karasawa, and W. A. Goddard, Atomic level simulations on a million particles: The cell multipole method for Coulomb and London nonbond interactions, *J. Chem. Phys. 97*:4309–4315 (1992).

166. J. A. Board, J. W. Causey, J. F. Leathrum, A. Windemuth, and K. Schulten, Accelerated molecular dynamics simulation with the parallel fast multipole algorithm, *Chem. Phys. Lett. 198*:89–94 (1992).

167. R. Zhou and B. Berne, A new molecular dynamics method combining the reference system propagator algorithm with a fast multipole method for sim-

ulating proteins and other complex systems, *J. Chem. Phys. 103*:9444–9459 (1995).

168. L. F. Greengard and V. Rokhlin, On the efficient implementation of the fast multipole algorithm, Tech. Rep. RR-602, New Haven, CT, Yale University, 1988.

169. J. Shimada, H. Kaneko, and T. Takada, Performance of fast multipole methods for calculating electrostatic interactions in biomolecular simulations, *J. Comput. Chem. 15*:28–43 (1994).

170. S. R. Lustig, S. Rostogi, and N. Wagner, Telescoping fast multipole methods using Chebyshev economization, *J. Comput. Phys. 122*:317–322 (1995).

171. H. G. Petersen, E. R. Smith, and D. Soelvason, Error estimates for the fast multipole method. II. The three-dimensional case, *Proc. R. Soc. Lond. A 448*: 401–418 (1995).

172. H. G. Petersen, D. Soelvason, J. W. Perram, and E. R. Smith, The very fast multipole method, *J. Chem. Phys. 101*:8870–8876 (1994).

173. A. Windemuth, Advanced algorithms for molecular dynamics simulation: The program PMD, *Parallel Computing in Computational Chemistry*, ACS Books, Washington DC, 1995.

174. H. Grubmüller, H. Heller, A. Windemuth, and K. Schulten, Generalized Verlet algorithm for efficient molecular dynamics simulations with long-range interactions, *Mol. Simul. 6*:121–142 (1991).

175. C. Niedermeier and P. Tavan, A structure adapted multipole method for electrostatic interactions in protein dynamics, *J. Chem. Phys. 101*:734–748 (1994).

176. M. E. Tuckerman, B. J. Berne, and G. J. Martyna, Reversible multiple time scale molecular dynamics, *J. Chem. Phys. 97*:1990–2001 (1992).

177. E. R. Smith, Electrostatic energy in ionic crystals, *Proc. R. Soc. Lond. A 373*:27–56 (1981).

178. J. A. Barker and R. O. Watts, Structure of water; a Monte Carlo calculation, *Chem. Phys. Lett. 3*:144–145 (1969).

179. A. Rahman and F. H. Stillinger, Molecular dynamics study of liquid water, *J. Chem. Phys. 55*:3336–3359 (1971).

180. F. H. Stillinger and A. Rahman, Molecular dynamics study of temperature effects on water structure and kinetics, *J. Chem. Phys. 57*:1281–1292 (1972).

181. F. H. Stillinger and A. Rahman, Improved simulation of liquid water by molecular dynamics, *J. Chem. Phys. 60*:1545–1557 (1974).

182. W. F. van Gunsteren and H. J. C. Berendsen, *Groningen Molecular Simulation (GROMOS) Library Manual*. BIOMOS, Nijenborgh 4, 9747 AG Groningen, The Netherlands, 1987.

183. G. Hummer, D. M. Soumpasis, and M. Neumann, Computer simulation of aqueous Na–Cl electrolytes, *J. Phys. Condens. Matt. 23A*:A141–A144 (1994).

184. G. Hummer and D M. Soumpasis, Computation of the water density distribution at the ice-water interface using the potentials-of-mean-force expansion, *Phys. Rev. E 49*:591–596 (1994).

185. L. Onsager, Electric moments of molecules in liquids, *J. Am. Chem. Soc.* 58:1486–1493 (1936).

186. C. Böttcher, *Theory of Electric Polarization*, Elsevier, Amsterdam, 1993.

187. G. Hummer, D. M. Soumpasis, and M. Neumann, Pair correlations in an NaCl–SPC water model simulations versus extended RISM computations, *Mol. Phys.* 77:769–785 (1992).

188. H. Alper and R. M. Levy, Dielectric and thermodynamic response of a generalized reaction field model for liquid state simulations, *J. Chem. Phys.* 99: 9847–9852 (1993).

189. P. E. Smith, W. F. von Gumsteren, I. G. Tironi, and R. Sperb, A generalized reaction field method for molecular dynamics simulations, *J. Chem. Phys.* 102:5451–5459 (1995).

190. B. A. Luty and W. F. van Gunsteren, Calculating electrostatic interactions using the particle–particle particle–mesh method with nonperiodic long-range interactions, *J. Phys. Chem.* 100:2581–2587 (1996).

191. C. Kittel, Introduction to Solid State Physics, John Wiley & Sons, New York, 1986.

192. B. Cichocki, B. U. Felderhof, and K. Hinson, Electrostatic interactions in periodic coulomb and dipolar systems, *Phys. Rev. A* 39:5350–5358 (1989).

193. G. H. Hardy, *A Course of Pure Mathematics*, Cambridge University Press, Cambridge, 1975.

194. U. Essmann, L. Perera, M. L. Berkowitz, T. Darden, H. Lee, and L. G. Pedersen, A smooth particle mesh Ewald method, *J. Chem. Phys.* 103: 8577–8593 (1995).

195. M. W. Deem, J. M. Newsam, and S. K. Sinha, The $h = 0$ term in coulomb sums by the Ewald transformation, *J. Phys. Chem.* 94:8356–8359 (1990).

196. E. R. Smith, Calculating the pressure in simulations using periodic boundary conditions, *J. Stat. Phys.* 77:449–472 (1994).

197. S. W. DeLeeuw, J. W. Perram, and H. G. Petersen, Hamilton's equations for contrained dynamical systems, *J. Stat. Phys.* 61:1203–1222 (1990).

198. J. P. Caillol, Comments on the numerical simulations of electrolytes in periodic boundary conditions, *J. Chem. Phys.* 101:6080–6090 (1994).

199. G. Hummer, L. R. Pratt, and A. E. Garcia, On the free energy of ionic hydration, *J. Phys. Chem.* 100:1206 (1996).

200. F. Figuerido, G. S. D. Buono, and R. M. Levy, On finite-size effects in computer simulations using the Ewald potential, *J. Chem. Phys.* 103:6133 (1995).

201. D. E. Williams, Accelerated convergence of crystal–lattice potential sums, *Acta Crystallogr.* A27:452–455 (1971).

202. D. Adams and G. Dubey, Taming the Ewald sum in the computer simulation of charged systems, *J. Comput. Phys.* 72:156–176 (1987).

203. J. W. Perram, H. G. Petersen, and S. W. DeLeeuw, An algorithm for the simulation of condensed matter that grows as the $3/2$ power of the number of particles, *Mol. Phys.* 65:875–893 (1988).

204. N. Karasawa and W. Goddard, Acceleration of convergence for lattice sums, *J. Phys. Chem.* 93:7320–7327 (1989).

205. J. Kolafa and J. W. Perram. Cutoff errors in the Ewald summation formulae for point charge systems, *Mol. Simul.* 9:351–368 (1992).

206. H. G. Petersen, Accuracy and efficiency of the particle mesh Ewald method, *J. Chem. Phys.* 103:3668–3679 (1995).

207. G. Hummer, The numerical accuracy of truncated Ewald sums for periodic systems with long-range coulomb interactions, *Chem. Phys. Lett. 235*: 297–302 (1995).

208. A. Toukmaji and J. A. Board, Ewald sum techniques in perspective: A survey, *Comput. Phys. Commun.* 95:75–91 (1996).

209. V. Natoli and D. M. Ceperley, An optimized method for treating long-range potentials, *J. Comput. Phys.* 117:171–178 (1995).

210. P. Procachi and M. Marchi, Taming the Ewald sum in molecular dynamics simulations of solvated proteins via a multiple time scale algorithm, *J. Chem. Phys. 104*:3003 (1996).

211. H. Q. Ding, N. Karasawa, and W. A. Goddard, The reduced cell multipole method for coulombic interactions in periodic systems with million-atom unit cells, *Chem. Phys. Lett. 196*:2 (1992).

212. C. G. Lambert, T. A. Darden, and J. A. Board, A multipole-based method for efficient calculation of forces and potentials in macroscopic periodic assemblies of particles, *J. Comput. Phys.* 126:274–285 (1996).

213. R. W. Hockney and J. W. Eastwood, *Computer Simulation Using Particles*, McGraw-Hill, New York, 1981.

214. J. Shimada, H. Kaneko, and T. Takada, Efficient calculations of coulombic interactions in biomolecular simulations with periodic boundary conditions, *J. Comput. Chem.* 14:867–878 (1993).

215. B. A. Luty, M. E. Davis, I. G. Tironi, and W. F. van Gunsteren, A comparison of particle–particle particle–mesh and Ewald methods for calculating electrostatic interactions in periodic systems, *Mol. Simul.* 14:11–20 (1994).

216. B. A. Luty, I. G. Tironi, and W. F. van Gunsteren, Lattice-sum methods for calculating electrostatic interactions in molecular simulations, *J. Chem. Phys. 103*:3014–3012 (1995).

217. T. A. Darden, D. M. York, and L. G. Pedersen, Particle mesh Ewald: An *N* log(*N*) method for Ewald sums in large systems, *J. Chem. Phys. 98*: 10089–10092 (1993).

218. P. Procachi, T. Darden, and M. Marchi, A very fast molecular dynamics method to simulate biomolecular systems with realistic electrostatic interactions," *J. Phys. Chem. 100*:10464–10468 (1996).

219. D. York and W. Yang, The fast Fourier Poisson (FFP) method for calculating Ewald sums, *J. Chem. Phys. 101*:3298 (1994).

220. Ajay and M. A. Murcko, Computational methods to predict binding free energy in ligand–receptor complexes, *J. Med. Chem.* 38:4953–4967 (1995).

12

Metals in Molecular Mechanics Force Fields and Simulations

Libero J. Bartolotti

*North Carolina Supercomputing Center, Research Triangle Park,
North Carolina*

Lee G. Pedersen

*National Institute of Environmental Health Sciences, Research Triangle
Park, North Carolina and University of North Carolina, Chapel Hill,
Chapel Hill, North Carolina*

I. INTRODUCTION

Metal atoms can form a broad range of ionic or covalent bonds in molecular systems. Providing adequate energy functions that properly describe the interactions across a broad class of chemistry poses a major challenge. In this chapter we will focus on actual work done in the past several years (to mid-1995).

The recent literature has been reviewed [LR1–LR4]. The review by Hay [LR1] provides a particularly interesting classification for potential energy functions (or "force fields") involving central metal atoms [M = metal, L = ligand, X = any other atom type]: (a) the valence force field form in which explicit interactions terms include *M-L* (distance), *M-L-X* (bond angle), *L-M-L* (bond angle), *M-L-X-X* (torsion), and terms such as *L-M-L-X*, and *M . . . X* (nonbonded) are either included or excluded; (b) points on a sphere form, which is the same as (a) except that the *L-M-L* terms are excluded; and (c) ionic form, which excludes all metal terms in

(a) and (b), but adds ionic and van der Waals nonbond terms for $M \ldots L$ and $M \ldots X$ (Fig. 1 shows common geometries found in simple to complex systems. The metal coordination geometries in biological systems are rarely exact matches to these examples.) Almost all empirical molecular mechanics or molecular dynamics calculations that include metals use one of these three schemes, perhaps modified to fit the specific situation. The review by Zimmer [LR4] lists recent applications to metalloproteins, including systems with polynuclear metallic sites. Zimmer emphasizes "there are no MM programs with reliable bioorganic force fields" [LR4]. There is, however, optimism for the future that the metal atom and its surrounding atoms can be treated quantum mechanically, while the distant atoms are treated classically [M12].

II. IONIC FORM

A. Several Ways to Compute the Ionic Interaction Terms for a Metal Ion and Its Ligands

It is perhaps instructive to indicate several approaches to obtaining parameters for the ionic case [LR1]. In the Aqvist [MF1] technique the interaction between the metal ion (M) and ligands (L = j) is written as

$$V_{\text{M,L}} = \sum_{j=1}^{n} \left[\frac{Q_{\text{M}} \cdot q_j}{r_{\text{M},j}} + \frac{A'_{\text{M}} \cdot A'_j}{r_{\text{M},j}^{12}} - \frac{B'_{\text{M}} \cdot B'_j}{r_{\text{M},j}^{6}} \right] \tag{1}$$

where $r_{\text{M},j}$ is the distance between metal ion and ligand, Q and q are the charges, and n is the number of metal–ligand interactions. Free-energy perturbation (FEP) calculations are performed using this potential energy function and the fixed SPC model for water (A'_j, B'_j, and q_j fixed). Assuming the charge of the metal ion, only the values of A'_{M} and B'_{M} remain to be determined. The procedure involved first computing the free energy to create either a Na^+ or Ca^{2+} ion in water by summing the FEP for this step, with the cavity and Born-charging corrections added. This procedure was iterated until a set of parameters (A'_{M}, B'_{M}) were found that gave the experimental hydration energy. With parameters for these two metal ions in hand, the parameters for the other group I and group II metals were determined by permuting the Na^+ and Ca^{2+} parameters into the desired ions until agreement with experimental data for the hydration energies was reached.

A somewhat different approach was taken by Bartolotti et al. [MQ1]. The hydrodynamic formulation of quantum mechanics couched in the methods of the time-dependent Kohn–Sham equations [MQ1] was used to compute the London dispersion attraction constant (C_6) between two iden-

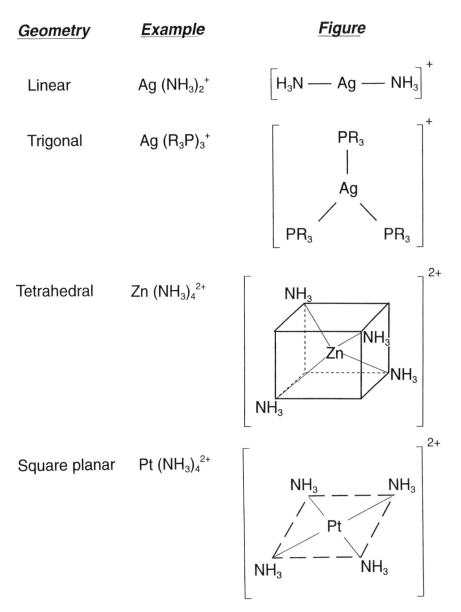

Figure 1 Some observed geometric forms of metal complexes.

Trigonal bipyramid $CuCl_5^{3-}$

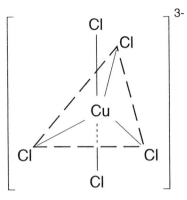

Tetragonal pyramid $VO\,(acac)_2$

$$acac = CH_3 - \overset{\overset{\displaystyle O^-}{|}}{C} = \overset{\overset{\displaystyle O}{\|}}{CHC} - CH_3$$

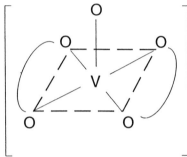

Octahedral $Co\,(NH_3)_6^{3+}$

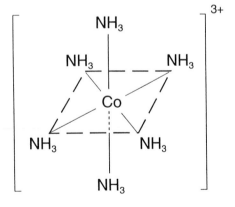

Figure 1   (Continued)

Pentagonal bipyramid ZrF_7^{3-}

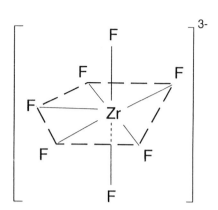

Square antiprism TaF_8^{3-}

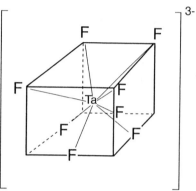

Cubic PaF_8^{3-}

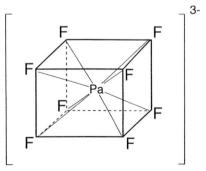

Dodecahedron   Mo $(CN)_8^{4-}$

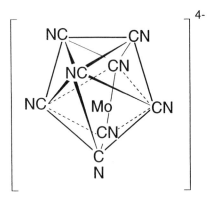

Figure 1   (Continued)

tical metal ions. Assuming a form similar to that used in AMBER [M1] for the interaction between a charged metal ion and ligand

$$V_{M,L} = \sum_{j=1}^{n} \left[\left(\frac{Q_M \cdot q_j}{r_{M,j}} \right) + \left(\frac{A_{M,j}}{r_{M,j}^{12}} - \frac{B_{M,j}}{r_{M,j}^{6}} \right) \right] \tag{2}$$

where $B = -2 \cdot \epsilon \cdot r_{min}^6$ and $A = -\epsilon \cdot r_{min}^{12}$

$\epsilon = [\epsilon_i \epsilon_j]^{1/2}$ and $r_{min} = r_{i0} + r_{j0}$

Since B is formally C_6, we then have that

$$\epsilon = \frac{-C_6}{[2 \cdot r_{min}^6]} = \frac{-C_6}{[2 \cdot (2 \cdot r_{i0})^6]} \tag{3}$$

Thus, a choice of r_{i0} (usually the covalent radius of the metal ion) suffices, and this allows the computation of ϵ_i (the Lennard-Jones potential well depth) from Eq. (3). Thus, it is clear that the last two terms of Eq. (2) can be written as a Lennard-Jones potential in terms of ϵ and r_{min}. If C_6 is computed in atomic units, it is necessary to multiply the right-hand side of Eq. (3) by $(627.5)(0.529)^6$ to obtain kilocalories per mole (kcal mol^{-1}) for ϵ_i. Finally, the values of ϵ and r_{min} (and, thus, $A_{M,j}$ and $B_{M,j}$) can be computed for any interaction of the metal ion with a ligand. The values thus computed for Mg^{2+}, Ca^{2+} and Sr^{2+} were used [MQ1] to evaluate the difference in hydration energies among these divalent metal ions by free-energy perturbation theory. Excellent agreement with experimental data was noted [MQ1].

Other simple models have been used to approximate $C_6 = B$. The polarizability α (which defines C_6) can be written as an expansion of the dipole spectra of the interacting atoms (i.e., the strengths of the transitions). London [MQ2] used an approximation for α in terms of the mean excitation energy E, arriving at the expression for the interaction between two atoms i and j,

$$C_6 = -\left(\frac{E_i \cdot E_j}{E_i + E_j}\right)\alpha_i\alpha_j$$

This expression can also be cast in terms of the ionization potentials and diamagnetic susceptibilities [MQ3]. Another simple model was proposed by Slater and Kirkwood [MQ4], namely

$$C_6 = \frac{3}{2}\left(\frac{\alpha_i\alpha_j}{(\alpha_i/n_i)^{1/2} + (\alpha_j/n_j)^{1/2}}\right)$$

where n_i is taken to be the number of electrons in the valence shell of atom i and likewise for n_j.

III. APPLICATIONS

Our own research applications have centered on the use of molecular dynamics simulations on large, charged systems, with neutralizing counterions for long periods [RM3,RM4,M10a,b]. In several of these systems, specifically bound metal ions were present [RM4a–c], in addition to the neutralizing counterions. It has been our experience for molecular systems involving charged proteins [M10b] or nucleic acids [RM3], that it is vitally important to employ a twin cutoff [RM4a–c] method or a particle mesh Ewald method [M10a,RM3] to accommodate the long-range interactions of coulombic charges. For instance, the H-*ras* *p*21 oncogene product protein [RM4a,b] binds GTP (charge -3 or -4, depending on the pH) and a magnesium ion (charge $+2$); the latter helps bridge the GTP to the protein. The overall ternary structure has a charge of -8. To provide for an electrically neutral simulation, eight sodium cations must be included. The placement of the counterions was accomplished by an arbitrary, but reasonable, procedure: (a) a large box of water was placed around the protein and energy-minimized; (b) the electrostatic potential was computed at each water oxygen; (c) sodium counterions were added sequentially by replacing the water molecules with the greatest negative potential. The system was re–energy-minimized with each sodium ion addition, followed by a recalculation of the electrostatic potential for placement of the ion. When we equilibrated in a large box of water, we found that the starting crystallographic system partially and unrealistically unfolded after approximately 100 ps using an 8-A cutoff for the nonbonded interactions. A key interaction of the protein (THR 35) with the magnesium ion was lost. Inclusion of long-range interactions to 22 A, however, using a twin cutoff procedure [RM4ab], provided for a stable folded protein for times up to 200 ps. A similar behavior was found for simulations that we performed for the Ca–prothrombin system. Prothrombin has ten γ-carboxyglutamic acid residues in the first 33 amino acids (NH_2-terminus) and seven Ca^{2+} ions bind to exactly charge-neutralize the first 145 amino acid segment at physiological pH. These calcium ions form a very tight network, with some of the calcium ions less than 4 A apart. When a simulation was performed with an 8-A cutoff, we found that the NH_2-terminus, which is actually attached to the body of the protein by three strong hydrogen bonds (and two calcium ions), dissociates unrealistically. This tight interaction is necessary for phospholipid binding and the subsequent catalytic release of thrombin. Accommodation of the long-range forces to 20 A, however, by use of the twin cutoff procedure, leads to a stable simulation in which the NH_2-terminus remains secure. In both the $p21$–H-ras and prothrombin simulations, the ions (Mg^{2+}, Ca^{2+}, and Na^+) were treated as simple ions by Eq. (1). Kollman's group [M10c] has also described the consequences of a short nonbond cutoff in a study of proteins and nucleic acids that employs the particle mesh Ewald method. The twin cutoff procedure, the particle mesh Ewald method [M10d] (or full Ewald), or the fast multipole expansion method [M10e], are becoming standard "equipment" in modern-modeling packages.

Molecular mechanics was clearly developed to provide a compromise for the need to perform accurate calculations and the need to do those calculations rapidly. As a consequence, quantum mechanical properties, such as charge exchange and polarization, are usually ignored. As numeric techniques and computer technology advance, one project ahead to the time when computations will be conducted completely by quantum mechanics. The recent calculations by the Ziegler [TS17] group using DFT methods with relativistic corrections for metal (Me = Ni, Pd, Pt, Fe, Ru, Os, Cr, Mo, W) carbonyls, and the ab initio calculations of the Morokuma group [RS4] for transition states involved in chelation-controlled carbonyl addition of specific ketones and aldehydes (metal = Mg) provide very recent examples of the rapidly advancing science. Of special interest is the development of intermediate techniques [M12] that treat the core of a molecular system (such as a metal center or a transition state of an active site) by ab initio or semiempirical quantum mechanical methods, and the outer (and thus less important) part of the system by molecular mechanics. These promising techniques have been applied to a transition metal organometallic system [TS18], and to the human carbonic anhydrase system that involves a central Zn coordination sphere [TM6].

Table 1 Abbreviations Used for the Following Description of the Recent Literature

AMB	AMBER [M1]
CHA	CHARMM [M2]
CFF	Consistent force field [M9]
DFT	Density functional theory
DIS	Discover [M8]
FEP/FE	Free energy perturbation calculations are performed or free energy profiles are determined.
GRO	Gromos force field [M7]
HG	"Home grown," not easily cataloged
IMOMM	Integrated molecular orbital molecular mechanics method [M12]
MAM	Macromodel [M4]
MD/MC	Molecular dynamics or Monte Carlo simulations are performed
MMI	Any of a number of MM2-based methods and extensions [M3]
MOB	MOBY [M5]
MOMEC	A HYPERCHEM molecular mechanics program [TS19]
PME	Particle–mesh Ewald [M10]
QM	A quantum mechanical method is used
QM/MD	A fully integrated quantum mechanical–molecular dynamics method (Car–Parrinello [M13])
QM/MM	A hybrid Hamiltonian is used that involves both quantum mechanics and molecular mechanics
STR	Molecular mechanics is used to determine structure and energy
SYB	SYBYL [M11]
TM	Transition metals
UFF	Universal force field [M6]

The foundation of a fully quantum mechanical molecular dynamics method was laid in 1985 by the seminal paper of Car and Parrinello [M13]. An interatomic potential is not necessary in this method. One proceeds by computing the needed forces at each integration step from the quantum mechanical (DFT) electronic structure. Implicit in this methodology is proper accommodation of time-dependent phenomena, such as charge exchange, polarization, dispersion, and so on. The current development of the theory, which is aimed at understanding the dynamic properties of first-row elements and transition metals, has been assessed [M14], as has an application of the methodology to H_2O absorbed to solid MgO [RQ2].

In the current chapter a partial, but representative list of papers from 1993 through early 1995 is provided. We have used a classification scheme

Table 2

Classification	Ref.	Metals	Force field	Comments
Methods				
STR	MS1	Li^+, Na^+, K^+	AMB	Discusses the inclusion of nonadditive effects for aromatic–cation systems.
STR	MS2	Alkali, alkali earth ions	MMI	Develops MM3 parameters using the "points on a sphere" approach of ions interacting with aliphatic ethers.
STR	MS3	Entire periodic table	UFF	Ambitious attempt to bring a single force field (based remotely on DREIDING) to all elements.
STR	MS4	Fe(II), Ru(II) Os(II), V(II) Co(II), Co(III) Fe(III), Ni(II)	CHA	Parameters are developed for a series of transition metal metallocenes: [Me[Cp]$_2$] where Cp is the cyclopentadienyl anion.
STR	MS5	Rh	HG	A force field is proposed for square planar transition metal complexes that involves an angular potential energy function about the metal ion.
STR	MS6	Zn	AMB	Zn binding in the carbonic anhydrase system is studied by accommodating valence bonding for the Zn atom.
STR	MS7	Al^{3+}	HG	A force field for aluminophosphates is proposed.
STR	MS8	Co, Zn	HG	A force field called "YETI" is proposed that includes parameters for the metal–ligand distance, the symmetry at the metal, ligand field stabilization, and ligand–metal charge exchange.

FEP	MF1	Alkali, alkali earth ions	GRO	Uses free energy calculations on ions that interact only by nonbonded (ionic/vdW) terms with solvent for calibration of parameters to hydration energies and radial distribution functions.
QM	MQ1	Alkali, alkali earth, transition, metal ions	AMB	A method is proposed for determining the C_6 van der Waals parameters for metal ions by use of the hydrodynamic analogy quantum mechanical approach.
QM/MM	M12	General metals	CHA (IMOMM)	A system is broken into a core and outer region. The core is treated quantum mechanically and the outer atoms are treated classically.

Main group metals

STR	RS1	Li$^+$, Na$^+$, K$^+$	CHA	Alkali metals interacting with peptide, fit to 6-31g* calculation.
STR	RS2	K$^+$	MMI	K$^+$ interacting with 11-hexadentate crown ether ligands.
STR	RS3	Many	UFF	Application of UFF to main group compounds.
STR	RS4	Mg^{2+}	QM	Accurate quantum mechanical calculations are used to locate transition states involving magnesium
MD	RM1	Alkalis	CHA	Ion transport in gramicidin channel; polarization added to standard function.
MC	RM2	Na$^+$	HG	Monte Carlo study of Na-23 distribution around cylinder of DNA to support NMR study.
MD	RM3	Na$^+$, Mg^{2+}	AMB	Use of particle mesh Ewald (PME) method to study dynamics of crystalline DNA.

Table 2 (continued)

Classification	Ref.	Metals	Force field	Comments
MD	RM4	Na^+, Mg^{2+}	AMB	Long dynamics on wild-type and mutant forms of $p21$–H-ras, twin cutoff found essential. Similar behavior is seen for the bovine prothrombin–calcium ion system.
MD	RM5	K^+	AMB	Dynamics of valinomycin and its K^+ complex.
MD	RM6	Na^+	DIS	Dynamics of salinomycin–Na^+ complex with and without $CHCl_3$ solvent, to support NMR.
MD	RM7	Al^{3+}, Li^+, K^+	HG	Dynamics simulations on periodic macrocells as function of pressure.
FEP	RF1	K^+	AMB	Free-energy perturbation study of K^+ and crown ether using the Ewald technique for coulombic interactions.
FEP	RF2	Alkalis	AMB	Free-energy perturbation study of the stability of antiparallel G-DNA quadruplexes as a function of metal ion size.
FEP	RF3	Alkalis	AMB	Application of free-energy derivative technique to study optimal size of ions in crown ether cavity.
FEP	RF4	Alkalis	AMB	Relative free energy study of alkali metal ions in 8-subunit cavitand molecules, methanol solvent.
FEP	RF5	Li^+, Cs^+, K^+	AMB	Free-energy perturbation study of $Li^+ \rightarrow Cs^+$ in water and K^+, ionophore potential of mean force to determine speedups in parallel computers.

FEP	RF6	Na⁺, K⁺	AMB	Solvation of ions in methanol using Åqvist parameters by free-energy simulations.
FE	RF7	Na⁺	CHA	Free-energy profile of Na^+ moving along gramicidin channel.
FEP	RF8	Ca^{2+}, Mg^{2+}	AMB	Free-energy calculations for $Ca^{2+} \rightarrow Mg^{2+}$ in solution and when bound to protein and lipid analogues. Solvent and cutoff options were investigated.
FEP	RF9	Li^+, Rb^+, Na^+	AMB	Mass spectroscopy and molecular dynamics studies on the relative stability of $M(H_2O)_{20}^+$.
QM/MM	RQ1	K^+	HG	Dynamics with hybrid Hamiltonian function for the interaction of K^+ with crown ethers.
QM/MD	RQ2	Mg^{2+}	DFT	Dynamics of H_2O interacting with solid MgO. No explicit interaction potential input.

Transition metals

STR	TS0	Zn^{2+}, $Cd^{,2+}$, Ca^{2+}	SYB/TAFF	Molecular mechanics calculations on divalents interacting with tetra-N-substituted cyclens. Points on a sphere approach.
STR	TS1	Ti, Zr, Hf	CHA-based	Structural study of $M(Cp)_2Cl_2$ complexes [M = metal, Cp = cyclopentadienyl], highly parameterized.
STR	TS2	Many TM, variable valence	CHARMM and UFF	Structural study of metal ion-macrocycle [1,4,7-trithiacyclononane] complexes.
STR	TS3	Co^{3+}	CFF modifications	Structural studies of Co^{3+} with sar [chlorinated hexaazabicyclo-[6.6.6]icosane] complexes.

Table 2 (continued)

Classification	Ref.	Metals	Force field	Comments
STR	TS4	Pd^{2+}	MAM(MM2*)	Structural study of allyl complexes of palladium.
STR	TS5	Os	MAM(MM2*)	Study of osmaoxetane intermediates.
STR	TS6	Fe^{3+}	AMB	Interaction of Fe^{3+}–transferrin complexes in vacuo and in water.
STR	TS7	Fe^{3+}	MAM(MM2*)	Study of orientation of axial pi-acceptors in Fe(III)–porphyrinates.
STR	TS8	Ni^{2+}	MMI	Study of Ni(II)–tetraaza macrocyclic complexes; many explicit parameters derived from calibration procedure.
STR	TS9	Zr	MOB	Study of zirconocene dichlorides; highly paramaterized to fit data from a large number of complexes.
STR	TS10	Ni(0)	MMI	Study of [4 + 4] cycloadditions, Ni(0) square planar pi-allyl metal complexes.
STR	TS11	Pd	MMI	Study of potential antiviral agents, palladium complexes with aminopyridines, and benzonitrile as ligands.
STR	TS12	Many	UFF	Application to classical coordination complexes and many other complexes of biological and organic systems. An attempt to accommodate backbonding and the *trans* influence is made.

STR	TS13	Ni^{2+}	MMI	A study if Ni(II)–tetraza annulenes on a graphite surface.
STR	TS14	Co, Hg, Sn	MMI	Several transition metals are ions studied in complex with 18-azo-crown-6 ethers.
STR	TS15	Zn^{2+}	MMI	A study of the tetrahedral complexes of Zn^{2+} with cysteine, histidine, and glutamic acid.
STR	TS16	Zn metal	HG	Zn atom clusters of 4–55 atoms are studied by the embedded atom method.
STR	TS17	Ni, Pd, Pt, Fe, Ru, Os, Cr, Mo, W	DFT	Metal carbonyl dissociation energies are computed by DFT with corrections for relativity.
STR	TS18	Pt	CH/IMOMM	The new IMOMM is applied to the addition of H_2 to a Pt complex.
STR	TS19	Cu(II)	MOMEC/(HYPERCHEM)	A new method for calculation of the structure of Jahn–Teller-distorted metal centers is presented.
STR	TS20	Cr, Rh	MMP2/BIOGRAPH	Calculation of ligand repulsive energy for 45 olefins in $Cr(CO)_5$ environment and 38 olefins in CpRh(CO) environment.
TR	TS21	Pt	AMBER-like	Correlated guanine–Pt interactions versus a number of experimental studies (NMR, X-ray).
STR	TS22	Fe(III)	AMBER	Parameters for a ferric transferrin environment were generated used model FE(III) chelates.
STR	TS23	Cr, Mo, Re, Os	MM2/EM0	Parameters developed for various electron configuration.
STR	TS24	Ti, Zr, Hf	CHA	Parameters for $M(C_p')_2$ and $M(Cp^*)_2$ developed/discussed: Cp' = cyclopentadienyl, Cp* = pentamethyl Cp'
STR	TS25	Cu(II)	MOMEC	A study of a dinuclear system.
MD	TM1	Fe^{2+}	HG	A systematic study of the effect of boundary condition of aqueous ionic solutions. Study includes use of Ewald summation techniques.

Table 2 (continued)

Classification	Ref.	Metals	Force field	Comments
Transition metals				
MD	TM2	Co^{2+}	MAM(MMI)	Study of cobalt bleomycin. Carried out a conformational search to determine a possible DNA-binding conformation.
MD	TM3	Fe^{2+}, Fe^{3+}	HG	Dynamics is used to develop a model for electron transfer between Fe^{2+} and Fe^{3+} using Kramer's and Grote–Hyne's theories.
MD	TM4	Zn^{2+}	AMB	A 200-ps simulation with electrostatics accommodated accurately for Zn^{2+} blocking the HIV-1 protease active site.
MD	TM5	Ru^{2+}, Ru^{3+}	CFF/mumod	A simulation study of ruthenium ion complexes in water. Some, but not all parameters are given.
MD	TM6	Zn	AMB	Four different simulation models are constructed to study the coordination of CN^- to Zn in human carbonic anhydrase.
QM/MD	TM7	Zn^{2+}	AMB	The Zn^{2+} coordination sphere in carbonic anhydrase is studied using a combined quantum mechanical (semiempirical) Hamiltonian function and classic mechanics for the outer-layer atoms.
MD	TM8	Fe^{3+}	CHA	Molecular dynamics of a model redox site in Rebredoxin ($Fe(SCH_2CH_3)_4^-$).
MD	TM9	Fe^{3+}	CHA	An extension of TM8 to the protein environment. Includes explicit solvent and counterions.
FEP	TF1	Fe^{2+}	AMB	CO and O_2 relative binding to myoglobin is simulated using a distance-dependent dielectric constant to substitute for solvent and neutralizing ions.
STR	LS1	Eu^{3+}	CHA	The molecular mechanics of Eu^{3+} in various multidentate complexes is studied.

of methods (including force fields), representative metals, and transition metals in this order. A list of abbreviations (Table 1) is used to classify the recent literature references (Table 2).

REFERENCES

Note: References code: XYI: X = [M, method; R, representative metal; T, transition metal; L, Lanthanide or actinide]; Y = [S, structural or energy; M, molecular dynamics or Monte Carlo; F, free-energy perturbation, profile or derivative; Q, quantum mechanical]; I = [no. in chronological order by date]; * = especially useful references. A subclassification gives the metal, the force field used, and a comment about the work.

Reviews

*LR1. B. P. Hay, Methods for molecular mechanics modeling of coordination compounds, *Coord. Chem. Rev. 126*:177 (1993).
LR2. C. R. Landis, D. M. Root, and T. Cleveland, Molecular mechanics force fields for modeling inorganic and organometallic compounds, *Reviews in Computational Chemistry*, Vol. 6 (K. B. Lipkowtiz and D. B. Boyd, eds.), VCH Publishing, New York, 1995, p. 73.
LR3. E. Osawa and K. B. Lipkowtiz, Published force field parameters, *Reviews in Computational Chemistry*, Vol. 6 (E. Osawa and K. B. Lipkowitz, eds.), VCH Publishers, New York, 1995, p. 355.
*LR4. M. Zimmer, Bioinorganic molecular mechanics, *Chem. Revs. 95*:2629 (1995).

Methods, Force Fields

*M1. W. Cornell, P. Ciepiak, C. I. Bayly, I. R. Gould, K. M. Merz, Jr., D. M. Ferguson, D. C. Spellmeyer, T. Fox, J. W. Caldwell, and P. A. Kollman, A second generation force field for the simulation of proteins, nucleic acids and organic molecules, *J. Am. Chem. Soc. 117*:5179 (1995) and references therein.
*M2. B. R. Brooks, R. E. Bruccoleri, B. D. Olafson, D. J. States, S. Swaminathan and M. Karplus, CHARMM: A program for macromolecular energy, minimization and dynamics calculations, *J. Comput. Chem. 4*:187 (1983) as well as references in [M1].
M3. (a) U. Burkert and N. L. Allinger, *Molecular Mechanics, ACS Monograph 177*, Washington DC, 1982 and references in [M1].
(b) N. L. Allinger, X. Zhou, and J. Bergsma, Molecular mechanics parameters, *J. Mol. Struct. 312*:69 (1994).
M4. F. Mohamadi, N. G. J. Richards, W. C. Guida, R. Liskamp, M. Lipton, C. Caufield, G. Chang, T. Hendrickson, and W. C. Still, MacroModel—C.

An integrated software system for modeling organic and bioorganic molecules using molecular mechanics, *J. Comput. Chem. 11*:440 (1990).

M5.　U. Howeler, MAXIMOBY 3.1; CHEOPS: Munster, Germany, 1992.

M6.　see Ref. MS3

M7.　W. F. van Gunsteren, H. J. C. Berendsen, Groningen molecular simulations (GROMOS) library manual, Groningen, 1987.

M8.　A. T. Hagler, P. S. Stern, S. Lifson, and S. Ariel, *J. Am. Chem. Soc. 101*: 813 (1979). see also J. R. Maple, M.-J. Hwang, T. P. Stockfish, U. Dinur, M. Waldman, C. S. Ewig, and A. T. Hagler, Derivation of class II force fields. I. Methodology and quantum force field for the alkyl functional group and alkane molecules, *J. Comput. Chem. 15*:162 (1994), and references therein.

M9.　K. Rasmussen, Potential energy functions in conformational analysis, *Lecture Notes in Chemistry*, Vol. 37, Springer, Berlin, 1985.

*M10.　*(a) T. Darden, D. York, and L. Pedersen, Particle mesh Ewald: An $N \log(N)$ method for Ewald sums in large systems, *J. Chem. Phys. 98*: 10089 (1993).

(b) D. M. York, A. Wlodawer, L. G. Pedersen, and T. A. Darden, Atomic-level accuracy in simulations of large protein crystals, *Proc. Natl. Acad. Sci. USA 91*:8715 (1994).

*(c) T. E. Cheatham III, J. L. Miller, T. Fox, T. A. Darden, and P. A. Kollman, Molecular dynamics simulations on solvated biomolecular systems: The particle mesh Ewald method leads to stable trajectories of DNA, RNA and proteins, *J. Am. Chem. Soc. 117*:4193 (1995).

*(d) U. Essmann, L. Perera, M. Berkowitz, T. Darden, H. Lee, and L. G. Pedersen, A smooth particle mesh Ewald method, *J. Chem. Phys. 103*: 8577 (1995).

(e) H. Q. Ding, N. Karasawa, and W. Goddard, Atomic level simulations on a million particles: The cell multipole method for Coulomb and London nonbond interactions, *J. Chem. Phys. 97*:4309 (1992).

M11.　SYBYL Program, available from TRIPOS Associates, 1699 South Hanley Road, St. Louis MO 63144.

*M12.　F. Maseras and K. Morokuma, IMOMM: A new integrated ab initio + molecular mechanics geometry optimization scheme of equilibrium structures and transition states, *J. Comput. Chem. 16*:1170–1179 (1995).

*M13.　R. Car and M. Parrinello, Unified approach for molecular dynamics and density functional theory, *Phys. Rev. Letts. 55*:478 (1985).

M14.　J. Hutter, M. Tuckerman, and M. Parrinello, Integrating the Car–Parrinello equations. III: Techniques for ultrasoft pseudopotentials, *J. Chem. Phys. 102*:859 (1995).

Methods, Specific

MS1.　J. W. Caldwell and P. A. Kollman, Cation–pi interactions, nonadditive effects are critical in their accurate representation, *J. Am. Chem. Soc. 117*: 4177 (1995).

MS2. B. P. Hay and J. R. Rustad, Structural criteria for the rational design of selective ligands: Extension of the MM3 force field to aliphatic ether complexes of the alkali and alkaline earth cations, *J. Am. Chem. Soc. 116*: 6316 (1994).

*MS3. A. K. Rappé, C. J. Casewit, K. S. Colwell, W. A. Goddard III, W. M. Skiff, UFF, A full periodic table force field for molecular mechanics and molecular dynamics simulations, *J. Am. Chem. Soc. 117*:10024 (1992).

MS4. T. N. Doman, C. R. Landis, and B. Bosnich, Molecular mechanics force fields for linear metallocenes, *J. Am. Chem. Soc. 114*:7264 (1992).

MS5. V. Allured, C. M. Kelly, and C. R. Landis, SHAPES empirical force field: New treatment of angular potentials and its application to square planar transition-metal complexes, *J. Am. Chem. Soc. 113*:1 (1991).

MS6. S. C. Hoops, K. W. Anderson, and K. M. Merz, Jr., Force field design for metalloproteins, *J. Am. Chem. Soc. 113*:8262 (1991).

MS7. G. J. Kramer, N. P. Farragher, and B. W. H. van Beest, Interatomic force fields for silicas, aluminumphosphates and zeolites: Derivations based on ab initio calculations, *Phys. Rev. B 43*:5068 (1991)

MS8. A. Vedani and D. W. Huhta, A new force field for modeling metalloproteins, *J. Am. Chem. Soc. 112*:4759 (1990).

*MF1. J. Aqvist, Modelling of ion–ligand interactions in solutions and biomolecules, *J. Mol. Struct. (Theochem.) 256*:135 (1992).

*MQ1. L. Bartolotti, L. G. Pedersen, and P. S. Charifson, Long range nonbonded attractive constants for some charged atoms, *J. Comput. Chem. 12*:1125 (1991); see also L. Bartolotti and Q. Xie, Dipole Cauchy moments of the atoms H through Ar: An application of Kohn–Sham theory with the atomic gradient expansion of the exchange–correlation energy density functional, *Theor. Chim. Acta 77*:239 (1990).

MQ2. F. London, *Z. Phys. Theor. System. Mol. 63*:245 (1930).

MQ3. See for instance, J. Goodisman, *Diatomic Interaction Potential Theory*, Vol. 2 Academic Press, New York, 1973, pp. 370–374

MQ4. J. G. Kirkwood, Polarizabilities, susceptibilities and van der Waals forces of atoms with several electrons. *Physik Z. 33*:57–60 (1932); J. C. Slater and J. G. Kirkwood, The van der Waals forces in gases. *Phys. Rev. 37*: 682 (1931).

Applications, Representative Metals

RS1. B. Roux and M. Karplus, Potential energy function for cation–peptide interactions: An ab initio study, *J. Comput. Chem. 16*:690 (1995).

RS2. B. P. Hay, J. R. Rustad, and C. J. Hostetler, Quantitative structure–stability relationship for potassium complexation by crown ethers. A molecular mechanics and ab initio study, *J. Am. Chem. Soc. 115*:11158 (1993).

*RS3. C. J. Casewit, K. S. Colwell, and A. K. Rappé, Application of a universal force field to main group compounds, *J. Am. Chem. Soc. 114*:10046 (1992).

RS4. S. Mori, M. Nakamura, E. Nakamura, N. Koga, and K. Morokuma, Theoretical studies on chelation-controlled carbonyl addition. Me_2Mg addition to α- and β-alkoxy ketones and aldehydes, *J. Am. Chem. Soc. 117*:5055 (1995).

RM1. B. Roux, B. Prod'hom, and M. Karplus, Ion transport in the gramicidin channel: Molecular dynamics study of single and double occupancy, *Biophys. J. 68*:876 (1995).

RM2. V. M. Stein, J. P. Bond, M. W. Capp, C. F. Anderson, and M. T. Record, Jr, Importance of coulombic end effects on cation accumulation near oligoelectrolyte B-DNA: A demonstration using 23-Na NMR, *Biophys. J. 68*:1063 (1995).

*RM3. H. Lee, T. A. Darden, and L. G. Pedersen, Molecular dynamics simulation studies of a high resolution Z-DNA crystal, *J. Chem. Phys. 102*:3830 (1995).

RM4. (a) M. Frech, T. A. Darden, L. G. Pedersen, C. K. Foley, P. S. Charifson, M. W. Anderson, and A. Wittinghofer, Role of glutamine-61 in the hydrolysis of GTP by *p*21-H-*ras*: An experimental and theoretical study, *Biochemistry 33*:3237 (1994).
(b) C. K. Foley, L. G. Pedersen, T. A. Darden, P. S. Charifson, A. Wittinghofer and M. W. Anderson, Molecular dynamics studies of H-*ras p*21-GTP, *Handbook of Experimental Pharmacology*, Vol 108/I, *GTPases in Biology* (B. F. Dickey and L. Birnbaumer, eds), Springer, Berlin, 1993.
(c) N. Hamaguchi, P. Charifson, T. Darden, L. Xiao, K. Padmanabhan, A. Tulinsky, R. Hiskey, and L. Pedersen, Molecular dynamics simulations of bovine prothrombin fragment 1 in the presence of calcium ions, *Biochemistry 31*:8840 (1992).

RM5. T. R. Forester, W. Smith, and J. H. R. Clarke, A molecular dynamics study of valinomycin and the potassium–valinomycin complex, *J. Phys. Chem. 98*:9422 (1994).

RM6. S. Mronga, G. Muller, J. Fischer, and F. Riddell, A model for ion transport across membranes: Solution structure of the ionophore metal complex salinomycin–Na determined by NMR and molecular dynamics calculation, *J. Am. Chem. Soc. 115*:8414 (1993).

RM7. S. L. Chaplot and S. K. Sikka, Molecular-dynamics simulation of pressure-induced crystalline to amorphous transition in some corner-linked polyhedral compounds, *Phys. Rev. B 47*:5710 (1993).

RQ1. M. A. Thompson, E. D. Glendening, and D. Feller, The nature of K^+/ crown ether interactions: A hybrid quantum mechanical–molecular mechanical study, *J. Phys. Chem. 98*:10465 (1994).

RQ2. W. Langel and M. Parrinello, Ab initio molecular dynamics of H_2O absorbed on solid MgO, *J. Chem. Phys. 103*:3240 (1995).

*RF1. L. X. Dang and P. A. Kollman, Free energy of association of the K^+:18-crown-6 complex in water: A new molecular dynamics study, *J. Phys. Chem. 99*:55 (1995).

RF2. W. S. Ross and C. C. Hardin, Ion-induced stabilization of the G-DNA quadruplex: Free energy perturbation studies, *J. Am. Chem. Soc. 116*: 6070 (1994).

RF3. P. Ciepiak, D. A. Pearlman, and P. A. Kollman, Walking on the free energy hypersurface of the 18-crown-6 ion system using free energy derivatives, *J. Chem. Phys. 101*:627 (1994).

RF4. B. E. Thomas IV and Peter A. Kollman, Free energy perturbation calculations of the relative binding affinities of an 8-subunit cavitand for alkali ions in methanol, *J. Am. Chem. Soc. 116*:3449 (1994).

*RF5. S. E. DeBolt, D. A. Pearlman, and P. A. Kollman, Free energy perturbation calculations on parallel computers: Demonstrations of scalable linear speedup, *J. Comput. Chem. 15*:351 (1994).

RF6. T. J. Marrone and K. M. Merz, Jr., Transferability of ion models, *J. Phys. Chem. 97*:6524 (1993).

RF7. B. Roux and M. Karplus, Ion transport in the gramicidin channel: Free energy of the solvated right-handed dimer in a model membrane, *J. Am. Chem. Soc. 115*:3250 (1993).

RF8. P. S. Charifson, R. G. Hiskey, L. G. Pedersen, and L. F. Kuyper, Free energy calculations on calcium and magnesium complexes: Protein and phospholipid model systems, *J Comput. Chem. 12*:899 (1991).

RF9. E. A. Steel, K. M. Merz, Jr., A. Selinger, and A. W. Castleman, Jr., Mass spectral and computational free energy studies of alkali metal ion-containing water clusters, *J. Phys. Chem. 99*:7829 (1995).

Applications, Transition Metals

TS1. T. N. Doman, T. K. Hollis, and B. Bosnich, Molecular mechanics for bent metallocenes of the type [M(Cp)$_2$Cl$_2$]. *J. Am. Chem. Soc. 117*:1352 (1995).

TS2. J. Beech, P. J. Cragg, and M. G. B. Drew, Conformational study of the macrocyle 1,4,7-trithiacyclononane in metal complexes, *J. Chem. Soc. Dalton Trans.* p. 719 (1994).

TS3. I. Creaser, T. Komorita, A. M. Sargeson, A. C. Willis, and K. Yamanari, New macrocyclic complexes derived from cobalt(III) cage complexes, *Aust. J. Chem. 47*:529 (1994).

TS4. P. Pregosin, H. Ruegger, R. Salzmann, A. Albinati, F. Lianza, and R. W. Kutz, X-ray diffraction, multidimensional NMR spectroscopy and MM2* calculations on chiral allyl complexes of palladium(II), *Organometallics 13*:83 (1994).

TS5. P.-O. Norrby, H. C. Kolb, and K. B. Sharpless, Toward an understanding of the high enantioselectivity in the osmium-catalyzed asymmetric dihydroxylation. 2. A qualitative molecular mechanics approach, *J. Am. Chem. Soc. 116*:8470 (1994).

TS6. W. Lin, W. Welsh, and W. R. Harris, Molecular mechanics studies of model iron (III) tranferrin complexes in vacuo and in aqueous solution, *Inorg. chem. 33*:884 (1994).

TS7. M. K. Safo F. A. Walker, A. M. Raitsimring, W. P. Walter, D. P. Dolata, P. G. Debrummer, and W. R. Scheidt, Axial ligand orientation in iron(III) porphyrinates: Effect of axial pi-acceptors. Characterization of the low-spin complex [Fe(TPP)(4-CNPy)$_2$]ClO$_4$, *J. Am. Chem. Soc. 116*:7760 (1994).

TS8.   K. R. Adam, I. M. Atkinson, M. Antolovich, L. G. Brigden, and L. F. Lindoy, Comparative molecular mechanics study of the high-spin Ni(II) complexes of an extended series of tetraaza macrocycles, *J. Mol. Struct. 323*:223 (1994).

TS9.   U. Howeler, R. Mohr, M. Knickmeier, and G. Erker, A valence force field for zirconocene dichlorides, *Organometallics 13*:2380 (1994).

TS10. M. M. Gugelchuk and K. N. Houk, Stereoselective organometallic reactions: A force field study of pi-allyl intermediates in nickel(0)-catalyzed cycloadditions, *J. Am. Chem. Soc. 11*:330 (1994).

TS11. P. C. Yates, Use of the MM2 force field to model palladium complexes with nitrogen-containing aromatic ligands, *J. Mol. Struct. (Theochem.) 303*:55 (1994).

*TS12. A. K. Rappé, K. S. Coldwell, and C. J. Casewit, Application of a universal force field to metal complexes, *Inorg. Chem. 32*:3438 (1993).

TS13. M. G. B. Drew, N. J. Jutson, P. C. H. Mitchell, R. J. Potter, and D. Thompsett, Experimental and computer modelling studies of carbon-supported metal complexes, *J. Chem. Soc. Faraday Trans. 89*:3963 (1993).

TS14. M. G. B. Drew and M. Amelia Santos, Molecular mechanics studies of the conformations of metal complexes of 1,4,7,10,13,16-hexaazacyclooctadecane: Calculations of macrocyclic cavity size, *Struct. Chem. 4*:5 (1993).

TS15. P. C. Yates, Molecular mechanics and semiempirical molecular orbital calculations on zinc complexes with amino acid derivatives, *J. Mol. Struct. (Theochem.) 281*:275 (1993).

TS16. R. Ramprasad and R. G. Hoagland, Thermodynamic properties of small zinc clusters based on atomistic simulations, *Model. Simul. Mater. Sci. Eng. 1*:189 (1993).

TS17. J. Li, G. Schreckenbach, and T. Ziegler, A reassessment of first metal–carbonyl dissociation energy in M(CO)$_4$ (M = Ni, Pd, Pt), M(CO)$_5$ (M = Fe, Ru, Os), and M(CO)$_6$ (M = Cr, Mo, W) by a quasi-relativistic density functional method, *J. Am. Chem. Soc. 117*:486 (1995).

*TS18. T. Matsubara, F. Maseras, N. Koga, and K. Morokuma, Application of the new "integrated MO + MM" (IMOMM) method to the organometallic reaction: Pt(PR$_3$)$_2$ + H$_2$(R = H, Me, *t*-Bu and Ph), *J. Phys. Chem. 100*:2573 (1996).

TS19. P. Comba and M. Zimmer, Molecular mechanics and the Jahn–Teller effect, *Inorg. Chem. 33*:5368 (1994).

TS20. D. P. White and T. L. Brown, Molecular orbital model of ligand effects. 7. Binding of η^2 ligands to Cr(CO)$_5$ and CpRh(CO): E_R values for olefins, *Inorg. Chem. 34*:2718 (1995).

TTS21. S. Yao, J. P. Plastaras, and L. G. Marzilli, A molecular mechanics AMBER-type force field for modeling Pt complexes of guanine derivatives, *Inorg. Chem. 33*:6061 (1994).

TS22. W. Lin, W. J. Welsh, and W. R. Harris, Molecular mechanics studies of model Fe(III) transferrin complexes in vacuo and in solution, *Inorg. Chem. 33*:884 (1994).

TS23. B. Blaive, G. Legsai, and R. Lai, Utilization of d^0, d^1, d^2 electron configurations to obtain parameters for transition metals in the molecular mechanics of dioxo- or diimido-tetrahedral complexes, *J. Mol. Struct. 354*: 245 (1995).

TS24. B. Bosnich, Molecular mechanics force fields for cyclopentadienyl complexes, *Chem. Soc. Rev. 23*:387 (1995).

TS25. P. Comba, A. Fath, and D. T. Richens, Double helical dinuclear copper (II) complexes of macrocyclic bis(dithiadiimine) ligands, *Angew. Chem. 34*:1883 (1995).

*TM1. J. E. Roberts and J. Schnitker, Boundary conditions in simulations of aqueous ionic solutions, *J. Phys. Chem. 99*:1322 (1995).

TM2. J. L. Tueting, K. L. Spence, and M. Zimmer, Binding geometry of cobalt bleomycin, an empirical force-field analysis, *J. Chem. Soc. Dalton Trans.* p. 551 (1994).

TM3. D. A. Rose and I. Benjamin, Molecular dynamics and nonadiabatic electron transfer, *J. Chem. Phys. 100*:3545 (1994).

TM4. (a) D. M. York, L. J. Barolotti, T. A. Darden, L. G. Pedersen, and M. W. Anderson, Simulations of the solution structure of HIV-1 protease in the presence and absence of bound zinc, *J. Comput. Chem. 15*:61 (1994).
(b) D. M. York, T. A. Darden, L. G. Pedersen, and M. W. Anderson, Molecular modeling studies suggest that zinc ions inhibit HIV-1 protease by binding at catalytic aspartates, *Environ. Health Perspect. 101*:246 (1993).

TM5. A. Broo, The dynamics of some metal–organic and organic molecules in water solution studied by molecular mechanical and molecular dynamical methods, *Chem. Phys. 174*:127 (1993).

TM6 Z. Peng, K. M. Merz, Jr., and L. Banci, Binding of cyanide, cyanate, and thiocyanate to human carbonic anhydrase II, *Proteins Struct. Funct. Genet. 17*:203 (1993).

*TM7. D. Hartsbough and K. M. Merz, Jr., Dynamic force field models: Molecular dynamics simulations of human carbonic anhydrase. II. Using a quantum mechanical/molecular mechanical coupled potential, *J. Phys. Chem. 99*:11266 (1995).

TM8. Y. Yang, B. W. Beck, V. S. Shenoy, and T. Ichiye, Aqueous solvation of a rubredoxin redox site analog. A molecular dynamics simulation, *J. Am. Chem. Soc. 115*:7439 (1993).

TM9. R. B. Yelle, N. S. Park, and T. Ichiye, Molecular dynamics simulations of rubredoxin from *Clostridium pasteurianum*: Changes in structure and electrostatic potential during redox reactions, *Proteins 22*:154 (1995).

TF1. M. A. Lopez and P. A. Kollman, Application of molecular dynamics and free energy perturbation methods to metalloporphyrin–ligand systems II: CO and dioxygen binding to myoglobin, *Protein Sci. 2*:1975 (1993).

LS1. S. T. Frey, C. A. Chang, J. F. Carvalho, A. Varadarajan, L. M. Schultze, K. L. Pounds, and W. D. Horrocks, Jr., Characterization of lanthanide complexes with a series of amide-based macrocycles, potential MRI contrast agents, using Eu^{3+} luminescence spectroscopy and molecular mechanics, *Inorg. Chem. 33*:2882 (1994).

13

New Vistas In Molecular Mechanics

J. Phillip Bowen and Guyan Liang
University of Georgia,
Athens, Georgia

I. INTRODUCTION

Molecular mechanics is a mathematical approach that has been success-fully applied to the calculation of diverse groups of organic structures —ranging from simple hydrocarbons to complex multifunctional com-pounds and biologically important macromolecules [1,2]. More recently, efforts are being made to extend the methodology to inorganic structures. Unlike quantum mechanics, molecular mechanics calculations do not treat electrons explicitly. The neglect of the electronic distribution and the focus on the nuclei can be justified by the Born–Oppenheimer approximation [3]. It can safely be said that molecular mechanics has become a standard tool for studying and designing molecular structure, and the accuracy in calculating molecular properties frequently rivals the results that can be obtained experimentally [4–15].

The combination of the equations and parameters in the mathematical formulation that define the potential energy surface of a molecule is re-ferred to as the *force field*. The development of more sophisticated molec-ular mechanics equations is an active area of research, which has led to some interesting new programs. Obviously, there has always been a com-promise between the mathematical rigor of molecular mechanics (or any computational method for that matter) and the speed of computers used to carry out the calculations. In general, molecular mechanics calculations are much faster than those methods based on quantum mechanics, because the former does not worry about optimal electron distribution.

Over the years, the literature outlining molecular mechanics calculations has grown rapidly [16]. There are numerous papers specifically devoted to force field development, and many more papers have applied molecular mechanics to various research problems, from conformational analysis to drug design. The vast amount of reported calculations and methods have focused primarily on ground-state organic structures. This is entirely understandable, given that the underlying concepts of bonding and molecular interactions inherent to the molecular mechanics approach are ideally suited for the classic bonding interactions found in most organic structures. In recent years, calculations have been extended to inorganic structures, molecular complexes, and excited-state structures [17–20]. Great caution should be exercised in using any present-day molecular mechanics program to determine transition-state structures that result from chemical reactions, in which bonds are broken and generated. Transition-state modeling involving a significant shift of electron density should properly fall under the domain of quantum chemistry, in which electron distributions are rigorously calculated.

Interestingly, molecular mechanics calculations are playing a larger role in college and university undergraduate and graduate education [21,22] The incorporation of computational chemistry into the curriculum at all levels makes sense because so many structural concepts and reactivity rationalizations can be explained easily with molecular mechanics. Often, specialized courses devoted entirely to computational chemistry have been developed. With proper instruction, students can rapidly tackle intricate problems of research quality in a classroom setting. Continuing education short courses and workshops devoted to molecular mechanics applicable to organic or biomedical research are now widespread and highly popular [23–25].

From the wealth of published calculations using the many different molecular mechanics programs now available, various trends concerning the reliability of the equations and adjustable parameters have been established. From this growing body of data, comparisons of the accuracy and capabilities of different programs can be made, as well as comparisons with experimental data or high-level ab initio calculations. Importantly, molecular mechanics development will continue (just as any other discipline) with new and better force fields. Much of this chapter will focus on the MM3 and MM4 force field development, parameterization, and performances.

Today, a modern molecular mechanics calculation should be able to provide from a single mathematical formalism accurate structural, thermodynamic, and spectral information simultaneously, without ad hoc adjustments. Approximately a decade ago, expectations were much lower. During this time, one could expect a molecular mechanics program to be able to calculate either structure or spectra reasonably well, but typically not both. Over the years, with advances in computer technology and greater understanding of the essential force field terms, the molecular mechanics methods have steadily improved. The mid-1990s marked a period when a new generation of force fields have been introduced, which is an exciting time for those scientists involved in the development; but perhaps it may be an even more exciting time for those researchers and educators who have awaited the availability of these improvements.

There are now several different force fields, ranging in availability, prices, and capabilities. Traditionally, most of the currently used force fields were developed in academic laboratories with a specific purpose in mind, and they quite naturally reflected the interests of the developer. Originally, most molecular mechanics programs could be grouped into specific categories: those that dealt with small molecules and those that dealt with large molecules. For example, the MM3 program [26–28] has been more closely associated with the calculation of small molecules (e.g., about the size of steroids or smaller) while CHARMM [29–31] and AMBER [32–35] are usually thought of in the context of macromolecules. Characteristically, programs more suitable for small molecules have more complex mathematical functions to reproduce well-known and highly accurate experimental data and ab initio results, whereas the molecular mechanics routines that deal with large molecules use less rigorous force field terms in an effort to minimize the extensive computer time required. Presently, the division between small molecule and large molecule force fields is blurring as the programs are expanded and the necessarily more complex equations become implemented.

This chapter will focus on the newly published MM4 force field [36–40]. There will be a brief discussion of the history and background of molecular mechanics calculations and the fundamentals involved in the mathematical formalisms. The important area of parameter generation [2] along with associated novel trends, emerging today will be outlined [41]. A single chapter cannot cover all aspects of molecular mechanics, which is the main objective, and we have only surveyed a limited number of topics. Nevertheless, we hope the material that was selected will stimulate researchers and educators to delve deeper into this subject, which continues to serve as a fundamental method for understanding molecular structure.

II. BACKGROUND AND HISTORY

Many scientists have just recently discovered the power that computers can bring to their research. For some scientists, molecular mechanics—the driving computational engine for essentially all molecular-modeling graphics display programs—is a new and exciting method that may be used to examine structures. Exciting, certainly, but not new. The basis for molecular mechanics has been understood for at least half a century, whereas the mathematical foundations have existed since the days of Sir Isaac Newton. Several excellent reviews on this subject have been written. [1–15].

The genesis of molecular mechanics can be traced back to the earlier part of the 20th century when Andrews outlined some of the fundamental principles that set the stage [42]. During the 1920s and 1930s, a flurry of scientific discoveries and new theoretical developments occurred. It was during this period that quantum mechanics was introduced to describe molecular and subatomic behavior. Unfortunately, only a very few selected problems of interest to chemists could be calculated readily at that time. Many of the problems of chemical relevance had to await the development of approximate methods and powerful commercially available computers.

It was not until the years immediately following the end of World War II (1946–1950) that three independent papers appeared outlining molecular mechanics applications [43–48]. Primarily because of the subject nature of the problem undertaken by one of these papers, the work by Westheimer and Mayer [44] was more convincing than the others. These investigations demonstrated that the structural characteristics of a series of optically active halogenated biphenyl derivatives could be rationalized on the basis of simple calculations. The biphenyl work investigated was probably the only real chemistry problem that could be calculated effectively by hand at that time. Because of the success of Westheimer, this approach was referred to early on as the Westheimer method, but almost everyone today uses the term *molecular mechanics* to describe this approach. Although the potential usefulness of this method had been demonstrated independently by all three research groups, there was very little progress that could be made without the aid of computers.

When computers became commercially available in the 1950s, it became possible to apply force fields to problems of interest to chemists. In the 1960s, early molecular mechanics programs were developed [6,7,49–53]. Many of the ideas for modern force field development can be traced to these early efforts. Unfortunately, many of the early molecular mechanics programs were specifically written for compounds of interest and not generalized for generic cases.

In the developmental history of molecular mechanic, there have been a number of noteworthy accomplishments. Clearly, the MM1 [52], MM2 [54], and MM3 [26–28] programs developed by Allinger and co-workers have made a lasting impression on the researchers in this field. Many of the concepts incorporated into the Allinger MM series have influenced the development of other molecular mechanics codes. MM2 and MM3 are the standards in the field to which other developers compare the performances of their programs. It is important to recognize that the widespread availability of MM1 in the 1970s, and particularly MM2 in the 1980s, made it possible for a generation of chemists, both experimentalists and theoreticians, to apply molecular mechanics methods routinely to research problems. Chemists with little formal training in computational chemistry were applying molecular mechanics to a variety of problems and reporting their results. In the 1990s, the application of molecular mechanics is so common that one would be hard pressed to find a chemical journal that does not have numerous articles wherein molecular mechanics calculations play an integral part in the study or have been used. Many of the advances enjoyed today by computational chemists (molecular modelers) would not have been possible without the willingness of the aforementioned pioneers in the field to make these early programs widely available. The new MM4 program [36–40] represents a plateau in molecular mechanics development in terms of incorporating many mechanical and chemical properties of molecules.

There are many imitations of MM2 and MM3 incorporated into various molecular-modeling packages. The quality of these force field implementations is highly dependent on the specific program, but caution should be exercised by anyone using these imitations. Important force field terms have frequently been omitted, and the full functionality of the original program is not present.

III. THEORY AND FORMULATION

A. Overview

Molecular mechanics consists of a series of mathematical steps used to calculate molecular geometry, energy, vibrational spectra, and other physical properties. The molecular mechanics method was originally based on a ball-and-spring model, that assumed the total energy of a molecular system was divided into various energy components. These individual energy terms may be attributed to mechanical, structural, and chemical effects. Typically, as can be seen with Eq. (1), the basic force field equation has the total energy E_{total} divided into standard parts associated with the energy for stretching or compressing a bond E_{str}; the energy necessary for bending or compressing an angle, E_{bnd}; the energy necessary for mimicking van der Waals interactions E_{vdW}; the energy required to describe torsional strain involving dihedral rotations E_{tors}; and the energy required to describe electrostatic interactions E_{ele}. The individual energy terms are summed over all appropriate bonds, bond angles, nonbonded atom pairs, and unique dihedrals. Unlike quantum mechanics, where the energy is a summation of various integrals that are usually unrecognizable or foreign to most experimentalists, the fundamental molecular mechanics energy equation has a logical separation of energy components that chemists recognize and with which they feel comfortable. The intuitive nature of the energy distribution as well as the speed of the calculations makes molecular mechanics an attractive and useful method.

$$E_{total} = \sum E_{str} + \sum E_{bnd} + \sum E_{vdW} + \sum E_{tors} + \sum E_{ele} \tag{1}$$

Each one of these energy terms can, for the most part, be represented by simple potential energy functions, which is another appealing feature of the molecular mechanics approach.

MM3

The MM3 hydrocarbon force field was introduced in a series of papers in 1989 and subsequently expanded in later years to other functional groups (Table 1). The MM3 force field was not just a simple upgrade of the popular MM2 program. The force field equations were significantly modified and expanded, which led to a major reparameterization effort. The MM3 project was undertaken because various assumptions made in MM2 were based on experimental data available at the time. The need for modifications arose as new experimental data became available. For example, MM2 was unable to calculate the nonbonded distances between the hydrogens on the one-carbon bridges of *exo, exo*-tetracyclo[6.2.1.1^{3,6}.$O^{2,7}$]dodecane, which were measured by accurate low-temperature neutron diffraction studies to be 1.75 Å [55]. Because of a van der Waals potential that was *too hard* (i.e., steep or repulsive), MM2 gave values in the order of 2 Å [2]. A list of known deficiencies in MM2 was studied and compiled [56]. For the most part, through the introduction of cross-terms and the modification of existing terms, MM3 was able to correct the known deficiencies. See Table 2 for a comparison of the MM2 and MM3 energy expressions. One major difference between MM3 and its predecessor was the ability to calculate vibrational frequencies.

Table 1 Selective Publications for MM1/MM2/MM3/MM4 Packages

Functional groups	Refs.
Silanes	Tribble, M. T.; Allinger, N. L., *Tetrahedron*, 1972, *28*, 2147.
Hydrocarbons	Allinger, N. L.; Sprague, J. T., *J. Am. Chem. Soc.* 1973, *95*, 3893.
Alkanethiols	Allinger, N. L.; Hickey, M. J., *J. Am. Chem. Soc.* 1975, *97*, 5167.
Alkynes	Allinger, N. L.; Meyer, A. Y., *Tetrahedron* 1975, *31*, 1807.
Organic halides	Meyer, A. Y.; Allinger, N. L., *Tetrahedron* 1975, *31*, 1971.
Alcohols and ethers	Allinger, N. L.; Chung, D. Y., *J. Am. Chem. Soc.* 1976, *98*, 6798.
Disulfides	Allinger, N. L.; Hickey, M. J.; Kao, J., *J. Am. Chem. Soc.* 1976, *98*, 2741.
Sulfoxides	Allinger, N. L.; Kao, J., *Tetrahedron* 1976, *32*, 529.
Hydrocarbon (MM2)	Allinger, N. L., *J. Am. Chem. Soc.* 1977, *99*, 8127.
Charge distribution	Allinger, N. L.; Wuesthoff, M. T., *Tetrahedron* 1977, *33*, 3.
Phosphines	Allinger, N. L.; Voithenberg, H. v., *Tetrahedron* 1978, *34*, 627.
Heats of hydrogenation of linear alkynes	Rogers, D. W.; Dagdagan, O. A.; Allinger, N. L., *J. Am. Chem. Soc.* 1979, *101*, 671.
Thermodynamic parameters for hydrocarbons	Wertz, D. H.; Allinger, N. L., *Tetrahedron* 1979, *35*, 3.
Alcohols and ethers	Allinger, N. L.; Chang, S. H.-M.; Glaser, D. H.; Honig, H., *Isr. J. Chem.* 1980, *20*, 51.
Heats of hydrogenation	Allinger, N. L.; Dodziuk, H.; Rogers, D. W.; Naik, S. N., *Tetrahedron* 1982, *38*, 1593.
Methyl vinyl ether	Dodziuk, H.; Voithenberg, M. v.; Allinger, N. L., *Tetrahedron* 1982, *38*, 2811.
Pentaprismane and hexaprismane	Allinger, N. L.; Eaton, P. E., *Tetrahedron Lett.* 1983, 3697.
Deuterium compounds	Allinger, N. L.; Flanagan, H. L., *J. Comput. Chem.* 1983, *4*, 399.
Electrostatic effects	Dosen-Micovic, I. L.; Jeremic, D.; Allinger, N. L., *J. Am. Chem. Soc.* 1983, *105*, 1716.
	Dosen-Micovic, L.; Jeremic, D.; Allinger, N. L. *J. Am. Chem. Soc.* 1983, *105*, 1723.

Table 1 (Continued.)

Functional groups	Refs.
Anomeric effect	Nørskov-Lauritsen, L.; Allinger, N. L., *J. Comput. Chem.* 1984, *5*, 326.
Alkyl radicals	Imam, M. R.; Allinger, N. L., *J. Mol. Struct.* 1985, *126*, 345.
Aliphatic amines	Profeta, S. J.; Allinger, N. L., *J. Am. Chem. Soc.* 1985, *107*, 1907.
Electronegativity	Allinger, N. L.; Imam, M. R.; Frierson, M. R.; Yuh, Y. H.; Schafer, L., *Mathematics and Computational Concepts in Chemistry* (N. Trinajstic, ed.), E. Horwood, London, 1986.
Supra-annular effect	Bowen, P.; Allinger, N. L., *J. Org. Chem.* 1986, *51*, 1513.
Aromatic molecules	Allinger, N. L.; Lii, J.-H., *J. Comp. Chem.* 1987, *8*, 1146.
Allenes and for nonlinear acetylenes	Allinger, N. L.; Pathiaseril, A., *J. Comp. Chem.* 1987, *8*, 1225.
Organophosphines	Bowen, P.; Allinger, N. L., *J. Org. Chem.* 1987, *52*, 2937.
β-Heteroatom-substituted cyclohexanones	Bowen, P.; Allinger, N. L., *J. Org. Chem.* 1987, *52*, 1830.
Aldehydes and ketones	Bowen, P.; Pathiaseril, A.; Profeta, S. J.; Allinger, N. L., *J. Org. Chem.* 1987, *52*, 5162.
MMP2	Sprague, J. T.; Tai, J. C.; Y. Yuh; Allinger, N. L., *J. Comput. Chem.* 1987, *8*, 581.
Hydrogen bonding in MM2	Allinger, N. L.; Kok, R. A.; Imam, M. R., *J. Comput. Chem.* 1988, *9*, 591.
Divinyl ethers and aromatic halide derivatives	Bowen, J. P.; Reddy, V. V.; Patterson, D. G. J.; Allinger, N. L., *J. Org. Chem.* 1988, *53*, 5471.
Silanes and polysilanes	Frierson, M. R.; Imam, M. R.; Zalkow, V. B.; Allinger, N. L., *J. Org. Chem.* 1988, *53*, 5248.
Conjugated nitrogen-containing heterocycles	Tai, J.; Allinger, N. L., *J. Am. Chem. Soc.* 1988, *110*, 2050.
Organoselenium and tellurium	Allinger, N. L.; Allinger, J. A.; Yan, L., *J. Mol. Struct. (Theochem)* 1989, *201*, 363.
Organometallanes of germanium, tin, and lead	Allinger, N. L.; Quinn, M. I.; K. Chen; Thompson, B., *J. Mol. Struct.* 1989, *194*, 1.

Norbornane and dodecahedrane	Allinger, N. L.; Geise, H. J.; Pyckhout, W.; Paquette, L. A.; Gallucci, J. C., *J. Am. Chem. Soc.* 1989, *111*, 1106.
Hydrocarbons (MM3)	Allinger, N. L.; Yuh, Y. H.; Lii, J.-H., *J. Am. Chem. Soc.* 1989, *111*, 8551.
Vibrational frequencies and thermodynamics (MM3)	Lii, J. H.; Allinger, N. L., *J. Am. Chem. Soc.* 1989, *111*, 8566.
van der Waals potentials and crystal data for aliphatic and aromatic hydrocarbons (MM3)	Lii, J.-H.; Allinger, N. L., *J. Am. Chem. Soc.* 1989, *111*, 8576.
Siloxanes	Frierson, M. R.; Allinger, N. L., *J. Phys. Org. Chem.* 1989, *2*, 573.
Aliphatic nitriles	Goldstein, E.; Allinger, N. L., *J. Mol. Struct.* 1989, *188*, 149.
Peptides	Lii, J.-H.; Gallion, S.; Bender, C.; Wikstrom, H.; Allinger, N. L.; Flurchick, K. M.; Teeter, M. M., *J. Comp. Chem.* 1989, *10*, 503.
Furan, thiophene, and related compounds	Tai, J. C.; J.-H. Lii; Allinger, N. L., *J. Comput. Chem.* 1989, *10*, 635.
Aliphatic and aromatic nitro compounds	Allinger, N. L.; Kuang, J.; Thomas, H., *J. Mol. Struct. (Theochem.)* 1990, *209*, 125.
Alkenes (MM3)	Allinger, N. L.; Li, F.; Yan, L., *J. Comput. Chem.* 1990, *11*, 848.
Conjugated hydrocarbons	Allinger, N. L.; Li, F.; Yan, L.; Tai, J. C., *J. Comput. Chem.* 1990, *11*, 868.
Alcohols and ethers	Allinger, N. L.; Rahman, M.; Lii, J.-H., *J. Am. Chem. Soc.* 1990, *112*, 8293.
Cyclononane	Dorofeeva, O. V.; Mastryukov, V. S.; Allinger, N. L.; Almenningen, A., *J. Phys. Chem.* 1990, *94*, 8044.
Aliphatic amines	Schmitz, L. R.; Allinger, N. L.; *J. Am. Chem. Soc.* 1990, *112*, 8307.
Aldehydes and ketones	Allinger, N. L.; Chen, K.; Rahman, M.; Pathiaseril, A., *J. Am. Chem. Soc.* 1991, *113*, 4505.
Sulfides	Allinger, N. L.; Quinn, M.; Rahman, M.; Chen, K., *J. Phys. Org. Chem.* 1991, *4*, 647.
Disulfides	Chen, K.; Allinger, N. L., *J. Phys. Org. Chem.* 1991, *4*, 659.
Electrostatic effects (double bonds and conjugated systems)	Dosen-Micovic, L.; Li, S.; Allinger, N. L., *J. Phys. Org. Chem.* 1991, *4*, 467.
Amides, polypeptides, and proteins	Lii, J.-H.; Allinger, N. L., *J. Comput. Chem.* 1991, *12*, 186.
Conjugated ketones	Allinger, N. L.; Rodriguez, S.; Chen, K. S., *J. Mol. Struct. (Theochem)* 1992, *92*, 161.

503

Table 1 (Continued.)

Functional groups	Refs.
Heats of formation	Allinger, N. L.; Schmitz, L. R.; Motoc, I.; Bender, C.; Labanowski, J. Am. Chem. Soc. 1992, 114, 2880.
Carboxylic acids and esters	Allinger, N. L.; Zhu, Z. Q.; Chen, K. H., J. Am. Chem. Soc. 1992, 114, 6120.
Cyclopropanes	Aped, P.; Allinger, N. L., J. Am. Chem. Soc. 1992, 114, 1.
Alkylphosphines	Fox, P. C.; Bowen, J. P.; Allinger, N. L., J. Am. Chem. Soc. 1992, 114, 8536.
Intensities of infrared bands	Lii, J. H.; Allinger, N. L., J. Comput. Chem. 1992, 13, 1138.
Ureas and amide	Kontoyianni, M.; Bowen, J. P., J. Comput. Chem. 1992, 13, 657.
Imine derivatives	Kontoyianni, M.; Hoffman, A. J.; Bowen, J. P., J. Comput. Chem. 1992, 13, 57.
Oxocarbenium ions	Woods, R. J.; Andrews, C. W.; Bowen, J. P. J. Am. Chem. Soc. 1992, 114, 850.
Sulfones	Allinger, N. L.; Fan, Y., J. Comput. Chem. 1993, 14, 655.
Furan, vinyl ethers	Allinger, N. L.; Yan, L. Q., J. Am. Chem. Soc. 1993, 115, 11918.
Alkyl peroxides	Chen, K. S.; Allinger, N. L., J. Comput. Chem. 1993, 14, 755.
Cyclopentane (MD)	Cui, W. L.; Li, F. B.; Allinger, N. L., J. Am. Chem. Soc. 1993, 115, 2943.
Bicycloalkyl hydrocarbons	Mastryukov, V. S.; Chen, K.; Yang, L. R.; Allinger, N. L., J. Mol. Struct. (Theochem.) 1993, 99, 199.
Nitrogen-containing aromatic heterocycles	Tai, J. C.; Yang, L. R.; Allinger, N. L., J. Am. Chem. Soc. 1993, 115, 11906.
Hydroxylamine	Liang, G. Y.; Bowen, J. P.; Bentley, J. A., J. Comput. Chem. 1994, 15, 866.
Glyoxal, quinones	Allinger, N. L.; Fan, Y., J. Comput. Chem. 1994, 15, 251.
Enamines and aniline derivatives	Allinger, N. L.; Yan, L. Q.; Chen, K. H., J. Comput. Chem. 1994, 15, 1321.
Azoxy compounds	Fan, Y.; Allinger, N. L., J. Comput. Chem. 1994, 15, 1446.
Directional hydrogen-bonding	Lii, J. H.; Allinger, N. L., J. Phys. Org. Chem. 1994, 7, 591.
Alkyl radicals	Liu, R. F.; Allinger, N. L., J. Comput. Chem. 1994, 15, 283.
1,3-Cycloheptadiene	Nevins, N.; Stewart, E. L.; Allinger, N. L.; Bowen, J. P., J. Phys. Chem. 1994, 98, 2056.
C–H bond lengths and stretching frequencies	Thomas, H. D.; Chen, K. H.; Allinger, N. L., J. Am. Chem. Soc. 1994, 116, 5887.
	Timofeeva, T. V.; Allinger, N. L.; Buehl, M.; Mazurek, U., Russ. Chem. Bull. 1994, 43, 1795.

Metallocarborane molecules — Timofeeva, T. V.; Allinger, N. L.; Buehl, M.; Mazurek, U., *Russ. Chem. Bull.* 1994, *43*, 1795.

Alkyl iodides — Zhou, X. F.; Allinger, N. L., *J. Phys. Org. Chem.* 1994, *7*, 420.

Nucleic acid bases — Stewart, E. L.; Foley, C. K.; Allinger, N. L.; Bowen, J. P., *J. Am. Chem. Soc.* 1994, *116*, 7282.

Unconjugated N⁺-containing compounds — McGaughey, G. B.; Stewart, E. L.; Bowen, J. P., *J. Comput. Chem.* 1995, *16*, 1250.

Derivatives of triptycene — Sakakibara, K.; Allinger, N. L., *J. Org. Chem.* 1995, *60*, 4044.

Hyperconjugative effects — Allinger, N. L.; Chen, K. S.; Katzenellenbogen, J. A.; Wilson, S. R.; Anstead, G. M., *J. Comput. Chem.* 1996, *17*, 747.

Sulfoxides — Allinger, N. L.; Fan, Y.; Varnali, T., *J. Phys. Org. Chem.* 1996, *9*, 159.

Nitriles and alkynes — Goldstein, E.; Ma, B. Y.; Lii, J. H.; Allinger, N. L., *J. Phys. Org. Chem.* 1996, *9*, 191.

Anomeric effect — Kneisler, J. R.; Allinger, N. L., *J. Comput. Chem.* 1996, *17*, 757.

Hydrazines — Ma, B. Y.; Lii, J. H.; Chen, K. S.; Allinger, N. L., *J. Phys. Chem.* 1996, *100*, 11297.

Parameterization toolkit, alkylphosphines — Liang, G. Y.; Fox, P. C.; Bowen, J. P., *J. Comput. Chem.* 1996, *17*, 940.

Conjugated N⁺-containing compounds — McGaughey, G. B.; Stewart, E. L.; Bowen, J. P., *J. Comput. Chem.* 1996, *17*, 1395.

Propargyl alcohol — Stewart, E. L.; Mazurek, U.; Bowen, J. P., *J. Phys. Org. Chem.* 1996, *9*, 66.

Sulfonamides — Liang, G. Y.; Bays, J. P.; Bowen, J. P., *J. Mol. Struct. (Theochem.)*, in press.

Ammonium ions — Liang, G. Y.; Chen, X. N.; Dustman, J. A.; Lewin, A. H.; Bowen, J. P., *J. Comput. Chem.* in press.

Saturated hydrocarbons (MM4) — Allinger, N. L.; Chen, K. S.; Lii, J. H., *J. Comput. Chem.* 1996, *17*, 642.

Alkenes — Nevins, N.; Chen, K. S.; Allinger, N. L., *J. Comput. Chem.* 1996, *17*, 669.

Conjugated hydrocarbons — Nevins, N.; Lii, J. H.; Allinger, N. L., *J. Comput. Chem.* 1996, *17*, 695.

Vibrational frequency calculations for alkenes and conjugated hydrocarbons — Nevins, N.; Allinger, N. L., *J. Comput. Chem.* 1996, *17*, 730.

Alkylphosphines — Liang, G. Y.; Bowen, J. P., submitted.

505

Table 2 Potential Energy Equations of MM2 and MM3

Energy terms	MM2	MM3
Bond-stretching	$143.88 \dfrac{K_s}{2} (\Delta l)^2 (1 - C_s \, \Delta l)$	$143.88 \dfrac{K_s}{2} (\Delta l)^2 \left[1 - C_s \, \Delta l + \dfrac{7}{12} C_s^2 \, (\Delta l)^2 \right]$
Angle-bending	$0.043828 \dfrac{K_b}{2} (\Delta \theta)^2 [1 + S_F (\Delta \theta)^4]$	$0.043828 \dfrac{K_b}{2} (\Delta \theta) 2 [1 + C_F \Delta \theta + C_F \Delta \theta + Q_F (\Delta \theta)^2 + P_F (\Delta \theta)^3 + S_F (\Delta \theta)^4]$
Torsion	$\dfrac{V_1}{2} (1 + \cos \omega) + \dfrac{V_2}{2} (1 - \cos 2\omega) + \dfrac{V_3}{2} (1 + \cos 3\omega)$	$\dfrac{V_1}{2} (1 + \cos \omega) + \dfrac{V_2}{2} (1 - \cos 2\omega) + \dfrac{V_3}{2} (1 + \cos 3\omega)$
van der Waals	$(\varepsilon_i \varepsilon_j)^{1/2} \left[2.9 \times 10^5 \exp \left(-12.5 \, \dfrac{r_i + r_j}{R} \right) - 2.25 \left(\dfrac{r_i + r_j}{R} \right)^6 \right]$ $\text{if } \dfrac{r_i + r_j}{R} \leq 3.311$ $(\varepsilon_i \varepsilon_j)^{1/2} \, 336.176 \left(\dfrac{r_i + r_j}{R} \right)^2$ $\text{if } \dfrac{r_i + r_j}{R} > 3.311$	$(\varepsilon_i \varepsilon_j)^{1/2} \left[1.84 \times 10^5 \exp \left(-12.0 \, \dfrac{r_i + r_j}{R} \right) - 2.25 \left(\dfrac{r_i + r_j}{R} \right)^6 \right]$ $\text{if } \dfrac{r_i + r_j}{R} \leq 3.02$ $(\varepsilon_i \varepsilon_j)^{1/2} \, 192.270 \left(\dfrac{r_i + r_j}{R} \right)^2$ $\text{if } \dfrac{r_i + r_j}{R} > 3.02$

Dipole–dipole	$\dfrac{F\mu_i\mu_j(\cos\chi - 3\cos\alpha\cos\beta)}{R^3D}$	$\dfrac{F\mu_i\mu_j(\cos\chi - 3\cos\alpha\cos\beta)}{R^3D}$
	χ is the angle between the dipoles. α and β are the angles between the dipole axes and the lines along which the R is measured. R is the distance between the midpoints of the bonds. D is the dielectric constant	χ is the angle between the dipoles. α and β are the angles between the dipole axes and the lines along which the R is measured. R is the distance between the midpoints of the bonds. D is the dielectric constant
Charge–dipole	N/A	$69.12\,\dfrac{q\mu\cos\alpha}{r^2D}$
Charge interaction energy for ions	$14.39418 \times 4.80298^2\,\dfrac{q_iq_j}{rD}$	$14.39418 \times 4.80298^2\,\dfrac{q_iq_j}{rD}$
Stretch–bend	$2.51118k_{sb}\Delta\theta(\Delta l_{ab} + \Delta l_{bc})$	$2.51118k_{sb}\Delta\theta(\Delta l_{ab} + \Delta l_{bc})$
Bend–bend	N/A	$-0.02191418k_{bb}\Delta\theta_1\Delta\theta_2$
Torsion–stretch	N/A	$\dfrac{k_{ts}}{2}\Delta l_{jk}(1 + \cos 3\omega_{ijkm})$

Note: K_s, k_{sb}, k_{bb}, and k_{ts} are force constants for stretching, stretch–bend, bend–bend, and tors–stretch energy equations. Δl refers to the difference between the measured bond length and the equilibrium bond length, and $\Delta\theta$ refers to the difference between the measured bond angle and the equilibrium bond angle.

MM4

In 1996, Allinger and co-workers introduced a new hydrocarbon force field. Again, as with the introduction of MM3, the new program was not a simple upgrade. Since the time MM3 was published, new experimental data have become available, as well as a greater understanding of the role the cross-terms played in calculating structure and spectra. A greatly expanded collection of potential energy functions have been added to correct known deficiencies in MM3.

Force Field Classifications

Hagler recently divided molecular mechanics force fields into two broad categories, type 1 and type 2, based on the sophistication of the mechanical description of the force field [57–60]. Type 1 force fields contain only the diagonal force constant elements in the mechanical treatment of the ball-and-stick model. This approach works reasonably well as a first approximation to describe structure and energy. MM2 was basically a type 1 force field. A type 2 force field includes many of the off-diagonal force constant elements. Allinger [36] has defined an additional force field level, type 3. In addition to all the mechanical effects taken into account in a type 2 force field there are "chemical" effects included, such as the electronegativity, Bohlmann, and anomeric effects. These chemical effects are explicitly considered when developing parameters. The new MM4, discussed in detail in Section V, represents a type 3 force field. Before undertaking a detailed description of MM4, some general comments about molecular mechanics are examined in the following sections.

B. Mechanical Effects

Bond-Stretching Potentials

If molecular vibrations were similar to an ideal spring, which is governed by Hooke's law, then the simplest mathematical approximation to bond stretching may be achieved by a quadratic term. This approach is known as the harmonic approximation, in which a bond is assumed to have a natural bond length l_0. Any deviation from l_0, whether due to bond stretching or bond compression, results in an energy increase [Eq. (2)]. This idea would be reasonable if molecular vibrations were identical to classic *ideal* spring, but molecules do not behave in this simple way. More complete higher-order mathematical expansions lead to more accurate force fields (Fig. 1). In the case of MM2, a cubic expansion more readily reproduced the anharmonic behavior of chemical bonds and is described by a Morse curve.

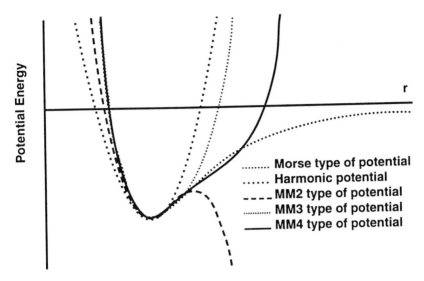

Figure 1 Different types of stretching potential functions used in molecular mechanics calculations.

$$E_{str} = \frac{1}{2} k_{str}(l - l_0)^2 \tag{2}$$

The use of a cubic term as a mathematical approximation to describe the anharmonicity of bond stretching works well if the bond is not stretched too far, or if the molecular structure does not have significant bonding distortions [Eq. (3)]. As a bond is stretched to longer and longer distances, the cubic term will dominate; the energy will drop precipitously to negative infinity (see Fig. 1). The catastrophic result of excessive bond stretching causes bonds to break. When viewing this strained structure on a computer graphics terminal, the molecular system will seem to explode, which is not particularly comforting for serious studies on the nature of the chemical bond. In MM2, for example, the cubic term is not activated until the structure is close to the bottom of the potential energy well, which was a programming workaround.

$$E_{str} = \frac{1}{2} k_{str}(l - l_0)[1 + C_1(l - l_0) + C_2(l - l_0)^2 + \cdots] \tag{3}$$

This bond-stretching problem can be avoided altogether through the introduction of higher-ordered, even terms, such as a quartic expansion.

For example, Allinger's MM3 and Halgren's MMFF94 molecular mechanics programs [61–65] each have quartic terms, which compensate for the cubic term, as shown in Table 2 and Eq. (4). The cubic and quartic force constants in the expansion are related to the quadratic force constants. The incorporation of higher terms in the stretching potentials of MM3, MMFF94, and MM4 not only avoids negative infinity energies caused by excessive stretching, but it also gives better overall agreement with experimental data.

$$
\begin{aligned}
E_{\text{str}}^{\text{MM4}} = 71.94 k_{\text{str}}(l - l_0)^2 &\left[1 - C_s(l - l_0) + \frac{7}{12} C_s^2(l - l_0)^2 \right. \\
&\left. - \frac{1}{4} C_s^3(l - l_0)^3 + \frac{31}{360} C_s^4(l - l_0)^4 \right]
\end{aligned}
\tag{4}
$$

Angle-Bending Potentials

Similar to bond stretching, simple Hooke's law-type potential energy functions may be used to mimic angle bending. Usually, a quadratic term is sufficient for an accuracy of approximately 10°. The MM4 force field uses the same mathematical form as its predecessor MM3. As can be seen by inspecting Eq. (5), terms higher than quadratic proved to be important (The terms of CF, QF, PF, and SF are constants that scale the bending constants parameter, $K_{\text{bnd.}}$). In MM3, the bending motions were divided into two categories: (a) in-plane bending and (b) out-of-plane bending. The latter was introduced to reproduce the geometry of trigonal planar systems. For example, to keep C_{sp2} centers flat and not distorting, such as with aldehydes, ketones, and alkenes, a force constant was introduced between the C_{sp2} center and an imaginary point in a plane defined by the three attached atoms. This stratagem worked well, for the most part; but owing to programming difficulties, this approach to out-of-plane bending was dropped in MM4 and substituted with an improper torsion angle method. The improper torsion angle approach leads to an accuracy similar to that of the out-of-plane method used in MM2 and MM3, without the aforementioned programming difficulties.

$$
\begin{aligned}
E_{\text{bnd}}^{\text{MM3}} = 0.043828 \frac{k_{\text{bnd}}}{2} (\theta - \theta_0)^2 &[1 + CF(\theta - \theta_0) \\
&+ QF(\theta - \theta_0)^2 + PF(\theta - \theta_0)^3 + SF(\theta - \theta_0)^4)]
\end{aligned}
\tag{5}
$$

Torsional Potentials

It has long been recognized that torsional strain must be included in molecular mechanics calculations to reproduce the ethane, butane, and homologous acyclic hydrocarbon potential energy curves [7,54,66,67]. Originally, it was hoped that stretching and nonbonding terms might do the trick, but this was unreasonable, given the physical nature of the underlying curves. The 2.9 kcal mol^{-1} energy barrier in ethane does not arise from classic nonbonded interactions, where the van der Waals radii of the vicinal hydrogens are banging into one another in the eclipsed conformation. In reality, although various explanations have been offered, there is a repulsion between the C–H bonds. One can imagine that the C–H bond electron density is causing ethane to adopt a staggered conformation. The net result of this repulsion between the C–H bonds can readily be demonstrated by quantum mechanics calculations that give a threefold barrier for ethane. To reproduce this bond-density repulsion effect in molecular mechanics, a truncated three-term Fourier series has been used effectively in MM3. Through the careful selection of V_1, V_2, and V_3 coefficients, the various torsional contributions to the overall potential energy curves can be approximated [Eq. (6)].

$$E_{tors}^{MMS} = \frac{V_1}{2}(1 + \cos \omega) + \frac{V_2}{2}(1 - \cos 2\omega) + \frac{V_3}{2}$$
$$(1 + \cos 3\omega) \tag{6}$$

The judicious selection of a combination of V_1, V_2, and V_3 will reproduce most energy profiles with reasonable accuracy. Figure 2 shows the curves generated for each of the three torsional terms. The third term found in Eq. 6 is important for structures with threefold barriers, and the second term is important for structures with twofold barriers, such as ethylene. The first term in Eq. (6) has been interpreted as dipole–dipole term, and is the most difficult to understand [68].

Nonbonded Potentials

To reproduce many fundamental physical properties that are attributed to London dispersion forces and van der Waals interactions, molecular mechanics must incorporate nonbonded potentials. Several possible formulations have been proposed. Traditionally, the Lennard-Jones 6–12 potential has been widely used, but the repulsive part of the 6–12 potential has been too hard (too steep) for organic molecules [69]. Lifson and co-workers demonstrated that to soften the nonbonded interactions, a power of 9 or 10 was more reasonable [70]. Most molecular mechanics codes use variations of Lennard-Jones potentials owing to the simplicity of the function and the speed of such calculations.

$$E(r) = 4\varepsilon \left[\left(\frac{\sigma}{r}\right)^{12} - \left(\frac{\sigma}{r}\right)^{6} \right] \tag{7}$$

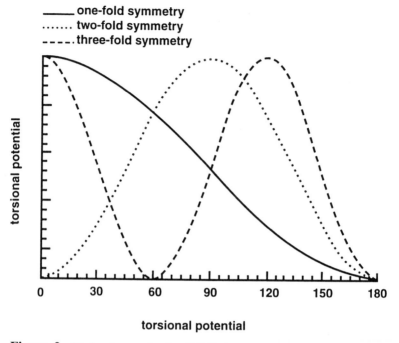

Figure 2 Molecular mechanics (MM2, MM3, MM4) torsional energy potential and its components.

In the MM2, MM3, and MM4 series of programs, the nonbonded interactions are treated by replacing the repulsive part of the 6–12 potential with an exponential. This "exponential-6" equation is a better theoretical treatment of the repulsion between electron clouds in organic structures. Table 2 shows that MM3 has a reduced exponential part (from 12.25 to 12.0). This softening was necessary to reproduce very close nonbonded distances, as described in the foregoing. The MM4 nonbonded terms are identical in their mathematical form with those of MM3.

Electrostatic Potentials

It is absolutely essential to have a self-consistent description of electrostatic interactions. In reality, molecules are simply nuclei dispersed in clouds of electrons. Concepts such as bonds may be considered as theoretical abstracts or models useful for picturing molecular structure. Most of our bonding ideas work extremely well, but there are situations for which the concepts break down. In molecular mechanics, covalent bonds must be defined. In addition to the nonbonded terms, explicit bonding terms are required for each of the defined bonds because the approach does not employ wave mechanics. Various approaches have been used to map explicit formal charges onto specific atoms within a molecule. Most typically, point charges using Coulomb's law have been used. In Eq. (8), q_i and q_j represent the charges on two atoms i and j, respectively, which are separated by a distance r. In this equation, C is a proportionality constant, and D is the dielectric constant. The advantages of using a point charge method are most apparent in terms of faster computer speeds. The most serious disadvantages, however, focus on the nature of having a localized point charge of an assigned magnitude. How can these charges be determined? Charge determination for individual atoms is not experimentally accessible, and formal charges are not quantum mechanics eigenvalues. Charges derived from quantum mechanics are calculated most commonly through population analysis schemes, and there are many such methods, most noticeably the Mulliken population [71]. There are well-known deficiencies in the various population analysis algorithms that have led to the introduction of ab initio electrostatically fit charges [72].

$$E(r) = \frac{C \cdot q_i q_j}{D \cdot r_{ij}} \tag{8}$$

For historical reasons, the Allinger MM series of programs have used a dipole–dipole scheme for calculating electrostatic interactions. Each uniquely defined bond was assigned a dipole. The interactions of the assigned bond dipoles produce a net dipole for a molecule. Because the net dipoles for many molecules are known, it was possible to adjust the bond dipoles to fit the experimental data. The method works very well, particularly for small, uncharged organic structures. See Table 2 for the mathematical expressions used in MM2 and MM3, which are carried over into MM4.

The disadvantage of using a dipole–dipole electrostatic approach is immediately apparent if one considers charged structures and macromolecules. For charged species, two additional terms need to be introduced for charge–dipole interactions and charge–charge interactions. This leads to additional parameterization (see Table 2). For macromolecules, such as proteins, with extensive charges and numerous polar covalent bonds, the dipole formulation is extremely time-consuming.

Is one approach better than the other in terms of accuracy? In principle, either the point charge or bond dipole methods work reasonably well [2]. There are advantages and disadvantages to both, as briefly outlined in the foregoing. If both methods are correctly formulated, the electrostatic picture should be essentially identical. In MM3 and MM4 an overall net charge for each atom can be obtained if the dipole terms are reduced to point charges and summed with any assigned charge. If this procedure is carried out, then there will be general agreement with ab initio data. For ammonium ion derivatives, the charge on nitrogen will indeed be negative if the formally assigned charge and the bond dipoles are summed.

Perhaps the biggest drawback in molecular mechanics at this time is the inability of assigned dipole or assigned charges to be modified according to conformation or induction effects by other groups. The ability to induce polarization by modifications of assigned charges or dipoles will be one of the next improvements seen in the coming years. Work is ongoing in many laboratories worldwide, including our own, on this problem. Kollman recently reported progress in this area [73].

Cross-Term Potentials

Unfortunately, the E_{str}, E_{bnd}, E_{vdW}, E_{tors}, and E_{elec} potential energy terms, described in the foregoing and shown in Eq. (1), do not, of themselves, provide the accuracy required to reproduce experimental data or higher-level ab initio calculations. Additional terms that couple one or more of the basic energy expressions are necessary. For example, it is well known that when a bond angle is compressed, the bond lengths stretch to relieve the introduced strain. This is a simple mechanical effect, during which bond stretching and angle compression are coupled. To reproduce this effect mathematically within a molecular mechanics framework, it is necessary to introduce an energy term (often referred to as a cross-term) that couples the bending and stretching behavior. Other ways are possible, such as introducing specific interaction terms between atoms in a 1,3-relation, such as Urey–Bradley terms. Cross-terms are not ad hoc additions. They are a natural mathematical consequence of expanding a potential function into a power series. The introduction of cross-terms allows better reproduction of molecular behavior. Equation (9) shows the complete fundamental equation used in modern molecular mechanics treatments.

$$E_{total} = \sum E_{str} + \sum E_{bnd} + \sum E_{vdW} + \sum E_{tors}$$
$$+ \sum E_{ele} + \sum E_{cross\text{-}terms} \tag{9}$$

Parameter Transferability

Another central assumption is made in molecular mechanics: the parameters are transferable from one molecule to the next. What this means is that if one determines, for example, the stretching parameters for the C_{sp3}–C_{sp3} bond in ethane, it may then be used for all other C_{sp3}–C_{sp3} bonds in different molecular structures. This is recognized as a first-approximation, but the scheme works out reasonably well for most structures. Otherwise molecular mechanics calculations would not work. If a new set of parameters had to be developed for every new structure that needed to be studied, then the method would be unappealing and without wide applicability.

One of the most cumbersome, but necessary, tasks in molecular mechanics is to identify the constants within the potential energy functions. There are literally hundreds of these constants or parameters that need to be determined to describe molecular behavior. The process of developing the parameters is referred to as molecular mechanics parameterization, which is both a science and an art. More will be aid about this subject later in Section VIII.

C. Chemical Effects

Molecular mechanics is a model for chemical behavior. Simple mechanical effects, such as stretching, bending, and torsion supplemented with an electrostatic scheme, are not sufficient alone to reproduce some well-known structural or spectroscopic phenomena, such as the electronegativity [74], anomeric [75,76], and Bohlmann effects [40]. These effects and other phenomena might be classified as *chemical effects*, and they are more readily explained by molecular orbital theory. Therefore, various programming and mathematical modifications must be made to incorporate molecular orbital effects into a molecular mechanics formalism. (Torsional interactions, as presented earlier, could very well be classified as resulting from quantum mechanical effects.) MM4, which incorporates diagonal and off-diagonal elements into its mechanical representation of molecular behavior, as well as chemical effects, provides a new generation of the molecular mechanics' codes, defined as a type 3 force field.

Electronegativity Effect

An examination of chemical-bonding effects indicates that the length of a particular bond is highly dependent on the electronegativity of the attached substituents. For example, the C_{sp3}–C_{sp3} in ethane has a bond length of 1.534 Å. What happens if a hydrogen is replaced by an electronegative atom? In ethyl chloride, the C_{sp3}–C_{sp3} bond shrinks to 1.528 Å. This is a general observation [74]; the bond shrinkage also depends on the number of electronegative atoms directly attached to the bond in question. An electropositive atom causes a similar, but opposite, effect whereby bonds lengthen.

In molecular orbital terms, the above described bond shrinkage can be explained. When an electronegative atom, such as chlorine, replaces a hydrogen, there is more p character present on the carbon forming the

C–Cl bond, which is a result of the tendency for chlorine to attract electrons relative to carbon. In turn, because there must be conservation of s and p orbitals, the hybrid orbital of the same carbon bearing the electronegative atom must have more s character when forming the C_{sp3}–C_{sp3} bond. This loss of p-character leads to a shorter observed bond length. The effect depends on the electronegative atom itself (e.g., F, Cl, Br, or other) and how many atoms are present. This is referred to as the *primary electronegativity effect*; but the effect is also observed for bonds not directly attached to the electronegative center, such as the C2–C3 bond of propyl chloride. This "through-bond" effect is quickly diminished, but is pronounced enough to be considered structurally important and is classified as the *secondary electronegativity effect*. The secondary electronegativity effect is proportional to the primary electronegatively effect.

Both a primary and secondary electronegativity effect are taken into account in MM3 and MM4. This electronegativity effect may be reproduced without resorting to molecular orbital hybridization effects: a simple solution has been achieved. The program examines the connectivity of every bond. If an electronegative atom is present, the default natural bond length, l_0, is shortened by a specified amount Δl_e^{ij}. The shortening depends on the electronegativity of the atom and the number of electronegative atoms included, according to Eqs. (10) and (11) for the primary and secondary electronegativity effects [J. Y. Shim and J. P. Bowen, unpublished data], respectively.

$$\Delta l_{e-\text{primry}}^{ij} = \Delta l_{e-\text{sub1}}^{ij} + 0.62 \Delta l_{e-\text{sub2}}^{ij} + 0.62^2 \Delta l_{e-\text{sub3}}^{ij} + \dots \tag{10}$$

$$Dl_{e-\text{secondary}}^{ij} = 0.40 Dl_{e-\text{primary}}^{ij} \tag{11}$$

The equilibrium bond length l_0^{ij} depends on the substituents attached to the bonded atoms i and j. When a substituent is significantly more electronegative than the atom to which it is attached, the bond length is reduced according to the electronegativity parameters. For multiple substituents, they all contribute to the overall electronegativity correction, as seen in Eq. (10), in which the individual terms are sorted according to decreasing absolute value of Δl_e^{ij}. The secondary electronegativity effect is proportional to the primary effect, as can be seen in Eq. (11).

Anomeric Effect

For dimethoxymethane and related systems of the type CH_3–O–CH_2–X, there is an unusual conformational preference that cannot be rationalized by steric arguments alone. It turns out that the *gg* conformation is the most stable. This conformational preference falls into a general category of stereoelectronic effects. The generalized anomeric effect, as it is sometimes referred to in example, is best known in cyclic carbohydrate compounds and derivatives. Various arguments about the origin of the anomeric effect have been suggested, ranging from unfavorable dipole–dipole interactions to n–σ^* MO interactions [77,78]. Most likely, both effects are operating simultaneously to various degrees.

If we look at 2-methoxytetrahydropyran, the more stable conformation exists where the methoxy group is axial. The anomeric effect can be rationalized easily in terms of nonbonded resonance arguments. From this depiction, one would anticipate bond lengthening of the axial C–O bond and bond shortening of the internal C–O bond, which is observed for systems of this type both by experiment and quantum mechanics. To make the *gauche* conformation more stable for a X–O1–C–O2–Y atomic arrangement, MM2 used special torsional terms [79]. In MM3 and MM4, this has been specifically programmed into the code [75] The bond stretching and contractions of the various C–O bonds are calculated by Eq. (12).

The bond parameter l_0 for a bond I–K changes by an amount Δl_a, when A and E are lone pairs of electrons for a string of three atoms I, K, and D, giving the A-I-K-D-E system, where ω is the torsion angle A-I-K-D, ω' is the torsion angle I-K-D-E, and k, c, d are anomeric effect parameters.

$$l'_{)0} = l_0 - \Delta l_a \tag{12}$$

$$\Delta l_a = 0.5k[(1 + \cos2\omega) - c(1 + \cos2\omega')] + d \tag{13}$$

longer bond length

Bohmann Effect

The length of C–H bonds adjacent to atoms bearing at least one lone pair of electrons (e.g., amines, alcohols, ethers, and fluorides) is a function of the orientation of the C–H bond relative to the lone pair of electrons. The differences in C–H bond lengths can be detected readily in IR spectra. C–H bands have been observed as low as 2700 cm^{-1}. When a C–H bond adjacent to the nitrogen in an amine, for example, is located *anti* to the lone pair of electrons, resonance arguments similar to those used in the foregoing to describe the anomeric effect can be invoked.

D. Atom Types

Unlike quantum mechanics, in which the bonds and atom hybridizations are determined by the calculations, in molecular mechanics one must explicitly specify the chemical bonds between atoms and the atomic hybridization states. An atom type is a concept used in molecular mechanics to indicate the hybridization of the various elements of the periodic chart. In MM3(96), for example, there are approximately 200 atom types. Typically, in all molecular mechanics programs atom types are numbers designating a particular atom, geometry, and bonding state (e.g., C_{sp3}, C_{sp2}, and C_{sp} are atom types 1, 2, and 4, respectively, in MM3). Occasionally, depending on the bonding environment, multiple atom types may be assigned to a single hybridization state. For example, C_{sp2} centers are divided into atom types 2 and 3, depending on whether the C_{sp2} is an alkene carbon or a carbonyl carbon, respectively. The MM3(94) program was modified to accept a less complex input. Instead of communicating with the program by atom type numbers, one can simply enter the element symbol. The program will determine what is the most appropriate atom type and assign the appropriate number, which is used internally to setup the correct parameters. Specifying the element is much simpler than having to keep track with a number of different atom types. Use of a sophisticated molecular-modeling program, such as SYBYL, that interfaces successfully to MM3 or has the complete, authentic force field incorporated within, avoids the atom-type problem as well.

IV. OTHER WIDELY USED MOLECULAR MECHANICS PROGRAMS

A. AMBER

The very popular AMBER program, developed by Kollman and co-workers is widely used by chemists in industry and academia for macromolecular calculations [Eq. (14)]. In 1978, when they first started the program, the goal was to develop a complete general molecular mechanics program, capable of energy component calculation and computer graphics display [32–35,72,73]. Since then, improvements have been made to the force field and its implementation. Additionally, new modules have been added that expand the functionality to include the following:

SANDER: for energy minimization, molecular dynamics, and NMR refinement
GIBBS: free energy simulations
SPASMS: molecular dynamics/free energy calculations
NMODE: normal mode analysis
LEaP: graphic molecular builder.

As a force field focused on macromolecular calculations, it mainly employs harmonic terms in its potential energy equations and avoids using cross-terms to reduce the computational load. The AMBER program has been expanded to include the Ewald sums representation of electrostatic interactions [see Eqs. (15–26)] 80].

$$
\begin{aligned}
V = &\sum_{\text{bonds}} K_r(r - r_{\text{eq}})^2 + \sum_{\text{angles}} K_\theta(\theta - \theta_{\text{eq}})^2 \\
&+ \sum_{\text{dihedrals}} \frac{V_n}{2} [1 + \cos(n\phi - \gamma)] \\
&+ \sum_{i<j} \left(\frac{A_{ij}}{R_{ij}^{12}} - \frac{B_{ij}}{R_{ij}^6} + \frac{q_i q_j}{\epsilon R_{ij}} \right) + \sum_{\text{H-bonds}} \left(\frac{C_{ij}}{R_{ij}^{12}} - \frac{D_{ij}}{R_{ij}^6} \right)
\end{aligned}
\tag{14}
$$

B. CFF93

The CFF93 force field, developed by Hagler and co-workers [57–60,81], is a product of the Biosym consortium (now MSI) on potential energy functions. It is one of the first molecular mechanics programs to use extensive cross-terms, and thus is an example of a type 2 force field. Additionally, it added anharmonicity corrections for stretching and bending energy terms by including the cubic and quartic terms in their potential energy equations.

$$
E_b = {}^2K_b(l - l_0)^2 + {}^2K_b(l - l_0)^3 + {}^4K_b(l - l_0)^4
\tag{15}
$$

$$
E_\theta = {}^2K_\theta(\theta - \theta_0)^2 + {}^3K_\theta(\theta - \theta_0)^3 + {}^4K_\theta(\theta - \theta_0)^4
\tag{16}
$$

$$
E_\phi = {}^1K_\phi(1 - \cos\phi) + {}^2K_\phi(1 - \cos2\phi) + {}^3K_\phi(1 - \cos2\phi)
\tag{17}
$$

$$E_{\text{nonbonded}} = \frac{q_i q_j}{r} + \epsilon \left[2\left(\frac{r^*}{r}\right)^9 - 3\left(\frac{r^*}{r}\right)^6 \right] \tag{18}$$

where the combination rules are

$$r^* = \left[\frac{r_j^{*6} + r_j^{*6}}{2} \right]^{1/6} \tag{19}$$

$$\varepsilon = (\varepsilon_i \varepsilon_i)^{1/2} \frac{2(r_i^* r_j^*)^2}{r_i^{*6} + r_j^{*6}} \tag{20}$$

The q, ε, r symbols represent partial charge, well-depth, and diameter parameters of the atom, respectively. There are several cross-terms that should be noted.

1. Bond–bond

$$\sum_l \sum_{l'} K_{ll'}(l - l_0)(l' - l_0') \tag{21}$$

2. Angle–angle

$$\sum_\theta \sum_{\theta'} K_{\theta\theta'}(\theta - \theta_0)(\theta' - \theta_0') \tag{22}$$

3. Bond–angle

$$\sum_l \sum_\theta K_{l\theta}(l - l_0)(\theta - \theta_0) \tag{23}$$

4. Bond–torsion

$$\sum_l \sum_\phi (l - l_0)({}^1K_{l\phi} \cos \phi + {}^2K_{l\phi} \cos 2\phi + {}^3K_{l\phi} \cos 3\phi) \tag{24}$$

5. Angle–torsion

$$\sum_\theta \sum_\phi (\theta - \theta_0)({}^1K_{\theta\phi} \cos \phi + {}^2K_{\theta\phi} \cos 2\phi + {}^3K_{\theta\phi} \cos 3\phi) \tag{25}$$

6. Angle–angle–torsion

$$\sum_\theta \sum_{\theta'} \sum_\phi K_{\theta\theta'\phi}(\theta - \theta_0)(\theta' - \theta_0')\cos \phi \tag{26}$$

CFF93 was developed based on sampling quantum mechanics surfaces of representative molecules, which include energy as well as the first and second derivatives.

C. CHARMM

Similar to AMBER, CHARMM, developed in Karplus' laboratory at Harvard [29,31,82], is another molecular mechanics package focused on biomacromolecules (nucleic acids, proteins, and carbohydrates). Because CHARMM targets biomolecules, similar to AMBER, harmonic energy potentials are used to enhance the computational speed, as outlined in Eq. (27).

$$V = \sum_{\text{bonds}} K_r(r - r_0)^2 + \sum_{\text{angles}} K_\theta(\theta - \theta_0)^2 + \sum_{\text{dihedrals}} K_\chi[1 + \cos(n\chi - \delta)]$$

$$+ \sum_{\text{Urey-Bradley}} K_{\text{UB}}(S - S_0)^2 + \sum_{\text{ipropers}} K_{\text{imp}}(\varphi - \varphi_0)^2$$

$$+ \sum_{i<j} \varepsilon \left[\left(\frac{R_{\text{min},ij}}{r_{ij}} \right)^{?12} - 2\left(\frac{R_{\text{min},ij}}{r_{ij}} \right)^6 \right] + \sum_{i<j} \frac{q_i q_j}{4\pi e r_{ij}} \tag{27}$$

The Urey–Bradley term in Eq. (27) can offer a limited anharmonicity correction version of the force. The latest version of force field parameters (CHARMM-23) was developed based on both experimental data and ab initio calculations. During the force field development, the TIP3P water model [83] was used. According to the authors, the balance between the solvent–solvent, solvent–solute, and solute–solute interactions was emphasized to maximize its performance during molecular dynamics simulations.

D. MMFF94

MMFF94 is the first published version of the Merck molecular mechanics force field (MMFF). MMFF94 was designed for application to condensed-phase processes in molecular dynamics simulations. The authors' stated goal was to achieve the same level of accuracy as MM3, while being applicable to proteins. MMFF94 has primarily been derived from high-level ab initio calculations. According to the author (T. Halgren) the training set from which the parameters were derived included 500 molecular structures optmized at the HF/6-31G* level of theory, 475 structures optimized at MP2/6-31G* (in which, 380 structures were further evaluated at MP4SDQ/TZP), and 1450 structures that were derived partly from the MP2/6-31G* geometries with subsequent evaluation at MP2/TZP. MMFF94 extensively uses anharmonic corrections, as well as a few cross-terms, to ensure the accuracy for both molecular geometry and vibrational frequencies and is also another example of a type 2 force field. The potential functions are outlined below in Eqs (28), through (35).

1. Bond-stretching

$$E_b = 143.9325 \frac{k_b}{2} \Delta l^2 \left(1 + c_s \Delta l + \frac{7}{12} c_s^2 \Delta l^2 \right) \tag{28}$$

2. Angle-bending

$$E_a = 0.043844 \frac{k_a}{2} \Delta\theta^2(1 + c_b\Delta\theta) \tag{29}$$

$$E_a = 143.9325k_a(1 + \cos \delta\Theta) \text{ for near-linear bond angles} \tag{30}$$

3. Torsion

$$E_t = \frac{V_1}{2}(1 + \cos \phi) + \frac{V_2}{2}(1 - \cos 2\phi) + \frac{V_3}{2}(1 + \cos 3\phi) \tag{31}$$

4. Out-of-plane bending

$$E_{OOP} = 0.043844 \frac{k_{OOP}}{2} \chi^2 \tag{32}$$

where χ is the Wilson angle between the bond and the plane

5. van der Waals (buffered-14-7 form)

$$E_{vdW} = \varepsilon_{ij}\left(\frac{1.07R_{ij}^*}{R_{ij} + 0.07R_{ij}^*}\right)^7\left(\frac{1.07R_{ij}^{*7}}{R_{ij}^7 + 0.07R_{ij}^{*7}} - 2\right) \tag{33}$$

R^* is the minimum energy separation and ε is dependent on the atomic polarizability.

6. Electrostatic interaction

$$E_q = 332.0716 \frac{q_iq_j}{D(R_{ij} + \delta)^n} \tag{34}$$

$\delta = 0.5$ Å is the "electrostatic buffering" constant, D is the dielectric constant, n can be 1 or 2 (distance-dependent dielectric constant).

7. Cross-term
    A cross-term stretch-bend is also employed in MMFF94. Notice that two constants, k_{ba}^{ij} and k_{ba}^{jk}, are defined to address the two bond lengths separately.

$$E_{ba} = 2.51210(k_{ba}^{ij}\Delta l_{ij} + k_{ba}^{jk}\Delta l_{jk})\Delta\theta \tag{35}$$

V. MM4 FORMATION

The MM4 force field is the latest evolution of the MM series of programs developed by Allinger and co-workers. Many of the parameters and functional form of the MM3 force field have been retained. The MM4 total energy equation may be divided into three parts, outlined in Eq. (36), where there are retained MM3 terms, new MM4 terms, and modified MM3 terms.

$$E_{total}^{MM4} = \sum E_{retained\ MM3\ terms} + \sum E_{new\ MM4\ terms} \qquad (36)$$
$$+ \sum E_{modified\ MM3\ terms}$$

For the most part, as shown in Eq. (37), the potential energy terms that treat only one type of distortion (diagonal elements of the force constant matrix) have been retained, such as the stretching energy (E_{str}), bending energy (E_{bend}), torsional energy (E_{tors}), nonbonded van der Waals interactions (E_{vdW}), dipole–dipole electrostatic interactions (E_{dipole}), as well as bend–bend ($E_{bend-bend}$) and stretch–bend ($E_{str-bend}$) cross-terms.

$$E_{retained\ MM3\ terms} = \sum (E_{str} + E_{bend} + E_{tors} + E_{vdW} + E_{dipole} \qquad (37)$$
$$+ E_{bend-bend(one\ center)} + E_{str-bend})$$

There are several new cross-terms that have been added to MM4, including the following: stretch–stretch ($E_{str-str}$), torsion–bend ($E_{tors-bend}$), bend–torsion–bend ($E_{bnd-tor-bnd}$), torsion–torsion ($E_{tors-tors}$), torsion–improper torsion ($E_{tors-impt}$), and improper torsion–torsion–improper torsion ($E_{impt-tors-impt}$). These new terms are mainly responsible for the greater flexibility and accuracy that can be achieved with this new program [see Eq. (38)]. Each of these terms is discussed in Section VI.

$$E_{new\ MM4\ terms} = \sum (E_{str-str} + E_{tors-bend} + E_{bend-tors-bend} \qquad (38)$$
$$+ E_{tors-tors} + E_{tors-impt} + E_{impt-tors-impt})$$

Two potential energy terms, improper torsion (E_{impt}) and torsion–stretch ($E_{tors-str}$) outlined in Eq. (39), present in MM3 have been modified in MM4.

$$E_{modified\ MM3\ terms} = \sum (E_{impt} + E_{tors-str}) \qquad (39)$$

VI. NEW TERMS

A. Overview

The MM4 force field has in the terms of Allinger reached a level in which future simple improvements do not seem obvious [36–40]. The addition of new off-diagonal matrix terms (the cross-terms) are responsible for the improved accuracy. These cross-terms, however, make parameterization of the new force fields all the more difficult and complex. Outlined in the following sections is a description of each new MM4 cross-term (stretch–stretch, torsion–bend, bend–torsion–bend, torsion–torsion, torsion–improper torsion, improper torsion–torsion–improper torsion) and its effects on the force field.

B. Stretch–Stretch

The stretch–stretch term affects stretching motions that are coupled to each other with a common atom at the center. Isobutene and benzene are especially affected by this term. The significance of this cross-term appears in vibrational frequencies.

$$E_{ss}^{MM4} = 143.88 K_{ss} \Delta l_1 \Delta l_2 \tag{40}$$

C. Torsion–Bend

Another newly introduced cross-term in MM4 is torsion–bend. It has been recognized for many years now that a torsion–bend term would improve the fit between experiment and molecular mechanics. This cross-term enables the bond angle (A–B–C or B–C–D) to adjust its values with the change of torsion angle A–B–C–D [see Eq. (41)]. Two sets of parameters $(K_{tb1}, K_{tb2}, K_{tb3}, \text{and } K_{tb1}', K_{tb2}', K_{tb3}')$ control the interactions among bond angles of A–B–C or B–C–D and the torsion angle of A–B–C–D. While these parameters are heavily coupled with one another, K_{tb1}, K_{tb2}, and K_{tb3} parameters mainly describes the dependency of bond angle A–B–C on the torsion angle A–B–C–D. K_{tb1}', K_{tb2}', and K_{tb3}', in turn, affect the behavior of the bond angle B–C–D. MM4 uses three cosine terms, similar to what is used in the pure torsional energy equation, to address the coupling between any bond angle–torsion angle pair. The onefold term K_{tb1} represents the bond angle difference between a torsion angle of 0° and 180°. The twofold term K_{tb2} addresses the difference of a bond angle between a torsion angle of 0° and 180° and between of 90° and 270°. The last parameter K_{tb3} describes the bond angle change between the threefold staggered conformations (torsion angles of 60°, 180°, and 300°) and eclipsed conformations (torsion angles of 0°, 120°, and 240°). Taken together, these torsion–bend cross-term parameters can offer a great deal of freedom for torsion–bending interactions under different chemical environments. For example, for K_{tb1}, a negative value decrease the bond angle when the torsion angle changes from 0° to 180°, whereas a positive parameter increases the bond angle during the same process.

$$E_{tb}^{MM4} = 2.51124\{[K_{tb1}(1 + \cos \omega) + K_{tb2}(1 - \cos 2\omega)$$
$$+ K_{tb3}(1 + \cos 3\omega)]\Delta\theta_1$$
$$+[K'_{tb1}(1 + \cos \omega) + K'_{tb2}(1 - \cos 2\omega)$$
$$+ K'_{tb3}(1 + \cos 3\omega)]\Delta\theta_2\}$$

(41)

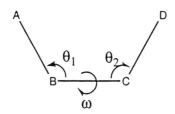

The torsion–bend cross-term was applied in the MM4 force field development for phosphine and its alkyl derivatives. It played an important role in increasing the performance of calculations involving ethylphosphine and ethyldimethylphosphine. For convenience during parameterization, the torsion angle was defined as C–C–P–L.P. (L.P. = lone-pair electrons). MM3, without torsion–bend cross-terms, underestimated the C–C–P bond angle by 3.9° when the torsion angle of C–C–P–L.P. was 180° (*trans* conformation), and it overestimated the same bond angle by 0.2° when the torsion angle was 60° (*gauche* conformation) [84]. With the contribution of torsion–bend cross-terms, MM4 reduced these two deviations to 0.0° and 0.1°, respectively. [G. Y. Liang and J. P. Bowen, unpublished data]. For ethyldimethylphosphine, the torsion angle was defined in the same fashion. Although MM3 (without torsion–bend interaction) carried C–C–P bond angle deviations of 8.9° and 0.6° for the *trans* and *gauche* conformations, MM4 (with torsion–bend cross-terms) virtually eliminated the deviations (both below 0.1°) for both of these two conformers.

gauche

trans

D. Bend–Torsion–Bend

Primarily, this cross-term contributes to the improvement in reproducing the vibrational frequencies, especially for certain modes in the hydrogen-terminated (A or D, or both are hydrogens) molecules (e.g., ethylene).

$$E_{btb}^{MM4} = 0.043828K_{btb} \cos \omega \Delta\theta_1 \Delta\theta_2 \tag{42}$$

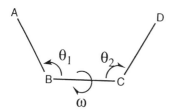

E. Torsion–Torsion

K_{tt1} is a torsion–torsion cross-term constant for torsion angle 1. K_{tt2} is a torsion–torsion cross-term constant for torsion angle 2, and P_{ij} and P_{jk} are bond orders for bonds ij and jk, respectively. The introduction of a torsion–torsion-coupling term has two consequences.

1. It increases the frequencies of the out-of-plane bending of C_{sp2}–C_{sp2}–C_{sp2}, atom triples, especially for benzene.

2. It also lowers the relative energy of the compounds that are highly aromatic which, in turn, yields a better heat of formation agreement with experimental data.

$$E_{tt}^{MM4} = -K_{tt1}(1 - P_{ij})(1 + \cos 3\omega_1)K_{tt2}(1 - P_{jk})(1 + \cos 3\omega_2) \tag{43}$$

F. Torsion–Improper Torsion

Consider the torsion angle A–B–C–D, where ω_1 is the improper torsion B–A–E–C, and ω_2 is the improper torsion C–F–D–B. This term "flattens" the C_{sp2} groups of ethylene and similar molecules. It contributes to attaining both the correct geometry and vibrational frequencies.

$$E^{MM4}_{tors-impt} = (1 - \cos^2 \omega)[K_{timpt1}(1 - \cos \omega_1) \qquad (44)$$
$$+ K_{timpt2}(1 - \cos \omega_2)]$$

ω is the torsion angle A–B–C–D, ω_1 is the improper torsion angle B–A–E–C, ω_2 is the improper torsion angle C–F–D–B.

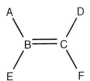

G. Improper Torsion–Torsion–Improper Torsion

This term decreases the deviations of two out-of-plane bending modes (B_{1u} and B_{2g}) for ethylene, where K_{ittit} is the force constant, ω_1 and ω_2 are the improper torsion angles, and ω is the torsion angle.

$$E^{MM4}_{ittit} = K_{ittit} \cos \omega_1 \cos \omega \cos \omega_2 \qquad (45)$$

VII. MODIFIED MM3 TERMS USED IN MM4

A. Overview

Many of the equations in MM3 are excellent approximations to molecular behavior. As more experimental data became available, the functional forms of MM3 needed modification and reparameterization. Although some functional forms have been retained in MM4 in their entirity, others have been modified, and new terms have been added together.

B. Improper Torsion

Previously, in Section III.B, the mathematical approach used in MM2 and MM3 to keep trigonal planar centers flat was discussed. The out-of-plane–bending terms are good ways to incorporate molecular geometry into a ball-and-stick mechanical model. Nevertheless, the programming involving complex interactions between the out-of-plane–bending method and other mechanical effects was difficult. One way to circumvent these problems was to eliminate the out-of-plane model and use an equivalent improper torsion scheme. Overall, the final molecular geometries were essentially identical whether an out-of-plane–bending or improper torsion method was used.

C. Torsion–Stretch

There are two types of torsion–stretch interactions in the MM4 program. A type 1 torsion–stretch designation refers to the effect of the interaction on the central bond length, whereas type 2 applies to the terminal bond lengths. The latter mainly applies to compounds with lone-pair electrons (Bohlmann effect) and compounds with double bonds (hyperconjugation). The bond lengths of C–C or C–H are mainly affected. See Eq. (46), where K_{ts1}, K_{ts2}, and K_{ts3} are force constants, Δl is the bond length deviation from the equilibrium value, and ω is the torsion angle; and Eq. (47), where K_{V1} and K_{V2} are force constants, Δl is the bond length deviation from the equilibrium value, and ω is the torsion angle.

Type 1

$$E_{ts1}^{MM4} = -k\Delta l[K_{ts1}(1 + \cos \omega) \tag{46}$$
$$+ K_{ts2}(1 - \cos 2\omega) + K_{ts3}(1 + \cos 3\omega)]$$

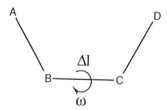

Type 2

$$E_{ts2}^{MM4} = -0.5\Delta l 11.995[K_{V1}(1 + \cos \omega) + K_{V2}(1 - \cos 2\omega)] \tag{47}$$

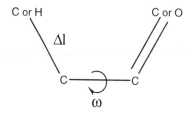

VIII. MOLECULAR MECHANICS PARAMETERIZATION

A. Overview

Although the accuracy of molecular mechanics calculations often rivals experimental data, it is critical that all the parameters for each unique combination of atoms be rigorously determined. There are various ways in which this may be achieved. More commonly, the "functional group" approach has been taken, whereby each single functional group is independently studied and parameters are developed based either on experimental value or theoretical results. The multitude of functional group combinations are then studied.

The reliability of force field calculations is strongly dependent on the previously discussed idea of transferable parameters. Transferability in the early days of molecular mechanics was hotly debated. There is no underlying theoretical reasons supporting the concept. The chemists' intuition that organic structures behave in similar ways, however, implies that the force constant parameters may be used within the same force field for similar structures. This does not mean that the parameters can be transferred from one program to another—i.e., from AMBER to MM3 or vice versa.)

Molecular mechanics parameterization is both an art and a science, and the groups developing parameters must be experienced with understanding the meaning of experimental data obtained from many different sources. During molecular mechanics parameterization, a set of training molecules needs to be assembled that covers all the properties for a class of compounds. The training set should be as large as possible to sample enough molecular structures to generate meaningful parameters. The contributions of each training molecule often need to be weighted differently. A molecule that has more reliable experimental data is more important than others for which the experimental data are of questionable quality. Even in the same molecule, one part of the data may be more reliable than others.

There is no single "right way" to develop molecular mechanics parameters as long as the force field is self-consistent. Occasionally, two or more sets of parameters may be developed that can reproduce experimental data equally well [85], although one set may have better physical meaning and appeal to the intuitive insight of chemists. Historically, the various groups involved in molecular mechanics development have used different data criteria, weighing some classes of compounds more heavily than others, which makes a direct comparison somewhat problematic. MM3 and MM4 were designed to reproduce experimental structures and energies in the gas phase, primarily based on electron diffraction data.

There are two traditional parameterization approaches that have been employed with varying degrees of success: (a) Parameters may be determined by inspection on a trial-and-error basis; or (b) alternatively, at the other extreme, least–squares-fitting methods have been used to optimize the parameters to the best-fit between the calculated and experimental data or *ab initio* calculations [41].

B. Inspection Method

The trial-and-error method usually leads to better agreement overall between calculated and target properties; but it is extremely time-intensive, laborious, and requires a great deal of knowledge about chemical principles and the specific class of compounds of interest. The trial-and-error method focuses exclusively with parameterizing on a functional group basis. It may take months or years to produce a set of accurate molecular mechanics parameters. Certainly, a significant amount of time is expended on judging the experimental reliability of the data used, but it still takes considerable time to adjust the parameters on a one-by-one basis to minimize the deviations between the calculations and experimental results. Presumably, if the chemist is familiar with structural aspects of the data set, large systematic errors can be eliminated. Nevertheless, small random errors still remain because of human limitations.

C. Least-Squares Methods

Computerized least-squares–fitting methods have difficulty in evaluating the overall performance of a set of molecular mechanics force field parameters. The deviations between the calculated results and target values (experimental or theoretical), including bond lengths, bond angles, torsion angles, dipole moments, moments of inertia, and vibrational frequencies, are the criteria used to evaluate the effectiveness of the force field. In general, these criteria are not equally important for all the parameters. For example, the deviations of bond lengths are more important than those of bond angles and vibrational frequencies for the development of equilibrium bond length parameters; consequently, they should be weighted more heavily in the parameterization process. The deviations of vibrational frequencies should be weighted more heavily than other deviations during the optimization of stretching and bending force constants.

D. Automated Methods

The performance of a force field involves an intricate balance of the parameters. Force field parameters are highly coupled with one another, and they are dependent on the calculated geometries of the structures in a training set. Any property generated by a molecular mechanics calculation, such as dipole moments, moments of inertia, or vibrational frequencies, are a function of the final optimized geometry and the specific parameters and equations used. The final optimized geometry depends on all the force field parameters that are included. Also, the parameters in the force field are not a complete set of orthogonal variables in mathematics, which is a requisite of most least-squares–fitting routines. The very nature of this complex coupling makes setting up a direct mathematical relation among the variables a least-squares–fitting nightmare. The overall root-mean-square (rms) deviation expression for any target molecule in the training set composed of m atoms may be written as a function of the parameters and the geometry as shown in Eq. (48), where $P_1, P_2, P_3, \cdots, P_n$ represent the complete set of force field parameters required for the molecular mechanics calculation of this structure and $x_1, y_1, z_1, x_2, y_2, z_2, \cdots, x_m, y_m, z_m$ are the optimized Cartesian coordinates.

$$\text{rms} = f(P_1, P_2, P_3, \cdots, P_n, x_1, y_1, z_1, x_2 y_2, z_2, \cdots, x_m, y_m, z_m) \tag{48}$$

Taking the partial derivatives of Eq. (48) is straightforward in a general sense, but leads to reasonably complex equation in practice [see Eq. (49)]. In molecular mechanics the terms that relate the partial derivative of one parameter to another throughout the entire set of parameters $\partial(P_2)/\partial P_1$, $\partial(P_3)/\partial P_1, \cdots, \partial(P_n)/\partial P_1, \partial(x_1)/\partial P_1, \partial(y_1)/\partial P_1, \cdots,$ and $\partial(z_m)/\partial P_1$ cannot be described analytically. Moreover, these expressions are too difficult and time-intensive to be routinely calculated numerically, and most typically these terms are ignored. This results in the equation of the derivative being truncated after the first term. In the molecular mechanics force field, $\partial(P_2)/\partial P_1, \partial(P_3)/\partial P_1, \cdots, \partial(P_n)/\partial P_1$ describe the correlation between the force field parameters, and $\partial(x_1)/\partial P_1, \partial(y_1)/\partial P_1, \cdots, \partial(z_m)/\partial P_1$ represent the correlation between the geometries of a training set of molecules and the force field parameters. Truncation of these terms in Eq. (49), after the first derivative of the root-mean-square deviation, indicates that these important correlations are excluded entirely from consideration by the least-squares–fitting method. In summary, the least-squares–fitting method may eliminate small local random errors, but introduce large systematic errors.

$$\frac{\partial(\text{rms})}{\partial P_1} = \left(\frac{\partial(\text{rms})}{\partial P_1} \right)_{P_2, P_3, \cdots, P_n, x_1, y_1, z_1, x_2, y_2, z_2, \cdots, x_m, y_m, z_m}$$

$$+ \left(\frac{\partial(\text{rms})}{\partial P_2} \right)_{P_1, P_3, \cdots, P_n, x_1, y_1, z_1, x_2, y_2, z_2, \cdots, x_m, y_m, z_m} \cdot \frac{\partial(P_2)}{\partial P_1}$$

$$+ \left(\frac{\partial(\text{rms})}{\partial P_3} \right)_{P_1, P_2, \cdots, \langle P_n \rangle, x_1, y_1, z_1, x_2, y_2, z_2, \cdots, x_m, y_m, z_m} \cdot \frac{\partial(P_3)}{\partial P_1}$$

$$+ \cdots + \left(\frac{\partial(\text{rms})}{\partial P_n} \right)_{P_1,P_2,P_3,\cdots,,x_1,y_1,z_1,x_2,y_2,z_2,\cdots,x_m,y_m,z_m} \cdot \frac{\partial(P_n)}{\partial P_1}$$

$$+ \left(\frac{\partial(\text{rms})}{\partial x_1} \right)_{P_1,P_2,P_3,\cdots,P_n,y_1,z_1,x_2,y_2,z_2,\cdots,x_m,y_m,z_m} \cdot \frac{\partial(x_1)}{\partial P_1}$$

$$+ \left(\frac{\partial(\text{rms})}{\partial y_1} \right)_{P_1,P_2,P_3,\cdots,P_n,x_1,z_1,x_2,y_2,z_2,\cdots,x_m,y_m,z_m} \cdot \frac{\partial(y_1)}{\partial P_1}$$

$$+ \cdots + \left(\frac{\partial(\text{rms})}{\partial z_m} \right)_{P_1,P_2,P_3,\cdots,P_n,x_1,y_1,z_1,x_2,y_2,z_2,\cdots,x_m,y_m} \cdot \frac{\partial(z_m)}{\partial P_1} \quad (49)$$

In contrast to both the least-squares–fitting and trial-and-error inspection methods, a new computer-assisted multiparameter multistep relaxation (MPMSR) method has been developed in our laboratories [41]. The MPMSR approach simulates the trial-and-error method on a computer, which reduces both systematic and random errors, and produces better molecular mechanics force field parameters in significantly less time.

IX. CONCLUSION AND PROGNOSIS

Modeling molecular structure and chemical reactions has been one of the goals chemists have pursued. For many years, hand-held mechanical models were of sufficient accuracy to satisfy experimentalists. Unfortunately, these mechanical ball-and-stick structures were not flexible enough to take into account subtle bond distortion effects, such as electronegativity, nonbonded interactions, and charge distributions. Moreover, the energy differences between different conformations could not be determined. Molecular mechanics calculations can account for all of these parameters and provide additional information.

Since the inception of using classical mechanics functions to describe molecular behavior in the 1920s and 1940s, followed by the impressive developments in the 1960s by the groups of Hendrickson, Lifson, Ermer, Bartell, Allinger, Schleyer, and Wiberg, molecular mechanics has developed into a highly successful method. All modern molecular mechanics calculations should be able to calculate molecular structure, vibrational frequencies, and thermodynamic properties to reasonable accuracy from a set of self-consistent potential energy functions and their associated parameters. More recent work in the 1990s by Allinger, Hagler, Halgren, and Kollman, among others, has ushered in a new age of molecular mechanics calculations, for which the results are more reliable, less expensive, and of greater applicability.

The future for molecular mechanics calculations looks promising. Molecular mechanics is as yet the only method that can allow for the reasonably accurate calculation of large, biologically important molecules. In general, large macromolecules cannot be calculated using quantum mechanically based programs. Also, force fields are the mathematical basis for molecular dynamics, free-energy perturbation, and related simulation methods. Many of the relationships between the potential energy functions and structure are now well understood and are being implemented. The force fields of today, for the most part, are becoming better and are able to handle more diverse functional groups.

Accurate parameterization still remains a time-consuming problem, but new automated methods, such as PARTS, are making this easier. In some instances, molecular mechanics programs can even estimate missing parameters. MM3 and MM4, for example, have artificial intelligence routines that will automatically generate missing parameters for complex atomic arrangements found in heterocyclic compounds that are of interest to the pharmaceutical industry. This estimation approach is a first approximation to rigorous parameterization, but it is far superior to using predetermined generalized parameters.

Overall, the state of molecular mechanics development may be considered to be in good order. In the next decade, many of the unresolved problems, such as polarizability and nonbonded interactions, will be resolved. The use of molecular mechanics calculations continues to rise in popularity in both the research and educational arenas. The progress in molecular mechanics is exciting, and there will be many new developments in the coming years.

REFERENCES

1. U. Burkert and N. L. Allinger, *Molecular Mechanics,* American Chemical Society, Washington DC, 1982.
2. J. P. Bowen and N. L. Allinger, Molecular mechanics: The art and science of parameterization, *Reviews in Computational Chemistry*, Vol. 2 (K. Lipkowitz and D. Boyd, eds.), VCH, New York, 1991, pp. 81–97.
3. N. L. Allinger, Calculation of molecular structure and energy by force field methods, *Adv. Phys. Org. Chem. 13*:1 (1976).
4. O. Ermer, Calculation of molecular properties using force field. Applications in organic chemistry, *Struct. Bonding (Berlin) 27*:161 (1976).
5. C. L. Altona and D. H. Faber, Empirical force field calculations. A tool in structural organic chemistry, *Top. Curr. Chem. 45*:1 (1974).
6. E. M. Engler, J. D. Andose, and P. v. R. Schleyer, Critical evaluation of molecular mechanics, *J. Am. Chem. Soc. 95*:8005 (1973).

7. L. S. Bartell, Representations of molecular force fields, 3. On *gauche* con-
    formational energy, *J. Am. Chem. Soc. 99*:3279 (1977).
8. D. N. J. White and M. Bovill, Molecular mechanics calculations on alkanes
    and nonconjugated alkenes, *J. Chem. Soc. Perkin Trans. 2*:1610 (1977).
9. J. D. Dunitz and H. B. Bürgi, Non-bonded interactions in organic molecules.
    International Review of Science: Physical Chemistry, Series Two, 1975–1976
    Vol. II (A. D. Buckingham and J. M. Robertson, eds.), Butterworths, London,
    1975, p. 81.
10. S. R. Niketic and K. Rasmussen, *The Consistent Force Field*, Springer, New
    York, 1977.
11. A. Warshel, The consistent force field and its quantum mechanical extension,
    Semiempirical Methods of Electronic Structure Calculation Vol. 7 (G. A. Se-
    gal, ed.), Plenum, New York, 1977, p. 133.
12. D. N. J. White, Molecular mechanics calculations, *Mol. Struct. Diffr. Methods*
    6:38 (1978).
13. K. Mislow, D. A. Dougherty, and W. D. Hounshell, Some applications of the
    empirical force field method to stereochemistry, *Bull. Soc. Chem. Belg. 87*:
    555 (1978).
14. J. E. Williams, P. J. Stang, and P. v. R. Schleyer, Physical organic chemistry:
    Quantitative conformational analysis; calculation methods, *Annu. Rev. Phys.
    Chem. 19*:531 (1968).
15. U. Dinur and A. T. Hagler, New approaches to empirical force field, *Reviews
    in Computational Chemistry* Vol. 2 (K. Lipkowitz and D. Boyd, eds.), VCH,
    New York, 1991, pp. 99–184.
16. N. L. Allinger and P. v. R. Schleyer, Editorial, *J. Comput. Chem. 17*:489
    (1996).
17. B. E. Thomas, R. J. Loncharich, and K. N. Houk, Force field modeling of
    transition structures of intramolecular ENE reactions and ab initio transition
    structures for an activated neophile, *J. Org. Chem. 57*:1354 (1992).
18. L. Raimondi, F. K. Brown, J. Gonzalez, and K. N. Houk, Empirical force-
    field models for the transition-states of intramolecular Diels–Alder reactions
    based upon ab initio transition structures, *J. Am. Chem. Soc. 114*:4796 (1992).
19. K. P. Eurenius and K. N. Houk, Rational vs random parameters in transition-
    state modeling—MM2 transition-state models for intramolecular hydride
    transfers, *J. Am. Chem. Soc. 116*:9943 (1994).
20. B. Depascualteresa, J. Gonzalez, A. Asensio, and K. N. Houk, ab initio-based
    force-field modeling of the transition states and stereoselectivities of Lewis-
    acid catalyzed asymmetric Diels–Alder reactions, *J. Am. Chem. Soc. 117*:4347
    (1995).
21. J. P. Bowen, Team effort by industry and academia results in new modeling
    center for North Carolina, *Chem. Design Autom. News*, June, 4–5 and 11
    (1988).
22. New molecular modeling lab is multidisciplinary effort, *Chem. Eng. News*,
    May 9, 44 (1988).

23. J. P. Bowen, UNC hosts ACS Short Course in Molecular Modeling, *Chem. Design Autom. News* October, 4 and 9–11 (1989).

24. S. Borman, Firms lend computers for ACS course, *Chem. Eng. News*, August 21, 22 (1989).

25. D. Williams, MACCS-3D becomes part of ACS short course, *Mol. Connect. 11*:1,6 (1992).

26. N. L. Allinger, Y. H. Yuh, and J.-H. Lii, Molecular mechanics. The MM3 force field for hydrocarbons. 1., *J. Am. Chem. Soc. 111*:8551 (1989).

27. J. H. Lii and N. L. Allinger, Molecular mechanics. The MM3 force field for hydrocarbons. 2. Vibrational frequencies and thermodynamics, *J. Am. Chem. Soc. 111*:8566 (1989).

28. J.-H. Lii and N. L. Allinger, Molecular mechanics. The MM3 force field for hydrocarbons. 3. The van der Waals potentials and crystal data for aliphatic and aromatic hydrocarbons, *J. Am. Chem. Soc. 111*:8576 (1989).

29. B. R. Brooks, R. E. Bruccoleri, B. D. Olafson, D. J. States, S. Swaminathan, and M. Karplus, CHARMM: Program for macromolecular energy, minimization, and dynamics calculations, *J. Comput. Chem. 4*:187–217 (1983).

30. S. N. Ha, A. Giammona, M. Field, and J. W. Brady, A revised potential-energy surface for molecular mechanics studies of carbohydrates, *Carbohydr. Res. 180*:207–221 (1988).

31. A. D. MacKerell, J. Wiórkiewicz-Kuczera, and M. Karplus, An all-atom empirical energy function for the simulation of nucleic-acids, *J. Am. Chem. Soc. 117*:11946 (1995).

32. S. J. Weiner, P. A. Kollman, D. A. Case, U. C. Singh, C. Ghio, G. Alagona, S. Profeta, Jr., and P. J. Weiner, A new force field for molecular mechanical simulation of nucleic acids and proteins, *J. Am. Chem. Soc. 106*:765–784 (1984).

33. S. J. Weiner, P. A. Kollman, D. T. Nguyen, and D. A. Case, An all atom force field for simulation of protein and nucleic acids, *J. Comput. Chem. 7*:230–252 (1986).

34. D. A. Pearlman, D. A. Case, J. W. Caldwell, W. S. Ross, T. E. Cheatham, S. Debolt, D. Ferguson, G. Seibel, and P. Kollman, AMBER, a package of computer-programs for applying molecular mechanics, normal-mode analysis, molecular-dynamics and free-energy calculations to simulate the structural and energetic properties of molecules, *Comput. Phys. Commun. 91*:1 (1995).

35. W. D. Cornell, P. Cieplak, C. I. Bayly, I. R. Gould, K. M. Merz, D. M. Ferguson, D. C. Spellmeyer, T. Fox, J. W. Caldwell, and P. A. Kollman, A 2nd generation force-field for the simulation of proteins, nucleic-acids, and organic-molecules, *J. Am. Chem. Soc., 117*:5179 (1995).

36. N. L. Allinger, K. S. Chen, and J. H. Lii, An improved force-field (MM4) for saturated-hydrocarbons, *J. Comput. Chem. 17*:642 (1996).

37. N. Nevins, K. S. Chen, and N. L. Allinger, Molecular mechanics (MM4) calculations on alkenes, *J. Comput. Chem. 17*:669 (1996).

38. N. Nevins, J. H. Lii, and N. L. Allinger, Molecular mechanics (MM4) calculations on conjugated hydrocarbons, *J. Comput. Chem. 17*:695 (1996).

39. N. Nevins and N. L. Allinger, Molecular mechanics (MM4) vibrational frequency calculations for alkenes and conjugated hydrocarbons, *J. Comput. Chem. 17*:730 (1996).

40. N. L. Allinger, K. S. Chen, J. A. Katzenellenbogen, S. R. Wilson, and G. M. Anstead, Hyperconjugative effects on carbon–carbon bond lengths in molecular mechanics (MM4), *J. Comput. Chem. 17*:747 (1996).

41. G. Y. Liang, P. C. Fox, and J. P. Bowen, Parameter analysis and refinement toolkit system and its application in MM3 parameterization for phosphine and its derivatives, *J. Comput. Chem. 17*:940 (1996).

42. D. H. Andrews, The relation between the Raman spectra and the structure of organic molecules, *Phys. Rev. 36*:544 (1930).

43. T. L. Hill, Steric effects, *J. Chem. Phys. 14*:465 (1946).

44. F. H. Westheimer and J. E. Mayer, The theory of the racemization of optically active derivatives of biphenyl, *J. Chem. Phys. 14*:733 (1946).

45. F. H. Westheimer, The calculation of the energy of the activation for the racemization of 2,2'-dibromo-4,4'-dicarboxybiphenyl, *J. Chem. Phys. 15*:252 (1947).

46. M. Rieger and F. H. Westheimer, The calculation and determination of the buttressing effect for the racemization of 2,2'3,3'-tetraiodo-5,5'-dicarboxybiphenyl, *J. Am. Chem. Soc. 72*:19 (1950).

47. F. H. Westheimer, Calculation of the magnitude of steric effects, *Steric Effect in Organic Chemistry* (M. S. Newman, ed.), Wiley, New York, 1956.

48. I. Dostrovsky, E. D. Hughes, and C. K. Ingold, XXXII. The role of steric hindrance. G. Magnitude of steric effect, range of occurrence of steric and polar effects, and place of the Wagner rearrangement in nucleophilic substitution and elimination, *J. Chem. Soc.* p. 173 (1946).

49. J. B. Hendrickson, Molecular geometry. I. Machine computation of the common rings, *J. Am. Chem. Soc. 83*:4537 (1961).

50. S. Lifson and A. Warshel, Consistent force field calculations of conformations, vibrational spectra, and enthalpies of cycloalkane and n-alkane molecules, *J. Chem. Phys. 49*:5116 (1968).

51. O. Ermer and S. Lifson, Consistent force field calculations. III. Vibrations, conformations, and heats of hydrogenation of nonconjugated olefins, *J. Am. Chem. Soc. 95*:4121 (1973).

52. N. L. Allinger and J. T. Sprague, The calculation of the structures of hydrocarbons containing delocalized electronic systems by the molecular mechanics method, *J. Am. Chem. Soc. 95*:3893 (1973).

53. K. B. Wiberg, A scheme for strain energy minimization. Application to the cycloalkanes, *J. Am. Chem. Soc. 87*:1070 (1965).

54. N. L. Allinger, Conformational analysis. 130. MM2. A hydrocarbon force field utilizing V_1 and V_2 torsional terms, *J. Am. Chem. Soc. 99*:8127 (1977).

55. O. Ermer and S. A. Mason, Extremely short non-bonded H $\cdots$ H distance in two derivatives of *exo, exo*-tetracyclo[6.2.1.1^{3,6}.O^{2,7}]dodecane, *J. Chem. Soc. Chem. Commun.* p. 53 (1983).

56. K. B. Kipkowitz and N. L. Allinger, Some computational deficiencies in MM2, *QCPE Bull. 7*:19 (1987).

57. A. T. Hagler and C. S. Ewig, On the use of quantum energy surfaces in the derivation of molecular-force fields, *Comput. Phys. Commun. 84*:131 (1994).

58. J. R. Maple, M. J. Hwang, T. P. Stockfisch, U. Dinur, M. Waldman, C. S. Ewig, and A. T. Hagler, Derivation of class-II force-fields. 1. Methodology and quantum force-field for the alkyl functional-group and alkane molecules, *J. Comput. Chem. 15*:162 (1994).

59. M. J. Hwang, T. P. Stockfisch, and A. T. Hagler, Derivation of class-II force-field. 2. Derivation and characterization of a class-II force-field, CFF93, for the alkyl functional-group and alkane molecules, *J. Am. Chem. Soc. 116*:2515 (1994).

60. J. R. Maple, M. J. Hwang, T. P. Stockfisch, and A. T. Hagler, Derivation of class-II force-fields. 3. Characterization of a quantum force-field for alkanes, *Isr. J. Chem. 34*:195 (1994).

61. T. A. Halgren, Merck molecular-force field. 1. Basis, form, scope, parameterization, and performance of MMFF94, *J. Comput. Chem. 17*:490 (1996).

62. T. A. Halgren, Merck molecular-force field. 2. MMFF94 van-der-Waals and electrostatic parameters for intermolecular interactions, *J. Comput. Chem. 17*: 520 (1996).

63. T. A. Halgren, Merck molecular-force field. 3. Molecular geometries and vibrational frequencies for MMFF94, *J. Comput. Chem. 17*:553 (1996).

64. T. A. Halgren and R. B. Nachbar, Merck molecular-force field. 4. Conformational energies and geometries for MMFF94, *J. Comput. Chem. 17*:587 (1996).

65. T. A. Halgren, Merck molecular-force field. 5. Extension of MMFF94 using experimental-data, additional computational data, and empirical rules, *J. Comput. Chem. 17*:616 (1996).

66. N. L. Allinger, D. Hindman, and H. Honig, Conformational analysis. 125. The importance of 2-fold barriers in the conformational analysis of saturated molecules, *J. Am. Chem. Soc. 99*:3282 (1977).

67. S. Fitzwater and C. S. Bartell, Representations of molecular force field. 2. A modified Urey–Bradley field and an examination of Allinger's *gauche* hydrogen hypothesis, *J. Am. Chem. Soc. 98*:5107 (1976).

68. L. Radom, W. J. Hehre, and J. A. Pople, Molecular orbital theory of the electronic structure of organic compounds. XIII. Fourier component analysis of internal rotation potential functions in saturated molecules, *J. Am. Chem. Soc. 94*:2371 (1972).

69. J. E. Lennard-Jones, Cohesion, *Proc. Phys. Soc. (Lond.), Ser. A 43*:461 (1931).

70. A. Warshel and S. Lifson, Consistent force field calculations. II. Crystal structures sublimation energies, molecular and lattice vibrations, molecular conformations and enthalpies of alkanes, *J. Chem. Phys. 53*:582 (1970).

71. W. J. Hehre, L. Radom, P. v. R. Schleyer, and J. A. Pople, *Ab Initio Molecular Orbital Theory*, Wiley, New York, 1986.

72. W. D. Cornell, P. Cieplak, C. I. Bayly, and P. A. Kollman, Application of RESP charges to calculate conformational energies, hydrogen bond energies, and free energies of solvation, *J. Am. Chem. Soc. 115*:9620 (1993).

73. P. A. Kollman, Advances and continuing challenges in achieving realistic and predictive simulations of the properties of organic and biological molecules, *Acc. Chem. Res. 29*:461–469 (1996).

74. N. L. Allinger, M. R. Imam, M. R. Frierson, Y. H. Yuh, and L. Schafer, The effect of electronegativity on bond lengths in molecular mechanics calculations, *Mathematics and Computational Concepts in Chemistry* (N. Trinajstic, ed.), E. Horwood, London, 1986, p. 8.

75. L. Nørskov-Lauritsen and N. L. Allinger, A molecular mechanics treatment of the anomeric effect, *J. Comput. Chem. 5*:326 (1984).

76. J. R. Kneisler and N. L. Allinger, Ab initio and density-functional theory study of structures and energies for dimethoxymethane as a model for the anomeric effect, *J. Comput. Chem. 17*:757 (1996).

77. W. A. Szarek, *Anomeric Effect: Origin and Consequences*, American Chemical Society, Washington DC, 1979.

78. C. W. Andrews, B. Fraser-Reid, and J. P. Bowen, Involvement of $n\sigma^*$ interactions in glycoside cleavage, *Am. Chem. Soc. Ser. 539, The Anomeric Effect and Associated Stereoelectronic Effects* (G. R. J. Thatcher, eds.), American Chemical Society, Washington DC, 1993.

79. T. Liljefors, J. C. Tai, S. Li, and N. L. Allinger, On the out-of-plane deformation of aromatic rings, and its representation by molecular mechanics, *J. Comput. Chem. 8*:1051 (1987).

80. D. M. York, A. Wlodawer, L. G. Pedersen, and T. A. Darden, Atomic-level accuracy in simulations of large protein crystals, *Proc. Natl. Acad. Sci. USA 91*:8715 (1994).

81. H. Sun, S. J. Mumby, J. R. Maple, and A. T. Hagler, An ab-initio CFF93 all-atom force-field for polycarbonates, *J. Am. Chem. Soc. 116*:2978 (1994).

82. J. C. Smith and M. Karplus, Empirical force-field study of geometries and conformational transitions of some organic-molecules, *J. Am. Chem. Soc. 114*:801 (1992).

83. W. L. Jorgensen, J. Chandrasekhar, J. D. Madura, R. W. Impey, and M. L. Klein, Comparison of simple potential functions for simulating liquid water, *J. Chem. Phys. 79*:926–935 (1983).

84. P. C. Fox, J. P. Bowen, and N. L. Allinger, MM3 molecular mechanics study of alkylphosphines, *J. Am. Chem. Soc. 114*:8536 (1992).

85. F. M. Menger and M. J. Sherrod, Origin of high predictive capabilities in transition-state modeling, *J. Am. Chem. Soc. 112*:8071–8075 (1990).

INDEX